FOUNDATIO

Rural Public Health

IN AMERICA

Joseph N. Inungu, MD, DrPH, MPH

Professor and Director
Master of Public Health Program
School of Health Sciences
Central Michigan University

Mark J. Minelli, PhD, MA, MPA

Professor
School of Health Sciences
Central Michigan University

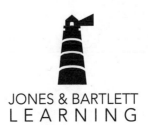

JONES & BARTLETT
LEARNING

World Headquarters
Jones & Bartlett Learning
5 Wall Street
Burlington, MA 01803
978-443-5000
info@jblearning.com
www.jblearning.com

Jones & Bartlett Learning books and products are available through most bookstores and online booksellers. To contact Jones & Bartlett Learning directly, call 800-832-0034, fax 978-443-8000, or visit our website, www.jblearning.com.

22518-1

Production Credits
VP, Product Development: Christine Emerton
Director of Product Management: Laura Pagluica
Product Manager: Sophie Fleck Teague
Content Strategist: Sara Bempkins
Project Manager: Kristen Rogers
Digital Project Specialist: Rachel DiMaggio
Director of Marketing: Andrea DeFronzo
Senior Marketing Manager: Susanne Walker
Production Services Manager: Colleen Lamy
VP, Manufacturing and Inventory Control: Therese Connell
Composition: Exela Technologies
Project Management: Exela Technologies
Cover Design: Theresa Manley
Text Design: Kristin E. Parker
Media Development Editor: Faith Brosnan
Rights & Permissions Manager: John Rusk
Rights Specialist: Liz Kincaid
Cover Image (Title Page, Part Opener, Chapter Opener):
    © Noppawat Tom Charoensinphon/GettyImages
Printing and Binding: McNaughton & Gunn

Library of Congress Cataloging-in-Publication Data
Names: Minelli, Mark J., author. | Inungu, Joseph N., author.
Title: Foundations of rural public health in America / Mark J. Minelli, Joseph N. Inungu.
Description: First edition. | Burlington, MA : Jones & Bartlett Learning,
    [2022] | Includes bibliographical references and index.
Identifiers: LCCN 2020033817 | ISBN 9781284182453 (paperback)
Subjects: MESH: Rural Health | Rural Health Services | Public Health
    Administration | Health Status Disparities | Vulnerable Populations | United States
Classification: LCC RA395.A3 | NLM WA 390 | DDC 362.10973–dc23
LC record available at https://lccn.loc.gov/2020033817

6048

Printed in the United States of America
25 24 23 22 21   10 9 8 7 6 5 4 3 2 1

Brief Contents

PART 4 Health Disparities Among Special Populations   301

PART 5 Advancing Rural Health: Assessment, Planning, and Interventions   381

Contents

PART 1 Understanding Rural Communities   1

PART 3 Health Disparities in Rural Communities 103

CHAPTER 11 **Oral Health in Rural Areas. 205**

Livingstone Aduse-Poku, MPH
Joseph N. Inungu, MD, DrPH, MPH

CHAPTER 12 **Cancers in Rural Areas in the United States 217**

Anuli Njoku, DrPH, MPH
Fathima Wakeel, PhD, MPH

CHAPTER 13 **Environmental Health in Rural Regions of the United States 235**

Salma Haidar, PhD, MPH
Rebecca Uzarski, PhD
Ruben Juarez, MPH

CHAPTER 17 Adolescent Health in Rural Areas..............327

Joseph N. Inungu, MD, DrPH, MPH
Livingstone Aduse-Poku, MPH

CHAPTER 18 Aging Populations in Rural United States 337

Eileen E. MaloneBeach, PhD
Han-Jung Ko, PhD
Mikiyasu Hakoyama, PhD

CHAPTER 19 **Rural Public Health for the LGBTQ Community 359**

Chun-Fang Frank Kuo, PhD, MS

Kathleen Khong Hor Yan, BS

PART 5 **Advancing Rural Health: Assessment, Planning, and Interventions 381**

CHAPTER 20 **Community Needs and Asset Assessment 383**

Mary L. Kushion, MSA

Reviewers

Kyle Brezinski, PhD
Assistant Professor
Bellevue University
Omaha, NE

Stephanie M. Chalupka, EdD, RN, PHCNS, FAAOHN, FNAP
Professor and Program Director
Worcester State University
Worcester, MA

Adrian Israel Martinez Franco, MD, MHA
Associate Professor at Abraham Baldwin
  Agricultural College
Tifton, GA

Andrew Intagliata, PhD
Assistant Professor
John Carroll University
University Heights, OH

Anuli Njoku, DrPH, MPH
Associate Professor
Ferris State University
Big Rapids, MI

Pam Slagle MSN, RN
Assistant Clinical Professor, RN to BSN
  Program Coordinator
Sam Houston State University
Conroe, TX

David X. Swenson, PhD LP
Director of the MBA in Rural Health at the
  College of St. Scholastica
Duluth, MN

Theresa Turick-Gibson, EdD candidate, MA, PPCNP-BC, RN-BC
Professor
Hartwick College
Oneonta, NY

Contributors

Rasheedat Adelabu, MPH candidate

Livingstone Aduse-Poku, MPH

Osayande Agbonlahor, MD, MPH

Tunde M. Akinmoladun, PhD, DAAS, FRSPH

Heather Craig Alonge, PhD, MPH, CHES

Governor Ameh, BDS

Stephanie J.S. Baiyasi-Kozicki, DVM, MPH, HSAC

Donald J. Breckon, PhD, MPH

Wei Wen Megan Chow, BA

Marybeth Denton

Carly Glunz, MPH candidate

Meredith Goodwin, MD

Richard G. Greenhill, DHA, PMP, FACHE

Salma Haidar, PhD, MPH

Mikiyasu Hakoyama, PhD

Carrie Henning-Smith, PhD, MPH, MSW

Roschelle Heuberger, PhD, RD

Monica Hill, MPH candidate

Shayesteh Jahanfar, PhD

James A. Johnson, PhD, MPA, MSc

Ruben Juarez, MPH

Andrew Kim, PhD, MPH

Jerome Kinard, DrPH

Han-Jung Ko, PhD

Zigmond A. Kozicki, DHA, MSHA, MA, LLP

Chun-Fang Frank Kuo, PhD, MS

Mary L. Kushion, MSA

Siew Li Ng, PhD, MA

Marty Malcolm, MA

Eileen E. MaloneBeach, PhD

Vincent Mumford, EdD

Rachael Nelson, PhD

Anuli Njoku, DrPH, MPH

Chimamanda Okafor, MPH

Angela Okonji, MPH

Busakorn Satipanya, MPH candidate

Naveen Sharma, PhD

Frank Synder, PhD, MPH

Maurice Tawil, MPH

Jemaneh Temesgen, DrPH

Rebecca Uzarski, PhD

Fathima Wakeel, PhD, MPH

Xiao Shiang Lee, MA

Kathleen Khong Hor Yan, BS

Micah Zuhl, PhD

Foreword

This book could not be more timely than now, as public health has risen to become central to national survival and the well-being of the world. During the worst pandemic in 100 years, we are seeing communities, both urban and rural, being severely stressed. These stressors are medical, economic, and social as they affect every aspect of society, including every individual and family as they seek to live through this period of uncertainty. The systemic challenge of a pandemic is compounded by political events that are reshaping the social and cultural landscape.

In times of great change, such as our current era, the need for informed and steady leadership could not be greater. As we head into a post-COVID-19 era, there is promise for more effective leadership. We are likely to see better informed health policy and more investment in public health infrastructure, including testing capacity, telehealth, health professions education, and human resources development and safety. However, as with many improvements of the past, rural communities are too often the last to benefit. Just this year, the National Rural Health Association summarizes the challenge as follows, "the obstacles faced by people in rural areas are vastly different than those in urban areas. Economic factors, cultural and social differences, shortage of health professionals, educational shortcomings, lack of recognition by legislators and sometimes the sheer isolation of living in remote areas all conspire to create health disparities and impede rural Americans in their struggle to lead healthier lives." (NRHA, 2020).

For this book, *Foundations of Rural Public Health in America*, the very capable editors

Joseph Inungu, MD, DrPH, MPH and Mark Minelli, PhD, MA, MPA both long-term colleagues of mine, have enlisted expert contributors from a range of public health disciplines and organizations to address critical topics important to rural public health. These carefully selected chapter authors bring together numerous professional experiences and perspectives that facilitate a deeper understanding of both challenges and opportunities. The book is well organized into five parts that cluster chapters thematically in a way that guides the reader through the rural health social, professional, and organizational landscape. In short, this systematic analysis and commentary provides a population perspective to a significant and too often neglected segment of American society.

Part I is titled "Understanding Rural Communities" and begins with the fundamentals such as defining rurality and discussing social determinants of health. Part II focuses on "Public Health Systems and Policies" while tracing the history of rural health in the United States through today with the development of federal agencies tasked with improving health in these populations. The book proceeds in Part III with a focus on "Health Disparities in Rural Communities" addressing cardiovascular disease, stroke, cancer, obesity, diabetes, maternal/child health, and associated lifestyle factors such as physical activity and dietary options and choices. Furthermore, critical issues around the environmental health, occupational health, and mental health are discussed. Part IV goes deeper into the "Health Disparities of Special Populations" by addressing the health needs and challenges of migrant workers, adolescents, the elderly, and LGBTQ individuals living in rural areas. The final cluster of chapters, Part V is titled "Advancing Rural Health–Assessment, Planning, and Interventions." As with most public health books, this set of chapters provides a focus on tools and concepts that supports to work of public health professionals in the field as they provide services aimed at improving health of the broad population. As is common in public health, whether urban, suburban, or rural there is a need for effective community assessment, program planning, policy development, and leadership.

This *Foundations* book provides the breadth and depth needed for students, policy makers, and practitioners seeking to become more knowledgeable on a topic area that is always dynamic and evolving. With the co-occuring epidemics of COVID-19 and SUD (substance use disorder) and a rise in suicide and domestic violence, the need for comprehensive public health intervention couldn't be greater. Fortunately, public health has many successes that span as far back as the beginning of the country and even further if we look globally. At every point in America's over 200 years history when crises arise, the public health professions and related organizations have been there to respond, often having anticipated the crisis or event. Due to political, economic, technological, and cultural barriers, some challenges take longer to mitigate and resolve than others. However, with knowledge and the will to assure health for all, regardless of geography, we do tend to find a way forward. This timely book adds to this much demanded knowledge and hopefully will inspire the willpower we need.

James A. Johnson, PhD, MPA, MSc
Medical Social Scientist and
Public Health Analyst

Preface

Rural public health issues span a wide variety of topics including consumer and family health, environmental and occupational health, mental health, substance abuse, disease prevention and control, rural healthcare delivery systems, health disparities, and more. These topics are covered in nationally used textbooks on rural public health. From a review of the literature, there appears to be no textbook or manual devoted to student interactive learning methods that instructors can use to enhance the classroom learning experience. Due to this shortcoming, the editors created this manual, which is strictly devoted to student interactive learning methods that teachers can utilize to better engage their pupils in these important topics.

Foundations of Rural Public Health in America is the culmination of contributions of many individuals. When developing this manual, the editors thought it would be an excellent strategy to challenge graduate students to be a part of this effort. Central Michigan University, located in Mount Pleasant, Michigan, is home to both the College of Health Professions and the College of Medicine focused on training public health leaders and physicians to serve in rural and underserved populations.

The editors (who have extensive experience in working with rural public health and underserved populations) have reached out to engage students, faculty, and working professionals to assist in developing the content of this textbook. Hands-on individual and group classroom learning gets students past a passive role in the learning experience. Many of the activities, case studies, and other material have already been tested in the classroom environment. Our goal was to provide the most up-to-date information on rural public health in America and engage students in the learning process. The COVID-19 pandemic has changed how education is being provided and this is a tool that can be used to help reach students in an ever-changing world. The editors hope you find this manual effective in reaching your students.

—Joseph N. Inungu and Mark J. Minelli

Dedication

I dedicate this textbook to my parents who inspired me,
to my brothers and sisters who encouraged me, to my wife Lucy,
my children (Lassal, Lys, and Danielle), and my granddaughters
(Nicholette and Gaby) who love me, and finally to the readers who
will use it to make the world a better place for all.

—Dr. Joseph N. Inungu

I would like to dedicate this book with love to my grandchildren
Owen, Benjamin, Emily, Isabelle, Evalyn, Heidi, Thomas,
and Henry.

—Dr. Mark J. Minelli

About the Authors

Dr. Joseph "Jeff" N. Inungu, MD, DrPH, MPH

Joseph N. Inungu is a professor in the School of Health Sciences at Central Michigan University (CMU). He is currently the Director of the Master of Public Health Program. Before joining CMU, he served as the Director of socio-behavioral research and was responsible for the development of the socio-behavioral research (SBR) program at International AIDS Vaccine Initiative (IAVI), a non-governmental organization based in New York. Prior to joining IAVI, he worked as the Regional Researchers for Population Services International, a U.S.-based ONG, for four years to provide technical assistance and oversee the design and implementation of social marketing research in West and Central Africa and conduct capacity building trainings in research in participating countries. He brings several years of experiences in global health and program monitoring and evaluation. He holds a Masters and a Doctor of Public Health degree from Tulane University and a Doctor of Medicine degree from the University of Kinshasa, DR Congo.

Mark J. Minelli, PhD, MA, MPA

Mark J. Minelli is currently a professor at Central Michigan University (CMU) and Adjunct Professor at Capella University. In 1986, CMU became the first institution within the National Collegiate Athletic Association (NCAA) to mandate that all student-athletes take a drug education course and this manual is now used as the course syllabus. Dr. Minelli was previously the past director of Substance Abuse Services, Inc., in Ludington, Michigan, and has extensive experience in both outpatient counseling and prevention services. He is nationally published in many health-related journals, including the *U.S. Journal of Drug and Alcohol Dependence, Addiction and Recovery, Journal of Physical Education, Recreation and Dance, Eta Sigma Gamma, Journal of College and Student Development, Topics in Clinical Nutrition,* and the *Journal of Alcohol and Drug Education.* His other books include: *Beyond Beer Googles: Interactive Teaching Methods for Alcohol, Other Drugs and AIDS Prevention* (4th edition), *The Art of Living: Pathways to Personal Growth* (3rd edition), *Community Health Education: Settings, Roles, and Skills* (5th edition), and *Drugs of Abuse: A Quick Information Guide.* Dr. Minelli is an active consultant for films, school districts, national radio talk shows, newspapers, and businesses. He and his wife, Debra, have four children, eight grandchildren, and reside in Mt. Pleasant, Michigan. Dr. Minelli was recently named Capella University Professor of the Year 2020.

Acknowledgments

This textbook would not have been possible without the commitment and contributions of so many people.

The editors owe an enormous debt of gratitude to those who contributed one or more chapters to this textbook. They gave freely of their time to complete this project. We would like to recognize and thank them: Carrie Henning-Smith, Chimamanda Okafor, Donald Breckon, Roschelle Heuberger, James A. Johnson, Eileen E. MaloneBeach, Han-Jung Ko, Mikiyasu Hakoyama, Shayesteh Jahanfar, Salma Haidar, Mary Kushion, Rebecca Uzarski, Rachael Nelson, Naveen Sharma, Anuli Njoku, Fathima Wakeel, Micah Zuhl, Maurice Tawil, Lee Xiao Shiang, Zigmond Kozicki, Stephanie Baiyasi-Kozicki, Siew Li Ng, Chun Fang "Frank" Kuo, Andrew Kim, Megan Chow Wei Wen, Ruben Juarez, Richard Greenhill, Heather Alonge, Osayande Agbonlahor, Governor Ameh, Livingstone Aduse-Poku, Jerome Kinard, Marty Malcolm, Jemaneh Temesgen, and Vincent Mumford.

We are immensely grateful to Marybeth Denton for her valuable contributions to the timely completion of this textbook. She coordinated the communication among various stakeholders, organized the work for the authors and kept them on task to meet the deadlines, and reviewed and edited the different chapters before submission to the publishers. She oversaw the team of MPH graduate assistants who worked tirelessly to prepare the faculty materials including the PowerPoint slides and the test bank. We hereby express our special gratitude to the MPH graduate assistants who worked hard to see this project through. We would like thank Rasheedat Adelabu, Carly Glunz, Monica Hill, Angela Okonji, and Busakorn Satipanya.

We are deeply indebted to Jones and Bartlett's team, including Sara Bempkins, Ramprasath Sridharan, and Liz Kincaid to name a few for their wonderful editorial support and guidance.

Finally, we cannot express enough thanks to our spouses for their continued support and encouragement. It was a great comfort and relief to know that they stood by us throughout this tedious process.

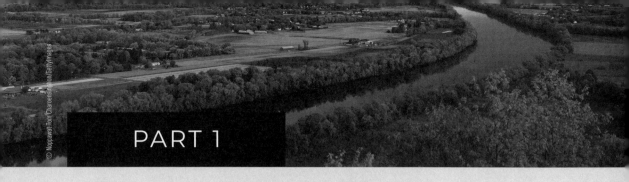

PART 1

Understanding Rural Communities

CHAPTER 1

Defining Rurality

Joseph N. Inungu, MD, DrPH, MPH

LEARNING OBJECTIVES

At the end of this chapter, readers will be able to:

1. Define and contrast the different definitions of the term "health."
2. Discuss the limitations of the World Health Organization's (WHO) definition of the term "health."
3. Review the contributions of the Ottawa Charter to the definition of Health.
4. Discuss the Meikirch Model definition of health.
5. Define and contrast the different definitions of "rurality."
6. Discuss the history of rural public health in the United States.

KEY TERMS

Health
Rural
Rural area
Metropolitan area
Meikirch Model
Urbanized area (UA)
Urban cluster (UC)
The Rural-Urban Continuum Codes, (RUCC)
Metropolitan counties

CHAPTER OVERVIEW

First, this chapter will begin by explaining the seemingly simple, yet complicated definitions of "health" and "rural," and introducing the primary organizations and their roles in contributing to rural health in America. Second, the chapter will provide an overview of the general state of rural public health in the United States. And finally, the chapter will describe the improvements made in rural public health in recent years and which obstacles health professionals still face in meeting the health needs of residents in rural areas.

Defining "Health" and "Rural"

Naming things is one of the first activities that human beings undertake to organize their surroundings (Brüssow, 2013). Properly defining a term or a concept allows people to gain a better understanding of their surroundings. People have the same understanding when speaking about or using a term or a concept. A good understanding of the textbook on the foundation of rural health hinges on clear definition of the terms "health" and "rural."

Definitions of Health

Ancient Time

Although men have always strived to define the term "health," the definition of this term has been changing as the levels of scientific and medical understanding have evolved over time (Badash et al., 2017). Illnesses and diseases have long been regarded as a celestial punishment for moral failings. In ancient Egypt, illnesses were attributed to the actions of demons and supernatural forces that had to be appeased to be cured (Žuškin et al., 2008). Health was perceived to be endowed by deities.

Hippocrates, the "Father of Modern Medicine," was the first person to describe the relationship between environmental, personal cleanliness, and the origin of diseases. Based on his teachings, diseases resulted from imbalances between four bodily fluids—black bile, yellow bile, phlegm, and blood. He considered health a state of physical balance (Yapijakis, 2009). His teaching contributed to the separation of the Greek medicine from the ancient supernatural concepts of health.

The Oxford Dictionary, on the other hand, defines "health" as *"the state of being free from illness and injury."* The concern with this definition is that it inherently suggests that medical professionals are the ones who can declare an individual healthy. The second concern with this definition is that advances in technology and medicine allow us to detect conditions in individuals who were considered healthy yesterday (Sartorius, 2006). These limitations called for a new definition for health.

The World Health Organization

During the establishment of the World Health Organization (WHO) in 1948, a new definition of the term "health" was added to its Constitution. Dr. Andrija Štampar, a Croatian scholar in social medicine and public health and one of the founders of the WHO, proposed a new definition (Svalastog, Donev, Kristoffersen, & Gajovic`, 2017). He defined

health as *a state of complete physical, mental and social well-being and not merely the absence of disease or infirmity* (WHO, 1946). The WHO definition of health was groundbreaking because of its breadth and ambition. It overcame the negative definition of health as absence of disease and included the physical, mental, and social domains (Huber et al., 2011). The new definition set out aspired to provide guidance on how these goals would be realized. However, the WHO definition of health has been facing mounting criticisms over the years (Jadad & O'Grady, 2008; Larson, 1999).

Huber and colleagues (2011) leveled important criticisms. First, the absoluteness of the word "complete" in relation to well-being poses problems. The requirement for "complete health" would leave most people unhealthy most of the time considering that the majority of individuals suffer from a physical ailment or mild mental disorder. The second criticism is the lack of operationalization of the definition of health. Although WHO developed several systems to classify diseases and describe aspects of health, disability, functioning, and quality of life, the *"state of complete physical, mental and social well-being"* is neither operational nor measurable.

The Search for a Universally Valid Definition of Health

The Ottawa Health Promotion

The first international conference on health promotion, held in Ottawa, Canada, on the 21st of November, 1986, focused on actions to achieve the objectives of the WHO *Health for All by the year 2000* initiative, launched in Alma Ata in 1981. The document that resulted from the conference, the Ottawa Charter (WHO, 1986), recognized that health was a resource for everyday life, not the objective of living. Therefore, health promotion is not just the responsibility of the health sector but goes beyond healthy lifestyles to well-being (Kickbusch, 2003). It defined prerequisites for health, including peace, shelter, education, food, income, stable ecosystems, sustainable resources, social justice, and equity. *"Health Promotion* was defined as the *process* of enabling people to increase control over and to improve their health." Dennis Raphael expands on that definition—"Health promotion provides a framework for efforts to improve the quality of life of individuals, communities, and societies by applying a wide range of activities and approaches to achieve desired outcomes (Raphael, 2010). It is also about citizen engagement; an important part of how democratic processes can improve quality of life." Five action areas for health promotion were identified in the charter:

- Build healthy public policy
- Create supportive environments
- Strengthen community action
- Develop personal skills
- Reorient health services

Conceptual Framework of Health

Instead of developing a new definition to replace the WHO definition of health, a consensus was reached among health experts to develop a conceptual framework of health instead. At the international conference in 2010, experts recommended that a definition of health should include: *"the resilience or capacity to cope and maintain and restore one's integrity, equilibrium, and sense of wellbeing."* (Boers & Jentoft, 2015). While the conference identified these useful principles, the participants stopped short of formulating a new definition of health (Bircher & Kuruvilla, 2014).

The Meikirch Model of Health

Although several definitions of health have subsequently been suggested (Bircher & Kuruvilla, 2014), none has been accepted and successfully applied to determine the health of individuals and the public. Dr. Johannes

Bircher, former Dean of the Medical Faculty at the University Witten/Herdecke in Germany and Dr. Shyama Kuruvilla, Senior Strategic Advisor, World Health Organization, proposed a new definition of health using the *Meikirch Model of Health* that views health as a Complex Adaptive System.

Based on the **Meikirch model**, *"Health is a dynamic state of wellbeing emergent from conducive interactions between individuals' potentials, life's demands, and social and environmental determinants."*

The Meikirch model consists of five components and 10 complex interactions, shown in **Figure 1-1**, where the five components are depicted and the interactions are exhibited as double-edged arrows.

Like the WHO definition, the Meikirch model uses the term "state" in its definition of health. For some people, the term "state" conveys the idea of permanency or immovability (Frenk & Gómez-Dantés, 2014). Because this model emphasizes the importance of social determinants and the environment, it offers opportunities to self-motivated individuals to improve their health-supporting behavior and; therefore, promote preventive approaches. (see Figure 1-1).

Definitions of Rurality

For many people, the term "rural" is reminiscent of pastoral landscapes, isolated areas, or farmlands away from large, noisy cities. These aspects of rurality are not sufficient by themselves to completely define "rural" (Hart, Larson, & Lishner, 2005). Generations of rural sociologists, demographers, and geographers struggled with these concepts (Miller & Luloff, 1980). Because the term "rural" means different things to many people and governments, a standardized definition is critical for government functions, regulation, and program administration to guide research, policy analysis, and the implementation of federal and state programs. For example, it can assist government officials in delineating eligible communities when

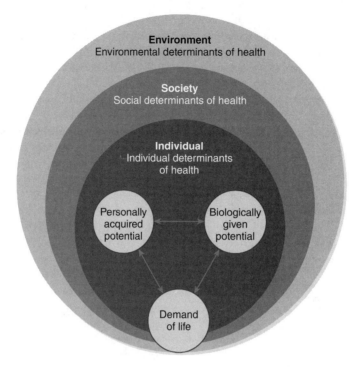

Figure 1-1 The Meikirch Model of Health.

Reproduced from Bircher, J., & Kuruvilla, S. (2014). Defining health by addressing individual, social, and environmental determinants: New opportunities for health care and public health. *Journal of Public Health Policy, 35*(3), 363–386. doi:10.1057/jphp.2014.19, Copyright © 2014 Palgrave Macmillan, a division of Macmillan Publishers Ltd. Retrieved from https://www.ncbi.nlm.nih.gov/pmc/articles/PMC4119253/figure/fig1/

implementing federal rural grant programs. When conducting research, government agencies and investigators will be able to assign data collected to rural versus urban communities.

The need for a proper definition of rurality to meet the unique needs of policymakers, researchers, and policy analysts led to the development of different definitions. The next section will address the five most commonly used definitions of the term rurality. They include:

- The urban-rural definition by the U.S. Census Bureau
- The metropolitan-nonmetropolitan classification by the Office of Management and Budget
- The Rural-Urban Continuum Code and the Rural-Urban Commuting Area by the Economic Research Service of the U.S. Department of Agriculture (USDA)
- The Index of Relative Rurality by Purdue University

U.S. Census Bureau

The Census Bureau began identifying urban places in reports following the 1870, 1880, and 1890 censuses. When identifying urban territory, the Census Bureau used a definition based on population density and other measures of dense development. In 2000, the Census Bureau defined two types of urban areas: *urbanized areas and urban clusters.*

- An **urbanized area (UA)**. An UA comprises one or more places ("central place") and the adjacent, densely settled surrounding territory ("urban fringe") that have a population of 50,000 or more people combined. The urban fringe generally consists of contiguous territory with a total land area of less than two square miles and a population density of at least 1,000 persons per square mile.

- An **urban cluster (UC)** is an area that encompasses a population of at least 2,500 but less than 50,000 persons.
- **Rural area**. The Census Bureau's classification of "**rural**" consists of all territory, population, and housing units located outside of UAs and UCs. While the definition of urban has continued to evolve to include more people and territory in the United States, the rural definition remains as all territory, persons, and housing units not defined as urban (Ratcliffe, Burd, Holder, & Fields, 2016).

Based on the 2010 census, there were 486 *urbanized areas* and 3,087 *urban clusters* in the United States. Urbanized areas contained 71.2% of the population, while 9.5% of the population was within urban clusters. The rural areas of the United States contained 19.3% of the population. Urban areas and urban clusters, which contained the majority of the population, only occupied about 3.0% of the land area of the country.

Office of Management and Budget (OMB)

OMB (2013) classified individual counties as metropolitan counties ("urban") and nonmetropolitan counties ("rural"). The OMB's taxonomy delineates metropolitan and micropolitan counties according to published standards that are applied to Census Bureau data. The federal government most frequently uses the county-based OMB metropolitan and nonmetropolitan classifications as policy tools.

The general concept of a metropolitan or micropolitan statistical area is that of a core area containing a substantial population nucleus, together with adjacent communities having a high degree of economic and social integration with that core (Ratcliffe, 2006).

- **Metropolitan counties**, or metro areas, are defined as central counties with one or more urbanized areas (cities with a population of at least 50,000) and outlying counties that are economically tied to the core [either 25% of workers living in the outlying county commute to the central counties, or 25% of the employment in the county consists of workers coming from the central counties—the so-called "reverse" commuting pattern.]
- **Nonmetropolitan counties:** Nonmetropolitan counties consist of some combination of open countryside, rural towns (places with fewer than 2,500 people), and urban areas with populations ranging from 2,500 to 49,999. Two types of nonmetropolitan counties are:
  - **Micropolitan counties:** Micropolitan counties have at least one urban cluster of at least 10,000 but less than 50,000 population, plus adjacent territory that has a high degree of social and economic integration with the core as measured by commuting ties.
  - **Noncore counties:** Noncore counties are those that do not have an urban core population of 10,000 or more. These counties are considered the most rural of this designation.

Based on the OMB classification, there are 381 *metro areas* and 536 *micro areas* in the United States. Metro and micro areas account for approximately 94% of the population, while the remaining 6% is nonmetro. The amount of land area in metro and micro areas is approximately 47% and the remaining 53% is nonmetro.

Comparison Between the Two Classifications

OMB's definition of metropolitan and nonmetropolitan populations and the Census Bureau's definition of rural and urban do not always identify the same area as rural. When the two definitions were cross-tabulated for the 2000 census, Hart, Larson, and Lishner (2004) found that 72% of the population was classified as both metropolitan (OMB definition) and urban (Census

Bureau definition), while 10% was classified as nonmetropolitan and rural. However, nearly 18% of the nation's population was divided between the two taxonomies: 11% were metropolitan but rural, and 7% were nonmetropolitan but urban.

Consequently, one could argue that the Census Bureau standard includes an overcount of the rural population; whereas the OMB standard represents an undercount. The lack of a strong correlation between the two definitions of urban and metropolitan areas underscores the need for a new definition.

The Rural-Urban Continuum Codes (RUCC) were created in 1975 by David L. Brown, Fred K. Hines, and John M. Zimmer, of the Economic Research Service (ERS), for their report, *Social and Economic Characteristics of the Population in Metro and Nonmetro Counties: 1970-80* (McGranahan, Hession, Mines, & Jordan, 1986).

ERS's 2013 Rural-Urban Continuum Codes is a classification scheme built on the OMB metropolitan and nonmetropolitan dichotomy. This classification scheme distinguishes metropolitan counties by the population size and nonmetropolitan counties by degree of urbanization and adjacency to a metro area or areas. To qualify as adjacent to a metropolitan county, a nonmetropolitan county must share a boundary with a metropolitan county and must meet a minimum work commuting threshold.

The Office of Management and Budget's 2013 metro and nonmetro categories have been subdivided into three metro and six nonmetro groupings, resulting in a nine-part county classification. Each county in the United States is assigned one of the nine codes.

The benefit of the RUCC is to provide researchers working with county data with a more detailed residential classification, beyond a simple metro-nonmetro dichotomy, for the analysis of trends related to degree of rurality and metro proximity. Although the name

(Rural-Urban Continuum Code) as well as the numeric coding suggests a "continuous" and monotonic increase of rurality on a nine-point scale, this suggestion is actually deceptive as it hides the initial distinction between metro (code 1 to 3) and nonmetro counties (code 4 to 9) (Waldorf, 2006).

To address the shortcomings outlined above, Isserman (2005) recently offered an alternative classification system, the so-called "Rural-Urban Density Typology" (Isserman, 2005).

The Rural-Urban Commuting Area System (RUCAs)

The Rural-Urban Commuting Area Codes (RUCA) are a new census tract-based classification scheme that uses the standard Bureau of Census Urbanized Area and Urban Cluster definitions in combination with work commuting information to characterize all of the nation's Census tracts regarding their rural and urban status and relationships.

The Federal Office of Rural Health Policy (FORHP), the Rural Research Center at the University of Washington, and the USDA's Economic Research Service created the RUCA IN 1998. The classification contains two levels. Whole numbers (1–10) delineate metropolitan, micropolitan, small town, and rural commuting areas based on the size and direction of the primary (largest) commuting flows. These 10 codes are further subdivided based on secondary commuting flows, providing flexibility in combining levels to meet varying definitional needs and preferences. A total of 33 separate codes allow demographers, healthcare researchers, policy makers, and others to aggregate these codes according to their needs.

RUCAs are flexible and can be grouped in many ways to suit particular analytic or policy purposes (Hart et al., 2005). The RUCAs are widely used for policy and research purposes (e.g., by the Centers for Medicare and

Medicaid Services and many researchers). RUCAs can identify the rural portions of metropolitan counties and the urban portions of nonmetropolitan counties.

The RUCA codes have been updated several times since its inception. RUCA codes (2010) by state census tracts can be downloaded from the USDA-ERS website. A ZIP code approximation of RUCAs is available from the University of North Dakota Center for Rural Health.

The Index of Relative Rurality

The Index of Relative Rurality (IRR) is a new classification introduced recently to measure a county's degree of rurality instead of delineating a county into rural or urban. The IRR is based on four dimensions of rurality: size, density, remoteness, and built-up area (Waldorf, 2006).

The first two dimensions, size and density, are represented in almost all existing taxonomies of rurality. There is a general agreement that places with small populations or low density are more rural than places with large populations or high density. Remoteness is a less frequently used dimension in existing taxonomies. It is based on the idea that remote places are more rural than less-remote places. The last dimension, built-up area, captures the idea that places with few built-up areas are more rural than heavily built-up places.

The index is scaled from 0 to 1, where 0 is the most urban place and 1 is the most rural place. The index is continual and thus does not suffer from problems that arise when using arbitrary thresholds to separate discrete categories (metro/nonmetro or urban/rural). This shift away from often ill-defined categories of rural and urban, to measuring the degree of rurality will shed new light on a wide array of rural issues ranging from rural poverty to economic growth as shown in **Table 1-1** (Waldorf, 2006).

Rural Public Health in the United States
Development of Rural Public Health

Rural health refers to the health status of people living in rural areas and the policies that guide the healthcare delivery system that serves them (Suh & Heady, 2013). The history of governmental public health in America dates back to the late 1700s. Early public health efforts in the United States focused on either specific populations, such as merchant seamen and the urban poor, or specific outbreaks of disease, such as cholera, smallpox, tuberculosis, yellow fever, malaria, and typhoid (Phillips & McLeroy, 2004). The *Marine Hospital Service* was established with the July 16, 1798, signing by President John Adams of an act for the relief of sick and disabled seamen. The first permanent Marine Hospital was authorized on May 3, 1807, to be built in Boston. The Marine Hospital Service, reorganized a decade earlier under the leadership of the nation's first surgeon general, Dr John M. Woodworth, would eventually take over national authority for issues of quarantine and public health from the National Board of Health in 1882. By the end of the 1800s, the Marine Hospital Service was solidly recognized as the chief health agency of the United States (Duffy, 1992).

Not until the Civil War was there a good understanding of proper sanitation in preventing diseases. With this understanding came the development of municipal health departments, with numbers expanding into the late 1880s (Meit & Knudson, 2009). The first city to establish a board of health was Philadelphia in 1794, followed by Baltimore in 1797, Boston in 1799, Washington, DC, in 1802, New Orleans in 1804, and New York City in 1805 (Fee & Brown, 2002). With the social and health challenges created by the burgeoning industrial machine that dominated the

Table 1-1 Key Characteristics of Commonly Used Rural Taxonomies

Definition	Agency	Geographic Unit	Number of Classes	Elements Used for Classification	Strengths	Weaknesses
Urban–Rural areas	U.S. Census Bureau	Census tract	3 Urban areas, clusters, and rural areas	Population size, population density	Census tract represents the smallest and most precise geographic unit.	A deficiency of classifying at the census tract level is that the boundaries of these areas are not well known. The only three classes, urban, cluster, and rural are not enough to adequately model variability in mobility need and available services.
Metropolitan and nonmetropolitan	OMB	County	3 Metropolitan, micropolitan, and noncore	Urbanized areas based on population density, population size, adjacency and commuting ties with the core	County boundaries represent political jurisdictions and remain stable over time.	The only two classes metropolitan and nonmetropolitan, are not enough to capture the variability in mobility needs and transportation services; county size varies substantially across the United States, and larger counties may dilute or mask the rural population given their geographic size and influence.

Rural–Urban Continuum Codes (RUCC)	ERS Economic Research Service	County	9 Metro and nonmetro categories are subdivided into three metro and six nonmetro groups. Each U.S. county is assigned to one of nine codes.	Population size, degree of urbanization, and adjacency to metropolitan areas	The system allows the identification of areas with significant economic integration.	County-based designations are not the optimum approach because large counties may dilute or mask rural population given their geographic size and influence.
Rural–Urban Commuting Areas (RUCAs)	Developed by the economic Research Service (ERS) of the United States Department of Agriculture, the University of Washington, and the Office of Rural Health Policy	Census tract, ZIP code	10 primary 21 secondary	Population density, urbanization, and daily commuting	It constitutes a vast improvement in rural/urban definitions based on counties; use of work commuting data differentiates rural areas.	Rely on work commuting patterns. The times and distances are actually estimates measured along the fastest road to the closest type of geographic unit.
The Index of Relative Rurality (IRR)	Indiana University	Aggregate of index: size, density, remoteness, and built-up area	N/A	Population size, population density, remoteness, and built-up area	"Is a county rural or urban?" but instead addresses the question "What is a county's degree of rurality?"	Complexity

Data from Guidelines for Using Rural-Urban Classification Systems for Community Health Assessment. Retrieved from https://www.doh.wa.gov/Portals/1/Documents/1500/RUCAGuide.pdf.

late 19th and early 20th centuries, the emphasis of public health was on epidemic control in poor populations in urban slums.

Prior to the establishment of local public health department, district nurses, later known as public health nurses, delivered much of the rural public health services. District nursing societies were established in the 1880s and eventually changed their names to Visiting Nurses Associations. The focus of these voluntary organizations was to provide care for the sick in their homes. As governmental public health expanded in the late 1800s, urban health departments began hiring nurses'to provide a wider array of public health services, beginning with Los Angeles and New York City (Meit & Knudson, 2009).

The Hospital Survey and Construction Act was signed into law by President Harry S. Truman on August 13, 1946. The law is commonly known as the Hill-Burton act, a reference to the names of its two principal sponsors, Sens. Lister Hill (D-Ala.) and Harold Burton (R-Ohio). The idea was to build hospitals where they were needed and where they would be sustainable once their doors were open. Subsequent decades witnessed the construction of new facilities in the 40% of U.S. counties that lacked hospitals in 1945 and by 1975, Hill-Burton had been responsible for construction of nearly one-third of U.S. hospitals.

Rural Public Health Challenges

Approximately 62 million people—nearly one in five Americans—live in rural America. (Bureau, n.d.) Although rural America is perceived to be a clean, pristine, and healthy environment, people living in rural America, from Appalachia and the Deep South to the Midwest and western states to Alaska and Hawaii, face several challenges, including poverty and lack of access to care due to limited number of healthcare practitioners and lack of health insurance (Kirby, 2014).

Farmers, people who live in ranches, reservations, and frontier areas lack access to

public health infrastructures such as district or county public health departments. They must travel long distances to reach the nearest healthcare provider. This requires taking hours off from work for an initial appointment or follow-up, forcing many people to delay or avoid seeking medical care. The United States' rural public health system remains ill equipped to respond to the health disparities experienced by its people. The system tends to be understaffed or to employ staff with little formal public health training (NRHA, 2016).

Recent rural hospital and clinic closures have compounded the problem. In the past decade, nearly 100 rural hospitals across the country have closed and another 600 are at risk of shutting down in the near future, leaving many rural Americans without easy access to essential medical service. (Stateline et al., 2019) The causes of rural hospital closures are multifactorials. Out-migration of educated young adults to urban areas leaving older and poor people behind is one factor. With the declining populations, rural hospitals often have empty beds, which means less revenue.

A rural public health system not only includes governmental agencies working to ensure population health but also a wide array of partners such as hospitals, healthcare providers, nonprofit organizations, cooperative extension agents, volunteers, and many more. For rural communities that otherwise lack public health capacities, these partners are of the utmost importance. To organize rural public health to reduce inefficiencies and improve the health of rural residents, state legislatures continually seek innovative ways to improve access to doctors and to better coordinate care. Considering that most existing public health principles and practices were developed and tested in urban settings, these "urban-centric" principles and practices require adjustment for them to be effective in rural areas.

The continued out-migration of increasingly educated young adults, in-migration of ethnic minorities, and growing numbers of retirees, have transformed rural American populations. The increasing diversity of rural America deserves a closer look at the racial-ethnic populations making up the rural landscape (*USDA ERS—Rural Population Trends*, n.d.) While Hispanics were the fastest-growing segment of the rural population, they account for only 9% of the rural population (20% in urban areas). African Americans made up 8% of the rural population (13% in urban areas). Native Americans were the only minority group with a higher rural (2%) than urban share (0.5%). Although rural communities share common challenges, the residents are often racially and ethnically varied and present distinct health inequities. Whether because of historical racism or language, cultural, or other barriers, racial-ethnic minorities often fare worse on several indicators than whites. The lack of cooperation and understanding between all segments of the rural population will threaten the viability of rural areas and lead to increased rates of poverty and social tension. (Kirschner, Berry, & Glasgow, 2006).

Despite the recognition of the breadth of challenges facing rural populations, remarkably little progress in eliminating rural health disparities has been done. Although much research and action assumed that theories, practices, and programs developed in urban settings will be translatable into rural settings, this simply is not the case. Rural-focused research is needed to improve rural public health.

Conclusion

Rural health refers to the health status of people living in rural areas and the policies that guide the healthcare delivery system that serves them. Although there is no consensus around a standardized definition of rurality, experts agreed to use a conceptual framework to define "health." The U.S. Census Bureau, the Office of Management and Budget, and the Economic Research Service (ERS) of the United States Department of Agriculture have developed different taxonomies to define the concept of rurality. End users of these methods must familiarize themselves with the existing methods to determine when to use them appropriately.

The development of rural public health is ongoing. It started with the development of local board of health to prevent epidemics among poor urban residents. The federal government became involved with the creation of the Marine Hospital to protect the health of seamen. The enactment of the Hill Burton Act in 1946 contributed to the construction of 40% of community hospitals. It improved access to care in rural areas.

The incidence of poverty is greatest in America's rural areas and central cities. Approximately 10 million persons, or 16.3% of the rural and small-town population, live in poverty. Nearly one-quarter of people in poverty live in rural areas (Kirby, 2014). People in poverty lack health insurance and often travel long distances to access health services. The ongoing wave of rural hospital and clinic closures have compounded the problem of access to care in rural areas. The in-migration of ethnic minorities and the growing numbers of retirees have changed the racial and ethnic make-up of rural residents creating a new challenge.

Chapter Summary

The term rural is vague. Two principal definitions of rural have been used by the federal government. The first definition is the "urban-rural" classification of populations developed by the Census Bureau. The Census Bureau identifies two types of urban areas: Urbanized Areas (UAs) of 50,000 or more people and Urban Clusters (UCs) of at least 2,500 and less than 50,000 people. The Census does not actually define "rural." Whatever is not urban is considered rural. The second definition is the "metropolitan/

nonmetropolitan" classification of counties developed by the OMB. **Metropolitan areas** contain core counties with one or more central cities of at least 50,000 population or with a Census Bureau defined urbanized area and a total area population of 10,000 or more, as well as fringe counties that are economically tied to the core counties.

Discussion Questions

1. Discuss the major differences between rural and urban areas?
2. List the different methods used to define rurality and explain the differences between these methods.
3. Of the different methods discussed above, which one would you use to define rurality and why.
4. Briefly discuss the benefits of using the *Index of Relative Rurality over the Census or OMB approach* to define rurality.
5. Discuss the future of rural area in America in terms of population and development.

Student Activities and Worksheets are available inside the Navigate eBook, included with the printed text. Simply redeem the access code found at the front of the book at www.jblearning.com.

References

Badash, I., Kleinman, N. P., Barr, S., Jang, J., Rahman, S., & Wu, B. W. (2017). Redefining health: The evolution of health ideas from antiquity to the era of value-based care. *Cureus, 9*(2), e1018.

Bircher, J., & Hahn, E. G. (2016). Understanding the nature of health: New perspectives for medicine and public health. Improved wellbeing at lower costs. *F1000Research, 5*, 167.

Bircher, J., & Kuruvilla, S. (2014). Defining health by addressing individual, social, and environmental determinants: New opportunities for health care and public health. *Journal of Public Health Policy, 35*(3), 363–386.

Boers, M., & Jentoft, A. J. C. (2015). A new concept of health can improve the definition of frailty. *Calcified Tissue International, 97*(5), 429–431.

Brüssow, H. (2013). What is health? *Microbial Biotechnology, 6*(4), 341–348.

Duffy, J. (1992). *The sanitarians: a history of American public health.* University of Illinois Press.

Fee, E., & Brown, T. M. (2002). The unfulfilled promise of public health: déjà vu all over again. *Health Affairs, 21*(6), 31–43.

Frenk, J., & Gómez-Dantés, O. (2014). Designing a framework for the concept of health. *Journal of Public Health Policy, 35*(3), 401–406.

Hart, L. G., Larson, E. H., & Lishner, D. M. (2005). Rural definitions for health policy and research. *Am J Public Health, 95*(7), 1149–1155.

Huber, M., Knottnerus, J. A., Green, L., van der Horst, H., Jadad, A. R., Kromhout, D., . . . Smid H. (2011). How should we define health? *British Medical Journal, 343*, d4163.

Isserman, A. M. (2005). In the national interest: Defining rural and urban correctly in research and public policy. *International Regional Science Review, 28*(4), 465–499.

Jadad, A. R., & O'Grady, L. (2008). How should health be defined? *British Medical Journal (Online), 337*, a2900.

Kickbusch, I. (2003). The contribution of the World Health Organization to a new public health and health promotion. *American Journal of Public Health, 93*(3), 383–388.

Kirby, S. (2014). Taking stock: Rural people, poverty, and housing in the 21st Century. *Housing and Society, 41*(2), 345–348. https://doi.org/10.1080/08882746.2014.11430636

Kirschner, A., Berry, E. H., & Glasgow, N. (2006). The changing faces of rural America *Population change and rural society* (pp. 53–74): Springer.

Larson, J. S. (1999). The conceptualization of health. *Medical Care Research and Review, 56*(2), 123–136.

McGranahan, D. A., Hession, J. C., Mines, F. K., & Jordan, M. F. (1986). Social and economic characteristics of the population in metro and nonmetro counties, 1970-80. *Economic Research, 800*, 336–4700.

Meit, M., & Knudson, A. (2009). Why is rural public health important? A look to the future. *Journal* of *Public Health Management & Practice, 15*(3), 185–190.

Miller, M. K., & Luloff, A. E. (1980). Who Is Rural? A Typological Approach to the Examination of Rurality. *ERIC Institution of Education Services.*

NRHA. (2016). *Rural public health policy paper.* Retrieved April 6, 2020, from https://www.ruralhealthweb.org /getattachment/Advocate/Policy-

Phillips, C. D., & McLeroy, K. R. (2004). Health in rural America: Remembering the importance of place. *American Journal of Public Health, 94*(10), 1661–1663.

Raphael, D. (2010). *Health promotion and quality of life in Canada: Essential readings.* Canadian Scholars' Press.

Ratcliffe, M., Burd, C., Holder, K., & Fields, A. (2016). Defining rural at the U.S. Census Bureau. *American Community Survey and Geography Brief*, 1–8.

Ratcliffe, M. R. (2006). Creating metropolitan and micropolitan statistical areas. *Measuring Rural Diversity, 3*(1).

Stateline, reporting, E. P. provides daily and analysis on trends in state policy. (2019). *Here's Why Rural Hospitals Are Shutting Down More Quickly in These States. HuffPost.* https://www.huffpost .com/entry/rural-hospitals-close-medicaid-aca_b _5c4734d8e4b09dd3f0cb1f08

Sartorius, N. (2006). The meanings of health and its promotion. *Croatian Medical Journal, 47*(4), 662–664.

Suh, R., & Heady, H. R. (2013). *Rural Health in the United States:* Oxford University Press.

Svalastog, A. L., Donev, D., Kristoffersen, N. J., & Gajović, S. (2017). Concepts and definitions of health

and health-related values in the knowledge landscapes of the digital society. *Croatian Medical Journal, 58*(6), 431–435.

United States Census Bureau. (2017). *What is Rural America?* One in five Americans live in rural areas. https://www.census.gov/library/stories/2017/08/rural -america.html

United States Department of Agriculture. Economic Research Service. (2019). Rural population trends. https://www.ers.usda.gov/amber-waves/2019 /february/rural-population-trends/

Waldorf, B. (2006). *A continuous multi-dimensional measure of rurality: Moving beyond threshold measures.* Paper presented at the annual meeting of the American Agricultural Economics Association, Long Beach, CA.

World Health Organization. (1946). Constitution of the World Health Organization. *Geneva: World Health Organization.*

World Health Organization, (1986). The Ottawa Charter for Health Promotion World Health Organization: Geneva.

Yapijakis, C. (2009). Hippocrates of Kos, the father of clinical medicine, and Asclepiades of Bithynia, the father of molecular medicine. *In Vivo, 23*(4), 507–514.

Žuškin, E., Lipozenčić, J., Pucarin-Cvetković, J., Mustajbegović, J., Schachter, N., Mučić-Pučić, B., & Neralić-Meniga, I. (2008). Ancient medicine–a review. *Acta Dermatovenerologica Croatica, 16*(3), 149–157.

CHAPTER 2

Determinants of Health in Rural Communities

Carrie Henning-Smith, PhD, MPH, MSW

LEARNING OBJECTIVES

At the end of this chapter, readers will be able to:

1. Understand the importance of social determinants of health in impacting population health outcomes.
2. Discuss key differences between rural and urban areas in the social determinants of health.
3. Identify salient determinants of health for rural populations.
4. Describe ways in which environmental, economic, and socio-demographic characteristics of rural areas are associated with population health outcomes.

KEY TERMS

Acute
Chronic
Environmental context
Poverty
Social determinants of health
Structural racism

CHAPTER OVERVIEW

There are countless factors that influence health outcomes. These include factors that appear very proximal to health, including health behaviors and health care. However, individual and population health are influenced more by what happens outside of the health care arena than what happens in the doctor's office (Rettenmaier & Wang, 2013) As a result, one's context is vitally important in determining one's health outcomes. This includes **environmental context**, economic landscape, and the population's socio-demographic characteristics. Collectively, these are often referred to as "social determinants of health." Rural and urban areas differ in each of those characteristics (Henning-Smith, Evenson, Corbett, Kozhimannil, & Moscovice, 2018a; Henning-Smith, Evenson, Kozhimannil, & Moscovice, 2017a; Henning-Smith, Kozhimannil, Casey, Prasad, & Moscovice, 2017; USDA, 2016, 2017), and it is important to understand ways in which social determinants of health uniquely impact health in rural areas. This chapter will explore social determinants of health for rural residents and will also provide an overview of the unique characteristics of rural health behaviors and health care. Subsequent chapters in this book will go into greater detail on specific determinants of health for rural populations as well as differences within rural areas and populations and potential policy and programmatic solutions to improve rural health by addressing the many factors that contribute to health.

Determinants of Health in Rural Communities

The health of individuals and populations is influenced by many factors, including genetics, behaviors, medical care, social and economic factors, and the physical environment (County Health Rankings & Roadmaps, 2019). Those factors that fall outside of traditional medical care and individual genetics are commonly referred to as the "**social determinants of health**" and, together, have the greatest impact on population health. For rural residents, this means that the environmental, economic, socio-demographic, and health care landscape of rural areas have a direct impact on health, causing health outcomes for rural residents to differ from those of urban residents. Additionally, all of those factors and a person's situation influence health behaviors, so, to the extent that health behaviors influence health outcomes, rural residents face a different set of variables and choices related to behaviors compared with urban residents. This could further differentiate the health of rural and urban populations. Each of these areas will be explored in more detail in this chapter, and many of them will be explored in depth in subsequent chapters throughout this book.

Environmental and Community Context

Rural areas are often portrayed as pastoral and pristine. This can be the case in many places; however, rural areas are also home to significant environmental factors that can seriously impact health, including issues related to air and water quality, toxic exposures, and impacts of climate change. Furthermore, rural areas differ from urban areas significantly when it comes to transportation and infrastructure and those differences lead to important differences in opportunities for health.

In general, rural areas, particularly non-core rural counties, have smaller amounts of particulate matter in the air, leading to better air quality and, potentially, better health outcomes as they relate to air quality (Strosnider, Kennedy, Monti, & Yip, 2017). However, rural areas have poorer water quality than urban areas, potentially because of rural-urban differences in water management practices and infrastructure capabilities (Strosnider et al., 2017). Access to clean water is essential for health, so differences in water quality may lead to health disparities for rural residents, relative to urban.

Even more than current conditions in the natural environment and their impact on rural health, the lasting impact of climate change threatens to greatly affect the vitality of rural places. While rural residents comprise less than one-fifth of the U.S. population, rural areas make up the vast majority (95%) of all land areas in the United States and are home to the majority of all agricultural and energy production (U.S. National Climate Assessment, 2014). The amount of land, coupled with fewer economic resources and limited infrastructure (described in detail below) puts rural residents at increased risk of the health effects of climate change (U.S. National Climate Assessment, 2014). Already, rural areas are seeing the devastating impact of increased natural disasters and extreme weather, such as severe heat, flooding, wildfires, and draught (U.S. National Climate Assessment, 2014). These have immediate effects on human health and can also have a long-lasting impact on entire ecosystems and environmental structures.

In addition to the natural environment and changing climate, rural areas differ from urban areas in significant ways related to infrastructure, which has both a direct and indirect impact on health. For example, rural areas have more limited access to broadband Internet and cellular connectivity (LaRose, Gregg, Strover, Straubhaar, & Carpenter, 2007; Whitacre, Wheeler, & Landgraf, 2017). This can make it more difficult for rural residents to actively participate in online economic activity, to connect with others, and to access health care and other services remotely. Policymakers are actively working to expand access to broadband Internet in many states, but more work is required to ensure universally equitable connectivity in all rural places.

Rural areas also have unique limitations related to transportation, including limited resources for building and maintaining roads and bridges, limited (and sometimes nonexistent) public transportation, and longer distances to travel between people, places, and services (Henning-Smith, Evenson, Corbett, Kozhimannil, & Moscovice, 2018a). All of these issues can impact health because people need to travel to reach health care and other resources and to connect with one another. In an era of declining populations in many rural areas, coupled with declining health care and other services, people need to travel even farther to get to where they need to go to meet their basic needs to ensure their own health. However, rural residents tend to have fewer financial resources (described below) to afford money for private vehicles, including gas and maintenance.

Addressing rural transportation issues is a multifaceted, complex problem, which involves working across multiple states and municipalities, each of which has its own transportation system and infrastructure, and thinking creatively about how to meet transportation needs of sparsely populated areas with limited means (Henning-Smith, Evenson, et al., 2018a). These issues are particularly **acute** for individuals with lower incomes or individuals who have health problems that make driving difficult. In fact, research suggests that rural residents with travel-limiting health problems are less likely than their urban counterparts to give up driving, likely because

there are fewer available options to get where they need to go (Henning-Smith, Evenson, Kozhimannil, & Moscovice, 2017b).

Issues around rural infrastructure also extend to housing, and safe housing is essential for human health (Taylor, 2018). Rural housing stock is, on average, older and in poorer shape than urban housing stock, and access to both safe, affordable housing and credit to afford housing equity can be difficult to obtain, especially for low-income, rural residents (National Rural Housing Coalition, 2018; White, 2015). Addressing issues of housing can be particularly challenging in rural areas, given the aforementioned limitations in other types of infrastructure and limited economic resources. Without access to high-quality, affordable housing, people are at risk of poor health outcomes, including asthma, lead poisoning, infections, and injuries, with a particular risk for young children living in substandard housing as their bodies and minds are still developing (National Rural Housing Coalition, 2018). Housing issues can also have an outsized impact on older adults who may want to "age in place" in rural communities, or remain in their homes and communities as they age. Doing so may require housing to be modified as individual's health and functional abilities change and this can be more difficult in rural areas, where housing tends to need more work to be fully accessible.(Henning-Smith & Blonigan, 2017).

A final important element of environmental characteristics relates to the characteristics of a person's immediate neighborhood and community and the extent to which it does—or does not—provide access to healthy behaviors and resources. This includes access to affordable, healthy food; access to safe and accessible opportunities for physical activity; and access to meaningful social interactions with others. Each of these is essential for health, as evidence shows that lack of access to nutritious food, exercise, and social connectedness are all related to higher risk of poor health outcomes (Corbett, Anglin, Evenson, & Moscovice, 2018; Holt-Lunstad, Smith, Baker, Harris, & Stephenson, 2015; Holt-Lunstad et al., 2010; Pate et al., 1995; Story, Kaphingst, Robinson-O'Brien, & Glanz, 2008; Walker, Keane, & Burke, 2010). As with the issues described above, each of these is different in rural environments compared with urban environments, and each requires unique approaches and solutions to addressing the underlying determinants of health in order to improve population health in rural areas.

For food access, many rural areas are home to "food deserts," or areas without adequate access to healthy, affordable food. In fact, many rural areas do not have grocery stores at all, or require lengthy drives to get groceries, which is made difficult by the transportation issues described above. In rural areas, lack of access to a grocery store is defined by needing to drive more than 10 miles to reach one, and sometimes lack of access to healthy food is further defined by focusing on food deserts specifically for rural residents with lower incomes, as issues of affording food and transportation impact them more severely (Remington, Catlin, & Gennuso, 2015; Wright Morton & Blanchard, 2007). Rural areas most likely to be food deserts are those where residents have lower socio-economic status, measured by educational attainment, incomes, and **poverty** rates (Wright Morton & Blanchard, 2007). Food deserts are also more common in the most sparsely populated rural areas, where people need to travel the farthest to access the resources needed for their daily lives (Wright Morton & Blanchard, 2007).

The "built environment," or ways in which towns and communities are designed and constructed, can promote or impede healthy behaviors. In the case of physical activity, rural areas are less likely than urban areas to have amenities like walking trails, bike paths, and sidewalks to promote daily physical activity (Brownson et al., 2000; Frost et al., 2010; Park, Eyler, Tabak, Valko, & Brownson,

2017). Access to indoor exercise opportunities (e.g., a gym or recreational facility) can also be difficult in sparsely populated areas, and, even if they do exist, they are not always affordable or accessible to all residents. When designing potential solutions to encourage physical activity among rural residents, it is essential to not assume that solutions that work in urban environments (e.g., designing strategies to encourage walking or bike commuting) would be feasible or even logical in rural areas; instead, unique solutions are required to meet the unique needs of individual rural areas and residents (Hansen, Umstattd Meyer, Lenardson, & Hartley, 2015).

Finally, the context of a person's community—combined with access to the connectivity, technology, and transportation described above—impact a person's social relationships and connectivity. There is ample evidence to show that loneliness and social isolation are detrimental to health, for both rural and urban residents (Cornwell & Waite, 2009; Holt-Lunstad et al., 2015, 2010). However, there are differences in the risk of social isolation by rurality, with some research showing rural residents reporting both more relationships (friends and family) and still greater feelings of loneliness (Henning-Smith, Moscovice, & Kozhimannil, 2019). Meeting the social needs of rural residents requires addressing the aforementioned infrastructure and environmental characteristics, and it also requires a unique approach to addressing the specific challenges and opportunities inherent in rural areas (Henning-Smith, Ecklund, et al., 2019). Furthermore, rural residents are heterogeneous, and the risk of social isolation differs not only by community context, but also by socio-demographic characteristics, such as gender, race, ethnicity, age, and socio-economic status (Henning-Smith, Ecklund, Moscovice, & Kozhimannil, 2018; Henning-Smith, Moscovice, et al., 2019), many of which are described in more detail below.

Economic Landscape

Access to economic and financial resources is essential for population and individual health. People need enough money to afford basic necessities like food, housing, transportation, and health care. Living in poverty, in particular, can be harmful to a person's health, especially if it is **chronic** (long-lasting) (Murray, 2006; Simon, 2013). This is because it is not only difficult to meet basic needs but also because of the chronic stress that accompanies living in poverty for long periods of time. Chronic stress, for any reason, can take a physical toll on the body and raise the person's allostatic load, increasing the risk of poor health outcomes (Beckie, 2012). Furthermore, economic and occupational opportunities provide access to other resources and to social and positional power, which are essential for health (Ravesteijn, Van Kippersluis, & Van Doorslaer, 2013).

People in rural areas feel these issues acutely because rural areas are, on average, worse-off economically than urban areas. Rural areas tend to have lower median incomes than urban areas, coupled with higher rates of poverty (USDA ERS, 2020). Rural areas also recovered more slowly from the Great Recession of the 2000s, seeing slower job growth in the years since (Hertz, Kusmin, Marré, & Parker, 2014). Like all issues related to rural health, these are not universally true across all rural areas; there are certainly rural places that are thriving economically. However, on average, the economic disadvantage faced by rural residents, relative to urban, places rural residents at a higher risk of poor health outcomes because of economic hardship and lack of occupational opportunities. With that said, rural areas have also seen economic improvement since 2013, with declining unemployment rates and rising income levels (Cromartie, 2018). Again, there is considerable variation from place to place.

The types of jobs that are available in rural areas also differ in meaningful ways from those available in urban areas. While not universally true, highly-skilled (and highly-paid) jobs tend to be concentrated in urban areas, while rural areas are home to some of the most labor-intensive and potentially dangerous jobs in the U.S. economy, including agriculture, mining, logging and forestry, and energy production and extraction (Abel, Gabe, & Stolarick, 2012; Laughlin, 2016). Certainly, not all rural residents work in those industries; in fact, the most common jobs in rural areas are similar to the most common jobs in urban areas, including education, health care, retail, manufacturing, and social services (Laughlin, 2016). Still, those jobs that are more common in rural areas than in urban areas tend to put employees at higher risk of workplace injuries and fatalities due to physically demanding work conditions and job requirements (Kim, Ozegovic, & Voaklander, 2012; Peek-Asa, Zwerling, & Stallones, 2004). Additionally, because the types of jobs tend to be different between rural and urban areas, so do the types and quality of benefits available to employees based on rurality, with rural residents tending to work at jobs with fewer benefits and less flexibility (Henning-Smith & Lahr, 2018b; Larson & Hill, 2004). Because of constrained economic environments and limited job choices, described above, rural residents may also have fewer available employment opportunities, which will limit their ability to choose a job based on safety, health, and quality of life benefits.

Socio-Demographic Characteristics

At the outset, it is important to note that socio-demographic characteristics (e.g., race, ethnicity, gender, immigration status) on their own should not determine health outcomes for rural residents. Rather, the ways in which society is structured with institutionalized systems of discrimination can lead to poorer health outcomes for some rural residents over others. Additionally, there are important ways in which rural and urban areas differ along socio-demographic lines that lead to differences in the health needs and profile of residents based on rurality.

First of all, rural areas differ in meaningful ways from urban areas because they tend to have a high proportion of older adults. This is partly due to out-migration of younger adults from some rural areas, leaving older adults to "age in place" (Henning-Smith & Blonigan, 2017) while younger adults seek other opportunities in more urban areas (Kumar, 2018). It is also due to declining fertility rates among rural residents (and across the United States) (Cromartie & Vilorio, 2019). As a result, on average, rural areas are also experiencing declining populations overall. This is exacerbated by increasing mortality rates among some rural residents (Case & Deaton, 2015; Cromartie & Vilorio, 2019; Garcia et al., 2017). Beyond changing aging structures, declining populations can have enormous consequences for rural communities, with direct impacts on health, such as diminishing tax revenues, limited workforce (for health care and all other sectors), and declining property values (Kumar, 2018). Again; however, it is important to note that not all rural areas are losing populations, nor are all rural areas aging more rapidly than urban areas. And, there is some limited evidence that rural population loss is slowing—or even reversing—as of the 2010s (Cromartie & Vilorio, 2019).

Because a disproportionate share of older adults live in rural areas, the health needs of rural populations tend to be different, with higher rates of disability, chronic conditions, and need for long-term services and supports (Henning-Smith & Blonigan, 2017; Skoufalos, Clarke, Ellis, Shepard, & Rula, 2017). However, rural older adults face constraints in accessing health care, financial resources, and other services necessary to support them in aging in rural communities (Henning-Smith,

Casey, Prasad, & Kozhimannil, 2017; Henning-Smith, Kozhimannil, Casey, & Prasad, 2018; Skoufalos et al., 2017). Additionally, given that the vast majority of care provided to older adults and others with functional limitations is provided by loved ones ("informal" or "unpaid" caregivers), and given that rural areas face unique constraints in accessing formal services, rural caregivers may have unique impacts on their own health as a result of their rural environment (Henning-Smith & Lahr, 2018a, 2018b; Henning-Smith, Lahr, & Casey, 2018). Still, not all older adults have functional impairments (aging and disability should not be synonymous); furthermore, even those who do are important members of their communities. As rural communities struggle with changing demographics, opportunities to engage and involve older adults in intergenerational community efforts will be essential to ensuring community vitality (Henning-Smith & Blonigan, 2017).

Beyond age, any discussion of rural socio-demographic characteristics and health needs should include a comprehensive exploration of race and ethnicity. Too often, rural areas are portrayed as largely white, which is inaccurate and does a disservice to the current and historical diversity present in rural areas. (Kozhimannil & Henning-Smith, 2017, 2019) Indeed, rural areas have always been racially and ethnically diverse, and some rural populations, including rural African Americans and rural Native Americans have deep historical roots in rural places, often dating back to well before their white neighbors. Rural areas are also increasingly racially and ethnically diverse; today, approximately one in five rural Americans is a person of color or Native American/American Indian. This percentage continues to increase with immigration, coupled with outmigration of some white rural residents (Kozhimannil & Henning-Smith, 2017; Lichter, 2012). Today (and throughout our history), there are rural areas where the majority of the population is not white, but rather is African American, Native American, Hispanic/Latino, or a heterogeneous group with no racial or ethnic majority group (Henning-Smith, Hernandez, Ramirez, Hardeman, & Kozhimannil, 2019).

People of color and Native Americans/American Indians experience poorer health outcomes, on average, than white Americans (Bailey et al., 2017; Gee & Ford, 2011). This is due to **structural racism**, where groups of people are systematically treated differently through both overt and covert policies, programs, and behaviors (Bailey et al., 2017; Gee & Ford, 2011). These may take the form of housing discrimination, employment discrimination, inequitable policing and criminal justice enforcement and imprisonment, and segregated neighborhoods with unequal access to resources. It may also take the form of macroaggressions in interpersonal interactions, even within the health care setting (Hardeman, Medina, & Kozhimannil, 2016). Living in a society with institutionalized racism can increase one's stress, leading to a higher allostatic load and compounding health disadvantages (Peters, 2006). These issues are present across levels of geography but are compounded in rural areas by the other issues discussed above. As a result, rural people of color, especially African Americans and Native Americans, are particularly at risk of poorer health outcomes, including mortality (Henning-Smith et al., 2019; James et al., 2017).

Countless other socio-demographic characteristics and identities are related to health outcomes for rural residents, including gender, sexual orientation, and immigration status. Each of those are associated with health outcomes and health disparities and each of them plays out uniquely in rural settings, with individuals facing the additional issues discussed earlier in this chapter. For example, rural women face more limited access to health care and have poorer health outcomes than urban women (American College of Obstetricians and Gynecologists., 2014). For

rural individuals who are recent immigrants or who self-identify as lesbian, gay, bisexual, or transgender (LGBT), it may be particularly difficult to find health care providers with appropriate training and exposure to appropriately meet their needs (Rosenkrantz, Black, Abreu, Aleshire, & Fallin-Bennett, 2016). They may also find themselves facing discrimination in rural communities, with more difficulty finding an "affinity community" within their local area that they feel safe within. Once again; however, it is important to emphasize that rural residents and rural places are heterogeneous; there are certainly places that are more welcoming than others. More work is needed, however, to ensure equitable access to good health for all rural residents.

Health Behaviors

One's health behaviors, or the behaviors and activities that one engages in to achieve (or not) good health outcomes, have an important impact on a person's physical and mental health (Cockerham, 2014). Health behaviors include activities like physical activity, diet and nutrition, social engagement, safety, avoiding tobacco and other harmful substances, and other actions that contribute to general health and quality of life (Cockerham, 2014). Engaging in poor health behaviors, like smoking or sedentary behavior, can lead to higher risk of poor health outcomes and mortality, both for individuals and entire populations (Cutler, Glaeser, & Rosen, 2007; De Rezende, Lopes, Rey-López, Matsudo, & Luiz, 2014).

In understanding the impact of health behaviors on health outcomes, it is essential to understand context, such as those environmental, neighborhood, and socio-economic features described earlier in this chapter. Individuals' behaviors are strongly influenced by their context, as is their set of choices and opportunities to engage in healthy (or not so healthy) behaviors. Therefore, in addressing the relationship between health behaviors and health outcomes, it is important to address structural, systemic-level policies and context and to avoid blaming individuals for their particular choices. Changing the physical, social, and policy environment within which individuals make choices will have a much greater impact on improving health behaviors and health (Cohen, Scribner, & Farley, 2000; Housemann, Bacak, Brownson, Brennan, & Baker, 2008).

Given the unique characteristics of rural environments, it is probably no surprise that there are rural-urban differences in health behavior. On average, rural residents have poorer health behaviors in several domains, including higher smoking rates, higher rates of sedentary (e.g., not active) behavior, and lower rates of maintaining healthy body weight (Matthews, 2017; Weaver, Palmer, Lu, Case, & Geiger, 2013). Rural residents also experience higher rates of motor vehicle fatalities (Henning-Smith & Kozhimannil, 2018), which may indicate less safe driving behaviors; as with the other behaviors discussed here, though, it also relates to differences in the environment for rural residents.

Health Care

Much more will be said about health care in the subsequent chapters of this book, especially in Part II; however, any discussion of the determinants of rural health should at least include a mention of health care. Although medical care does not contribute the most toward health, it is inarguably an important component of health, via preventive care, ongoing care for chronic and long-lasting conditions, and care for acute and emergency situations. Access to appropriate and high-quality health care for each of those types of care is important for ensuring timely, efficient, and effective treatment to achieve the best possible outcomes. Both access to care and quality of care are more challenging in rural areas (Martin et al., 2013; Henning-Smith, Prasad, Casey, Kozhimannil, & Moscovice, 2017; Merwin, Snyder, & Katz,

2006; Nayar, Yu, & Apenteng, 2013), which can have the negative effect of leading to poorer health outcomes for rural residents who are not able to receive the care they need.

Access to care is more difficult for rural residents for a myriad of reasons. One of these is shortages in the health care workforce (Daniels, Vanleit, Skipper, Sanders, & Rhyne, 2007; Fields, Bigbee, & Bell, 2016). These shortages occur at all levels of health care practice but are particularly challenging for specialty care. Access is also compromised by closures of entire hospitals, or units within hospitals, nursing homes, and other facilities (Hung, Kozhimannil, Henning-Smith, & Casey, 2017; North Carolina Rural Health Research Program, 2019). This causes rural residents to need to drive longer distances to get the care they need (Henning-Smith, Kozhimannil, et al., 2018). Such increased distances may compromise health and put rural residents in danger of poorer outcomes, especially in emergent situations, or of using emergency care rather than routine primary care (Haggerty, Roberge, Lévesque, Gauthier, & Loignon, 2014; Kozhimannil, Hung, Henning-Smith, Casey, & Prasad, 2018). Rural residents are less likely than their urban counterparts to receive recommended preventive care services (Casey, Thiede Call, & Klingner, 2001; Loftus, Allen, Call, & Everson-Rose, 2018). Access is also challenging because of financial barriers to care. This is true for health care providers, who may struggle to remain viable in the face of low patient volume coupled with high-overhead costs and potentially inadequate reimbursement rates. It is also true for individual rural residents, especially those with limited incomes, as discussed above in the section on economic characteristics of rural communities.

All of the other characteristics of rural places and populations described in the previous sections contribute to the complexities of providing health care in rural settings. Ensuring timely, appropriate, and high-quality care in the midst of long distances and sparse populations is a consistent challenge and one that will require creative solutions. Researchers, providers, and policymakers are actively working to address these issues in various ways, including workforce incentives, telemedicine and technology, integrated care, and increased collaboration across systems and geography. For any solution to be effective in a rural setting; however, it will need to take into account all of the other determinants of health for rural residents.

Conclusion

A wide variety of factors contribute to the health of rural residents, including environmental, economic, and demographic characteristics; health behaviors; and health care. None of these operates independently and all of them need to be thought of simultaneously when considering the most effective way to support the health of rural populations. Furthermore, rural people and places are diverse; what works to improve the determinants of health in one rural area may be ineffective in another. While this chapter provided a brief overview of some of the most important determinants of rural health, many of these issues are discussed in much more detail in subsequent chapters, with specific examples of programs and policies working to improve the health of rural populations by addressing their underlying determinants of health.

Chapter Summary

Rural health is made up of several contributing factors, which work together to comprise overall population health outcomes. These include environmental characteristics such as air and water quality, climate change, neighborhood physical environment, and infrastructure; economic characteristics such as poverty, income, and access to employment; socio-demographic characteristics such as structural racism and aging populations; health behaviors, which are influenced by the other factors described above; and the health care landscape of rural areas. In each of these, there are unique challenges and opportunities in rural areas, and solutions to improve health must address those distinct needs rather than applying a one-sized-fits-all approach to both rural and urban areas. Furthermore, rural areas are heterogeneous and these factors will look different from one community to the next, with different implications for health. Policy and programmatic solutions should be mindful of this diversity and should incorporate rural residents into any efforts to improve health.

Discussion Questions

1. What determinant or determinants of health stand out to you as being the most influential for rural health?
2. In considering determinants of rural health, does it seem more important to consider rural vs. urban differences? Or differences between rural residents? Or both? How does this vary depending on the health determinant or health outcome in question?
3. Considering the broad array of determinants that impact rural health, what would be your top three priorities for policy and programmatic change to improve rural health? What stakeholders would you need at the table to implement those changes?
4. Are there determinants that you can think of for rural health that were not included in this chapter?

Additional Reading

- County Health Rankings & Roadmaps. What is Health? https://www.county healthrankings.org/what-is-health
- Rural Health Information Hub. Social Determinants of Health for Rural People. https://www.ruralhealthinfo.org/topics /social-determinants-of-health

- Rural Health Research Gateway. *Social Determinants of Health.* (List of research projects by federally-funded Rural Health Research Centers on this topic.) https:// www.ruralhealthresearch.org/topics /social-determinants-of-health

---

Student Activities and Worksheets are available inside the Navigate eBook, included with the printed text. Simply redeem the access code found at the front of the book at www.jblearning.com.

References

Abel, J. R., Gabe, T. M., & Stolarick, K. (2012). *Workforce Skills across the Urban-Rural Hierarchy.* Retrieved from https://www.newyorkfed.org/medialibrary /media/research/staff_reports/sr552.pdf

American College of Obstetricians and Gynecologists. (2014). *Health Disparities in Rural Women.* Retrieved from American College of Obstetricians and Gynecologists website: https://www.acog.org/clinical/clinical -guidance/committee-opinion/articles/2014/02 /health-disparities-in-rural-women

Bailey, Z. D., Krieger, N., Agénor, M., Graves, J., Linos, N., & Bassett, M. T. (2017). Structural racism and health inequities in the USA: Evidence and interventions. *The Lancet (London, England), 389*(10077), 1453–1463. https://doi.org/10.1016/S0140-6736(17)30569-X

Beckie, T. M. (2012). A systematic review of allostatic load, health, and health disparities. *Biological Research for Nursing, 14*(4), 311–346. https://doi.org/10.1177 /1099800412455688

Brownson R. C., Baker E. A., Housemann, R. A., Brennan, L. K., & Bacak, S. J. (2001). Environmental and Policy Determinants of Physical Activity in the United States. *American Journal of Public Health.* https://doi .org/10.2105/ajph.91.12.1995

Brownson, R. C., Housemann, R. A., Brown, D. R., Jackson-Thompson, J., King, A. C., Malone, B. R., & Sallis, J. F. (2000). Promoting physical activity in rural communities: walking trail access, use, and effects. *American Journal of Preventive Medicine, 18*(3), 235–241. Retrieved from http://www.ncbi.nlm.nih.gov /pubmed/10722990

Case, A., & Deaton, A. (2015). Rising morbidity and mortality in midlife among white non-Hispanic Americans in the 21st century. *Proceedings of the National Academy of Sciences of the United States of America, 112*(49), 15078–15083. https://doi.org /10.1073/pnas.1518393112

Casey, M. M., Thiede Call, K., & Klingner, J. M. (2001). Are rural residents less likely to obtain recommended preventive healthcare services? *American Journal of Preventive Medicine, 21*(3), 182–188. https://doi.org /S0749-3797(01)00349-X [pii]

Cockerham, W. C. (2014). Health Behavior. In *The Wiley Blackwell Encyclopedia of Health, Illness, Behavior, and Society* (pp. 764–766). https://doi.org/10.1002 /9781118410868.wbehibs296

Cohen, D. A., Scribner, R. A., & Farley, T. A. (2000). A structural model of health behavior: A pragmatic approach to explain and influence health behaviors at the population level. *Preventive Medicine. 30*(2), 146–154. https://doi.org/10.1006/pmed.1999 .0609

County Health Rankings & Roadmaps. (2019). What is Health? Retrieved July 9, 2019, from https://www .countyhealthrankings.org/what-is-health

Corbett, A., Anglin, A., Evenson, A., & Moscovice, I. (2018) *Rural Food Access Toolkit.* Retrieved from https://www.ruralhealthinfo.org/toolkits/food-access

Cornwell, E. Y., & Waite, L. J. (2009). Social disconnectedness, perceived isolation, and health among older adults. *Journal of Health and Social Behavior, 50*(1), 31–48. https://doi.org/10.1177/002214650905000103

Cromartie, J. (2018). *Rural America at a Glance, 2018 Edition.*

Cromartie, J., & Vilorio, D. (2019). *Rural Population Trends.* Retrieved from https://www.ers.usda.gov /amber-waves /2019/february/rural-population-trends/

Cutler, D. M., Glaeser, E. L., & Rosen, A. B. (2007). *Is the US Population Behaving Healthier?* https://doi.org /10.3386/w13013

Daniels, Z. M., Vanleit, B. J., Skipper, B. J., Sanders, M. L., & Rhyne, R. L. (2007). Factors in recruiting and retaining health professionals for rural practice. *The Journal of Rural Health: Official Journal of the American Rural*

Health Association and the National Rural Health Care Association, 23(1), 62–71. https://doi.org/JRH69 [pii]

De Rezende, L. F. M., Lopes, M. R., Rey-Lopez, J. P., Matsudo, V. K. R., & Luiz, O. D. C. (2014). Sedentary behavior and health outcomes: An overview of systematic reviews. *PLoS ONE.* https://doi.org/10.1371/journal.pone.0105620

Fields, B. E., Bigbee, J. L., & Bell, J. F. (2016). Associations of Provider-to-Population Ratios and Population Health by County-Level Rurality. *The Journal of Rural Health. 32*(3), 235–244. https://doi.org/10.1111/jrh.12143

Frost, S. S., Goins, R. T., Hunter, R. H., Hooker, S. P., Bryant, L. L., Kruger, J., & Pluto, D. (2010). Effects of the built environment on physical activity of adults living in rural settings. *American Journal of Health Promotion, 24*(4), 267–283. https://doi.org/10.4278/ajhp.08040532

Garcia, M. C., Faul, M., Massetti, G., Thomas, C. C., Hong, Y., Bauer, U. E., & Iademarco, M. F. (2017). Reducing potentially excess deaths from the five leading causes of death in the rural United States. *Morbidity and Mortality Weekly Report (MMWR). Surveillance Summaries, 66*(2), 1–7. https://doi.org/10.15585/mmwr.ss6602a1

Gee, G. C., & Ford, C. L. (2011). Structural racism and health inequities: Old issues, new directions. *Du Bois Review: Social Science Research on Race, 8*(1), 115–132. https://doi.org/10.1017/S1742058X11000130

Haggerty, J. L., Roberge, D., Lévesque, J.-F., Gauthier, J., & Loignon, C. (2014). An exploration of rural–urban differences in healthcare-seeking trajectories: Implications for measures of accessibility. *Health & Place, 28*, 92–98. https://doi.org/10.1016/j.healthplace.2014.03.005

Hansen, A. Y., Umstattd Meyer, M. R., Lenardson, J. D., & Hartley, D. (2015). Built Environments and active living in rural and remote areas: A review of the literature. *Current Obesity Reports. 4*, 484–493. https://doi.org/10.1007/s13679-015-0180-9

Hardeman, R. R., Medina, E. M., & Kozhimannil, K. B. (2016). Structural racism and supporting black lives—the role of health professionals. *New England Journal of Medicine, 375*(22), 2113–2115. https://doi.org/10.1056/NEJMp1609535

Henning-Smith, C., Ecklund, A., Moscovice, I., & Kozhimannil, K. (2018). *Gender differences in social isolation and social support among rural residents. The University of Minnesota Rural Health Research Center.* Minneapolis, MN. Retrieved from https://rhrc.umn.edu/publication/gender-differences-in-social-isolation-and-social-support-among-rural-residents/

Henning-Smith, C, Evenson, A., Corbett, A., Kozhimannil, K., & Moscovice, I. (2018a). *Rural transportation: challenges and opportunities. The University of Minnesota Rural Health Research Center.* Minneapolis, MN.

Retrieved from https://rhrc.umn.edu/publication/rural-transportation -challenges-and-opportunities/

Henning-Smith, C, Hernandez, A., Ramirez, M., Hardeman, R., & Kozhimannil, K. (2019). *Dying too soon: County-level disparities in premature death by rurality, race, and ethnicity.* Retrieved from https://rhrc.umn.edu/publication/dying-too-soon-county-level-disparities-in-premature-death-by-rurality-race-and-ethnicity/

Henning-Smith, C., & Blonigan, S. (2017). *Rural Aging in Place Toolkit.* Retrieved from https://www.ruralhealthinfo.org/toolkits/aging

Henning-Smith, C., Casey, M., Prasad, S., & Kozhimannil, K. (2017). *Medical Barriers to Nursing Home Care for Rural Residents | The University of Minnesota Rural Health Research Center.* Retrieved from https://rhrc.umn.edu/publication/medical-barriers-to-nursing-home-care-for-rural-residents/

Henning-Smith, C., Ecklund, A., Lahr, M., Evenson, A., Moscovice, I., & Kozhimannil, K. (2018). *Key informant perspectives on rural social isolation and loneliness.* Retrieved from https://rhrc.umn.edu/publication/key-informant-perspectives-on-rural-social-isolation-and-loneliness/

Henning-Smith, C., Evenson, A., Kozhimannil, K., & Moscovice, I. (2017a). Geographic variation in transportation concerns and adaptations to travel-limiting health conditions in the United States. *Journal of Transport & Health. 8*, 137–145. https://doi.org/10.1016/J.JTH.2017.11.146

Henning-Smith, C., Evenson, A., Kozhimannil, K., & Moscovice, I. (2018). Geographic variation in transportation concerns and adaptations to travel-limiting health conditions in the United States. *Journal of Transport & Health. 8*, 137–145. https://doi.org/10.1016/j.jth.2017.11.146

Henning-Smith, C., & Kozhimannil, K. B. (2018). Rural–urban differences in risk factors for motor vehicle fatalities. *Health Equity. 2*(1), 260–263. https://doi.org/10.1089/heq.2018.0006

Henning-Smith, C., Kozhimannil, K. B., Casey, M. M., & Prasad, S. (2018). Beyond clinical complexity: nonmedical barriers to nursing home care for rural residents. *Journal of Aging & Social Policy, 30*(2), 109–126. https://doi.org/10.1080/08959420.2018.1430413

Henning-Smith, Carrie, Kozhimannil, K., Casey, M., Prasad, S., & Moscovice, I. (2017). Rural-Urban differences in Medicare Quality Outcomes and the impact of Risk Adjustment. *Medical Care, 55*(9), 823–829. https://doi.org/10.1097/MLR.0000000000000761

Henning-Smith, C., & Lahr, M. (2018a). *Perspectives on Rural Caregiving Challenges and Interventions.* Retrieved from http://rhrc.umn.edu/wp-content/files_mf/1535633283UMNpolicybriefcaregivingchallenges.pdf

Henning-Smith, C., & Lahr, M. (2018b). Rural-urban difference in workplace supports and impacts for employed caregivers. *The Journal of Rural Health. 35*(1), 49–57. https://doi.org/10.1111/jrh.12309

Henning-Smith, C., Lahr, M., & Casey, M. (2019). A national examination of caregiver use of and preferences for support services: Does rurality matter? *Journal of Aging and Health. 31*(9), 1652–1670. 089826431878656.https://doi.org/10.1177/0898264 318786569

Henning-Smith, C., Moscovice, I., & Kozhimannil, K. (2019). Differences in social isolation and its relationship to health by rurality. *The Journal of Rural Health. 35*(4), 540–549. https://doi.org/10.1111 /jrh.12344

Henning-Smith, C., Prasad, S., Casey, M., Kozhimannil, K., & Moscovice, I. (2019). Rural-urban differences in Medicare quality scores persist after adjusting for sociodemographic and environmental characteristics. *The Journal of Rural Health. 35*(1), 58–67. https://doi .org/10.1111/jrh.12261

Hertz, T., Kusmin, L., Marré, A., & Parker, T. (2014). *Rural Employment in Recession and Recovery*. Washington, DC.

Holt-Lunstad, J., Smith, T. B., Baker, M., Harris, T., & Stephenson, D. (2015). Loneliness and social isolation as risk factors for mortality: A meta-analytic review. *Perspectives on Psychological Science, 10*(2), 227–237. https://doi.org/10.1177/1745691614568352

Holt-Lunstad, J., Smith, T. B., Layton, J. B., (2010). Social relationships and mortality risk: A meta-analytic review. *PLoS Medicine, 7*(7), e1000316. https://doi .org/10.1371/journal.pmed.1000316

Hung, P., Kozhimannil, K., Henning-Smith, C., & Casey, M. (2017). *Closure of Hospital Obstetric Services Disproportionately Affects Less-Populated Rural Counties | The University of Minnesota Rural Health Research Center*. Retrieved from https://rhrc.umn.edu/publication /closure-of-hospital-ob-services/

James, C. V, Moonesinghe, R., Wilson-Frederick, S. M., Hall, J. E., Penman-Aguilar, A., & Bouye, K. (2017). Racial and ethnic health disparities among rural adults—United States, 2012–2015. *Morbidity and Mortality Weekly Report (MMWR). Surveillance Summaries. 66*(3), 1–9.

Kim, K., Ozegovic, D., & Voaklander, D. C. (2012). Differences in incidence of injury between rural and urban children in Canada and the USA: A systematic review. *Injury Prevention, 18*(4), 264–271. https://doi .org/10.1136/injuryprev-2011-040306

Kozhimannil, K. B., & Henning-Smith, C. (2017). Racism and health in rural America. *Journal of Health Care for the Poor and Underserved, 29*(1), 35–43. Retrieved from https://preprint.press.jhu.edu/preprints/racism -and-health-rural-america

Kozhimannil, K. B., & Henning-Smith, C. (2019). Missing voices in America's rural health narrative. Retrieved April 25, 2019, from Health Affairs Blog website: https://www.healthaffairs.org/do/10.1377/hblog 20190409.122546/full/

Kozhimannil, K. B., Hung, P., Henning-Smith, C., Casey, M. M., & Prasad, S. (2018). Association between loss of hospital-based obstetric services and birth outcomes in rural counties in the United States. *JAMA, 319*(12), 1239–1247. https://doi.org/10.1001/jama.2018.1830

Kumar, D. (2018). *Rural America is losing young people: consequences and solutions*. Retrieved from https:// publicpolicy.wharton.upenn.edu/live/news/2393 -rural-america-is-losing-young-people-

LaRose, R., Gregg, J. L., Strover, S., Straubhaar, J., & Carpenter, S. (2007). Closing the rural broadband gap: Promoting adoption of the Internet in rural America. *Telecommunications Policy, 31*(6–7), 359–373. https://doi.org/10.1016/j.telpol.2007.04.004

Larson, S. L., & Hill, S. C. (2004). Rural-urban differences in employment-related health insurance. *The Journal of Rural Health. 21*(1), 21–30. https://doi.org/10.1111/j .1748-0361.2005.tb00058.x

Laughlin, L. (2016). Beyond the farm: Rural industry workers in America. In *Census Blog*. https://www .census.gov/newsroom/blogs/random-samplings /2016/12/beyond_the_farm_rur.html

Lichter, D. T. (2012). Immigration and the new racial diversity in rural America. *Rural Sociology, 77*(1), 3–35. https://doi.org/10.1111/j.1549-0831.2012.00070.x

Loftus, J., Allen, E. M., Call, K. T., & Everson-Rose, S. A. (2018). Rural-urban differences in access to preventive health care among publicly insured Minnesotans. *The Journal of Rural Health, 34*(S1), s48–s55. https:// doi.org/10.1111/jrh.12235

Martin, A. B., Torres, M., Vyavaharkar, M., Chen, Z., Towne, S., & Probst, J. C. (2013). *Rural Border Health Chartbook*. Retrieved from http://rhr.sph.sc.edu/report /SCRHRC Rural Border Health.pdf

Matthews, K. A., Croft J. B., Liu, Y., Lu, H., Kanny D., Wheaton, A. G., . . . Giles, W. H.(2017). Health-related behaviors by urban-rural county classification—United States, 2013. *Morbidity and Mortality Weekly Report (MMWR). Surveillance Summaries, 66*(5), 1–8. https://doi.org/10.15585 /MMWR.SS6605A1

Merwin, E., Snyder, A., & Katz, E. (2006). Differential access to quality rural healthcare: Professional and policy challenges. *Family & Community Health, 29*(3), 186–194. https://doi.org/00003727-200607000-00005 [pii]

Murray, S. (2006). Poverty and health. *Canadian Medical Association Journal, 174*(7), 923. https://doi.org/10 .1503/cmaj.060235

National Rural Housing Coalition (2018). Barriers to affordable rural housing. (2018). Retrieved July 10, 2019, from website: http://ruralhousingcoalition.org /overcoming-barriers-to-affordable-rural-housing/

Nayar, P., Yu, F., & Apenteng, B. A. (2013). Frontier America's health system challenges and population health outcomes. *The Journal of Rural Health,* *29*(3), 258–265. https://doi.org/10.1111/j.1748-0361 .2012.00451.x

North Carolina Rural Health Research Program. (2019). 171 Rural hospital closures: January 2005 - Present. Cecil G. Sheps Center for Health Services Research, The University of North Carolina at Chapel Hill. Retrieved from http://www.shepscenter.unc.edu /programs-projects/rural-health/rural-hospital -closures/

Park, T., Eyler, A. A., Tabak, R. G., Valko, C., & Brownson, R. C. (2017). Opportunities for promoting physical activity in rural communities by understanding the interests and values of community members. *Journal of Environmental and Public Health. 2017,* 1–5. https://doi.org/10.1155/2017/8608432

Pate, R. R., Pratt, M., Blair, S. N., Haskell, W. L., Bouchard, C., Macera, C. A., . . . Wilmore, J. H. (1995). Physical activity and public health: A recommendation from the Centers for Disease Control and Prevention and the American College of Sports Medicine. *JAMA. 273*(5), 402–407. https://doi.org/10.1001 /jama.1995.03520290054029

Peek-Asa, C., Zwerling, C., & Stallones, L. (2004). Acute traumatic injuries in rural populations. *American Journal of Public Health. 94*(10), 1689–1693. https:// doi.org/10.2105/AJPH.94.10.1689

Peters, R. M. (2006). The relationship of racism, chronic stress emotions, and blood pressure. *Journal of Nursing Scholarship. 38*(3), 234–240.

Ravesteijn, B., Van Kippersluis, H., & van Doorslaer, E. (2013). The contribution of occupation to health inequality. *Research on Economic Inequality. 21,* 311–332. https://doi.org/10.1108/S1049-2585(2013) 0000021014

Remington, P. L., Catlin, B. B., & Gennuso, K. P. (2015). The County Health Rankings: rationale and methods. *Population Health Metrics, 13,* 11-015-0044-2. eCollection 2015. https://doi.org/10.1186/s12963 -015-0044-2

Rettenmaier, A. J., & Wang, Z. (2013). What determines health: A causal analysis using county level data. *The European Journal of Health Economics, 14*(5), 821–834. https://doi.org/10.1007/s10198-012-0429-0

Rosenkrantz, D. E., Black, W. W., Abreu, R. L., Aleshire, M. E., & Fallin-Bennett, K. (2017). Health and health care of rural sexual and gender minorities: A systematic review. *Stigma and Health. 2*(3), 299–243. https:// doi.org/10.1037/sah0000055

Simon, D. (2013). *Poverty Fact Sheet: Poor and In Poor Health.* Retrieved from https://www.irp.wisc.edu /publications/factsheets/pdfs/PoorInPoorHealth.pdf

Skoufalos, A., Clarke, J. L., Ellis, D. R., Shepard, V. L., & Rula, E. Y. (2017). Rural aging in America: Proceedings of the 2017 Connectivity Summit. *Population Health Management. 20*(22), s1–s10. https://doi .org/10.1089/pop.2017.0177

Story, M., Kaphingst, K. M., Robinson-O'Brien, R., & Glanz, K. (2008). Creating healthy food and eating environments: Policy and environmental approaches. *Annual Review of Public Health. 29,* 253–272. https:// doi.org/10.1146/annurev.publhealth.29.020907 .090926

Strosnider, H., Kennedy, C., Monti, M., & Yip, F. (2017). Rural and urban differences in air quality, 2008– 2012, and community drinking water quality, 2010– 2015—United States. *Morbidity and Mortality Weekly Report (MMWR). Surveillance Summaries. 66*(13), 1–10. https://doi.org/10.15585/mmwr.ss6613a1

Taylor, L. (2018). Housing and Health: An overview of the literature. Health Affairs Health Policy Brief. *Health Affairs.* https://doi.org/10.1377/hpb20180313 .396577

USDA. (2020). USDA ERS - Rural Poverty & Well-Being. Retrieved September 1, 2020, from https:// www.ers.usda.gov/topics/rural-economy-population /rural-poverty-well-being/

United States Department of Agriculture Economic Research Service. (2019). Rural Poverty & Well-Being. Retrieved July 9, 2019, from Rural Economy & Population website: https://www.ers.usda.gov/topics /rural-economy-population/rural-poverty-well-being/

U.S. Census Bureau (2018). *Differences in Income Growth Across U.S. Counties.* Retrieved from https://www .census.gov/library/stories/2018/12/differences-in -income-growth-across-united-states-counties.html

U.S. National Climate Assessment. (2014). *Climate Change Impacts in the United States.* https://doi.org/10.7930 /J0Z31WJ2

Walker, R. E., Keane, C. R., & Burke, J. G. (2010). Disparities and access to healthy food in the United States: A review of food deserts literature. *Health & Place. 16*(5), 876–884. https://doi.org/10.1016/j.healthplace .2010.04.013

Weaver, K. E., Palmer, N., Lu, L., Case, L. D., & Geiger, A. M. (2013). Rural-urban differences in health behaviors and implications for health status among US cancer survivors. *Cancer Causes & Control. 24,* 1481–1490. https://doi.org/10.1007/s10552-013 -0225-x

Whitacre, B. E., Wheeler, D., & Landgraf, C. (2017). What can the national broadband map tell us about the health care connectivity gap? *The Journal of Rural Health, 33*(3), 284–289. https://doi.org /10.1111/jrh.12177

White, G. B. (2015, January). Rural America's silent housing crisis. *The Atlantic.* Retrieved from https:// www.theatlantic.com/business/archive/2015/01 /rural-americas-silent-housing-crisis/384885/

Wright Morton, L., & Blanchard, T. C. (2007). Starved for access: Life in rural America's food deserts. *Rural Realities. 1*(4). Retrieved from https://www.rural sociology.org/assets/docs/rural-realities/rural-realities -1-4.pdf

CHAPTER 3

Ethical Issues in Rural Communities

Chimamanda Okafor, MPH
Mark J. Minelli, PhD, MA, MPA

LEARNING OBJECTIVES

At the end of this chapter, readers will be able to:

Describe how the rural context influences healthcare ethics.

1. Identify the different types of ethical challenges that emerge and their potential impact.
2. List frequently encountered ethical challenges.
3. Identify the strengths and challenges of working in rural areas.
4. Discuss the importance of rural health ethics.

KEY TERMS

Confidentiality
Ethics
Privacy

CHAPTER OVERVIEW

According to the U.S. census bureau, 19.3% of the U.S. population live in rural areas with the median age for the adults being 51 years. People who live in rural areas tend to be older than those in urban counterparts (U.S. Census Bureau, 2016). By 2060, it is estimated that the number of Americans aged 65 and older will double from 46 million to approximately 100 million (Mark Mather, 2018). Those living in rural areas are already classified as the hard-to-reach groups. The social determinants of health are a major public health concern and it is important to note that these issues are more apparent in the rural communities than in the urban areas. This issue has been going on for decades and for almost every health issue, the rural population has it worse off, from substance abuse to mental health disorders (Erwin, 2017). Regarding mental health in rural communities, there is a shortage of mental health professionals and rural residents are less likely to recognize the illness as well as the stigma associated with it (National Rural Health Association, 2019). There are many factors that have an influence on this such as limited access to clinicians, health facilities, specialized services, and geographic and climatic barriers (W. A. Nelson & Schifferdecker, n.d.). In addition, these characteristics/factors influence ethical issues. With that said, it is important to outline the ethical considerations essential to clinical practice in these closely knit, tightly interdependent community settings.

Answering Ethical Questions

Sometimes in life, we are forced to make decisions that are confusing. **Ethics** are often discussed as value statements or codes of ethics. We read about companies that make poor business decisions based on the bottom line as opposed to sound ethical choices.

As consumers of health products and services, the public must be aware that sales methods like testimonials may not be based on scientific literature reviews. Even if studies for a product are cited, where did they come from? How many studies were cited? What was the number of test subjects performed?

Some models have been developed to help guide a path to making sound ethical decisions. From its basis of guiding principles, Rotary International has a list of questions one can pose: Is it the truth? Is it fair to all concerned? Will it build goodwill and better friendships? Will it be beneficial to all concerned? These are questions to consider when making ethical decisions and choices.

Another paradigm offered by MESSA (2002) poses four questions to the individual: (1) Is this activity legal? (2) If someone did this to us, would we think it is fair? (3) Would you like your parents to see you do this? (4) Would you feel good about having this activity reported on the front page of your local newspaper? The rating for this states that if you can answer yes to all four questions, it is probably ethical. Using these models can assist in making ethical decisions if a person is questioning a judgment or action to be taken. It is usually easier to prevent a problem than to fix one already in progress.

Ethical Issues in Rural Areas

In the United States, there are four main principles that define the ethical duties that healthcare professionals owe to patients. These principles are autonomy, beneficence, nonmaleficence, and justice (Vermont Ethics Network, 2017). These principles are a little bit more complicated to abide by in rural areas and are often considered as inapplicable by healthcare professionals in these areas. In rural areas, the line between practical and ethical is often blurred or nonexistent. This is due to the familiarity and interconnectedness that occurs between the clinicians and their patients (Shih & Goldman, 2011). Most of the clinicians' report that they were untrained and unprepared to deal with the ethical dilemmas in rural settings. It is important that separate clinical training is conducted for clinicians who need to practice in rural areas because the ethical dilemmas are quite different.

Some common rural ethics dilemmas are (W. A. Nelson & Schifferdecker, n.d.):

- Confidentiality and privacy
- Shared decision making
- Boundary issues and healthcare professional-patient relationship
- Limited resources and access to care
- Cultural and personal values in relation to professional standards
- Patient's inability to pay for care
- Disease stigma

Confidentiality and Privacy

Privacy is defined as the right of individuals to hold information about themselves in secret, free from the knowledge of others. **Confidentiality**, on the other hand, is the assurance that information about identifiable persons or release of it will not be disclosed without consent (Magnuson & Fu, 2014). Due to the overlapping relationships between the clinicians, the patients, and the community; the privacy and confidentiality of the patients are threatened. For example, a patient, relative, or friend could be a member of the healthcare professionals' staff or be the billing clerk increasing the likelihood of them knowing the patients' diagnoses.

Limited Resources and Access to Care

Some clinicians are forced to practice outside of their training, and this compromises the quality of care given. In addition, the shortage of health professionals willing to work in rural areas has led to the idea that substandard care given to rural communities is better than nothing, causing an unskilled physician to remain in the community (Shih & Goldman, 2011). This shouldn't be the case, as everyone deserves quality care. Lack of resources can also affect care; for example, there was an article in the New York Times that stated that in some rural areas of America, there are few people to drive the ambulances, which depend on volunteers to do the job (Kohrman, 2019).

Patients' Inability to Pay for Care

Health professionals working in rural areas do not have it as easy as their urban counterparts. Sometimes they must compromise and work with limited resources to ensure that their patients get the best care. Rural areas have higher rates of uninsured residents and unemployment (National Rural Health Association, 2019). When a patient is unable to pay for care, some of the clinicians make the decision to continue care because of their closeness in the community and the need to always put the patients' health first. This issue

happens frequently as a physician indicated that after practicing for 11 years in Jal, New Mexico, he was owed more than $45,000 in three-and four-dollar visit fees (p.103) (Klugman & Dalinis, 2008).

Boundary Issues and Professional Patient Relationship

The tight-knit community found in rural areas causes the issue of dual roles played by the physicians. Compared with the urban counterparts, the professionals get to see their clients outside of the professional boundaries leading to uncomfortable situations. For instance, in the urban areas, a professional can decide not to work with a client due to the close personal or professional relationship with the person. However, in the rural areas, when there is a limited option for referral of the patients or when the next professional is miles away, it is difficult to refuse treatment (Klugman & Dalinis, 2008). Another issue that can occur is some professionals feeling like they have to disengage from some community events or gatherings to prevent being kept in uncomfortable situations. This can lead to a sense of rejection, lack of trust, and less productive clinical environment (W. Nelson, Pomerantz, & Howard, 2007).

Telehealth

Health Resources and Services Administration (2019) defined telehealth as "the use of electronic communication and information technologies to provide or support long-distance clinical health care, patient and professional health-related education, public health, and health administration" (Health Resources and Services Administration, 2019). One of the causes of ethical dilemmas in rural areas is geographic barrier. The nearest hospitals or specialists are miles away leaving limited staffing in the community. Telehealth is an innovative approach that can address this barrier by giving the community access to specialists without them having to travel the distance. However, it has its limitations, it requires an Internet connection, and 53% of rural residents lack access to high-speed Internet. For health departments wanting telehealth services, there are some Medicare and Medicaid reimbursement restrictions. These restrictions make it harder to implement telehealth in certain areas/health departments (National Advisory Committee on Rural Health & Human Services, 2015).

Moving Forward

Recruitment of health professionals to rural communities should require comprehensive training. This could start with the education of the professionals in schools by making rural health a course people can specialize in, as this will allow for the right people who understand the dynamics of rural areas to work in these areas (settings). Programs will need to incorporate more information about the rural practice, especially on rural cultural norms and boundary negotiation, and providing training experiences on serving rural populations. There should be an understanding that no one professional is more important than another. For example, mental health professionals are just as important as physicians, as they play important roles in the community.

Additionally, programs could help clinicians in training to develop skills to assess the needs of small communities in order to identify any special areas of practice that would benefit those communities (Hastings & Cohn, 2013). Resource allocation is important in dealing with the health issues that rural areas face, most of which are preventable. Clinical rotations with medical school students can help with the recruitment of physicians to rural areas (Artnak, Mcgraw, & Stanley, 2011). Students and health professionals should be educated on the strengths of working in

rural areas to encourage satisfaction and willingness to work in these areas. Some strengths of working in rural areas include: the ability to be a generalist, integrated care, financial incentives, and similarity of beliefs and values (Hastings & Cohn, 2013). An example of a financial incentive is the National Health Service Corporation, which provides loan repayment of up to $25,000 a year if the health professional agrees to work in these areas (U.S. Department of Health and Human Services, 2019). This is a great option for the health professional to pay off student loan debt plus the benefit of a lower cost of living. In rural areas, there are possibilities of working with the members of the same family at the same time, which gives the professional a better understanding and an all-around perspective of the issue. Systems thinking can be applied to rural communities due to the close-knit culture of these areas and the ability for them to work as a team. For instance, physicians can communicate with the psychologist to get an understanding of the best medications to work for the client.

Conclusion

The older population is predicted to double by 2050, meaning that we are going to have more elderly people living in rural areas. This calls for more research and awareness on the importance of addressing the issues that these communities face. Current research on rural healthcare ethics is limited. Health professionals need to be aware of the ethical dilemmas of working in these communities. In addition, the strengths of these communities should be highlighted to encourage individuals and increase their willingness to work in rural areas.

Chapter Summary

- Rural residents are hard to reach groups facing a lot of health issues that are worse than their urban counterparts. This ranges from substance abuse to mental health disorders. They have a shortage of health professionals, health facilities, specialized services, and geographic barriers.

- Common ethical dilemmas in rural areas are confidentiality and privacy, Shared decision making, boundary issues and healthcare professional-patient relationship, limited resources and access to care, patient's inability to pay for care, and disease stigma.

- Recruitment of health professionals to rural communities should require comprehensive training. In addition, students and health professionals should be educated on the strengths of working in rural areas to encourage satisfaction and willingness to work in these areas. Some strengths of working in rural areas include: the ability to be a generalist, integrated care, financial incentives, and similarity of beliefs and values.

Discussion Questions

1. What types of ethical challenges face healthcare professionals in rural communities?
2. What examples of unethical behaviors do you know of or have read about in healthcare or the business environment?
3. Why is it important to have high ethical standards in health care?
4. How is ethical behavior developed?
5. How do we know what is the right thing to do in work and personal situations?

Student Activities and Worksheets are available for use inside the Navigate eBook, included with the printed text. Simply redeem the access code found at the front of the book at www.jblearning.com.

References

Artnak, K. E., Mcgraw, R. M., & Stanley, V. F. (2011). Health care accessibility for chronic illness management and end-of-life care: A view from rural America. *The Journal of Law, Medicine & Ethics. 39*(2), 140. https://doi.org/10.1111/j.1748-720X.2011.00584.x

Erwin, P. C. (2017). Despair in the American Heartland? A focus on rural health. *American Journal of Public Health. 107*(10), 1533–1534. https://doi.org/10.2105/AJPH.2017.304029

Hastings, S. L., & Cohn, T. J. (2013). Challenges and opportunities associated with rural mental health practice. *Journal of Rural Mental Health. 37*(1), 37–49. https://doi.org/10.1037/rmh0000002

Health Resources and Services Administration. (2019). Telehealth Programs. Retrieved February 27, 2019, from https://www.hrsa.gov/rural-health/telehealth/index.html

Klugman, C. M., & Dalinis, P. M. (2008). *Ethical issues in rural health care.* Craig M. Klugman and Pamela M. Dalinis (eds.). Baltimore, MD: Johns Hopkins University Press.

Kohrman, N. (2019). In Rural America, There Are Few People Left to Drive the Ambulances. *The New Yorker.* Retrieved January 30, 2019, from https://www.newyorker.com/news/dispatch/in-rural-america-there-are-few-people-left-to-drive-the-ambulances

Magnuson, J. A., & Fu, P. C. (2014). *Public Health Informatics and Information Systems.* (2nd ed.) London, U.K.: Springer.

Mather, M., Scommegna P., & Kilduff L. (2018). Fact Sheet: Aging in the United States – Population Reference Bureau. Retrieved January 18, 2019, from https://www.prb.org/aging-unitedstates-fact-sheet/

National Advisory Committee on Rural Health & Human Services. (2015). *A Review of Technologies and Strategies to Improve Patient Care with Telemedicine.* Retrieved from https://www.hrsa.gov/sites/default/files/hrsa/advisory-committees/rural/publications/2015-telehealth.pdf

National Rural Health Association. (2019). Rural Health Care. Retrieved January 2, 2019, from https://www

.ruralhealthweb.org/about-nrha/about-rural-health-care#_ftn1

Nelson, W. A., & Schifferdecker, K. E. (n.d.). *Rural Health Care Ethics A Manual for Trainers*. Retrieved from https://geiselmed.dartmouth.edu/cfm/resources/manual/manual

Nelson, W., Pomerantz, A., Howard, K., & Bushy A. (2007). A proposed rural healthcare ethics agenda. *Journal of Medical Ethics, 33*(3), 136–139. https://doi.org/10.1136/jme.2006.015966

Shih, T. L., & Goldman, J. J. (2011). Recognizing and Resolving Ethical Dilemmas in Rural Medicine. *Virtual Mentor, 13*(5), 291–294. https://doi.org/10.1001/virtualmentor.2011.13.5.jdsc1-1105

U.S. Department of Health and Human Services. (2019). *National Health Service Corps Loan Repayment Program Description*. Retrieved from https://nhsc.hrsa.gov/loan-repayment/nhsc-loan-repayment-program.html

U.S. Census Bureau. (2016). *New Census Data Show Differences Between Urban and Rural Populations. United States Census Bureau*. Retrieved from https://www.census.gov/newsroom/press-releases/2016/cb16-210.html.

Vermont Ethics Network. (2017). Medical Ethics: Overview of the Basics. Retrieved January 25, 2019, from http://www.vtethicsnetwork.org/ethics.html

PART 2

Public Health Systems and Policies for Rural Communities

CHAPTER 4

History of the Development of Rural Health in the USA

Andrew Kim, PhD, MPH

LEARNING OBJECTIVES

At the end of this chapter, readers will be able to:

1. Understand how rural health in the United States came into being.
2. Describe forces that have helped shaped rural health.
3. Define obstacles to rural health historically.
4. Identify major forces shaping rural health today.

KEY TERMS

Affordable Care Act
Hill-Burton Act
Medicaid
Medicare

CHAPTER OVERVIEW

Rural Health in the United States is a relatively new concept. In the Late 18th century, the industrial revolution took place from an agricultural society to mills, factories, and mines in urban centers. People migrated from rural areas into towns and cities. With the urbanization of people into city centers, public health came into being as problems began to emerge. Public health was mostly composed of combating infectious and communicable diseases, which was the main concern in urban areas. By the late 1800s, people began to move out of cities into rural areas. The migration of rural dwellers created a need for rural health. Resources, such as the creation of local health departments, allocated essential services to populations in rural areas. This chapter explores the historical roots and processes that have shaped rural health today.

History of Development of Rural Health in the United States

Early Rural Health History

Public health has been an urban phenomenon for much if its history. During the middle ages, a plague inflicted Europe and Asia. This was known as the Bubonic plague and it killed approximately 75% of the total population. There was little knowledge in medicine and public health and that partly contributed to the catastrophe. For example, they did not know communicable diseases were caused by bacteria, viruses, and parasites. Initially, cats were thought to be the cause of the disease. Furthermore, most of the population in the world lived in close proximity to one another, which contributed to the spread of diseases. Often, diseases were attributed to poor moral and spiritual conditions and resulted in isolation or quarantine (Goudsblom, 1986).

The adoption of the poor practice law, which was passed in England in 1601, continued with the American colonies (Chadwick & Flinn, 1965). Voluntary hospitals for the physically and mentally disabled were established in local communities.

The 1700s

At the time when the population saw innovations and advances due to the Industrial Revolution, plagues and diseases were rampant throughout towns and cities.

Thus, the need for public health was an important issue about which the government took responsibility. The increasing population, poor working conditions, and long working hours contributed to the development of urban areas known as slums. The spread of diseases originated in areas where people lived in close proximity to each other.

In the late 1700s, machines started to change the landscape of labor. Machines made an immediate impact on the textile industry, reducing the need and time for workers.

The 1800s

Edwin Chadwick was a lawyer from London who is best known for the sanitary reform movement. In 1838, he surveyed the living and working conditions, which eventually published the general report on the sanitary conditions of the laboring population of Great Britain. His work and the pressure applied by the health of towns association led to the Public Health Act of 1842. It allowed smaller towns to implement changes to sanitation.

Chadwick was the first to propose a national board of health that would oversee municipalities within the country (Chadwick, 1842). Later, John Snow (**Figure 4-1**) was the first to track the cholera outbreak in London in 1854. Although the germ theory came later, John Snow was able to recognize that communicable diseases spread by people's movements.

In the United States, similar studies were being conducted. Public health in the United States began as a largely urban phenomenon, dating back to the late 1700s. In much the same way as in history, public health was focused on urban populations. Dirty environmental conditions became common in working-class areas, and the spread of disease became rampant. Much of government agencies sought to improve public health by focusing on poor sanitation and close-proximity living quarters. Lemeul Shatuck published the *Massachusetts Sanitary Commission* in 1850. The publication included statistics on the Massachusetts population: differences in morbidity and mortality rates in different locations. The report recommended new census schedules; regular surveys of local health conditions; supervision of water supplies and waste disposal; and the establishment of a state board of health and local boards of health to enforce sanitary regulations. (Winslow, 1923; Rosenkrantz, 1972)

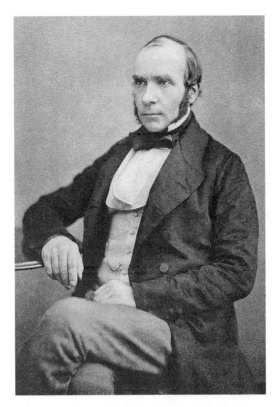

Figure 4-1 John Snow.

Much of public health in rural areas existed through local community organizations and nurses. There were no formal public health agencies that existed in rural areas; however, local public health boards were created voluntarily and as people began to migrate from urban centers to rural areas, so did the diseases. Outbreaks of typhoid, hookworm, and pellagra resulted in formalizing local health departments in rural areas. Health departments were heavily underfunded, so they relied on private donors.

1910 to the Mid 1940s

In 1945, Congress passed the **Hill-Burton Act**, which funded states to create hospitals and health centers in rural areas. This legislation became the foundation of rural public health. Where many rural communities lacked public health agencies, the creation of hospitals and clinics became the center of basic healthcare services that served the critical needs of rural communities.

There was additional legislation that prompted rural public health, which included the Public Health Service Act (1975), and the Rural Health Clinic Act of 1977. These acts sought to improve access and quality of services in rural communities.

In 1987, the Office of Rural Health Policy (ORHP) was created within the Health Resources and Services Administration to address issues in rural health. **Figure 4-2** showed the percentage of the Population in Rural Areas by State 2011–2015.

The ORHP has expanded to assist states with collecting and disseminating

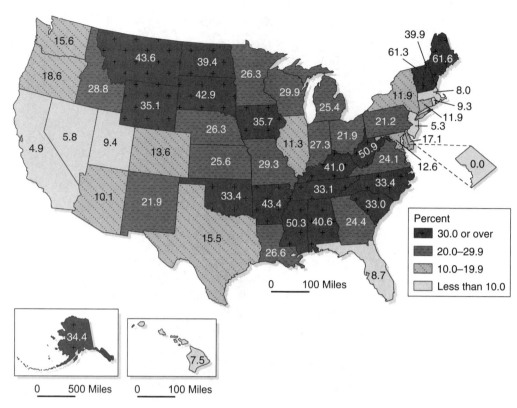

Figure 4-2 Percentage of the Population in Rural Areas by State 2011–2015.

U.S. Census Bureau, 2011-2015 American Community Survey, 5-year estimates.

health-related information; grant programs; conducting research; and offering technical assistance, policy, advocacy, and border health activities.

1965

On July 30, 1965, President Lyndon B. Johnson signed a set of laws that established the **Medicare** program. Funded only by the federal government, Medicare provides medical assistance to those individuals who are eligible. Although Medicare was established to aide those individuals who can't afford health insurance, it is now available to all people over the age of 65 years, end-stage renal disease (ERSD), and people under the age of 65 with certain disabilities (Medicare.gov, 2019). Although being over the age of 65 and being disabled are generally the main qualification for Medicare, other aspects are also taken into consideration when determining eligibility, depending on the plan.

Medicare, being the largest source of funding for medical and health-related services for America's elderly, has had many successes throughout its history. Medicare has provided supplemental health coverage for the country's people in need. With America's historical economic struggles, the Social Security Act has contributed to America's health status today (Medicare.gov, 2019). The Medicare program must offer medical assistance for certain basic services to most categorically needy populations (Mitchell & Cromwell, 1982). These services that contribute to better living conditions for those unable to provide are: inpatient/outpatient hospital services or skilled nursing care facilities (Part A), doctor care and services received as an outpatient, and some preventive care (Part B), or prescription drugs (Part D). Medicare advantage plans (Part C) combine Part A and Part B coverage, often combining drug coverage (Part D) into one plan (Kaiser, 2010). All of these plans have contributed to better lifestyles and assistance for those who are unable to provide for their family or for themselves. In essence, the main objective of Medicare is to provide access, better quality of care, specific benefits, and enhanced outreach programs for the elderly or disabled, with emphasis on the dependent under these provisions.

2010 to Present

Patient Protection Affordable Care Act

The Patient Protection and **Affordable Care Act** of 2010 (PPACA or ACA) is the first comprehensive health reform law enacted in U.S. modern history. Its passage was historic and is the most notable legislation of President Barack Obama (Stolberg and Pear, 2010). Ever since Franklin D. Roosevelt, every administration until Obama's has failed to pass comprehensive healthcare reform (Starr, 2011). The massive legislation consists of 10 titles, with 487 separate subsections, with a major focus on expanding insurance coverage for the United States citizens (McDonough 2011). The primary goal of the ACA is to increase access to affordable health insurance for the millions of Americans without coverage and to make health insurance more affordable for those already covered. In addition, the ACA made many revisions in how health care is financed, organized, and delivered. The ACA restructured the private health insurance market, set minimum standards for health coverages, created mandates, and enabled citizens to purchase private health insurance. Certain individuals and families may receive tax credits and federal subsidies to reduce the cost of purchasing health insurance. Some major provisions include the following: every U.S. citizen must have individual health insurance or pay a penalty; children are allowed to stay on their parents' plan until age 26 years, companies with over 50 full-time employees must provide employer health insurance; and insurance companies are prevented from denying coverage based on pre-existing conditions. The Congressional Budget Office (CBO) estimated that the ACA would reduce the number of nonelderly people who are uninsured by 32 million, thus increasing the proportion of legal residents under age 65 years with insurance from 83% to 94% (CBO 2010).

Medicaid is expanded from 100% to incomes below 138% of the federal poverty level (FPL); small businesses and individuals with incomes between 100% statutory threshold is 133% FPL; but 5% of an individual's income is disregarded, making it 138% of the practical threshold (KFF 2012). Additionally, 400% of the federal poverty level can receive subsidies to purchase private insurance through the health insurance exchange Market (HIX). **Figure 4-3** shows President Obama signing the ACA's passage on March 23, 2010 when he stated that "Health insurance reform becomes the law of the land in the United States of America" (White House, 2010). President Obama and the Democratic party managed and convinced some Republicans in Congress to vote for the Affordable Care Act. President Obama signed the ACA's passage on March 23, 2010, and stated that "Health insurance reform becomes the law of the land in the United States of America" (White House, 2010). However, opponents of the ACA

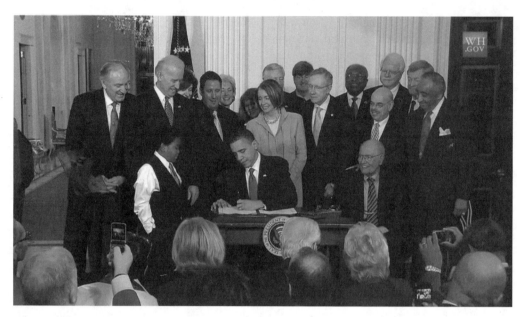

Figure 4-3 President Obama signing the Patient Protection and Affordable Care Act of 2010 into Law.

Courtesy Barack Obama Presidential Library.

attempted to repeal the legislation after more than 50 congressional attempts at repeal, a 5-4 decision by the U.S. Supreme Court on a lawsuit signed by 26 states, and during President Obama's re-election campaign in 2012. There were disagreements over whether to fund major parts of the law. Most of the ACA went into effect on January of 2014; however, key provisions of the law were up for contention by the courts. A majority of the states did not participate in the Medicaid expansion and negative press coverage of the ACA's implementation undermined President Obama's agenda. The ACA's implementation continues to be difficult. **Figure 4-4** shows the current status of state medical expansion decisions in the United States. The legislation gives an enormous responsibility to the states, the legislation is highly politicized and left open for repeal even though President Obama has left office, and billions of dollars are needed to fund the ACA's provisions before it can fully go into effect. The issue of federalism

plays a role as states are given enormous responsibility to implement major parts of the ACA (Weil, 2013). States play an important role in expanding Medicaid, developing health insurance exchanges, reviewing health insurance premium increases, and enforcing new market regulations. It is not a unique situation as states have expertise in administering and implementing federal programs from the past; however, the legislation comes in at a time when state budgets have been at their lowest since World War II and budget shortages total 136 billion dollars (National Governors Association & National Association of State Budget, 2010). Furthermore, managerial capacity, hiring freezes, mandatory furloughs, and the addition of 24 newly elected governors complicate matters. But even before states can begin to implement the legislation, Congress has to vote on the many provisions on how this task will be executed. The division of responsibility between levels of government has been contentious, with states resisting flexibility in some cases

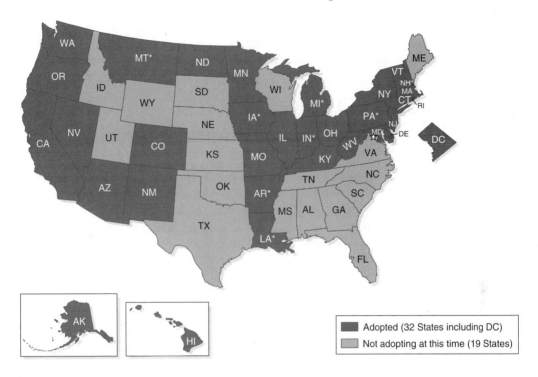

Figure 4-4 Current Status of State Medical Expansion Decisions.

Notes: Current status for each state is based on KCMU tracking and analysis of state executive activity. *AR, IA, IN MI, MT, NH and PA have approved Section 1115 waivers. Coverage under the PA waiver went into effect 1/1/15, but it has transitioned coverage to a state plan amendment. Coverage under the MT waiver went into effect 1/1/2016. LA's Governor Edwards signed an Exective order to adopt the Medicaid expansion on 1/12/2016, but coverage under the expansion is not yet in effect. WI covers adults up to 100% FPL in Medicaid, but did not adopt the ACA expansion. See source for more information on the states listed as "adoption under discussion."

Data from "Status of State Action on the Medicaid Expansion Decision," KFF State Health Facts, updated May 29, 2020. Retrieved from https://www.kff.org/health-reform/state-indicator/state-activity-around-expanding-medicaid-under-the-affordable-care-act/

and resenting perceived federal overreach in others. This is the essence of federalism, where power is vested between levels of government. Although the ACA is the law of the land, it is highly contested internally by its implementation complications and externally by the opposition party, states, and lobbyists.

Effects of Legislation on Rural Health

Understandably, rural health populations on average have relatively more elderly, children, unemployed, poor, and uninsured residents.

The primary purpose of Medicare, Medicaid, and the PPACA was to increase access, quality, and decrease cost of health care. Rural health has been impacted greatly by these legislations. For example, The Medicaid expansion helps reduce rural health disparities and supports rural hospitals. The Medicaid expansion has decreased the number of uninsured. Eighty-two percent of rural hospital closures has been in nonexpanded states (Cohen, 2019). Furthermore, after Kentucky expanded its Medicaid program, the uninsured rate for rural, low-income adults dropped from 40% in 2009 to 13% in 2016 (Cohen, 2019).

As millions apply for health insurance, the problem of primary care physicians grows. The Kaiser Family Foundation estimates that 8,073 additional primary care physicians were required to eliminate primary care health professional shortages in 2014. Rural areas are especially in critical need of primary care physicians.

Conclusion

The history of rural health in the United States provides a basis for understanding the factors that contribute to promoting health disparities and accomplishments that promote positive health outcomes. Public Health in the United States is committed to taking initiatives, such as Healthy People 2020, to improve health,

especially in rural areas. This would include eliminating health disparities, improving access and eliminating barriers to health, addressing primary care prevention, and providing new technologies.

Chapter Summary

This chapter explored the historical roots shaping rural health as people moved from cities to less-populated areas of the country. A historical timeline examined the development of rural health and legislation promoting the transformation to what we see today. As the population of many states have fairly large rural contingencies, public health professionals need to understand the unique challenges and service delivery components involved.

Discussion Questions

1. Which factors contribute to the promotion and adversity of rural health?
2. What are some of the challenges in rural health today?
3. Describe how innovations and legislations affected rural health.

Student Activities and Worksheets are available inside the Navigate eBook, included with the printed text. Simply redeem the access code found at the front of the book at www.jblearning.com.

References

An Act for the Relief of the Poor. 43 Elizabeth I, c. 2.

Chadwick, E., & Flinn, M. W. (1965). Report on the sanitary condition of the labouring population of Gt. Britain. (1842). (ed). with an introduction by Flinn, M. W. Edinburgh: University Press.

Cohen, M. (2019). Health communities and health workplaces. *Guest Speaker Healthcare Forum*. Raleigh, North Carolina.

Congressional Budget Office. (2016). The budget and economic outlook: 2016 to 2026. Retrieved from the CBO website: https://www.cbo.gov/sites /default/files/114th-congress-2015-2016/reports /51129-2016Outlook.pdf.

Goudsblom, J. (1986). Public health and the civilizing process. *The Milbank Quarterly.* 64(2), 161–188.

Henry J. Kaiser Family Foundation (2010e.) Medicare at a glance. Menlo Park, CA: Henry J. Kaiser Family Foundation.

Henry J. Kaiser Family Foundation (KFF). (2012). Quick take: Who benefits from the ACA Medicaid expansion. Kaiser Family Foundation.

McDonough, J. E. (2011). Inside national health reform. University of California Press: Berkeley, CA.

Medicare.gov. (2019). Medicare.gov: the official U.S. government site for Medicare. Available at: http:// medicare.gov. Accessed July 22, 2019.

Mitchell, J. B., Cromwell, J. (1982). Physician behavior under the Medicare assignment option. *Journal of Health Economics.* 1(3), 245–264.

National Governors Association and National Association of State Budget Officers. (2010). State fiscal update. Washington (DC): National Association of State Budget Officers.

Rosenkrantz, B. G. (1974). Cart before horse: Theory, practice, and professional image in American public health, 1870–1920. *Journal of History of Medicine and Allied Sciences.* 29(1), 55–73.

Starr, P. (2011). Remedy and reaction: The peculiar American struggle over health care reform. *Yale* University Press: New Haven.

Stolberg, S., & Pear, R. (2010, March 23). Obama Signed Overhaul Healthcare Into Law. The New York Times. Retrieved from http://www.nytimes.com

Weil, A. (2013). Promoting cooperative federalism through state shared savings. *Health Affairs.* 32(8).

Winslow, C. E. A. (1984). The evolution and significance of the modern public health campaign. *Journal of Public Health Policy.* South Burlington, VT.

CHAPTER 5

Federal Rural Health Organizations

Andrew Kim, PhD, MPH

LEARNING OBJECTIVES

At the end of this chapter, readers will be able to:

1. Understand the health policymaking process.
2. Identify rural health policy issues.
3. Describe the role of the federal government in health policy.
4. Provide an overview of federal agencies contributing to rural health.

KEY TERMS

Federal Government Agencies
Federal Health Policy
Policymaking

CHAPTER OVERVIEW

One of the main purposes of the federal government is to ensure that the rural population can receive affordable, high-access and high-quality health care. Health policies from the federal government can originate from the legislative, executive, and judicial branches. Legislations such as Medicare, Medicaid, and the Patient Protection Affordable Care Act ensure that the public receives health care equitably.

Federal rural health organizations have specific **federal government agencies** addressing different needs of the rural health population. The center of rural health in the federal government is the federal office of Rural Health Policy, which is located within the Health Resource and Services Administration. They are responsible for coordinating activities that pertain to rural health care within the Department of Health and Human Services.

Important matters pertaining to healthcare have come out of these branches and have affected rural health in significant ways. This chapter provides an overview of the process of health policymaking, the federal government's role in health care, and policies that affect rural health.

Federal Rural Health Organizations

Overview of Federal Agencies Contributing to Rural Health

The federal government's executive branch implements laws for which sole power lies in the hands of the President of the United States. Of the 15 departments in the executive branch, matters that pertain to health are headed by the Department of Health and Human Services. It is the federal government's principal agency for protecting the health of all Americans and providing essential human services, especially for those who are least able to help themselves. The secretary of Health and Human Services oversees a budget of approximately $700 billion and approximately 65,000 employees. The Department's programs are administered by 11 operating divisions, including eight agencies in the U.S. Public Health Service and three human services agencies. There are specific agencies under the Department of Health and Human Services that are responsible for specific areas of health care. These agencies are essential for providing aid to people living in rural areas.

Overview

Over the past century, public health in the United States has shifted from treating infectious diseases to chronic diseases (Fee, 2009). The germ theory brought communicable diseases to light and the role of public health was to prevent and control the spread of diseases.

The mortality rate declined from the turn of the century where the average life expectancy was 50 years of age (Roser, 2019).

An examination of the top causes of death in the 1900s highlights the progression of public health up to today. The most common infectious diseases at the turn of the century were pneumonia and tuberculosis (CDC, 1999a).

Many important advances contributed to the improvement and quality of health care. Improvements in sanitation, vaccinations, and medical treatments, such as antibiotics, led to the decline of infectious diseases. With that control, public health turned its attention to the effects of chronic diseases, which are now responsible for the 10 leading causes of death (Murphy et al., 2017). **Figure 5-1** shows the 10 leading causes of death. Although the shift has led a new frontier of diseases, the average life expectancy has increased to 80 years of age as a result of the advances of modern medicine and public health (Roser, 2019).

Currently, the public health paradigm has shifted toward social determinants and health disparities. Public health policies focus on the status of health from a diverse population that involves a variety of issues.

The Institute of Medicine periodically releases a report describing the state of public health in the past, present, and future. In 1988, the Institute released a report titled, *The future of public health*, where a large portion of public health services were in a state of "disarray." The report highlighted areas of major improvement, recommendations, and new innovations and advances on the horizon. The report is aimed at multiple sectors and these sectors comprise the country's public health system, which is defined as "governmental and nongovernmental organizations that contribute to the performance of essential public health services for a defined community or population" (Schutfield & Keck, 2009, p. 792).

The report focused on specific functions and responsibilities of the government that are essential to public health. The functions are assessment, policy development, and assurance as shown in **Figure 5-2**. Assessment is "regular and systematic collection, assembling, analyzing and making available information on the health of the community, including statistics on health status, community health needs, and epidemiologic and other studies of health problems."

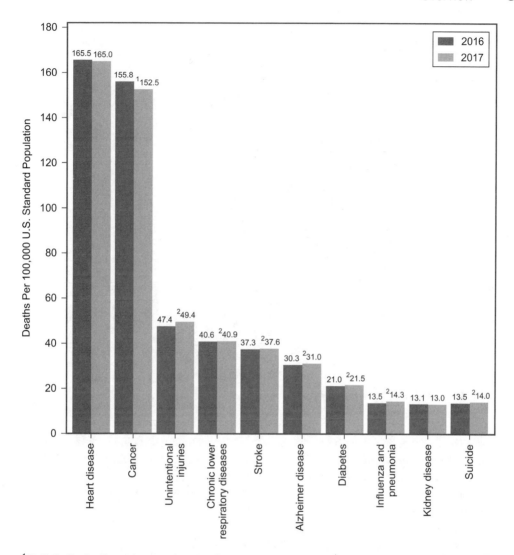

[1]Statistically significant decrease in age-adjusted death rate from 2016 to 2017 ($p < 0.05$).

[2]Statistically significant increase in age-adjusted death rate from 2016 to 2017 ($p < 0.05$).

NOTES: A total of 2,813,503 resident deaths were registered in the United States in 2017. The 10 leading causes accounted for 74.0% of all deaths in the United States in 2017. Causes of death are ranked according to number of deaths. Rankings for 2016 data are not shown. Data table for Figure 4 includes the number of deaths for leading causes. Access data table for Figure 4 at: https://www.cdc.gov/nchs/data/data-briefs/db328_tables-508.pdf#4.

Figure 5-1 Ten Leading Causes of Death.

CDC/NCHS, National Vital Statistics System, Mortality.

Policy development is understood best as public health agencies exercising their responsibility to serve the public interest in the development of comprehensive public health policies by promoting the use of the scientific knowledge base in decision making on public health and by leading in developing public health policy.

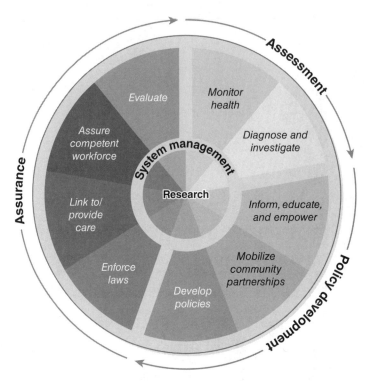

Figure 5-2 Public Health Core Essential Functions.
Retrieved from https://www.cdc.gov/nceh/ehs/ephli/core_ess.htm

Assurance is "public health agencies assuring their constituents the services necessary to achieve agreed upon goals are provided by encouraging actions by other entities (private or public sector), by requiring such actions through regulation, or by providing services directly" (Schutfield & Keck, 2009, p.39).

During the Clinton Administration, healthcare reform was a primary agenda item to provide health care for all American Citizens and legal residents. President Clinton appointed a healthcare reform task force to introduce a series of bills and legislations to improve healthcare delivery and services.

The Core Public health functions steering committee developed the 10 essential public health services in lieu of the International Organization for Migration's (IOM) recommendation of assurance, policy development, and assessment.

The committee included representatives from the Center for Disease Control and Prevention's (CDC) public health practice program office and the secretary of the Department of Health and Human Service's office of disease prevention and health promotion (CDC, 2013).

The 10 essential services are:

1. Monitor health status to identify and solve community health problems
2. Diagnose and investigate health problems and health hazards in the community
3. Inform, educate, and empower people about health issues
4. Mobilize community partnerships and action to identify and solve health problems
5. Develop policies and plans that support individual and community health efforts
6. Enforce laws and regulations that protect health and ensure safety

7. Link people to needed personal health services and assure the provision of health care when otherwise unavailable
8. Assure competent public and personal healthcare workforce
9. Evaluate effectiveness, accessibility, and quality of personal and population-based health services
10. Research new insights and innovative solutions to health problems

Role of Federal Health Policy

The role of the nation's government is to uphold the safety and well-being of its citizens. The means by which they do that is through health and health care. Health is not only essential to the physical and mental well-being of people but also to the nation's economy.

The United States spent 17.8% of its gross domestic product, which is approximately $3.6 trillion dollars in 2018. The Government accounts for half of this amount. Between 2018 and 2027, healthcare spending is projected to increase by 5.5% annually. By 2027, national health spending is expected to reach almost $6 trillion, when it is projected to represent 19.4% of gross domestic product. (Sisko et al., 2014).

Health and health care are expressed through public policy and mostly managed through the private sector in what is known as managed care. When the government is involved with the pursuit of health for its citizens, it often revolves around increased quality, decreased costs, and increased access. As discussed in the chapter on ethical issues in rural communities, Medicare, Medicaid, and the Patient Protection and Affordable Care Act are prime examples of understanding the **federal health policy** process through the federal government and its effect on health in the United States. The government's public **policymaking** process is essential to health.

Federal health policies take shape through laws, regulations, implementation decisions, executive orders, and judicial decisions.

Health Policies

It is imperative to understand what health policies are and how they function in the overall context of public policy. Policies are created in the government, not for profit or nongovernmental agencies, and the private sector. Policies are made at all levels of government (federal, state, and local), The American Public Health Association, the Institute of Medicine, and private organizations such as the Mayo Clinic and corporations such as Microsoft. By nature, policies are authoritative and binding because they are made by people who have the expertise to make those decisions. Presidents, CEOS, directors, and managers of companies make executive decisions because of the nature of their position.

In the public sector, certain people have the right to make policies because they were elected by the people to make decisions on their behalf. In the federal government, members of Congress, the president of the United States, and the Supreme Court justices all have the right to make policies.

The private sector makes health policies that are important and can affect health. Policy decisions are made by executives in healthcare organizations that pertain to regulation, marketing, quality improvement, and profit margins. The Joint Commission on accreditation of healthcare organizations (JCAHO), a private organization, a private accrediting body for healthcare organizations, and the committee for quality assurance are examples of private-sector health organizations that make important health policies.

Public Policy has many different meanings and there is no consensus on a definitive definition. "Anything a government chooses to do or not to do" (Dye, 1972: 2) is a widely known, simple definition of public policy stated by Thomas Dye. Another scholar, William Jenkins, states that public policy is "a set of interrelated decisions taken by a political actor or group of actors concerning the selection of goals and the means of achieving them" (Jenkins 1978).

Lastly, Anderson (1984) describes public policy as "a purposive course of action followed by an actor or a set of actors in dealing with a problem or a matter of concern."

For the purposes of this chapter, public policy is defined as the laws or decisions that are passed by the legislative, executive, and judicial branches of government that places incentives or disincentives to alter behavior, actions, and decisions of individuals.

Moreover, health policy is a subset of public policy, which is the responsibility of the government to ensure the safety of the public through health and to ensure high quality and access to health. Public-sector health policies are made in the legislative, executive, and judicial branches of government that are intended to influence the actions, behaviors, and decisions of individuals. Health policies are made at the federal, state, and local levels of government for different purposes. They are targeted toward different classes of people and organizations. For example, Medicaid targets low income people and Medicare targets the elderly.

Thus, health policy is made through the framework of public policy. People have been healthier due to the impact of policies passed in the United States; however, there are still significant challenges and issues that affect the health of the people and problems that plague the healthcare system. Although policies are made with good intentions, policies may not always have a positive effect and can have unintended consequences.

Federal Policy Related to Rural Health

Efforts to improve rural health from the federal government revolve around increasing access through health insurance, increasing quality of care, and decreasing costs. Before the ACA, the U.S. healthcare system had been a fee-for service, which paid physicians more for services. Studies have shown that paying more for health care does not necessarily translate to better health outcomes. As a result, a paradigm shift changed the focus from volumetric health care to quality metric health care. With the passing of the ACA, health care focused more on primary preventative measures and rating of healthcare services. The burden shifted on healthcare providers to focus on the quality of life rather than disease management.

Over the past 30 years, healthcare costs have quadrupled from 11 billion dollars to 44 billion dollars (AHA, 2012). Safety-net hospitals and hospitals struggle to meet the demand of patients without insurance. The problems were compounded with a shortage of primary care physicians, particularly in rural communities. There is also a disproportionate distribution of practitioners in rural communities living and working in isolated rural areas and/or willing and appropriately trained to serve low-income and uninsured individuals compared with their urban counterpart.

Millions of people are living in areas of the United States with insufficient basic care, as the nursing and primary care physician shortages grow (HRSA, 2009).

According to the Health Resources and Services Administration (HRSA), approximately 65 million people live in areas without adequate primary care services, 49 million people live in areas with shortages of basic dental care and 80 million people live in areas with shortages of mental health care.

Furthermore, there is an estimated shortage of over 400,000 nurses, projected to grow to 1 million nurses by 2020 (Derksen & Whelen, 2009).

The number of medical school graduates choosing primary care disciplines has been declining sharply, as more graduates are choosing to specialize (Petterson et al., 2012). As much as 60 to 65% of all medical graduates are in specialized fields. One major reason is rising medical tuition costs. The income for primary care physicians may not outweigh the debt and interest accrued after medical school. The federal government offers programs that exchange service in rural areas for subsidized loan repayment or loan forgiveness.

Overall, the federal government realizes the barriers of health care, especially in rural areas.

Many federal programs aim to improve health care in rural communities. The HRSA's Bureau of Health Professions addresses workforce shortages and insufficient diversity in the health work force by identifying areas of need and administering a variety of grants and other funding for health professional education and training. They also administer technical assistance and grants to federal health centers to low income and uninsured populations.

Before the ACA, President Obama signed the American Recovery and Investment Act of 2009 to stimulate the economy, create jobs, modernize infrastructure, become energy independent, and preserve and improve affordable health care. Some of those jobs were in health care to meet the demands of growing underinsured or uninsured populations. Approximately 200 million dollars was allocated for healthcare training through grants, scholarships, loans, and loan repayments (ARRA, 2009). An additional 300 million dollars is designated for the expansion of the National Health Service corps by providing scholarships and loan repayments for graduates who agree to practice primary care in rural and underserved areas.

A persistent shortage of skilled workers (nurses, lab technicians, and physicians) will have a cascading effect on the health system. For example, a shortage of lab technicians can create a backlog in processing lab diagnostic tests causing treatment delays. Innovative approaches are needed to address the labor imbalance in the healthcare systems.

Conclusion

Rural populations face growing challenges in the 20th century. The federal government's role in public health is essential to curtailing chronic diseases. It is imperative that the federal, state, and local levels of government address a growing need for healthcare services in rural areas. However, due to the widely differing power structure of the government, public health agencies encounter difficulty in the delivery and finance of health care. Growing health expenditures are a continuing source of budgetary pressure of the federal government. As growing health expenditures continue to consume the government resources, it is becoming more difficult for the government to support other programs.

Chapter Summary

Public health governmental agencies and larger public health systems are major, though overlooked, contributors to the community's health. Most, if not all, agencies are federally funded and provide a substantial portion of services in rural communities. Often, in rural communities, they become the last resort when patients require care. Public Health departments and public health systems represent a lifeline to many communities, especially in rural areas. The main purpose of these institutions are to provide health promotion and disease prevention on a population scale. In order to understand how best to approach rural health, it is essential to understand how the federal government is involved in public health. This chapter introduces governmental systems, rural health policy development, and federal health policies.

Discussion Questions

1. Discuss the role(s) of the federal government in health policy.
2. Discuss the impact of physician shortages in rural areas and how local public health

departments would cope under those circumstances?

3. Identify areas of need where the federal government can intervene.

> *Student Activities and Worksheets are available inside the Navigate eBook, included with the printed text. Simply redeem the access code found at the front of the book at www.jblearning.com.*

References

American Recovery and Reinvestment Act of 2009: law, explanation and analysis. (2009). P.L. 111-5, as signed by the President on February 17, 2009. Chicago, Ill.: CCH.

Anderson, James E. (1975). Public Policy-Making. New York: Praeger.

Centers for Disease Control and Prevention (CDC). (1999). Achievements in public health, 1900–1999: Control of infectious diseases. *Morbidity and Mortality Weekly Report (MMWR).* 48(29), 621–629.

Centers for Disease Control and Prevention (CDC). (2010). National Public Health Performance Standards Program (NPHPSP): 10 Essential Public Health Services. https://www.whitehouse.gov/about-the-white-house/the-executive-branch/

Derksen, D., & Whelan, E. M. (2009). *Closing the health care workforce gap: Reforming federal health care workforce policies to meet the needs of the 21st Century.* Retrieved from the American Progress website: https://www.americanprogress.org/wp-content/uploads/issues/2010/01/pdf/health_care_workforce.pdf

Dye, T. R. (1972). *Understanding-public policy.* Englewood Cliffs: Prentice-Hall.

Fee, E. (2009). History and development of public health principles of public health practice (pp. 12–35). Clifton Park, NY: Delmar.

Institute of Medicine. (1988). *The future of public health.* Washington, DC: National Academy Press.

Jenkins, W. I. (1978). *Policy Analysis: A Political and Organizational Perspective.* London: Martin Robertson.

Murphy S. L., Xu, J., Kochanek K. D., Arias, E. Mortality in the United States, 2017. (2018). *NCHS Data Brief,* No. 328. Hyattsville, MD: National Center for Health Statistics.

Petterson, S. M., Liaw, W. R., Phillips, R. L., Rabin, D. L., Meyers, D. S., & Bazemore, A. W. (2012). Projecting US primary care physician workforce needs: 2010–2025. *Annals of Family Medicine.* 10(6), 503–509. doi:10.1370/afm.1431

Roser, M. (2019). Life Expectancy. *OurWorldInData.org.* Retrieved from: https://ourworldindata.org/life-expectancy

Schutfield, F. D., & Keck, C. W. (2009). *Principles of public health practice.* Clifton Park, NY: Delmar. Available at strategic-plan/introduction/index.html

Sisko, A. M., Keehan, S. P., Cuckler, G. A., Madison, A. J., Smith, S. D., Wolfe, C. J., . . . Poisal, J. A. (2014). National health expenditure projections, 2013–23: Faster growth expected with expanded coverage and improving economy. *Health Affairs.* 33(10), 1841–1850.

CHAPTER 6

U.S. Rural Health Systems in Transition

Zigmond A. Kozicki, DHA, MSA, MA, LLP
Stephanie J.S. Baiyasi-Kozicki, DVM, MPH, HSAC

LEARNING OBJECTIVES

At the end of this chapter, readers will be able to:

1. Define rural America.
2. Identify the social determinants of rural health.
3. Understand the importance of access to care and health outcomes.
4. Consider the relationship of health insurance, sustainability, and access to care.
5. Examine value-based care and the importance of rural emergency services.
6. Understand rural hospital classification.
7. Consider the ongoing relationship between rural residents and rural healthcare providers.
8. Appreciate how technology is important to the rural healthcare delivery process.
9. Consider the alternative models of delivering health care in rural settings.

KEY TERMS

Access to Care
Allied Health
Artificial intelligence (AI)
Community Outpatient Hospital (COH)
Critical Access Hospital
Disproportionate Share Hospital
Frontier Community Health Integration Project
Health Information Technology
Medicaid
Medicare
Medicare-Dependent Hospital
Population Health
Population Health Centers
Quality-adjusted life year
Rural America
Rural Freestanding Emergency Departments
Rural Health Care
Rural Health Clinic
Rural Referral Center
Social Determinants
Sole Community Hospital
Telehealth services
Value-based programs

CHAPTER OVERVIEW

Rural health care is being transformed as a result of changes in reimbursement, the aging of the population, and decreasing economic resources. The **social determinants** of health are becoming increasingly more important in the effort to manage healthcare status in rural settings. Rural hospitals are facing a challenge to remain open. A transition from the existing delivery process is necessary and will require a greater emphasis on the use of technology and **population health** methods. Public policy regarding rural health care will change to provide value-based care.

Rural hospitals are an integral part of the rural healthcare system. Because of their significant contributions to overall community well-being, they are a critical component of communities across rural America. Rural hospitals provide services across the continuum of care from primary care to long-term care (Rural Health Information Hub, 2018).

Rural Health in America

- Approximately 62 million people—nearly one in five Americans—live in rural and frontier areas.
- Rural Americans reside in 80% of the total U.S. land area but only comprise 20% of the U.S. population.
- There are 4,118 primary care Health Professional Shortage Areas (HPSAs) in rural and frontier areas of all U.S. states and territories compared with 1,960 in metropolitan areas.
- The average median income for rural U.S. residents is $40,615 compared with $51,831 for urban residents.
- Approximately 15.4% of rural U.S. residents live in poverty compared with 11.9% of urban residents.

(National Organization of State Offices of Rural Health, NOSORH, 2019).

Social Determinants and Rural Health Status

Conditions in the places where people live, learn, work, and play affect a wide range of health risks and outcomes. These conditions are known as social determinants of health (SDOH). In particular, unstable housing, low income, unsafe neighborhoods, or substandard education is often linked to health risks and unfavorable health status (Centers for Disease Control and Prevention [CDC], 2018).

An example of how social determinants can affect health status can be identified in a population-based analysis of residents of Kentucky. Prostate cancer (PC) is considered the most common male cancer in the United States (Myint et al., 2019). A significant difference in (PC) survival exists between rural Appalachian and non-Appalachian Kentucky. The difference was not related to geographic location, but rather to high comorbidity score, high poverty rate, and low education. This study compared the incidence and mortality rates of PC.

The surveillance epidemiology results from 2005–2014 show that Appalachian Kentucky had a lower incidence (113/100,000 versus 137/100,000) but a higher mortality rate (23.8% versus 21.8%) compared with non-Appalachian Kentucky. In this population-based analysis, there was a significant difference in PC survival between men from Appalachian Kentucky and that of men from non-Appalachian Kentucky. This study supports the concept that patients from Appalachia generally present with later stage, more aggressive disease. "This is likely most impacted by the differences in socioeconomic and educational backgrounds of the Appalachian and non-Appalachian population that may delay diagnosis and care" (Myint et al., 2019). An earlier study (Coyne et al., 2006) explored cultural norms of people in rural Appalachia about health and concluded that "increased awareness of family cancer history, adopting a healthy lifestyle, securing social and familial support, and engaging in informed and shared decision making between PC patients and providers— along with alleviating fear and correcting misperceptions— can empower men to take control of their health."

The social determinants of health are becoming an increasingly important framework for understanding and taking into account the broad range of factors that affect health outcomes in the United States. The National Advisory Committee on Rural Health and Human Services (NACRHHS or the Committee) has examined individual social determinants of health, poverty, access to services, economic opportunity, rates of chronic disease, homelessness, intimate partner violence, and life expectancy. The Committee found that rural communities often fare worse than their urban and suburban counterparts (Health Resources & Service Administration, (HRSA), 2017).

In 2013, according to the Office of Management and Budget (OMB) definition, 62.8% of U.S. counties were considered rural, encompassing 15% of the total U.S. population. Rates of chronic disease such as diabetes, chronic obstructive pulmonary disease (COPD), heart disease, and obesity are all higher in rural areas than they are in other parts of the country (Meit, 2014). From 2005–2009, the mortality rate in rural counties was 13% higher than in metro counties and residents of metro counties lived two years longer on average than residents of rural counties (OMB, 2014). There appears to be a greater vulnerability for morbidity and mortality in **rural America** compared with nonrural America.

Access to Health Care in Rural Communities

U.S. rural communities—from Appalachia and the Deep South to the Midwest and western states to Alaska and Hawaii—face particular challenges related to accessing healthcare services. These challenges, including few local doctors, poverty, and remote locations, contribute to the risks for poorer health.

Rural areas—This section reviews the different healthcare facilities accessible to the 57 million Americans living in rural areas and how they were developed.

Facilities

While nearly 85% of U.S. residents can reach a Level I or Level II trauma center within an hour, only 24% of residents living in rural areas can do so within that time frame— this, despite the fact that 60% of all trauma deaths in the United States occur in rural areas.

Approximately 21.9% of residents in remote rural counties are uninsured, compared with 17.5% in rural counties adjacent to urban counties and 14.3% in urban counties. Rural residents spend more on health care out of pocket than their urban counterparts; on average, rural residents pay for 40% of their healthcare costs out of their own pocket compared with the urban share of one-third. One in five rural residents spends more than $1,000 out of pocket in a year (National Organization of State Offices of Rural Health, [NOSORH], 2019)

There are nearly 5,000 short-term, acute-care hospitals in the United States. Half of them are in urban areas and half are in rural areas. Most rural hospitals are located in large (39%) and small (39%) rural areas. Fewer (22%) are located in isolated rural areas (Freeman et al., 2015). Hospitals are considered to be rural if they are a) in a nonmetropolitan county or b) in a metropolitan county but in an area that has a Rural Urban Community Area (RUCA) code of 4 or greater according to the U.S. Department of Agriculture (USDOA, 2016).

Rural Hospitals

It has been suggested in the past that "The role of hospitals in the American healthcare system is changing rapidly, and some believe that hospitals may be replaced by networks of professionals and institutions tied together to coordinate care and promote health—the so-called virtual hospital" (Ricketts & Heaphy, 2000). This has not yet come to be the prevailing method of delivering health care to rural people. However, it will probably be considered, especially if funding for the existing rural hospital delivery process is inadequate.

- Rural hospitals are sources of innovation and resourcefulness that reach beyond geographic boundaries to deliver quality care. They are also typically the economic foundation of their communities— every dollar spent on rural hospitals generates about $2.20 for the local economy.

- Twelve percent of rural hospitals indicate they are not considering health information technology (HIT) investments because of cost concerns compared with 3% of urban hospitals.

- Critical Access Hospitals care for a higher percentage of Medicare patients than other hospitals because rural populations are typically older than urban populations.

(National Organization of State Offices of Rural Health, NOSORH, 2019).

Hill-Burton Hospitals

Federal Funding Many public and nonprofit facilities received financial assistance under Titles VI and XVI of the Public Health Service Act, commonly known as the Hill-Burton Act of 1946 (Health and Human Services, 2015). This U.S. Federal law provided funds to improve hospitals that had become obsolete because of lack of money during the Great Depression and World War II (i.e., 1929–1945). Hill-Burton hospitals received grants and were required to provide uncompensated services for 20 years to indigent patients. Most rural hospitals were built using Hill-Burton funding. Keep in mind that hospitals were initially considered public health centers. Staffing for hospitals was not funded through the Hill-Burton law. The program stopped providing funds in 1997, but approximately 140 healthcare facilities nationwide are still obligated to provide free or reduced-cost care (HRSA, 2019). Hill-Burton was the last and perhaps the most progressive expression of redistributive New Deal liberalism (Kruse, 2006).

"The Hill-Burton Act was signed into law by President Harry S. Truman on August 13, 1946. Known formally as the Hospital Survey and Construction Act, Hill-Burton started as a Truman initiative. Hill-Burton provided construction grants and loans to communities that could demonstrate viability, based on their population and per capita income, in the building of health care facilities. The Hill-Burton grants were used to build hospitals where they were needed and where they would be sustainable once their doors were open."

By 1975, Hill-Burton had been responsible for construction of nearly one-third of U.S. hospitals. That year Hill-Burton was rolled into bigger legislation known as the Public Health Service Act. By the turn of the century, approximately 6,800 facilities in 4,000 communities had in some part been financed by the law. These not only included hospitals and clinics but also rehabilitation centers and long-term care facilities. In 1997, this type of direct, community-based federal health care construction financing came to an end.

Hill-Burton introduced many ideas in health care financing that are still in use today. Chief among them is that hospitals receiving federal monies are obligated to provide free or subsidized care to a portion of their indigent patients. U.S. nonprofit hospitals (still the vast majority) must demonstrate evidence of "community benefit" to maintain tax-exempt status. Providing care to the uninsured is one of the most common ways to meet this obligation (Schumann, 2016). Tax-exemption is a form of federal assistance.

Hill-Burton recipient facilities include:

- Acute care general hospitals
- Special hospitals
- Nursing homes
- Public health centers
- Rehabilitation facilities

Every hospital or other facility that ever gave a Community Service Assurance in exchange for Hill-Burton funds under Title VI of the Public Health Service Act must:

- Provide emergency services to any person living in its service area who cannot afford those services
- Give each person living in its service area nonemergency medical treatment

at the facility no matter their race, color, national origin, creed, or any other factor unrelated to a person's ability to pay for a needed service and the facility's ability to provide the needed service

- Participate in the Medicare and Medicaid programs unless they are ineligible
- Make arrangements for reimbursement for services with principal state and local third-party payers that provide reimbursement that is not less than the actual cost of the services
- Post its community service obligations in English and Spanish, and any other language spoken by 10% or more of the households in the service area
- The Hill-Burton Act also applies to people working in the service area of the facility if it was funded under Title XVI of the Public Health Service Act
- The community service obligation does not require the facility to make nonemergency services available to persons unable to pay for them

A facility's Community Service Assurance obligations also extend to people working in its service area if the facility received funds under Title XVI of the Public Health Service Act (Health and Human Services, 2015).

Author's Opinion A rural community with a Hill-Burton hospital should negotiate continued care for the rural population with the owner of the facility even if the hospital is considered at risk of closing. From 1947 to 1971, Hill-Burton underwrote the creation of a modern healthcare infrastructure with $3.7 billion in federal funding and $9.1 billion in matches from state and local governments (Kruse, 2006). Communities essentially have a covenant with the federal government if they received Hill-Burton funding. If the community provided matching funds, it could seek continued support from the federal government to subsidize their community hospital.

Health Insurance

Residents of rural counties often encounter barriers to access healthcare services to obtain the care they need although they are still forced to pay insurance at higher rates than those living in urban areas. Even when an adequate supply of healthcare services exists in the community, many other factors hamper access to health care. These factors include poverty, lack of transportation, low health literacy, etc. Approximately 11.3% of people in mostly rural counties lacked health insurance compared with 10.1% for mostly urban counties. In this section, we will review the impact of selected federal programs (Medicare and Medicaid) to improve access to health care in rural areas.

Medicare

On July 30, 1965, President Lyndon B. Johnson signed into law the Congressional bill that led to Medicare and Medicaid. The original **Medicare** program included Part A (Hospital Insurance) and Part B (Medical Insurance). Today, these two parts are called "Original Medicare." Over the years, Congress has made changes to Medicare including adding Part C (coinsurance) and Part D (prescription drug benefit). Since 1965, more people have become eligible. In 1972, Medicare was expanded to cover the disabled and people with end-stage renal disease (ESRD). There are approximately 61 million people enrolled in Medicare in the United States (CMS, 2019, May).

Medicare is the federal health insurance program for:

- People who are 65 or older
- Certain younger people with disabilities
- People with end- stage renal disease (permanent kidney failure requiring dialysis or a transplant, sometimes called ESRD)

The Centers for Medicare & Medicaid Services, CMS, is part of the Department of Health and Human Services (HHS). CMS provides federal administrative oversight for Medicare and Medicaid. (CMS, 2019, Feb 20).

The different parts of Medicare help cover specific services, and these are:

- Medicare Part A (Hospital Insurance)

Part A covers inpatient hospital stays, care in a skilled nursing facility, hospice care, and some home health care.

- Medicare Part B (Medical Insurance)

Part B covers certain doctors' services, outpatient care, medical supplies, and preventive services.

- Medicare Part C (Co- insurance benefit)

The Medicare Prescription Drug Improvement and Modernization Act of 2003 (MMA) allowed private health plans approved by Medicare and became known as Medicare Advantage Plans. These plans are sometimes called "Part C" or "MA Plans." Medicare Part C is administered by private insurance companies contracted with Medicare. Medicare Part C covers everything that the original Medicare (Part A and Part B) cover and may cover extra benefits as well. The MMA also expanded Medicare to include an optional prescription drug benefit, "Part D," which went into effect in 2006.

Coinsurance plans are offered by insurance companies and other private companies approved by Medicare. Medicare Advantage Plans may also offer prescription drug coverage that follows the same rules as Medicare Prescription Drug Plans. https://www.medicare.gov/what-medicare-covers/your-medicare-coverage-choices/whats-medicare

- Medicare Part D (prescription drug coverage) was first available to the public in 2006. Part D adds prescription drug coverage to:
- Original Medicare
- Some Medicare cost plans
- Some Medicare private fee-for- service plans
- Medicare medical savings account plans
- Medicare Part D Prescription Drug benefit

The Medicare-for-All program being considered would cover all medically necessary services, with defined categories of benefits to be covered, as well as dental and vision services, a broader definition of benefits than is currently covered by Medicare or by the ACA essential health benefits (Neuman, Pollitz & Tolbert, 2019).

Medicaid

Medicaid provides health coverage to millions of Americans, including eligible low-income adults, children, pregnant women, elderly adults, and people with disabilities. Medicaid is administered by states, according to federal requirements. The program is funded jointly by states and the federal government. It provides coverage to approximately 65 million people (CMS, 2019, Apr).

Between 2013 and 2015, states that expanded Medicaid under the Affordable Care Act (ACA) saw their uncompensated care cost drop from 3.9% of operating costs to 2.3%. During this same time frame, operating costs remained fairly flat in nonexpansion states. Considering that the average operating margin for a nonprofit hospital is around 2.7%, even small reductions in the level of uncompensated care can represent the difference between them.

Children's Health Insurance Program

The Children's Health Insurance Program (CHIP) was created in 1997 to provide health insurance and preventive care for nearly 11 million, or 1 in 7, uninsured American children. Many of these children came from uninsured working families that earned too much to be eligible for Medicaid. All 50 states, the District of Columbia, and the territories have CHIP plans.

Affordable Care Act

The Patient Protection and Affordable Care Act, often shortened to the Affordable Care Act or nicknamed Obamacare, is a United States federal statute enacted by the 111th United States Congress and signed into law by President Barack Obama on March 23, 2010. The ACA created the Health Insurance Marketplace, a single place where consumers can apply for and enroll in private health insurance plans. It also offered new ways for the U.S. government to design and test how to pay for and deliver health care. Medicare and Medicaid have also been better coordinated to make sure people who have Medicare and Medicaid can get quality services.

The argument for supporting the ACA considers that uncompensated care in hospitals will not disappear as long as there remain low-income patients who cannot qualify for Medicaid or insurance premium subsidies. Supporting measures that increase insurance coverage for as many people as possible would improve the financial well-being of the U.S. hospital system. Helping U.S. hospitals means lowering the number of uninsured patients who get treated in them. Before the efforts throughout the summer of 2017 to undo the ACA, healthcare insurance markets were trending toward stabilization and potentially generating modest profits for 2017 (Weisman, et al., 2017).

Federal Public Plan Option

Three proposals that the U.S. Congress can consider would establish a federal public plan option to build upon, rather than replace, the current blend of private insurance and public coverage. These three proposals aim to address some of the shortcomings in ACA marketplaces by giving individuals and employers a new option that may provide more affordable coverage. Two of these proposals invoke Medicare in naming the public plan (Medicare Part E and Medicare-X); the Schakowsky bill incorporates many of Medicare's features in the public plan, without using its name. Under all three proposals, the public plan option would be offered alongside private insurance through the ACA

marketplace to individuals and small employers eligible to purchase coverage there. Two of the bills would also offer the public plan in the individual and small group markets outside of the marketplace. Under each of the three proposals, the new public plan would cover (at a minimum) all ACA essential health benefits. (Neuman, Pollitz & Tolbert, 2018).

In 2020, all health insurance plans offered in the Marketplace cover these 10 essential health benefits:

- Ambulatory patient services (outpatient care you get without being admitted to a hospital)
- Emergency services
- Hospitalization (like surgery and overnight stays)
- Pregnancy, maternity, and newborn care (both before and after birth)
- Mental health and substance use disorder services, including behavioral health treatment (this includes counseling and psychotherapy)
- Prescription drugs
- Rehabilitative and habilitative services and devices (services and devices to help people with injuries, disabilities, or chronic conditions gain or recover mental and physical skills)
- Laboratory services
- Preventive and wellness services and chronic disease management
- Pediatric services, including oral and vision care (but adult dental and vision coverage aren't essential health benefits) (HealthCare.gov, 2020).

Value-Based Health Care

The precedent of Hill-Burton is continued in the current era of federally funded, **value-based programs** and healthcare providers. These programs and providers are being rewarded with incentive payments for the quality of care they give to people covered by Medicare. These programs are part of a larger-quality strategy to reform how health care is delivered and paid for.

Value-based programs support a three-part aim:

1. Better health for the population
2. Better care for the individuals
3. Lower cost through improvement

There are six priorities that value-based programs are expected to consider. (CMS, 2019, May 17).

1. Making care safer by reducing harm caused in delivery of care
2. Ensuring that each person and family is engaged as partners in their care
3. Promoting effective communication and coordination of care
4. Promoting effective prevention and treatment practices for the leading causes of mortality, starting with cardiovascular disease
5. Working with communities to promote best practices to enable healthy living
6. Making quality care more affordable for individuals, families, employers, and governments by developing and spreading new healthcare delivery models

Value-based programs are important because they enable Medicare to move toward paying providers based on the quality, rather than the quantity, of care they provide to patients.

There are five original value-based programs; their goal is to link provider performance of quality measures to provider payment:

- End-Stage Renal Disease Quality Incentive Program (ESRD QIP)
- Hospital Value-Based Purchasing (HVBP) Program
- Hospital Readmission Reduction (HRR) Program
- Value Modifier (VM) Program (also called the Physician Value-Based Modifier or PVBM)
- Hospital Acquired Conditions (HAC) Reduction Program

There are other value-based programs:

- Skilled Nursing Facility Value-Based Program (SNFVBP)
- Home Health Value-Based Program (HHVBP)
- (CMS, 2019, May 17).

The timeline for these programs can be found in **Figure 6-1** on next page.

How do value-based programs, shown in **Figure 6-2**, work with other CMS quality efforts?

Quality-Adjusted Life Year

The quality-adjusted life year or quality-adjusted life-year (QALY) is a generic measure of disease burden, including both the quality and the quantity of life lived. It is used in economic evaluation to assess the value of medical interventions. One QALY equates to one year in perfect health. A **quality-adjusted life year** is a measure of both the quantity and quality of life lived used to assess the value for money of a medical intervention. It is based on the number of years that would be added to a patient's life by a particular medical intervention.

Value-based programs should consider the increase in QALY as a measure of effectiveness. When a program adds life years, it should be considered instrumental for promoting population health. Each intervention should be evaluated. In **Figure 6-3**, the intervention leads to QALY gains both by increasing or maintaining quality of life and by extending life. The main advantage of the QALY approach is that it provides one combined measure of the benefits of a program that both extends life and maintains quality of life (Australian Department of Health, 2002).

The diagram shows that without the program, as the quantity of life (years) increases the quality of life (weights) decreases from 1.0 to 0.0 (death). The diagram also shows that with the program, there is a gain in life years. (Australian Department of Health, 2002).

	2008	2010	2012	2014	2015	2018	2019
Legislation passed	MIPPA	ACA		PAMA	MACRA		
Program implemented			ESRD-QIP				APMs
			HVBP	HACRP	VM	SNFVBP	MIPS

Legislation
ACA: Affordable care act
MACRA: The medicare access and CHIP reauthorization act of 2015
MIPPA: Medicare improvement for patients and providers act
PAMA: Protecting access to medicare act

Program
APMs: Alternative payment models
ESRD-QIP: End-stage renal disease quality incentive program
HACRP: Hospital-acquired condition reduction program
HRRP: Hospital readmissions reduction program
HVBP: Hospital value-based purchasing program
MIPS: Merit-based incentive payment system
VM: Value modifier or physician value-based modifer (PVBM)
SNFVBP: Skilled Nursing facility value-based purchasing program

Figure 6-1 Value-Based Programs.

From U.S. Centers for Medicare & Medicaid. What are the value-based programs? Value Based Programs. Retrieved from https://www.cms.gov/Medicare/Quality-Initiatives-Patient-Assessment-Instruments/Value-Based-Programs/Value-Based-Programs

The Emergency Medical Treatment and Labor Act (EMTALA)

The Emergency Medical Treatment and Labor Act (EMTALA) is a U.S. federal law and unfunded mandate that requires anyone coming to an emergency department to be stabilized and treated, regardless of their insurance status or ability to pay. EMTALA was enacted by Congress in 1986 as part of the Consolidated Omnibus Budget Reconciliation Act (COBRA) of 1985 (42 U.S.C. §1395dd) (American College of Emergency Physicians (ACEP), 2020). The law benefits people without healthcare coverage but also increases unfunded services in rural and urban settings.

"The provisions of EMTALA apply to all individuals (not just Medicare beneficiaries) who attempt to gain access to a hospital for emergency care. The regulations define

"hospital with an emergency department" to mean a hospital with a dedicated emergency department (ED). In turn, the regulation defines "dedicated emergency department" as any department or facility of the hospital that either (1) is licensed by the state as an emergency department; (2) held out to the public as providing treatment for emergency medical conditions; or (3) on one-third of the visits to the department in the preceding calendar year actually provided treatment for emergency medical conditions on an urgent basis" (DHHS-CMS, 2019). Hospital-based outpatient clinics not equipped to handle medical emergencies are not obligated under EMTALA and can refer patients to a nearby emergency department for care (ACEP, 2020).

How does EMTALA define an emergency? According to the ACEP, an emergency medical condition is defined as "a condition manifesting itself by acute symptoms of sufficient

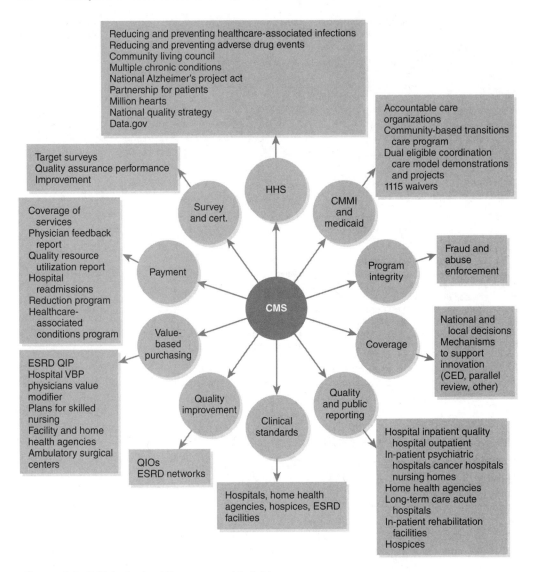

Figure 6-2 CMS Authorized Programs and Activities.

From U.S. Centers for Medicare & Medicaid. What are the value-based programs? Value Based Programs. Retrieved from https://www.cms.gov/Medicare/Quality-Initiatives-Patient-Assessment-Instruments /Value-Based-Programs/Value-Based-Programs

severity (including severe pain) such that the absence of immediate medical attention could reasonably be expected to result in placing the individual's health [or the health of an unborn child] in serious jeopardy, serious impairment to bodily functions, or serious dysfunction of bodily organs." An example could be a pregnant woman with an emergency condition that must be treated until delivery is complete,

unless a transfer under the statute is appropriate (ACEP, 2020).

According to the ACEP, the ongoing issue is that "the burden of uncompensated care is growing, closing many emergency departments, decreasing resources for everyone and threatening the ability of emergency departments to care for all patients." One of the suggested solutions to this funding

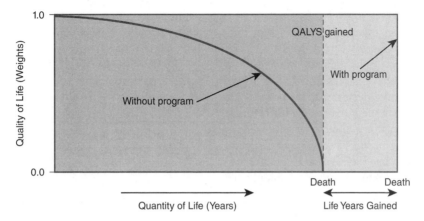

Figure 6-3 Quality-Adjusted Life Years.

Reproduced from Australian Department of Health. (2002). Quality-Adjusted-Life-Years (QALYs). Retrieved from https://www1.health.gov.au/internet/publications/publishing.nsf/Content/illicit-pubs-needle-return-1
-rep-toc~illicit-pubs-needle-return-1-rep-5~illicit-pubs-needle-return-1-rep-5-2

shortfall according to the ACEP is the recognition of uncompensated care as a legitimate practice expense for emergency physicians." (ACEP, 2020).

Hospitals have three main obligations under EMTALA:

1. "Any individual who comes and requests must receive a medical screening examination to determine whether an emergency medical condition exists. Examination and treatment cannot be delayed to inquire about methods of payment or insurance coverage. Emergency departments also must post signs that notify patients and visitors of their rights to a medical screening examination and treatment.
2. If an emergency medical condition exists, treatment must be provided until the emergency medical condition is resolved or stabilized. If the hospital does not have the capability to treat the emergency medical condition, an "appropriate" transfer of the patient to another hospital must be done in accordance with the EMTALA provisions.
3. Hospitals with specialized capabilities are obligated to accept transfers from hospitals who lack the capability to treat unstable emergency medical conditions.

- In addition, a hospital must report to CMS or the state survey agency any time it has reason to believe it may have received an individual who has been transferred in an unstable emergency medical condition from another hospital in violation of EMTALA" (ACEP, 2020).

Opioid Epidemic and Rural Health

Rural Americans are farther away from emergency care and treatment options, especially for mental health and substance abuse. In 55% of all U.S. counties, most of which are rural, there are no psychologists, psychiatrists, or social workers (Siegel, 2018).

In October of 2017, the Centers for Disease Control and Prevention (CDC) announced that the rates of drug overdose deaths are rising in rural areas, surpassing rates in urban areas. The opioid epidemic is devastating to its victims and their families. The impact of this issue on small towns and rural places has been particularly significant. In 2017, drug overdose in the United States accounted for 70,237 deaths (USDA, 2018). The age-adjusted rate of overdose deaths increased significantly by 9.6% from 2016

(19.8 per 100,000) to 2017 (21.7 per 100,000). Opioids—mainly synthetic opioids (other than methadone)—are currently the main driver of drug overdose deaths. Opioids were involved in 47,600 overdose deaths in 2017 (67.8% of all drug overdose deaths). At 197 people each day, this is more than the number of lives lost in car accidents or gun-related homicides. An overwhelming majority of these overdose deaths involved an opioid (Scholl et al., 2018).

There are solutions to the opiate epidemic:

- Protect Medicaid as a funding source to provide treatment.
- Expand access to substance abuse treatment services including medication-assisted treatment and traditional substance-abuse treatment.
- Develop evidence-based prevention programs tailored to the needs of rural communities.
- Increase the implementation of harm-reduction strategies.
- Promote use of evidence-based prescribing guidelines and strengthen prescription drug-monitoring programs.
- Expand use of substance-abuse treatment as an alternative to incarceration (Siegel, 2018).

Rural Hospital Classification

The rural-urban commuting area (RUCA) codes classify U.S. census tracts using measures of population density, urbanization, and daily commuting. The most recent RUCA codes are based on data from the 2010 decennial census and the 2006-10 American Community Survey. The classification contains two levels. Whole numbers (1-10) delineate metropolitan, micropolitan, small town, and rural commuting areas based on the size and direction of the primary (largest) commuting flows. These 10 codes are further subdivided based on secondary commuting flows, providing flexibility in combining levels to meet varying definitional needs and preferences (Freeman et al., 2015, U.S. Dept of Agriculture, 2016, Rural Health Information Hub, 2018).

Rural hospitals are further divided into three levels of rurality:

1. Large Rural Areas — hospitals in areas with a RUCA code less than 7
2. Small Rural Areas — hospitals in areas with a RUCA code of 7, 8, or 9
3. Isolated Rural Areas — hospitals in areas with a RUCA code of 10 (North Carolina Rural Health Research Program 2018, Freeman et al., 2015).

Rural Hospital Designations/ Provider Types

Government payment programs define rural hospitals (Rural Health Information, 2018). **Table 6-1** summarizes the various rural hospital designation types. These include the following:

- Critical Access Hospital (CAH)   53.5% of rural hospitals are designated as **Critical Access Hospitals** (Freeman et al., 2015). These rural hospitals maintain no more than 25 acute care beds. CAHs must be located more than 35 miles, or 15 miles by mountainous terrain or secondary roads, from the nearest hospital — unless designated by a state as a necessary provider prior to 2006. Unlike hospitals paid prospectively using IPPS, CAHs are reimbursed based on the hospital's Medicare allowable costs.
- Rural Referral Center (RRC)   Rural tertiary hospitals that receive referrals from surrounding rural acute care hospitals. An acute care hospital can be classified for Medicare purposes as an **Rural Referral Center** if it meets one of several qualifying criteria based on location, bed size, and/or referral patterns. In general, CMS classifies a Medicare participating acute care hospital as an RRC if it is in a rural area and it meets one of the following criteria:

Table 6-1 Rural Hospital Affiliations

Hospital Type	Hospital Beds	Part of a Group Purchasing Organization	Part of a Health System
Critical Access Hospital **(CAH)**	6 to 24	68%	46%
Disproportionate Share Hospital **(DSH)** Sole Community Hospitals (SCHs)	25 to 49	68%	57%
Medicare- dependent Hospital **(MDH)**	50 to 99	66%	68%
	100 to 199	70%	75%
Rural Referral Center (RRC)	200 to 299	77%	77%

Data from American Hospital Association (2016). Small and Rural Update. Retrieved from https://www.aha.org/2017-05-30-small-or-rural-update-0

1. It has 275 or more usable beds available during its most recently completed cost-reporting period.
2. It shows one of these elements: Non-staff physicians or other hospitals refer at least 50% of the hospital's Medicare patients At least 60% of the hospital's Medicare patients live more than 25 miles from the hospital The hospital furnishes at least 60% of all services to Medicare patients living more than 25 miles from the hospital.
3. If a hospital does not meet the criteria in numbers 1 or 2, it is classified as an RRC if located in a rural area, meets the criteria specified in a and b below, and meets at least one of the criteria specified in c or d below:
   a. Discharges during the most recent federal fiscal year ended at least one year prior to the beginning of the cost reporting period that the hospital is seeking RRC status, and its Case-Mix Index (CMI) equals one of these:
      - The lower of the median CMI value for all urban hospitals nationally
      - The median CMI urban hospital's value for urban hospitals in its region, excluding those hospitals receiving indirect

   medical education payments specified in 42 CFR 412.105.
   b. Its number of discharges is at least one of these:
      - 5,000 (3,000 for an osteopathic hospital)
      - The median urban hospital's number of discharges in the census region where it is located, set by CMS yearly in Acute Care Hospital IPPS rulemaking, according to 42 CFR 412.96(c)(2)
   c. Medical staff: More than 50% of its active medical staff are specialists who meet the conditions specified at 42 CFR 412.96(c)(3)
   d. Source of inpatients: At least 60% of all inpatient discharges reside more than 25 miles from the hospital
   e. Volume of referrals: Other hospitals or nonstaff physicians refer at least 40% of all inpatients treated.

- Sole Community Hospital (**SCH**) Designation as a **Sole Community Hospital** is based on a hospital's distance in relation to other hospitals, indicating that the facility is likely the only hospital serving a community. Distance requirements vary.
- Medicare-Dependent Hospital (**MDH**) A **Medicare-Dependent Hospital** designation from the CMS provides enhanced

Table 6-2 Average Hospital Patient Activity by Bed Size

Hospital Type	Hospital Beds	Average Admissions	Average Outpatient Visits
Critical Access Hospital **(CAH)**	6 to 24	379	24,839
Disproportionate Share Hospital **(DSH)** Sole Community Hospitals (SCHs)	25 to 49	917	47,656
Medicare-Dependent Hospital **(MDH)**	50 to 99	2,084	66,003
	100 to 199	5,838	141,842
Rural Referral Center (RRC)	200 to 299	11,035	220,826

Data from American Hospital Association (2016). Small and Rural Update. Retrieved from https://www.aha.org/2017-05-30-small-or-rural-update-0

payment to support small rural hospitals with 100 or fewer beds for which Medicare patients make up at least 60% of the hospital's inpatient days or discharges.

- Disproportionate Share Hospital **(DSH)** A special reimbursement designation under Medicare and Medicaid, called a **disproportionate share hospital**, is designed to support hospitals that provide care to a disproportionate number of low-income patients.
- Rural Community Hospital Demonstration Implements cost-based reimbursement in participating small rural hospitals that are not eligible for Critical Access Hospital designation.

Is There a Typical Rural Hospital?

The typical rural hospital is located in a county with a median population of 27,980, with 36 residents per square mile, with 16.8% of the population 65 years and older, with an average per capita income of $32,781, and with 17.5% of the population living below the federal poverty level (American Hospital Association, 2015).

The typical rural hospital offers inpatient care that includes surgical services, obstetric services, and swing bed services; but does not

include an intensive care unit, a skilled nursing facility, a psychiatric unit, or a rehabilitation unit. **Table 6-2** summarizes the average hospital patient activities by bed size.

The typical rural hospital offers outpatient care that includes outpatient surgical services, cardiac rehabilitation services, breast cancer screening/mammography, and a health fair; but does not include a rural health clinic, hospice services, home health services, chemotherapy services, dental services, or outpatient alcohol/drug abuse care. Staffing at rural hospitals is influenced by bed size (American Hospital Association). **Table 6-3** summarizes the average hospital staffing by bed size.

The typical rural hospital has a financial profile with total margin of 2.7%, current ratio of 2.2, outpatient care representing 69.3% of total revenue, charges for Medicare patients representing 31.0% of all charges, 58 days cash on hand, and patient deductions/allowances making up 52.0% per revenue dollar (Freeman et al., 2015).

Rural Health Clinics (RHCs)

The **Rural Health Clinic** (RHC) program is intended to increase access to primary care services for patients in rural communities. RHCs

Table 6-3 Average Hospital Staffing by Bed Size

Hospital Type	Hospital Beds	Number of Full-time Employees	Number of Part-time Employees
Critical Access Hospital **(CAH)**	6 to 24	101	50
Disproportionate Share Hospital **(DSH)** Sole Community Hospitals **(SCHs)**	25 to 49	182	83
Medicare-Dependent Hospital **(MDH)**	50 to 99	296	139
	100 to 199	672	276
Rural Referral Center **(RRC)**	200 to 299	1,232	468

Data from American Hospital Association (2016). Small and Rural Update. Retrieved from https://www.aha.org/2017-05-30-small-or-rural-update-00

can be public, nonprofit, or for-profit health-care facilities. To receive certification, they must be located in rural, underserved areas. They are required to use a team approach of physicians working with non-physician providers such as nurse practitioners (NP), physician assistants (PA), and certified nurse midwives (CNM) to provide services. The clinic must be staffed at least 50% of the time with a NP, PA, or CNM. RHCs are required to provide outpatient primary care services and basic laboratory services. The main advantage of RHC status is enhanced reimbursement rates for providing Medicare and Medicaid services (Rural Health Information Hub, 2019).

The Rural Healthcare Providers

Health professions' workforce shortages are exacerbated in rural areas, where communities struggle to attract and retain well-trained providers. While approximately 16% of the U.S. population lives in rural America, only approximately 11% of physicians practice in rural locations. Approximately 65% of primary care health professional shortage areas (HPSAs) are rural (HRSA, 2012).

There are multiple barriers to expanding the rural provider supply. Healthcare delivery is challenging in rural locations where patients tend to be poorer and often older, face transportation barriers, and have less health insurance than their urban counterparts. Challenges also include lower reimbursements for provider services, clinician lifestyle demands, spousal career needs, and the educational needs of families.

Workforce Shortage Problems

There is a shortage of physicians in rural communities (National Rural Health Association, 2019). The patient-to- primary care physician ratio in rural areas is only 39.8 physicians per 100,000 people, compared with 53.3 physicians per 100,000 in urban areas. This uneven distribution of physicians has an impact on the health of the population (American Academy of Family Physicians, 2015, Hing, & Hsiao, 2014). There are 30 generalist dentists per 100,000 residents in urban areas versus 22 per 100,000 in rural areas (Doescher et al., 2009). Access to oral health services is a problem for many segments of the U.S. population and is typically related to factors such as geography and maldistribution of providers, insurance status, and low income (HRSA, 2012).

Primary Care Providers

Since its introduction in 1961, the term primary care has been defined in various ways, often using one or more of the following categories to describe what primary care is or who provides it (Lee, 1992; Spitz, 1994). These categories include:

- The care provided by certain clinicians— some proposed legislation, for example, lists the medical specialties of primary care as family medicine, general internal medicine, general pediatrics, and obstetrics and gynecology. Some experts and groups have included nurse practitioners and physician assistants (OTA, 1986; Pew Health Professions Commission, 1994)
- A set of activities whose functions define the boundaries of primary care—such as curing or alleviating common illnesses and disabilities
- A level of care or setting—an entry point to a system that includes secondary care (by community hospitals) and tertiary care (by medical centers and teaching hospitals) (Fry, 1980); ambulatory versus inpatient care
- A set of attributes, as in the 1978 IOM definition—care that is accessible, comprehensive, coordinated, continuous, and accountable—or as defined by Starfield (1992)—care that is characterized by first contact, accessibility, longitudinality, and comprehensiveness
- A strategy for organizing the healthcare system as a whole—such as community-oriented primary care, which gives priority to and allocates resources to community-based health care and places less emphasis on hospital-based, technology-intensive, acute-care medicine (IOM, 1984).

Primary Care

The domain of primary care includes the primary care physician, other physicians who include some primary care services in their practices, and some non-physician providers. However, central to the concept of primary care is the patient. Therefore, such definitions are incomplete without including a description of the primary care practice (American Academy of Family Physicians [AAFP], 2019).

The patient-to- primary-care physician ratio in rural areas is only 39.8 physicians per 100,000 people, compared with 53.3 physicians per 100,000 in urban areas. This uneven distribution of physicians has an impact on the health of the population (Hing & Hsiao, 2014).

The recruitment of primary care physicians in rural America is a critical factor in sustaining rural health services. Challenges to overcome to attract physicians to rural practice include:

- Shortage of academic medical programs
- Lack of family and an established social network
- Fewer employment opportunities for spouse/significant other
- Fewer entertainment opportunities (e.g., concert venues and family attractions) and dining options (e.g., upscale restaurants and variety of ethnic foods) than in urban locales
- School systems with fewer offerings than those situated in metropolitan areas
- Less diversity in religion, which could impact provider's ability to practice his or her faith
- Inclination of newly trained physicians finishing residency and fellowship to remain close to where they have trained (Hall, 2017).

Incidentally, recruitment of women to work in rural settings is becoming more important because more women than men applied to U.S. medical schools, comprising 50.9% of applicants. The trend is that women are becoming the majority of matriculants (new enrollees) to medical school. There is a significant projected shortage of up to 121,300 physicians by 2030 (AAMC, 2018). To increase the number of female physicians practicing in rural communities' employers will need to be more supportive of the challenges in maintaining work-life balance.

Educators, employers, communities, and policymakers can adapt their practices to help female family physicians thrive in rural communities (Phillips et al., 2015).

Allied Health Rural Health Care

Allied health may be defined as those health professions that are distinct from medicine and nursing. Because of the shortage of primary care physicians, Allied Health professionals will need to fill the gap.

Allied Health professionals are involved with the delivery of health or related services pertaining to the identification, evaluation, and prevention of diseases and disorders; dietary and nutrition services; rehabilitation and health systems management; among others. Allied health professionals, to name a few, include dental hygienists, diagnostic medical sonographers, dietitians, medical technologists, occupational therapists, physical therapists, radiographers, respiratory therapists, and speech language pathologists.

Federal Definitions of Allied Health

Allied health is defined in the Federal Code and further defined in The Patient Protection and Affordable Care Act. Allied health is also included in eligibility criteria for participation in grant programs administered by the U.S. Department of Labor and the U.S. Public Health Service. The ACA (P.L. 111-148) defines allied health professionals as follows:

1. *ALLIED HEALTH PROFESSIONAL.—The term "allied health professional" means an allied health professional as defined in section 799B(5) of the Public Health Service Act (42 U.S.C. 295p(5)) who— (A) has graduated and received an allied health professions degree or certificate from an institution of higher education; and (B) is employed with a Federal, State, local or tribal public health agency, or in a setting or in a setting where*

patients might require health care services, including acute care facilities, ambulatory care facilities, personal residences, and other settings located in health professional shortage areas, medically underserved areas, or medically underserved populations, as recognized by the Secretary of Health and Human Services.

Title 42, Chapter 6A, Subchapter V, Part F, Sec. 295p of the Federal Code states that the term "allied health professionals" means a health professional (other than a registered nurse or physician assistant) who has not received a degree of doctor of medicine, a degree of doctor of osteopathy, a degree of doctor of dentistry or an equivalent degree, a degree of doctor of veterinary medicine or an equivalent degree, a degree of doctor of optometry or an equivalent degree, a degree of doctor of podiatric medicine or an equivalent degree, a degree of bachelor of science in pharmacy or an equivalent degree, a degree of doctor of pharmacy or an equivalent degree, a graduate degree in public health or an equivalent degree, a degree of doctor of chiropractic or an equivalent degree, a graduate degree in health administration or an equivalent degree, a doctoral degree in clinical psychology or an equivalent degree, or a degree in social work or an equivalent degree, or a degree in counseling or an equivalent degree.

Critical Rural Allied Health Providers

There are critical health providers who are necessary to manage the health issues in rural America. The emerging advanced-level practitioners (ACPs) come from a range of professional backgrounds such as nursing, pharmacy, paramedics, occupational therapy, healthcare science, and midwifery (NHS, 2019). In America, with the expected shortage of primary care physicians, advance practice providers such as physician assistants, nurse practitioners, pharmacists, dentists, physical therapists, and psychologists will become more important.

- Advance Practice Providers in Rural Population
- Physician Assistant (PA) and the Nurse Practitioner (NP)

Advanced Practice Provider (APP) Utilization and the Impact on Rural Medicine

There are multiple challenges to providing care to those who live in rural settings. One of the greatest hurdles to adequate care is the persistent shortage of primary care providers practicing in rural America. This shortage has been recognized for over 50 years and this disparity continues to worsen for a myriad of reasons including one key cause, the continued trend of physicians choosing specialty over primary care (Hart, 2012). This has led to an insufficient number of medical graduates to even cover retiring rural physicians (Ewing et al., 2013). One study indicates that only one in six medical school graduates chose a primary care residency in 2017, while APP growth in rural areas continues. It is projected that by 2030, demand for primary care will increase by 38% of those over 65 years old and by 55% of those over 75 years old (Heath, 2018). Other significant factors also threaten to worsen this maldistribution as well. These include an aging population of both rural clinicians and patients, threatened governmental programs, inadequate rural funding, and the increase in covered lives secondary to the Affordable Care Act enacted in 2010 (NCLS, 2019; Smith, 2018).

The introduction of the Physician Assistant (PA) and the Nurse Practitioner (NP) professions in the late 60s were in part created to address the need for more primary care

providers as well as increasing the numbers of clinicians in rural and frontier areas in the United States. Other countries (e.g., England, Canada, the Netherlands, Australia, etc.) have also addressed these needs and have modeled their own versions of non-physician providers (O'Connor, 2007). These problems appear to be global and how we continue to address these disparities will resonate internationally. As the pioneers in the realm of APP utilization, we are experts in ways to address these needs in rural America (Basen, 2017). It will take all of the tools we have, using them consistently and more effectively to meaningfully impact these disparities.

What are Physician Assistants and Nurse Practitioners?

Both professions are identified by multiple monikers including: midlevel providers (MLP), non-physician practitioner/provider (NPP), advanced practice provider (APP), etc. For this discussion, the acronym APP will be used, which although contested, seems to be the most acceptable one in use today. These clinicians are trained to provide services and care that are very similar to their physician counterparts but with limitations (Nurse Journal, 2019; O'Connor, 2007).

- Physician Assistants: PAs have been in existence since Duke University graduated their first class in 1967 with the mission of addressing the shortage of primary care physicians with the greatest disparity noted in the rural setting (AAPA, 2019; Ricketts, 2000). The PA education is based on the medical model and includes an intensive program of approximately 24 months, with both didactic and clinical training (approximately a year of each) and the majority of graduates receiving a master's degree. They are trained in all major areas of medicine and have career opportunities from primary care to tertiary care specialties. Their training includes a nationally recognized certification and recertification process that must be maintained throughout their career and includes extensive annual continuing medical education (CME). States license PAs differ in levels of autonomy and prescriptive rights. Physician assistants maintain a collaborative relationship with a physician, again defined by the individual state's medical board (USNLM-NIH, 1994).

- Nurse Practitioners: NPs were created in 1965 to address a shortage of primary care providers, especially in rural locations. The training of NPs is based on the nursing model and is approximately 24 months and also includes a year in didactic studies and a year spent clinically with a focus of study within a primary care field. Their education culminates in a master's or a doctoral degree. They, too, are nationally certified and state licensed with continuing education units also required for license maintenance. Nursing collaborative varies widely by state legislation and may range from fully collaborative to fully independent (Ewing et al., 2013).

Examining the Major Barriers to Rural Health Care and Outcomes Disparities

- Cost/decreased funding impacting the sustainability of rural medical infrastructure and clinicians as well as annual vulnerability
- Lack of medical doctors, both absolute numbers and those practicing in rural settings, exacerbated by "urban-centric" teaching in medical education (Rural Health Hub, 2018)
- Recruitment and retention — lower pay, professional isolation, lack of spousal job opportunities, longer hours, and high levels of responsibility, etc.

- Regulatory limitations to practice/limited scope of practice (NRHA, 2017; Heath, 2018)
- Community and medical community perceptions and acceptance (Auerbach, 2018; Baldwin, 2007)
- Rural patient demographics (older, more impoverished, more complex and present with more advanced disease (Rural Health Hub, 2018; Smith, 2018)

Review of APP Utilization Benefits in Addressing the Barriers

- Growth of the APP professions: It is predicted that in the coming decades, the scope of the provider shortage will increase to a deficit of thousands of primary care providers in rural areas. Between 2010 to 2016, the growth in APPs was greater than that of physicians while only representing 10% of the physician workforce. The number of NP/PA graduates during the same timeframe doubled, from approximately 15 APPs per 100 physicians to almost 30 (Auerbach, 2018).
- Cost of the APP: Compared with the costs of physician utilization, APPs cost less to recruit and are paid less in salaries and overall compensation. They are reimbursed by Medicare and Medicaid at a lower rate, usually around 85% of physician reimbursements. Some private insurers facing decreasing revenue view APPs as more cost-effective resources (Hart, 2012), cost-savings to both the employer and the healthcare systems themselves. Medicine, in general, is increasing in overall cost and decreasing in reimbursements, making it critical that cost-saving measures are instituted, and governmental support continues for the viability of rural healthcare systems.
- Accessibility to the supply of APPs vs MD/DOs: Physician education is substantially

longer and accordingly more expensive. Medical schools have limited abilities to expand their numbers in the long term and almost no meaningful expansions are possible in the short term. This is largely due to longer training times, medical schools' limited capacity for meaningful expansion, and the number of nationally accredited residencies (Buerhaus, 2018 & Auerbach, 2018). Conversely, APPs have two-year training programs and have continued to expand exponentially over the last 30 years with no projections of slowing down. Physician distribution has always been well underrepresented in rural areas and the trend is for even reduced numbers of graduates choosing to settle in rural America. It is important to note that an effective means to increase rural practice interest is to focus medical school and APP school recruitment on rural students. It is well documented that clinicians from rural locales are more likely to return to rural locales to practice (Furlow, 2012; USN-LM-NIH, 1994). So, a consideration of both rural exposure during rotations and a dedicated effort to recruit rural students to increase their enrollment and ultimately their return to rural communities to practice is an effective strategy to increase rural clinicians (Basen, 2017).

The creation of Rural Health Clinics (RHC) in 1977, which required these federally funded clinics to staff 50% or greater of their clinicians as APPs, was a giant step toward meeting rural clinician needs but was not then, and is not now, enough to bridge this ever widening gap of rural versus urban primary care clinician distribution (Rural Health Information Hub, 2018). APPs have had modest increases in rural areas, but with focused incentivization, these numbers could increase at a much higher rate, impacting the rural disparities in a more meaningful way.

Flexibility (rapid) of the professions (PA-specific): Physician assistants' training allows for them to practice in every setting.

This allows for better representation rurally, and also allows for duality in their roles within the primary care setting. This means that they are able to work in a family practice, pediatric, women's health or internal medicine practice but also have the knowledge foundation to spend time covering the emergency room or assist in the operating room (O'Connor, 2007). NPs are trained within the spectrum of primary care and could address these dire rural needs as well.

APP educational focus: (patient education, role in preventative and referral care). It is well established that APPs spend more time with patients, which means more time giving patient education and attending to the complex needs of these more complex patients. They are trained to perform most of the functions of physicians but with the added benefit of more time being spent with patients while handling much of the same patient profiles related to patient complexity and workload (Basen, 2017). With the expansion of healthcare coverage under the ACA, more patients are in need of primary care providers with a disproportionate burden on rural populations, although incentive programs are in place but have had a minimal impact on the maldistribution (Furlow, 2012; Smith, 2018). Physician expansion has been and will continue to be unable to meet these rural populations' needs. This will necessitate an expansion of the care team model to better incorporate a greater proportion of APPs in order to improve **access to care** (Ewing et al., 2013).

Barriers to Increasing APP Presence in Rural America

- Regulatory limitations on APP practice: APPs are bound to federal and state limitations on scope of practice. This includes the level of supervision/collaboration required, prescriptive authority, and referral functions. These restrictions can have a negative impact in an urban setting that translates to a devastating impact in a rural setting where they may be the only practitioner for many miles. There has been legislation for many years that addresses these restrictions and has led to multiple regulatory changes that have improved access to care provided by APPs in these underserved communities. Improvements in telemedicine utilization could substantially offset these restrictions by allowing a physician to more effectively supervise or collaborate from afar (Furlow 2012; Ricketts, 2000).

- Resistance to acceptance: Reimbursement for NPs and PAs is usually 85% of the customary reimbursement of a physician. Although this reduction in payment provides a modest reduction in governmental costs, in the rural setting, this can discourage the hiring of APPs when the narrow focus of incoming payments dominates. This mentality of reduced reimbursements alone reduces their utilization. The substantial cost savings of a salary package for an APP versus a physician should be stressed to motivate hiring of non-physician providers.

The view that APPs will compete for the jobs of physicians is an irrational but very real opposition in small-town America. The ability of NPs in some states with independent practice can exacerbate this perceived threat. As part of the same discussion, those opposed to APP practice will insist that APPs are not trained adequately to care for patients as well as physicians can, and that patient satisfaction is reduced. Both quality of care and patient satisfaction have been addressed in multiple studies with the conclusion that non-physician providers offer similar care with similar outcomes and with high patient satisfaction overall. Can APPs improve access? Outcomes? Quality of Care? Reduce cost to a struggling rural health infrastructure? Improve patient satisfaction? Improve physician retention and recruitment by reducing physician workload and allowing

them to focus on the more complex cases? There is strong evidence for over 50 years to support this.

APPs are uniquely situated to meaningfully impact the burgeoning healthcare disparities crisis facing rural America today. With thoughtful education of physicians and the public, their acceptance would be more fully embraced. With important changes to healthcare policies, they would be more supported, leading to improved utilization. Allowing APPs to function at the top of their licenses and skills would help alleviate provider shortages by taking away the practice limitations of a physician presence (improved use of telemedicine would help offset these limitations). With targeted grants, APP's presence would be encouraged, leading to improved recruitment and retention for both physicians and APPs. The challenges facing rural America will need to be met creatively and with persistence to tip the balances of our rural healthcare disparities and the whole world will be watching.

Rehabilitative Care for a Rural Population

Rehabilitative health care is necessary for many people who have unfavorable medical conditions. The quality of life and ability to manage ADLs and instrumental activities of daily living (IADLs) may depend on physical and/or occupational therapy. Rehabilitative services can be provided to hospital inpatients and in long-term care facilities, outpatient and home health settings.

Activities of Daily Living (ADLs)

Activities of daily living (ADLs) are basic tasks that must be accomplished every day for an individual to thrive:

- **Personal hygiene**
  Bathing, grooming, oral, nail, and hair care

- **Continence management**
  A person's mental and physical ability to properly use the bathroom
- **Dressing**
  A person's ability to select and wear the proper clothes for different occasions
- **Feeding**
  Whether a person can feed themselves or needs assistance
- **Ambulating**
  The extent of a person's ability to change from one position to the other and to walk independently

Instrumental Activities of Daily Living (IADLs)

IADLs are somewhat more complex but nevertheless also reflect on a person's ability to live independently and thrive.

- **Companionship and mental support**
  This is a fundamental and much needed IADL. It reflects on the help that may be needed to keep a person in a positive frame of mind
- **Transportation and shopping**
  How much a person can go around or procure their grocery and pharmacy needs without help
- **Preparing meals**
  Planning and preparing the various aspects of meals, including shopping and storing groceries
- **Managing a person's household**
  Cleaning, tidying up, removing trash and clutter, and doing laundry and folding clothes
- **Managing medications**
  How much help may be needed in getting prescriptions filled, keeping medications up to date, and taking meds on time and in the right dosages
- **Communicating with others**
  Managing the household's phones and mail and generally making the home hospitable and welcoming for visitors
- **Managing finances**
  How much assistance a person may need in managing bank balances and checkbooks and paying bills on time (Kindly Care, 2018).

Physical therapy is a wide-ranging practice in medicine with the primary goal of enabling individuals to achieve an optimal quality of life (Brody & Hall, 2011). Physical therapists largely focus on using clinical skills and knowledge to impact patients on a functional level. Composed of examining, evaluating, diagnosing, and treating (Brody & Hall, 2011), their role in patient care is both comprehensive and inclusive. To guide patients in rehabilitative exercises and to provide detailed education, therapists often need many resources to effectively perform their jobs as part of the medical team. For example, acute care therapists working in hospitals to provide short-term patient care and assist with discharge planning (American Physical Therapy Association, 2019) have short periods of time to treat patients. To do this, these therapists need quick access to the patient's electronic medical records, a multitude of assistive devices to trial and educate patients with (Smith, Fields, & Fernandez, 2010), and strengthening equipment for therapeutic exercises, among other things. While resources in many urban areas remain abundant, this is not the case across the entire country.

Providing rehabilitative services in long-term care facilities, in assisted living facilities, and or home settings also requires resources such as access to patient's medical records, a multitude of assistive devices to trial and educate patients and in many instances assistance from home health nurses, family members, friends of the patient, and/or home health aides. Durable medical equipment provided to home bound patients will require supportive and knowledgeable people. In rural America, rehabilitation is a challenge because of physical distances, inadequate technology such as available broad band and phone service as well as qualified people to form a rehabilitative team. Vulnerable people often depend on the availability of transportation. In rural settings, public transportation options may not be available.

As defined by the World Health Organization, *access to health care* refers to "the continuing and organized supply of its care that is geographically, financially, culturally and functionally within easy reach of the whole community" (World Health Organization, 1978). Unfortunately, not all locations in the United States can provide the same levels of care. While many urban settings continue to grow, access to rural health care is in danger and physical therapy is no exception to this. Troubling declines in the health of rural Americans have been seen recently, with reports suggesting such concerns as increased rates of chronic disease (Moy et al., 2017) and a widening difference between rural and urban life expectancy (Singh & Siahpush, 2014; National Advisory Committee on Rural Health and Human Services, 2015). According to the National Rural Health Association (2019), "Medical deserts are appearing across rural America, leaving many of our nation's most vulnerable populations without timely access to care" (National Rural Health Association, 2019). From a physical therapy standpoint, hospital closings are not helping an already need-filled area. There are already almost 48% more physical therapists per 10,000 individuals in urban areas compared with rural areas, according to the U.S. Department of Health and Human Services (2014). The mean annual wage of physical therapists working in general medical and surgical hospitals is significantly higher than those working in outpatient clinics (U.S. Department of Labor, 2018), which is a natural draw to the acute care, hospital-based setting. It is apparent that rural hospital closings are not only detrimental to population health but also to prospective rural health employees.

The United States is not alone when it comes to a lack of physical therapy opportunities in rural areas. Even Canada, a nation with a universal healthcare system (Government of Canada, 2018), has its problems with rural health. Ranked 30th out of 191 WHO member states in terms of overall health system performance in a widely cited 2000 report (Tandon, Murray, Lauer, & Evans, 2000), Canada's health care does many things well. Still, rural health is an area that could use improvement. Rural residents often have a greater need for health services but less opportunity to receive them, and physical therapy is no exception to this (Landy, Ricketts, Fraher, & Verrier, 2009; Wilson, Lewis, & Murray, 2009; Gupta, Castillo-Laborde, & Landry, 2011). For example, Saskatchewan has 11.2% of its physical therapy practices located in rural areas, while roughly 36% of the province's population live in such areas (Bath et al., 2015). Saskatchewan's population may only be approximately 1.1 million people, but this still makes it the sixth largest province in Canada in terms of population (Statistics Canada, 2019).

It is not just higher income nations like the United States and Canada that have problems regarding to physical therapy services in rural settings. It may come as no surprise that individuals in low-income countries in need of rehabilitation services have significantly challenged access to do so as well (World Health Organization, 2011). This begs the question: how can this problem be fixed? Opportunities for professional growth and the availability of and access to practice supports have been found to be more influential to physical therapists' decisions to locate, stay, or leave rural settings than the actual location itself (Roots & Li, 2013).

Without rehabilitative services, some patients may end up in assisted living, skilled care, or hospital settings. Home health services could be an alternative but have obvious facility limitations and also require increased staffing. Travel time for a limited number of specialty care professionals reduces the time spent with patients in rehabilitative treatment. Telehealth can be useful but also has limitations, especially if broadband services are inadequate or absent. Providing treatment at a hospital, population health center, or community center should be considered the preferred method unless the patient is homebound and unable to travel. Traveling long distances to receive physical therapy or any other specialty service creates an obstacle for patient compliance and rehabilitative optimization, especially if public transportation is not available. If there are greater incentives for physical therapists to locate in rural America, rehabilitative services for rural populations will increase.

Mental Health Services for a Rural Population

Mental Health Services in Rural America

According to most estimates, individuals living in rural locations experience mental and substance use disorders at rates that are similar to (and sometimes higher than) those of their urban counterparts (Cicero et al., 2007), (Meit, 2014), (Probst et al., 2006), (Rosenblum et al., 2007), (Substance Abuse and Mental Health Services Administration, 2012) & (Young et al., 2012). Recent estimates by the CDC show that approximately 25% of adults nationwide have a mental illness or diagnosable mental disorder (Bagalman & Napili, 2014). Problems with mental health are very common in the United States, with an estimated 50% of all Americans diagnosed with a mental illness or disorder at some point in their lifetime. Mental illnesses, such as depression, are the third most common cause of hospitalization in the United States for those aged 18–44 years old, and adults living with serious mental illness die on average 25 years earlier than others (CDC, 2018).

The following factors are challenges to the provision of mental health services (WICHE, 2018):

- Availability includes the staffing or service shortages limiting the receipt of services.
- Accessibility addresses the knowledge of when and where to obtain services,

including coordination of services across sectors of the health and social service system, as well as the travel issues that may be involved.

- Affordability involves the costs associated with receiving care and availability of benefits/insurance to offer services.
- Acceptability incorporates the persistent issues related to the negative perception and stigma attached to the need for services.

To build a comprehensive policy framework around rural behavioral health reform, expanding the availability, accessibility, affordability, and acceptability of behavioral health services must encompass all major components of a multipronged approach. (National Rural Health Association, 2015).

The measurement of mental health services in rural America is imprecise. Nevertheless, the estimate is that "60% of rural Americans live in mental health professional shortage areas, and more than 90% of all psychologists and psychiatrists and 80% of Masters of Social Work, work exclusively in metropolitan areas. More than 65% of rural Americans get their mental health care from a primary healthcare provider, and the mental health crisis responder for most rural Americans is a law enforcement officer" (NIH, 2018).

It is accepted that "behavioral health is not the exclusive purview of behavioral health professionals, especially in rural areas. This is especially true in frontier or rural areas where everyone depends on each other in a variety of ways. Behavioral health information and resources need to be promoted by all people of influence within the community." The key people in community behavioral health include but are not limited to attorneys, behavior health practitioners, faculty of behavioral health training programs, clergypeople, pharmacists, and primary care practitioners (SAMHSA, 2016).

The suggested intervention includes Telehealth, which has the potential to give rural and frontier patients access to primary care providers and medical specialists, improving the quality of care and health outcomes. Telehealth may also reduce the costs of both obtaining and providing health care (Rural Health Information Hub, n.d.).

Primary care practitioners should:

- Collaborate with other professionals including advance practice providers to develop expanded services.
- Become involved in telebehavioral health resources in the community.
- Consider developing an integrated practice (a practice that includes treatment for both medical issues and mental and substance use disorders).
- Identify mutual-help resources within the community and those that may be available online (such as Alcoholics Anonymous).
- Consider continuing education opportunities that offer training and mentorship in telebehavioral health (SAMHSA, 2016).

It is obvious that in rural America, more resources should be provided to encourage integrated care. In addition, there needs to be an increase in the number of behavioral health providers, such as licensed clinical social workers, licensed clinical counselors, and licensed psychologists, practicing in primary care settings. In addition, there is a need for well-developed referral mechanisms to specialists, inpatient behavioral service providers, and inpatient substance abuse providers in other communities with referrals back to local community outpatient providers. This referral network should include "community leaders and other healthcare professionals such as nurse practitioners, physician assistants, pharmacists, psychologists, social workers, and marriage and family therapists (Riding & Werth, 2014)."

Rural Healthcare Challenges

What are the most prominent challenges faced by rural hospitals?

- Remote geographic location— This barrier is at the root of the challenges that rural hospitals face. Low population density results in low volumes and relatively high operational costs.
- Modest budgets— Low population density tends to keep hospital size small and patient volume low, thereby keeping hospitals' budgets modest. Lean budgets with limited flexibility in cash flow make necessary capital investments in the facility or equipment difficult. This leaves facilities vulnerable, with little capacity to keep services and equipment up to current standards.
- Workforce recruitment and retention— The workforce is an ongoing challenge closely linked to the remote geographic location of the healthcare facility. Without an adequate workforce, it is difficult for hospitals to provide necessary and high-quality services to meet the needs of their communities.
- Demographics of Rural America— On average, rural residents are older, poorer, and have more chronic conditions. This can lead to additional challenges and unique pressures to the healthcare facility providing care for these individuals.
- Rural health disparities— Rural residents face various health disparities, and in particular, rural racial and ethnic minorities face challenges related to access and health status (CDC, 2017).
- Rapid changes within health care— Changes to reimbursement, quality reporting requirements, and the related transition from volume- to-value-based care and focus on population health are opening up new opportunities for rural hospitals but also require new approaches and adaptation. "Rural healthcare providers face significant challenges in a quickly transitioning healthcare environment. A network of special statutory designations has protected rural safety net providers for nearly 30 years but now proves to be a

significant obstacle blocking the rural transition from volume to value. Innovative quality measurement programs encourage improvement for most providers but exert little incentive for rural communities where low volume and varied service delivery limit their applicability." (National Advisory Committee on Rural Health and Human Services, 2015).

Challenges for Rural Healthcare Administrators

The authors of this chapter asked a rural hospital president to provide a glimpse into the ongoing challenges involved in keeping a hospital solvent today. The hospital is in Michigan. The name of the hospital and the administrator are being kept anonymous. This is a small, 45-bed, acute-care hospital, which is staffed by more than 350 employees and is served by 50 specialists. This community-based hospital provides high-quality medical care and advanced diagnostic services to residents in the surrounding communities. It is one of nine community hospitals in the healthcare system.

1. What are the biggest challenges that rural hospital administrators like yourself face today?
   Physician recruitment and retention is the biggest issue I've faced. My hospital is small enough that if I lose one specialist, our revenue can be negatively affected enough to cause us to miss annual financial budget goals.

2. What kind of patient care is typical in a rural hospital? In addition, what is the biggest challenge in delivering this care to patients?
   We are licensed for 45 inpatient beds. We no longer provide OB services or operate an ICU in the hospital. Our specialties include neurology, nephrology (visiting), cardiology (visiting), dermatology, gynecology, orthopedics, general surgery, urology, ENT, wound care
   with hyperbaric oxygen, ophthalmology, pediatrics, family practice and internal medicine. Pathology, emergency medicine, hospitalist, anesthesia, and radiology are contracted services with national companies. Our radiology department offers 3D mammography, ultrasound, computed tomography (CT), magnetic resonance imaging (MRI), nuclear medicine, positron emission tomography (PET) scans, and fluoroscopy. The biggest challenge in delivering care is the attitude of citizens who believe services are better at larger facilities.

3. Is capital for new projects difficult to find?
   When my hospital was not owned by a healthcare system, access to capital for building capital was difficult to obtain. Our parent company guaranteed $25 million over five years in capital improvements upon our joining the system.

4. In an ideal situation, what, as an administrator, would you wish for in order to provide a full range of services?
   We need to develop a gerontology line of services. The median age of residents in this county is over 51 years. With the addition of gerontology, we have to be more prepared to operate our facilities closer to Medicare reimbursement margins.

5. Has the Affordable Care Act helped or hindered rural hospital operations?
   It's hard to know what's left of the ACA.

6. What are the threats to hospital solvency today?
   Loss of programs like 340B drug pricing would be devastating to our hospital. Our budgeted net revenue for FY20 is $78 million, and the loss of that program on the savings and retail sides would be a $3.5 million loss.

7. Where are the shortages in professional people most prevalent?
   Physical therapy has been the hardest hospital-based position to recruit. We are not experiencing a nurse shortage in this region. Finding orthopedic surgeons tends to be a long search.

8. What do you think the rural hospital will look like in five years?

   When I became CEO of this hospital in January 2012, 65% of revenue was generated by outpatient services, and by the end of FY19, the percentage has grown to 90%. Payors continue to limit diagnosis that can be counted as admissions and have classified them as observation status. Our hospital continues to care for the same number of patients on our medical unit, but only 60% of them are now reimbursed as an admission, which is three to four times higher reimbursement than observation stays.

9. Is Medicare and Medicaid adequate to pay for services provided? If not, how much of an adjustment needs to be made? Percentage increase.

   Last month, we completed an extensive study to determine how much cost we'd have to take out of our operations to operate at Medicare reimbursement rates and found we'd have to eliminate 7.5% of our expenses. We are implementing a plan to operate at Medicare margins in four years. We've budgeted a 4.4% operating margin for FY20.

10. Is the margin (return on investment) improving, about the same, or getting worse?

    On average, it's held steady for my time here.

11. What else would you like to offer as an observation?

    Working in health care is rewarding and frustrating. The federal government has been deeply involved for decades and that isn't going to change.

    - The hospital president's responses represent one hospital and should not be used to make a claim to know what other rural hospital administrators are dealing with. However, it does demonstrate that rural hospitals are operating under ongoing economic and demographic pressures.

Preventing Hospital Closures

Hospitals in the United States that operate with 100 beds or fewer have unique economic challenges. The small hospitals are often the only healthcare facilities available in rural counties. The small hospitals most likely to be at risk of closing tend to have more patients that are poor, minorities, and elderly with chronic health conditions. The expected continuation of hospital closures provides an opportunity to transform hospitals into **population health centers** and provide an effective alternative.

More than 120 rural hospitals have gone out of business since 2005, and the trend has been accelerating since 2010 (Kaufman et al., 2016). Between 2010 and 2016, 80 rural hospitals closed, 27 of which were Critical Access Hospitals (Health Resources & Services Administration [HRSA], 2017); Critical Access Hospital is a designation by the Centers for Medicare and Medicaid Services for facilities that provide essential services in especially isolated communities.

Although half of the closed hospitals stopped providing health services altogether, the remainder have since converted to an alternative healthcare delivery model (Kaufman et al., 2016). At least 250 hospitals were at risk of closing in 2017 (North Carolina Rural Health Research and Policy Analysis Center, 2017).

A Morgan Stanley analysis concluded that after analyzing over 6,000 U.S. hospitals, nearly 20% were either weak or at risk of potential closure (Flanagan, 2018). A range of factors have squeezed hospital profit margins, including:

- New competition from alternative sites of care such as UnitedHealthcare and CVS-Aetna.
- "Merger indigestion" after a wave of deal activity in the hospital sector following the passage of the Affordable Care Act.

- The rise in the uninsured population.
- Higher healthcare costs are also putting pressure on hospital systems from patients, insurance companies, and policymakers.

U.S. Hospitals at Risk of Closure

There are 1,142 hospitals operating in the United States identified as having 100 or fewer beds (American Hospital Directory, 2017). The Federal Office of Rural Health Policy housed at HRSA has a number of programs designed to help these smaller hospitals improve quality and track their viability. Currently, 96% of the 1,340 access facilities in the United States are reporting rural-relevant quality measures (Health Resources and Services Administration, 2017). In the United States, there are 3,976 nonfederal, short-term, acute-care hospitals (American Hospital Directory, 2017).

Hospitals located in rural areas and those with fewer than 100 beds have been closing their doors more frequently and at higher rates than urban facilities in recent years. Hospital closures will continue and occur relatively more frequently in disadvantaged communities. Financial distress is a complex phenomenon. The number of rural hospitals at high risk of financial distress is growing. It is estimated that at least 9% of rural hospitals, approximately 120, are at high risk of financial distress (North Carolina Rural Health Research and Policy Analysis Center, 2017). There is emerging evidence that disadvantaged communities are more adversely affected by hospital closures (Kaufman et al., 2016). The expected continuation of small hospital closures provides an opportunity for population health models to become an effective alternative to no service.

Reasons identified for this increase in hospital closures include market factors such as declining populations, high unemployment, increasing uninsured patients, a large proportion of Medicare and Medicaid patients, and competition in close proximity. Hospital operational factors that contribute to closures include low daily census, lack of consistent physician coverage, a deteriorating facility, fraud, patient safety concerns, and poor management. Financial factors that lead to closures include high and increasing charity care and bad debt. The hospitals at risk of closing end up severely in debt with insufficient cash flow to cover current liabilities and a negative profit margin. The most likely U.S. hospitals at risk of closure because of financial distress continue to be in the South. States most at risk include: Florida, Alabama, Tennessee, Arkansas, Virginia, and Texas (Kaufman et al., 2016). Of the hospitals in the "at risk" pool, the highest concentration was found in Texas, Oklahoma, Louisiana, Kansas, Tennessee, and Pennsylvania (Hu, 2018).

Hospitals are often measured by benchmarks. Key ratios that are used to flag hospitals at potential risk include but are not limited to:

- Maintained bed occupancy less than 65.4%
- Operating margin less than 2.7%
- Operating cash flow margin less than 9.3%
- Return on assets less than 4.1% (Ellison & Cohen, 2018)

An S&P rating is a letter grade. The best is 'AAA.' That means it is highly likely that the borrower will repay its debt. The worst is 'D,' which means the issuer has already defaulted. Standard & Poor's uses multiple letters and pluses or minuses to indicate strength (Standard & Poor's [S & P], 2018). In health care, an operating margin of 4% is given the AA+ rating and is considered a very strong performer. A healthcare provider with a 2% operating margin is given a BBB+ rating, which is considered adequate (S & P, 2016). Organizations with a ROI of less than 2% receive a rating of BB+ and they are considered speculative. Organizations with this rating face major future uncertainties.

How U.S. Healthcare Policy Promotes Hospital Closings

- Medicare is the nation's largest insurer (Centers for Medicare & Medicaid Services [CMS], 2016).
- The federal anti-deficit law currently in effect could trigger automatic cuts from Medicare (Alonso-Zaldivar, 2017).
- The Centers for Medicare & Medicaid Services has reported that hospitals that treated large numbers of low-income patients tended to do worse (CMS, 2016).

Consider one example of how Medicare funding can impact hospital operations. Three dozen Michigan hospitals are being forced to adjust to the changes in reimbursement for certain drugs from 6% above the sales price to 22.5% under the sales price because of the Centers for Medicare and Medicaid Services 340B drug discount program. This took effect on January 1, 2018. It is estimated that 2,500 nonprofit hospitals nationally participate in the 340B program. In Michigan, 108 of the 130 nonprofit hospitals participate in the program (Greene, 2018). In Michigan, Ascension Health, the largest healthcare system in the United States, employs approximately 26,000 people in Michigan and Ascension recently laid off more than 500 workers, including 20 executives or managers, at its 14 hospitals in Michigan. At Ascension of Michigan, more layoffs are expected to cut operating expenses (Greene, 2018, March 12).

Ongoing efforts to reduce Medicare payments to hospitals are expected. CMS is planning to make payments for clinic visits site neutral. This will happen by reducing the payment rate for hospital outpatient clinic visits provided at off-campus, provider-based departments to 40% of the outpatient prospective payment system (OPPS) rate. This change, amid other revenue pressures, would further constrain hospital margins, according to a study conducted by Moody's Services (Ellison, 2018).

Other structural changes will reduce funding for hospitals. The Congressional Tax Cut and Jobs Act of 2017 eliminates the individual mandate penalty for not having health insurance starting in 2019. The ACA included a provision, generally called the individual mandate, which required most U.S. citizens and noncitizens who lawfully reside in the country to have health insurance meeting specified standards and imposes penalties on those without an exemption who do not comply. Further efforts to eliminate the ACA will likely create an additional burden on struggling hospitals.

"While the Trump administration and the Republican-led Congress failed to repeal and replace the Affordable Care Act, a number of ACA-weakening strategies put forward by the administration are already underway. These include inadequate enforcement of the individual mandate, imposition of work requirements on Medicaid recipients, and failure to promote enrollment through advertising and outreach. An unintended consequence of these strategies is likely to be an increase in the amount of uncompensated provided by America's hospitals (Weisman et al., 2017)."

The Congressional Budget Office (CBO) and Joint Committee on Taxation (JCT) estimate that repealing that mandate starting in 2019 and making no other changes to current law would have the following effects: 1) federal budget deficits would be reduced by about $338 billion between 2018 and 2027 2) the number of people with health insurance would decrease by 4 million in 2019 and 13 million in 2027 3) nongroup insurance markets would continue to be stable in almost all areas of the country throughout the coming decade and 4) average premiums in the nongroup market would increase by about 10% in most years of the decade (with no changes in the ages of people purchasing insurance accounted for) relative to CBO's baseline projections. Those effects would occur mainly because healthier people would be less likely to obtain insurance and because, especially in the nongroup market, the resulting increases in premiums would cause more people to not purchase insurance (CBO, 2017b).

The Tax Cut and Job Act of 2017 is projected to add $1.5 trillion to the deficit over the next decade. The Tax Cut and Jobs Act is expected to lead to 13 million Americans dropping their health insurance coverage (Long, 2017).

Under the 2010 "pay-as-you-go" law, also known as PAYGO, an increase to the deficit would have triggered automatic spending cuts to programs, including a $25 billion cut to Medicare in 2018 alone (CBO, 2017a). Congress has acted to prevent mandatory funding cuts to Medicare and other programs vital to millions of older Americans that were set to occur as a result of the new tax overhaul legislation in 2018. There is no guarantee that these automatic cuts will be waived in future years.

Medicare and other programs will continue to face budgetary pressure. Medicare, Social Security, and Medicaid are among the government's biggest programs. The government will spend approximately $700 billion on Medicare this year, a number the Congressional Budget Office projects will increase to nearly $1.4 trillion in 2027 (AARP, 2018).

In addition, should Congress decide to repeal the ACA in the future, additional threats to hospital operations would likely lead to more hospital closings. For example, the repeal in 2018 would create a loss of coverage with a net impact on hospitals of $165.8 billion due to the restoration of Medicare and Medicaid Disproportionate Share Hospital (DSH) reductions. With the ACA Medicare reductions, hospitals would also suffer additional losses of $289.5 billion from removal of their inflation updates (Dobson DaVanzo & Associates, LLC, 2016).

Michigan Hospitals at Risk of Closure

Michigan is a harbinger of possibilities for the rest of the U.S. hospital nation. A systematic review and quantitative analysis of 90 Michigan community hospitals listed in the 2017 American Hospital Directory was conducted using a ROI of 2% or less as a criterion for risk of closing. A follow-up systematic review and quantitative analysis of 90 Michigan community hospitals listed in the 2019 American Hospital Directory was conducted using a ROI of 2% or less as a criterion for risk of closing. The results show an increase in hospitals in both urban and rural settings at risk of closing. The implication is that the current healthcare market is seemingly becoming more of a risk for healthcare providers operating community hospitals.

In Michigan, 54 hospitals (36 urban and 18 rural hospitals) were considered at risk of closing because their ROI was 2% or less in 2017. In all, 54 (60%) of Michigan's hospitals were at-risk. If these 54 hospitals closed, this would cause the shifting of 1,832,268 patient days from these 54 at-risk hospitals to the remaining 36 Michigan hospitals. In 2018, 62 hospitals (39 urban and 23 rural) were considered at risk of closing because their ROI was 2% or less. In 2019, the number of Michigan hospitals at risk of closing increased from to 62% to 68%. This increase was both in urban and rural settings (see **Table 6-4**).

Smaller Michigan hospitals, 100 beds or fewer, are at even greater risk of closing. In Michigan, there are 35 hospital facilities that have fewer than 100 staffed beds (American Hospital Directory, 2017 & 2019). In 2017, of these 35 hospitals, 26 (74%) of them had an ROI of 2% or less and would be considered at-risk. In 2019, of these 35 hospitals, 25 (71%) of them had an ROI of 2% or less and would be considered at-risk. The change

Table 6-4 Michigan Hospitals at Risk of Closing by Location and Year

Hospitals at Risk	2017	2019
Urban	36	39
Rural	18	23

Table 6-5 Michigan Hospitals 100 Beds or Fewer by Location

Hospitals with 100 or Fewer Beds at Risk	2017	2019
Urban	14	13
Rural	12	12

between 2017 and 2019 is not considered significant. See **Table 6-5** for rural urban split.

This Michigan hospital closing scenario can be used to estimate potential at-risk hospitals in the United States. (Kozicki & Baiyasi-Kozicki, 2017 & 2019).

In 2019, a review of these Michigan hospitals took place to determine their operating status. Rural hospitals again showed weak economic performance. A second systematic review and quantitative analysis of 90 Michigan community hospitals listed in the 2019 American Hospital Directory was conducted using a ROI of 2% or less as a criterion for risk of closing. In 2019 in Michigan, the total number of hospitals at risk of closing increased. Most of these at-risk hospitals are part of a multi hospital system and have been merged into regional operations. They are often subsidized by the healthcare system. Despite the subsidies, most continue to have ROI shortfalls.

Rural Health Innovation

In 2016, an American Hospital Association (AHA) task force released its report on Ensuring Access to Care in Vulnerable Communities. The report offers hospital and health system leaders nine innovative ways to preserve access to essential health services in vulnerable communities. Each of these innovations moves away from the current community hospital model.

These nine strategies are:

1. Addressing the social determinants of health
2. Global budgets
3. Inpatient/outpatient transformation strategy
4. Emergency medical centers
5. Urgent care centers
6. Virtual care strategy
7. Frontier health system
8. Rural hospital-health clinic strategy
9. Indian health service strategy (American Hospital Association, 2016).

There are alternative models for rural communities. The following are some alternative rural health care models to be considered.

Rural Freestanding Emergency Departments (RFEDs): RFEDs can help maintain emergency services in a rural community. These facilities offer outpatient and emergency services and do not offer inpatient beds or surgical services. They may be affiliated with a hospital, allowing for Medicare reimbursement, or independent, with no facility Medicare reimbursement.

Frontier Community Health Integration Project (FCHIP): FCHIP is a CMS demonstration program to develop and test new models for the delivery of healthcare services in frontier areas. Ten Critical Access Hospitals in Montana, North Dakota, and Nevada are participating in the demonstration, which will provide enhanced payment for certain services with the aim of keeping patients in the community who might otherwise be transferred to distant providers.

Community Outpatient Hospital (COH): COH is a provider type that was proposed in legislation in the Save Rural Hospitals Act. This model has been proposed to help maintain services in rural communities. It would eliminate inpatient services while maintaining outpatient and emergency services.

Rural Emergency Acute Care Hospital (REACH): The Rural Emergency Acute Care Hospital Act would allow CAHs and small rural hospitals with 50 or fewer beds to convert to rural emergency hospitals and continue providing necessary emergency and observation services (at enhanced reimbursement rates) but stop inpatient services. The legislation also provides enhanced reimbursement rates for the transportation of patients to acute-care hospitals in neighboring communities. (American Hospital Association, 2016).

Population Health Program (PHP): The PHP model improves the health of the people after considering a full range of health determinants. The model draws on existing knowledge about health promotion. The PHP considers that comprehensive action strategies are needed to influence the underlying factors and conditions that determine health. The PHP can utilize existing national goals. PHP would provide the structure to guide health-service providers. A population health model would include the individual, family and friends, community (people linked by a common interest or geographic setting such as a neighborhood, school or workplace), sector/system (education, income support, housing, etc.), and society as a whole (Government of Canada, 2001).

Technology is Changing Rural Health Care

Technological advancements are increasing access to, and quality of, healthcare services in rural communities. The use of technology in rural settings is crucial to maintaining necessary services. The introduction of electronic health records, telehealth, and artificial intelligence are the most recognizable rural health technology advances. Technologies have advanced communication between physicians and patients and offer innovative methods of overcoming challenges with providing healthcare services to rural communities.

Health Information Technology (HIT)— HIT is the use of computers to store, protect, retrieve, and transfer healthcare information, enabling healthcare professionals to better provide care due to improved contextual awareness of the patient's health status. While rural hospitals and physicians have adopted HIT at the same, or greater, rates as their urban counterparts, meaningful-use attestation varies dramatically among rural providers. Rural hospitals have lower rates of patient viewing, downloading, and transmitting electronic health information; and rates similar to urban hospitals for electronic reporting to immunization information systems (Heisy-Grove, 2016).

Electronic Health Record

Electronic health records (EHRs) are especially beneficial to rural America. In rural areas where distances between clinics are great and specialists are often few and far between, EHRs can:

- Instantly provide **accurate, up-to-date, and complete information about patients** so rural healthcare organizations can make timely decisions and save lives.
- Enable rural healthcare providers to interface with HIT capabilities including telehealth to **access remote clinicians, pharmacists, and staff members**, improving and extending access for patients.
- Facilitate **efficient transfer to other facilities** for vital services not offered locally
- Help rural healthcare organizations offer **efficient local care** after intense care in a tertiary hospital, reducing costs for rural communities.
- Improve **specialty referrals** in communities where specialists are often limited (ONC, 2019).

Telehealth Services

Telehealth services allow for the remote delivery of health care and information via telecommunications technology. The Office for the Advancement of Telehealth (OAT) promotes the use of telehealth technologies for healthcare delivery, education, and health information services. Telehealth is especially critical in rural and other remote areas that lack sufficient healthcare services, including specialty care.

The range and use of telehealth services have expanded over the past decades, along with the role of technology, in improving and coordinating care. Traditional models of telehealth involve health care delivered to a patient at an originating (usually spoken) site from a specialist working at a distant (or hub) site. Most telehealth network consists of a series of originating sites receiving services from a collaborating distant site(s).

Telehealth is defined as "the use of electronic information and telecommunication technologies to support and promote long-distance clinical health care, patient and professional health-related education, public health, and health administration. Technologies include video conferencing, the internet, store-and-forward imaging, streaming media, and terrestrial and wireless communications" (HRSA, 2019).

Telehealth is different from telemedicine. Telehealth refers to a *broader scope of remote healthcare services* than telemedicine. While telemedicine refers specifically to remote clinical services, telehealth can refer to remote nonclinical services, such as provider training, administrative meetings, and continuing medical education, in addition to clinical services (ONC, 2019).

Artificial Intelligence

"Artificial intelligence" (AI) aims to mimic human cognitive functions. AI is a paradigm shift in health care. AI relies on healthcare data and rapid progress of analytics techniques. AI can use algorithms to 'learn' from a large volume of healthcare data, to assist clinical practice. It can be set up with self-correcting features to improve its performance. "An AI system can assist physicians by providing up-to-date medical information from journals, textbooks and clinical practices to inform proper patient care." (Jiang, Jiang, Zhi, et al., 2017). AI can also be used for home monitoring and intervention systems since it is based on intelligent agent methodology.

Rural health providers can reach more people, especially the elderly using AI smart technologies. "The use of ubiquitous in-home monitoring and smart technologies for aged people's care will increase their independence and the healthcare services available to them as well as improve frail elderly people's healthcare outcomes" (Sapci & Sapci, 2019). Leveraging AI smart technology can be useful to overcome distance and transportation issues. It can lead to timely action and also build a data base to further improve efforts to manage population health in rural settings. When supported by a capable home health nursing service and emergency medical service, AI smart technology can improve the quality of life for many people in rural settings. "Medical AI technology has the potential to both improve the availability of healthcare access and healthcare quality within rural areas (Guo & Li, 2018)."

Population Health Promotion (PHP)

Population health is the study of relationships among many health determinants and/or health outcomes in large populations. It sits at the intersection of medicine and public health, spanning basic and social sciences, enabling integrated research that encompasses virtually every domain of life and society (Stanford Medicine, 2019).

In the United States, health service administrators in communities with faltering hospitals should consider implementing a Population Health Promotion (PHP) model as one method of transforming their facility into a population health center. The PHP model improves the health of the people after considering a full range of health determinants. The model draws on existing knowledge about health promotion. The PHP should demonstrate that comprehensive action strategies are needed to influence the underlying factors and conditions that determine health. It can utilize existing national goals like Healthy People 2020 & 2030.

PHP can provide the structure to guide health service providers. Models like the Ottawa Charter for Health Promotion can be used to create community-based interventions that transform existing hospital-based healthcare services into population health centers. A population health model would include the individual; family and friends; community (people linked by a common interest or geographic setting such as a neighborhood, school or workplace); sector/system (education, income support, housing, etc.); and society as a whole (Government of Canada, 2001).

Population Health Centers

Many communities would benefit from a Population Health Center (PHC). A PHC helps to form a community-based solution that enables a system that holds "*everyone accountable*" (Klasko & Shea, 2018, p. 186). In this system, aggregate citizen well-being is an outcome. Well-being replaces health care as the focus for policy makers. Funding for health care is dynamic. In a population health model, well-being becomes a precondition for continued support (Klasko & Shea, 2018, p. 190). A PHC can be useful to shift health care from focusing only on individuals to focusing on individuals and the larger patient population.

Hospitals are already moving beyond their own institutions to provide preventive care and chronic disease management in the community, and primary care physicians and outpatient settings are becoming more central players in patients' health (Becker's Hospital Review,

2013). Population health centers could involve every agency and service in a community that would be useful to promote wellness.

PHC Example

The PHC model could be modified to serve unique rural communities. There are many PHC models that can be considered. It is not the case that one- size- fits-all communities. People should know that efforts to integrate healthcare services and efforts to improve health at the population level (e.g., beginning with the work of public health agencies) are already under way at the state and local levels (Institute of Medicine, 2013).

The University of Michigan in Ann Arbor, Michigan, operates a population health center (PHC). This is what the U of M PHC provides to the University of Michigan Health System:

- The PHC has access to content experts within the health system that guide the staff regarding the impact of health reform efforts and value-based payment models.
- The PHC manages all alternative payment arrangements with commercial and government payers.
- The PHC supports project managers and staff.
- The PHC is responsible for developing systems and support projects directed toward improving care coordination, practice and care delivery transformation, and deepening community partnerships to be successful in the ongoing shift to fee-for-value.

The staff at the PHC Staff focus on a diverse portfolio of projects including:

- Working collaboratively with skilled nursing facilities.
- Creating a culture of advanced care planning across the health system.
- Developing a value-based reimbursement model.
- Aligning internal medical group compensation models with external payment programs.

- Identifying strategies to reduce Emergency Department utilization.
- Establishing a vision for care management.
- Developing a governance structure across the health system.
- House Calls program for high-risk patients.
- Addressing social determinants of health through linkages between primary care and community-based resources (Michigan Medicine, 2019).

Accountable Care Collaborative (ACC) Example

Accountable Care Organizations (ACOs) are groups of doctors, hospitals, and other healthcare providers who come together voluntarily to give coordinated high-quality care to their Medicare patients (CMS, 2019, Mar 8).

ACC Examples

Austen BioInnovation Institute in Akron, Ohio (ABIA) is a 501(c)(3) nonprofit established to coordinate activities among three independent healthcare systems and two universities in northeastern Ohio. ABIA operates with a vision to improve the health of the community through a collaborative, integrated, multi-institutional approach that emphasizes shared responsibility for the health of the community. It includes the five core institutions and partners with public health and more than 65 additional social services and education entities, including the local faith community and Cuyahoga Valley National Park (ABIA, 2012).

The ABIA-led ACC includes a large grassroots component that aims to give an equal voice to all of the constituents in the community, not just those who have a particular health insurance policy or belong to a specific health system. Key components of the ABIA ACC include integrated, collaborative medical and public health models; interprofessional medical teams; a robust health information technology infrastructure that standardizes data across the multiple electronic health records (EHRs); a community health surveillance and data warehouse; and a dissemination infrastructure to share best practices. This data-driven system also includes a data analysis team to measure the impact of the ACC on community-wide health and a group dedicated to policy analysis and advocacy.

The system is based on the Healthy People 2020 framework of health promotion, disease prevention, improved access to care and services, and healthcare delivery. The first step to building this system involved conducting a community-wide inventory of assets and resources (Frieden, 2010).

ABIA took each of the metrics of Healthy People 2020 and conducted a broad-based examination of which resources were available that could address health priorities at the bottom of the community-wide health impact pyramid. Where the analysis identified gaps, the partners developed programs to address those gaps and shifted resources when needed. The partnership also established a set of benchmark metrics that include short-term process measures, intermediate outcome measures, and longitudinal measures of impact. It will use those measures to demonstrate the economic case for healthcare payment policies that lower the preventable burden of disease, reward improved health, and deliver cost-effective care across the broad community. The accountable care community involves cost avoidance and cost recovery models that will help reinvest savings in the coalition's work (Institute of Medicine, 2014).

Colorado is using an Accountable Care Collaborative (ACC) model to expand medical home services for their adult and pediatric Medicaid population. Using this model, primary care medical providers (PCMPs) contract with seven regional care collaborative organizations (RCCOs) to provide medical home services to Medicaid enrollees. The goal of the ACC is to have every member linked with a primary care medical provider (PCMP) as his or her central point of care, and the PCMPs are directly responsible for ensuring timely access to primary care for ACC members. These PCMPs essentially function as medical homes, a model that promotes comprehensive, coordinated, team-based, and client-centered care and enhances client experience and outcomes (Primary Care Collaborate, 2018).

These examples provide a framework for other community population health models.

Discussion

If Congress were to implement funding for a significantly improved production or delivery method in rural hospitals, this would be a form of "process innovation." If insurance companies shifted the incentives to well-being instead of illness treatment, process innovation would occur. The use of technology alone will not improve rural health. The support for the existing rural hospital model will continue to be reactive. A new healthcare strategy for rural America must be created. The Hill-Burton strategy has been useful but is no longer feasible. The social determinants of health must be considered in all meaningful solutions. Rural communities need to begin developing a strategy for process innovation. America needs something equivalent to the Hill-Burton Plan for the 21st century. The Institute of Medicine (IOM), in its Learning Healthy Systems Initiative and its Innovation Collaborative, promote process innovation. This process innovation incorporates:

- A participatory, team-based culture
- Patient anchored and tested processes
- Fully active and engaged patients and the public
- Informed, facilitated, shared, and coordinated decisions
- Care that starts with best practice every time
- Transparent and constantly assessed outcomes
- Incentives aligned for value

- Knowledge that is an ongoing, seamless product of service and research
- Health information that is reliable, secure, and reusable for the patient and the common good
- Leadership that is multi-focal, networked, and dynamic (McLaughlin & McLaughlin, 2019, p. 265)

Healthcare policy makers need to facilitate process innovation. This will need to be a community or bottom-up activity. Each community in America can and should begin this process as soon as possible. In doing so communities will define what people in rural America need to do promote wellness and improve the quality of life.

There are specific actions that can be initiated to transform at-risk hospitals and prevent the loss of healthcare services to hundreds of U.S. communities:

- Congress can rewrite The Tax Cut and Jobs Act to carve out small hospitals (100 or fewer beds) as being protected from Medicare cuts.
- Congress can offer Medicare to all Americans who are poor and minorities or with chronic health conditions.
- Congress and State governments can invest more in medical research aimed at managing chronic health.
- Third-party payers such as CMS can provide adequate compensation for population health services.
- State and community governments can increase taxes to subsidize small hospitals.
- Health Services Associations (HSAs) can continue to subsidize at-risk hospitals.
- HSAs can invest more resources into primary care & accountable care organization (ACO) models.
- Hospital administrators can increase the use of an evidence-based medicine standard.
- Hospital clinical staff can increase utilization of telemedicine and AI programs.

- Hospital strategic plans could emphasize population health promotion as a priority.
- Hospital administrators and their fiduciary boards can begin transforming their facility into a population health delivery model based on community needs.
- Communities can create their own local community population health advisory group.
- Community advisory groups who have a Hill-Burton Hospital in their community can demand that the federal government and hospital holding companies continue to honor the provisions of the Hill-Burton Act.
- Community population health advisory groups can begin to network and work together to create a coalition sharing ideas and concerns. (Kozicki, & Baiyasi-Kozicki, 2017).

Conclusion

In the United States, rural health service administrators in communities need to consider significant transformation to continue to provide necessary services to rural Americans. This is especially the case with at-risk hospitals. Healthcare administrators and policy makers should consider implementing alternative delivery methods as necessary. Alternatives to closing rural facilities should be designed with the community in mind. Several alternative models including a virtual hospital should be considered. All rural hospitals will require greater utilization of technology. The Population Health Promotion model would be useful to consider transforming at-risk hospital facilities into Population Health Centers.

Chapter Summary

- Approximately 62 million people — nearly one in five Americans — live in rural and frontier areas.

- There are 4,118 primary care Health Professional Shortage Areas (HPSAs) in rural and frontier areas of all U.S. states and territories compared with 1,960 in metropolitan areas.
- There is a shortage of physicians in rural communities (National Rural Health Association, 2019). The patient-to-primary-care- physician ratio in rural areas is only 39.8 physicians per 100,000 people compared with 53.3 physicians per 100,000 in urban areas.
- Allied health professionals will be more useful as healthcare providers.
- Technology will be used to create new paradigms.
- In rural America, more resources are needed to provide integrated care.

The social determinants of health are becoming an increasingly important framework for understanding and taking into account the broad range of factors that affect health outcomes in the United States. While nearly 85% of U.S. residents can reach a Level I or Level II trauma center within an hour, only 24% of residents living in rural areas can do so within that time frame — despite the fact that 60% of all trauma deaths in the United States occur in rural areas. Approximately 21.9% of residents in remote rural counties are uninsured. Three proposals that the U.S. Congress can consider would establish a federal public plan option to build upon, rather than replace, the current blend of private insurance and public coverage. These three proposals aim to address some of the shortcomings in ACA marketplaces

It has been suggested in the past that "The role of hospitals in the American healthcare system is changing rapidly, and some believe that hospitals may be replaced by networks of professionals and institutions tied together to coordinate care and promote health—the so-called virtual hospital." Technological advancements are increasing access to, and quality of, healthcare services in rural communities. The use of technology in rural settings is crucial to maintain necessary services. The full use of the EHR as well as telehealth and artificial intelligence will become essential to integrate services. Value-based programs should consider the increase in QALY as a measure of effectiveness.

Hospitals located in rural areas and those with fewer than 100 beds have been closing their doors more frequently and at higher rates than urban facilities in recent years. Hospital closures will continue and occur relatively more frequently in disadvantaged communities. The expected continuation of small hospital closures provides an opportunity for population health models to become an effective alternative to no service. Rural health care should reflect the need of the American rural population.

Discussion Questions

1. There are far more primary care Health Professional Shortage Areas (HPSAs) in rural and frontier areas of all U.S. states and territories compared with metropolitan areas. What do you propose that would increase the number of primary care professionals to in rural and frontier areas? Could your proposal also alleviate shortages in urban areas?

2. Can Congress develop a new version of the Hill-Burton Act to meet the needs of Rural Americans? If yes, what should this legislation specifically identify as the problem(s)? What is the action that healthcare policy experts and healthcare administrator's need to take to improve rural health care?

3. How has Medicare and Medicaid influenced access to care? Could Medicare provide universal coverage in the United States? Universal coverage refers to a system where all residents have health coverage.

4. What is the value-based program's three-part aim?

5. What are the six priorities of value-based programs?

6. How does the Center for Medicare and Medicaid Services authorize services?

7. Rural health care should reflect the need of the American rural population. Considering the following proposed models, which do you think will be successful? Provide a rationale for your choice.

8. Should some rural hospitals close? What should be the criteria for closing a rural facility? What can rural communities do to prevent the closure of rural hospitals?

9. Are virtual hospitals realistic? Provide an explanation for your answer.

10. What are the challenges people living in rural America experience in order to remain healthy?

Student Activities and Worksheets are available inside the Navigate eBook, included with the printed text. Simply redeem the access code found at the front of the book at www.jblearning.com."

References

AARP. (2018). Medicare spared from budget cuts in 2018. Retrieved from https://www.aarp.org/politics-society /advocacy/info-2017/medicare-paygo-cutsfd.html

Abramson, J.H., and Kark, S.L. (1983). Community-Oriented Primary Care: Meaning and Scope. Pp. 21–59 in: Community-Oriented Primary Care— New

Directions for Health Services. Washington, D.C.: National Academy Press.

Alonso-Zaldivar, R. (2017). Tax bill impacts on health law coverage and Medicare. Chicago Tribune. Retrieved from https://www.chicagotribune.com/business/ct-biz-tax-bill-impacts-health-care-medicare-20171205-story.html

American Academy of Family Physicians (AAFP). (2019). Primary Care. Retrieved from https://www.aafp.org/about/policies/all/primary-care.html#4

American Academy of Family Physicians. (2015). Rural Practice, Keeping Physicians In. Retrieved October 7, 2015, from AAFP.org.

American Academy of Physician Assistants. (2019). History. Retrieved from https://www.aapa.org/about/history/

American College of Emergency Physicians. (2020). The Emergency Medical Treatment and Labor Act. EMTLA Fact Sheet. Retrieved from https://www.acep.org/life-as-a-physician/ethics--legal/emtala/emtala-fact-sheet/

American Hospital Association (2016). Small and Rural Update. Retrieved from https://www.aha.org/2017-05-30-small-or-rural-update-0

American Hospital Directory. (2017). Hospital statistics by State: Nonfederal, short term, acute care hospitals summarized by state. Retrieved from https://www.ahd.com/state_statistics.html

American Physical Therapy Association. (2019). About physical therapist (PT) careers. Retrieved from https://www.apta.org/PTCareers/Overview/

Association of American Medical Colleges (AAMC). (2018). Women were majority of U.S. medical school applicants in 2018. Retrieved from https://www.aamc.org/news-insights/press-releases/women-were-majority-us-medical-school-applicants-2018

Auerbach, D. I., Staiger, D. O., & Buerhaus, P. I. (2018). Growing ranks of advanced practice clinicians - Implications for the physician workforce. Retrieved from https://pubmed.ncbi.nlm.nih.gov/29924944/

Australian Government Department of Health. (2002). Quality-Adjusted-Life-Years (QALYs). Retrieved from https://www1.health.gov.au/internet/publications/publishing.nsf/Content/illicit-pubs-needle-return-1-rep-toc~illicit-pubs-needle-return-1-rep-5~illicit-pubs-needle-return-1-rep-5-2

Bagalman, E., & Napili, A. (2015). Prevalence of mental illness in the United States: Data sources and estimates. Washington, DC: Congressional Research Service.

Baldwin, K. A., Sisk, R. J., Watts, P., McCubbin, J., Brockschmidt, B., & Marion, L. N. (1998). Acceptance of nurse practitioners and physician assistants in meeting the perceived needs of rural communities. *Public Health Nursing, 15*(6), 389–397. Retrieved from https://onlinelibrary.wiley.com/doi/abs/10.1111/j.1525-1446.1998.tb00365.x

Basen, R. (2017). NP, PA workforce growth could address physician shortage - Researchers report at AAMC conference. *MedPage Today*. Retrieved from https://www.medpagetoday.com/publichealthpolicy/workforce/65098

Bath, B., Gabrush, J., Fritzler, R., Dickson, N., Bisaro, D., Bryan, K., . . . Shah, T. I. (2015). Mapping the physiotherapy profession in Saskatchewan: Examining rural versus urban practice patterns. *Physiotherapy Canada, 67*(3), 221–231. http://dx.doi.org/10.3138/ptc.2014-53

Becker's Hospital Review. (2013). The evolution of Centers of Excellence in an era of population health. Retrieved from https://www.beckershospitalreview.com/hospital-key-specialties/the-evolution-of-centers-of-excellence-in-an-era-of-population-health.html

Bolin, J. N., Bellamy, G. R., . . . , Helduser, J. W. (2015). Rural healthy people 2020: New decade, same challenges. *Journal of Rural Health, 31*(3), 326–333. http://dx.doi.org/10.111/jrh.12116

Brody, L. T., & Hall, C. M. (2011). *Therapeutic exercise: Moving toward function* (3rd ed.). Philadelphia, PA: Lippincott Williams & Wilkins.

Buerhaus, P. (2018). Nurse practitioners: A solution to America's primary care crisis [Report]. Retrieved from https://www.aei.org/research-products/report/nurse-practitioners-a-solution-to-americas-primary-care-crisis/

Center for the Health Professions. (n.d.). UCSF. Retrieved from http://www.futurehealth.ucsf.edu/Public/Center-Research/Home.aspx?pid=88

Centers for Disease Control and Prevention (CDC). (2017). Racial/ ethnic health disparities among rural adults—United States, 2012–2015. *Surveillance Summaries, 66*(23), 1–9. Retrieved from https://www.cdc.gov/mmwr/volumes/66/ss/ss6623a1.htm?s_cid=ss6623a1_w

Centers for Disease Control and Prevention (CDC). (2018). Social determinants of health. Know what affects health. Retrieved from https://www.cdc.gov/socialdeterminants/index.htm

Centers for Disease Control and Prevention (CDC). (2018a). Mental Health. Data and Publications. Retrieved from https://www.cdc.gov/mentalhealth/data_publications/index.htm

Centers for Medicare and Medicaid Services (CMS). (2017). Data brief: Evaluation of national distributions of overall hospital quality star ratings. Retrieved from https://www.cms.gov/Newsroom/MediaRelease Database/Fact-sheets/2016-Factsheets-items/2016-07-21-2.html

Centers for Medicare and Medicaid Services (CMS). (2018). History. CMS' program history. Retrieved from https://www.cms.gov/About-CMS/Agency-information/History/

Centers for Medicare and Medicaid Services (CMS). (2019). Accountable Care Organizations (ACOs). Retrieved from https://www.cms.gov/Medicare/Medicare-Fee-for-Service-Payment/ACO/

Centers for Medicare and Medicaid Services (CMS). (2019). Medical enrollment dashboard. Retrieved from https://www.cms.gov/Research-Statistics-Data-and-Systems/Statistics-Trends-and-Reports/CMSProgramStatistics/Dashboard.html

Centers for Medicare and Medicaid Services (CMS). (2019). Medicare Enrollment. Medicare Dashboard. Retrieved from https://www.cms.gov/Research-Statistics-Data-and-Systems/Statistics-Trends-and-Reports/Dashboard/Medicare-Enrollment/Enrollment%20Dashboard.html

Centers for Medicare and Medicaid Services (CMS). (2019). Rural Referral Center (RRC) Program. ICN 006815 Page 11-18. Retrieved from https://sway.office.com/uvfAUb0V1e9cZuHw?ref=Link&fbclid=IwAR2NZ8HsyTe__4VqhmI2oyz8h6kKI-19zLn1uvX03FB-PG389inceHzaz9I

Cicero, T. J., Surratt, H., Inciardi, J. A., & Munoz, A. (2007). Relationship between therapeutic use and abuse of opioid analgesics in rural, suburban, and urban locations in the United States. *Pharmacoepidemiology & Drug Safety, 16*(8), 827–840. http://dx.doi.org/10.1002/pds.1452

CMS.gov. (2019). What are the value-based programs? Retrieved from https://www.cms.gov/medicare/quality-initiatives-patient-assessment-instruments/value-based-programs/value-based-programs.html

Congressional Budget Office. (2017a). Distributional analysis of the Tax Cuts and Jobs Act, as ordered reported by the Senate Committee on Finance on November 16, 2017, excluding the effects of eliminating the individual mandate penalty. Retrieved from https://www.cbo.gov/publication/53349

Congressional Budget Office. (2017b). Repealing the _individual health insurance mandate: An updated estimate. Retrieved from https://www.cbo.gov/system/files/115thcongress-2017-2018/reports/53300-individualmandate.pdf

Coyne, C. A., Demian-Popescu, C., & Friend, D. (2006). Social and cultural factors influencing health in southern West Virginia: A qualitative study. *Preventing Chronic Disease; 3*(4), A124. PMid: 16978499. Retrieved from https://www.ncbi.nlm.nih.gov/pubmed/16978499

Dobson, DaVanzo & Associates, LLC. (2016). Estimating the impact of repealing the Affordable Care Act on hospitals: Findings, assumptions and methodology. Retrieved from https://www.aha.org/system/files/2018-02/impact-repeal-acareport_0.pdf

Doescher, M. P., Keppel, G. A., Skillman, S. M., & Rosenblatt, R. A. (2009). The Crisis in Rural Dentistry. *Policy brief.* Retrieved from http://depts.washington.edu/uwrhrc/uploads/Rural_Dentists_PB_2009.pdf

Ellison, A. (2018). Proposed payment changes likely to ding hospital margins. *Becker's Hospital Review.* Retrieved from https://www.beckershospitalreview.com/finance/proposed-payment-changes-likely-to-ding-hospital-margins.html

Ellison, A. & Cohen, J. K. (2018). 224 hospital benchmarks: 2018. *Becker's Hospital Review.* Retrieved from https://www.beckershospitalreview.com/lists/224-hospital-benchmarks-2018.html

Ewing, J. & Hinkley, K. N. (2013). Meeting the primary care needs of rural America: Examining the role of non-physician providers. Retrieved from http://www.ncsl.org/documents/health/RuralBrief313.pdf

Flanagan, C. (2018). U.S. hospitals shut at 30-a-year pace, with no end in sight. *Bloomberg Business News.* Retrieved from https://www.bloomberg.com/news/articles/2018-08-21/hospitals-are-getting-eaten-away-by-market-trends-analysts-say

Floyd, D. (2017). Explaining the Trump Tax Reform Plan. Investopedia. Retrieved from https://www.investopedia.com/taxes/trumps-tax-reform-plan-explained/ Updated: Jan 20, 2020.

Freeman, V.A., Thompson, K., Howard, A., Randolph, R. & Holmes, M. (2015). The 21st Century Rural Hospital: A chart book March 2015. Retrieved from https://www.shepscenter.unc.edu/wp-content/uploads/2015/02/21stCenturyRuralHospitalsChartBook.pdf

Frieden, T. R. (2010). A framework for public health action: The health impact pyramid. *American Journal of Public Health, 100*(4), 590–595. https://www.ncbi.nlm.nih.gov/pmc/articles/PMC2836340/

Fry, J. (1980). Primary Care. London: Heineman, 1980. Primary Care: America's Health in a New Era. Institute of Medicine (US) Committee on the Future of Primary Care; Donaldson MS, Yordy KD, Lohr KN, et al., (eds). Washington (DC): National Academies Press (US); 1996.

Furlow, B. (2012). Filling the primary-care gap in rural, low-income clinics. Retrieved from https://www.clinicaladvisor.com/home/your-career/filling-the-primary-care-gap-in-rural-low-income-clinics/

Government of Canada. (2001). Population health promotion: An integrated model of population health and health promotion. Retrieved from https://www.canada.ca/en/public-health/services/health-promotion/population-health/population-health-promotion-integrated-model-population-health-health-promotion.html

Government of Canada. (2018). Canada's health care system. Retrieved from https://www.canada.ca/en/health-canada/services/health-care-system/reports-publications/health-care-system/canada.html

Greene, J. (2018). Ascension layoffs total 500, with more coming. *Crain's Detroit Business.* Retrieved from https://www.crainsdetroit.com/article/20180311/news/654911/ascension-layoffs-total-500-with-more-coming

Greene, J. (2018). Some hospitals feel impact of federal drug-discount cutbacks. *Crain's Detroit Business.* Retrieved from https://www.mha.org/Newsroom/ID/1279/Crains-Detroit-Business-Some-hospitals-feel-impact-of-federal-drug-discount-cutbacks

Guo, J. & Li, B. (2018). The application of medical artificial intelligence technology in rural areas of developing countries. *Health Equity, 2*(1), 174–181. http://dx.doi.org/10.1089/heq.2018.0037.

Gupta, N., Castillo-Laborde, C., & Landry, M. D. (2011). Health-related rehabilitation services: Assessing the global supply of and need for human resources. *BMC Health Services Research, 11*(1), 276. Retrieved from http://dx.doi.org/10.1186/1472-6963-11-276

Hall, K. (2017). Attracting and retaining physicians in rural America. *Becker's Hospital Review.* Retrieved from https://www.beckershospitalreview.com/hospital-physician-relationships/attracting-and-retaining-physicians-in-rural-america.html

Hart, G. (2012). Why NPs and PAs choose to work in rural settings. Retrieved from https://www.staffcare.com/why-nps-and-pas-choose-to-work-in-rural-settings/

HealthCare.gov (2020). Health benefits & coverage: What marketplace health insurance plans cover. 10 essential benefits. Retrieved from https://www.healthcare.gov/coverage/what-marketplace-plans-cover/

HealthIT.gov. (2019). *What are the advantages of electronic health records for rural health care organizations?* Retrieved from https://www.healthit.gov/faq/what-are-advantages-electronic-health-records-rural-health-care-organizations

HealthIT.gov. (2019). *What is telehealth? How is telehealth different from telemedicine?* Retrieved from https://www.healthit.gov/faq/what-telehealth-how-telehealth-different-telemedicine

Health Resources & Services Administration (HRSA). (2017). Social Determinants of Health National Advisory Committee on Rural Health and Human Services Policy Brief, January 2017. Retrieved from https://www.hrsa.gov/sites/default/files/hrsa/advisory-committees/rural/publications/2017-social-determinants.pdf

Health Resources & Services Administration (HRSA). (2019). Hill-Burton free and reduced-cost health care. Retrieved from https://www.hrsa.gov/get-health-care/affordable/hill-burton/index.html

Health Resources & Services Administration (HRSA). (2019). Telehealth programs. Retrieved from https://www.hrsa.gov/rural-health/telehealth/index.html

Health Resources & Services Administration. (2017). Rural hospital programs. Retrieved from https://www.hrsa.gov/rural-health/rural-hospitals/index.html

Heath, S. (2018). NPs, PAs could reduce primary care physician shortage nearly 70%. Retrieved from https://patientengagementhit.com/news/nps-pas-could-reduce-primary-care-physician-shortage-nearly-70

Heisey-Grove, D. M. (2016). Variation in rural health information technology adoption and use. *Health Affairs (Millwood), 35*(2). Retrieved from http://dx.doi.org/10.1377/hlthaff.2015.0861

Hing, E. & Hsiao, C. J. (2014). State variability in supply of office-based primary care providers: United States, 2012. U.S. Department of Health and Human Services. Centers for Disease Control and Prevention (CDC). NRHA, NCHS Data Brief, No. 151. Retrieved from https://www.ruralhealthweb.org/NRHA/media/Emerge_NRHA/PDFs/db151.pdf

Hu, C. (2018). Almost 20% of hospitals in US are in bad shape according to Morgan Stanley. *Business Insider.* Retrieved from https://www.businessinsider.com/almost-20-of-hospitals-in-the-us-are-in-bad-shape-according-to-morgan-stanley-2018-8

Hudson, D. L. & Cohen, M. E. (2016). Intelligent agent model for remote support of rural healthcare for the elderly. Published in 2006 International Conference of the IEEE Engineering in Medicine and Biology Society. August 30– September 3, 2006. New York, NY. Retrieved from https://ieeexplore.ieee.org/abstract/document/4463258/metrics#metrics

Institute of Medicine (IOM). (1984). *Community Oriented Primary Care: A Practical Assessment. Volume I.* The Committee Report. Washington, D.C.: National Academy Press. [PubMed] Primary Care: America's Health in a New Era. Institute of Medicine (US) Committee on the Future of Primary Care; Donaldson MS, Yordy KD, Lohr KN, et al., (eds). Washington (DC): National Academies Press (US); 1996.

Institute of Medicine. (1996). Primary Care: *America's Health in a New Era.* Washington, DC: The National Academies Press, http://doi.org/10.17226/5152

Institute of Medicine. (2013). Best care at lower cost: The path to continuously learning health care in America. Washington, D.C.: The National Academies Press. Retrieved from https://www.nap.edu/read/13444/chapter/1

Institute of Medicine. (2014). *Population Health Implications of the Affordable Care Act: Workshop Summary.* Washington, DC: The National Academies Press. Chapter: 3 Current Models for Integrating a Population Health Approach into Implementation of the Affordable Care Act. Retrieved from https://doi.org/10.17226/18546.

Jiang, F., Jiang, Y., Zhi, H., Dong, Y., Li, H., Ma, S., . . . & Wang, Y. (2017). Artificial intelligence in healthcare: Past, present and future. *Stroke and Vascular Neurology, 2*(4), 230–243. Retrieved from https://svn.bmj.com/content/2/4/230.full

Kaufman, B. G., Thomas, S. R., Randolph, R. K., Perry, J. R., Thompson, K. W., Holmes, G. M., & Pink, G. H. (2016). Rising rate of rural hospital closures. *The Journal of Rural Health, 32*(1), 35–43. Retrieved from https://www.ncbi.nlm.nih.gov/pubmed/26171848

Kindly Care. (2018). Activities of daily living. Retrieved from https://www.kindlycare.com/activities-of-daily-living/

Klasko, S. K., & Shea, G. P. (2018). We can fix healthcare. *Healthcare Transformation, 1*(2). New Rochelle, NY: Mary Ann Liebert, Inc.

Kozicki, Z. A., & Baiyasi-Kozicki, S. J. S. (2019). The New Michigan Rural Initiative. Submitted to The Michigan Academy of Sciences, Arts, and Letters. March 13, 2020 at Lawrence Technological University.

Kozicki, Z. A., & Bayasi-Kozicki, S. J. S. (2017). The effect of the 2017 Tax Cut and Jobs Act on Michigan hospital operations. *Michigan Academy of Sciences, Arts, and Letters*. Central Michigan University.

Kruse, T. K. (2006). The Hill-Burton Act and civil rights: Expanding hospital care for black southerners, 1939–1960. *Journal of Southern History, 72*(4). Questia. Retrieved from https://www.questia.com/library/journal/1G1-155039477/the-hill-burton-act-and-civil-rights-expanding-hospital

Landry, M. D., Ricketts, T. C., Fraher, E., & Verrier, M. C. (2009). Physical therapy health human resource ratios: A comparative analysis of the United States and Canada. *Physical Therapy, 89*(2), 149–161. http://dx.doi.org/10.2522/ptj.20080075

Larson, E. H., Hart, L. G., & Hummel, J. (1994). Rural physician assistants: A survey of graduates of MEDEX Northwest. *Public Health Reports, 109*(2), 266–274. Retrieved from https://www.ncbi.nlm.nih.gov/pmc/articles/pmc1403485/

Lee, P. (1992). The Problem: Assessing the Primary Care Paradigm. In Proceedings: Volume I. The National Primary Care Conference. Washington, D.C., March 29–31, 1992. Rockville, Md.

Long, H. (2017). The Senate just passed a massive tax bill. Here's what is in it. Washington Post. Retrieved from https://www.washingtonpost.com/news/wonk/wp/2017/12/15/the-final-gop-tax-bill-is-complete-heres-what-is-in-it/

McLaughlin, C. P., & McLaughlin, C. D. (2019). *Health Policy Analysis: An Interdisciplinary Approach* (3rd. ed.). Burlington, MA: Jones & Bartlett Learning.

McVicar, B. (2016). Michigan's urban and rural divide. MLive. Retrieved from http://www.mlive.com/news/index.ssf/2016/12/michigans_urban_rural_divide_o.html

Medicaid.gov. (2019). Medicaid Enrollment. Retrieved from https://www.medicaid.gov/medicaid/index.html

MedPAC Staff. (2019). Improving Medicare's payment policies for advanced practice registered nurses and physician assistants. Retrieved from http://www.medpac.gov/-blog-/the-commission-recommends-aprns-and-pas-bill-medicare-directly-/2019/02/15/improving-medicare's-payment-policies-for-aprns-and-pas

Meit, M., Knudson, A., Gilbert, T., Yu, A. T. C, Tanenbaum, E., Ormson, E., . . . , & Popat, S. (2014). The 2014 update of the rural-urban chartbook. Rural Health Reform Policy Research Center. Retrieved from https://ruralhealth.und.edu/projects/health-reform-policy-research-center/pdf/2014-rural-urban-chartbook-update.pdf

Michigan Medicine. (2019). Population health office. Retrieved from http://www.med.umich.edu/aco/index.html

Moy, E., Garcia, M. C., Bastian, B., Rossen, L. M., Ingram, D. D., Faul, M., . . . , & Iademarco, M. F. (2017). Leading causes of death in nonmetropolitan and metropolitan areas— United States, 1999–2014. *MMWR Surveillance Summaries, 66*(1), 1–8. doi:10.15585/mmwr.ss6601a1

Myers, A., Cain, A., Franz, B., & Skinner, D. (2019). Should hospital emergency departments be used as revenue streams despite needs to curb overutilization? *AMA Journal of Ethics*. Retrieved from https://journalofethics.ama-assn.org/article/should-hospital-emergency-departments-be-used-revenue-streams-despite-needs-curb-overutilization/2019-03

Myint, Z. W., O'Neal, R., Chen, Q., Huang, B., Vanderpool, R., & Wang, P. (2019). Disparities in prostate cancer survival in Appalachian Kentucky: A population-based study. *Rural and Remote Health*. Retrieved from https://www.rrh.org.au/journal/article/4989

National Advisory Committee on Rural Health and Human Services. (2015). Delivery system reform and implications for rural communities. Retrieved from https://www.hrsa.gov/sites/default/files/hrsa/advisory-committees/rural/publications/2015-delivery-system-reform.pdf

National Advisory Committee on Rural Health and Human Services. (2015, October). *Mortality and life expectancy in rural America: Connecting the health and human service safety nets to improve health outcomes over the life course* (Policy Brief). Retrieved from https://www.hrsa.gov/sites/default/files/hrsa/advisory-committees/rural/publications/2015-mortality.pdf

National Conference of State Legislatures. (2011). Closing the gaps in the rural primary care workforce. Retrieved from http://www.ncsl.org/Portals/1/documents/health/RHPrimary.pdf

National Institute of Health. (2018). *Mental Health and Rural America: Challenges and Opportunities*. Global Mental Health 2018 webinar series. Retrieved from https://www.nimh.nih.gov/news/media/2018/mental-health-and-rural-america-challenges-and-opportunities.shtml

National Organization of State Offices of Rural Health NOSORH (2012). About rural health in America. Retrieved from https://www.aapsus.org/wp-content/uploads/About-Rural-Health-in-America.pdf

National Rural Health Association (2015). The future of rural behavioral health. *National Rural Health Association Policy Brief*, 1–12. Retrieved from https://www.ruralhealthweb.org/NRHA/media/Emerge_NRHA/Advocacy/Policy%20documents/The-Future-of-Rural-Behavioral-Health_Feb-2015.pdf

National Rural Health Association. (2019). Medicare cuts hurt rural America. Retrieved from https://www.ruralhealthweb.org/advocate/medicare-cuts-hurt-rural

Neuman, T., Pollitz, K & Tolbert, J. (2018) Medicare-for-all and public plan buy-in proposals: Overview and key issues. Kaiser Family Foundation. Retrieved from https://www.kff.org/report-section/medicare-for-all-and-public-plan-buy-in-proposals-overview-and-key-issues-issue-brief/

NHS (2019). Advanced clinical practice. Retrieved from https://www.nhsemployers.org/your-workforce/plan/workforce-supply/education-and-training/advanced-clinical-practice

North Carolina Rural Health Research and Policy Analysis Center. (2017). *Rural hospital closures.* Retrieved from https://www.shepscenter.unc.edu/programs-projects/rural-health/rural-hospital-closures/

North Carolina Rural Health Research Program. (2019). *Definitions.* Retrieved from https://www.shepscenter.unc.edu/programs-projects/rural-health/

NurseJournal.org. (2019). *Nurse Practitioner vs. Physician Assistant.* Retrieved from https://nursejournal.org/nurse-practitioner/np-vs-physician-assistants/

Office of Management and Budget (2014). *Revised delineations of metropolitan statistical areas, micropolitan statistical areas, and combined statistical areas, and guidance on uses of the delineations of these areas.* White House Executive Office of the President. OMB Bulletin No. 15-01 Vol. Washington, DC: 2015.

Office of Technology Assessment (OTA). (1986). *Nurse Practitioners, Physician Assistants, and Certified Nurse-Midwives: A Policy Analysis* (Health Technology Case Study 37), OTA-HCS-37 (Washing, DC: US Government Printing Office, December 1986)

Original Citation: Largest tax cut in our country's history hikes most people's taxes. Retrieved from https://www.facebook.com/Investopedia/posts/1704804452884597 Chen, J., & Mansa, J. (2017). Return on investment (ROI). *Investopedia.* Retrieved from https://www.investopedia.com/terms/r/returnoninvestment.asp

O'Connor, T. M., & Hooker, R. S. (2007). Extending rural and remote medicine with a new type of health worker: Physician assistants. *The Australian Journal of Rural Health, 15*(6), 346–351. Retrieved from https://onlinelibrary.wiley.com/doi/full/10.1111/j.1440-1584.2007.00926.x

Pew Health Professions Commission. (1994). Nurse practitioners: Doubling the graduates by the year 2000. San Francisco: Pew Health Professions Commission.

Primary Care: America's Health in a New Era. Institute of Medicine (US) Committee on the Future of Primary Care; Donaldson MS, Yordy KD, Lohr KN, et al., (eds). Washington (DC): National Academies Press (US); 1994.

Phillips, J., Hustedde, C., Bjorkman, S., Prasad, R., Sola, O., Wendling, A., Bjorkman, K. & Paladine, H. (2016). Rural women family physicians: Strategies for successful work-life balance. *Annals of Family Medicine, 14*(3), 244–251. doi:10.1370/afm.1931Ann Fam

Primary Care Collaborate. (2018). *Colorado Medicaid Accountable Care Collaborative (ACC) statewide.* Retrieved from https://www.pcpcc.org/initiative/colorado-medicaid-accountable-care-collaborative-acc

Probst, J. C., Laditka, S. B., Moore, C. G., Harun, N., Powell, M. P., & Baxley, E. G. (2006). Rural-urban differences in depression prevalence: Implications for family medicine. *Family Medicine, 38*(9), 653–660.

Ricketts, T. C. (2000). The changing nature of rural health care. *Annual Review of Public Health, 21*, 639–657. Retrieved from https://www.annualreviews.org/doi/full/10.1146/annurev.publhealth.21.1.639

Ricketts, T. C. & Heaphy, P. (2000). Hospitals in rural America. *Western Journal of Medicine, 173*(6), 418–422. doi:10.1136/ewjm.173.6.418

Riding-Malon, R., & Werth, J. L., Jr. (2014). Psychological practice in rural settings: At the cutting edge. *Professional Psychology: Research and Practice, 45*(2), 85–91. https://doi.org/10.1037/a0036172

Roots, R. K., & Li, L. C. (2013). Recruitment and retention of occupational therapists and physiotherapists in rural regions: A meta-synthesis. *BMC Health Services Research, 13,* 59. doi:10.1186/1472-6963-13-59

Rosenblum, A., Parrino, M., Schnoll, S. H., Fong, C., Maxwell, C., Cleland, C. M., . . . & Haddox, J. D. (2007). Prescription opioid abuse among enrollees into methadone maintenance treatment. *Drug and Alcohol Dependence, 90*(1), 64–71.

Rural Health Information Hub. (2016). *Social determinants of health for rural people.* Retrieved from https://www.ruralhealthinfo.org/topics/social-determinants-of-health

Rural Health Information Hub. (2018). *Rural healthcare workforce.* Retrieved from https://www.ruralhealthinfo.org/topics/health-care-workforce

Rural Health Information Hub (2018). *Rural hospitals.* Retrieved from https://www.ruralhealthinfo.org/topics/hospitals

Rural Health Information Hub. (2019). *Rural health clinics (RHCs).* Retrieved from https://www.ruralhealthinfo.org/topics/rural-health-clinics

Rural Health Information Hub. (n.d.). *Health and healthcare in frontier areas.* Retrieved from www.ruralhealthinfo.org/topics/frontier#challenges

S&P Global Ratings. (2017). *U.S. not-for-profit health care children's hospital median financial ratios — 2016 vs. 2015*. Retrieved from https://www.spratings.com/documents/20184/908554/US_PF_Event_Webcast_hc91417_art5.pdf/465887db-278b-4fb2-adb2-3864ab613c1d

Sapci, A. H. & Sapci, H. A. (2019). Innovative assisted living tools, remote monitoring technologies, artificial intelligence-driven solutions, and robotic systems for aging societies: Systematic review. *JMIR Aging, 2*(2): e15429. doi:10.2196/15429.

Scholl, L., Seth, P., Kariisa, M., Wilson, N., & Baldwin, G. (2018). Drug and opioid-involved overdose deaths – United States, 2013–2017. *Morbidity and Mortality Weekly Report (MMWR), 67*(5152), 1419–1427. Retrieved from https://www.cdc.gov/mmwr/volumes/67/wr/mm675152e1.htm

Schumann, J. H. (2016). *A bygone era: When bipartisanship led to health care transformation. R National Public radio*. Retrieved from https://www.npr.org/sections/health-shots/2016/10/02/495775518/a-bygone-era-when-bipartisanship-led-to-health-care-transformation

Seigel, J. (2018). *Treating the opioid crisis in rural America*. Rural Health Voices. *NRHA*. Retrieved from https://www.ruralhealthweb.org/blogs/ruralhealthvoices/march-2018/treating-the-opioid-crisis-in-rural-america

Singh, G. K., & Siahpush, M. (2014). Widening rural-urban disparities in all-cause mortality and mortality from major causes of death in the USA, 1969–2009. *Journal of Urban Health, 91*(2), 272–292. doi:10.1007/s11524-013-9847-2

Smith, B. A., Fields, C. J., & Fernandez, N. (2010). Physical therapists make accurate and appropriate discharge recommendations for patients who are acutely ill. *Physical Therapy, 90*(5), 693–703.

Smith, N. (2018). *PAs in rural locations ready to meet primary care needs*. Retrieved from https://www.aapa.org/news-central/2018/06/pas-rural-locations-ready-meet-primary-care-needs/

Spitz, B. (1994). The architecture of reform, or how do we build our health care system around primary care when we don't know who a primary care provider is, how many we need, or what they do? Unpublished draft document. *Primary Care: America's Health in a New Era*. Institute of Medicine (US) Committee on the Future of Primary Care; Donaldson MS, Yordy KD, Lohr KN, et al., (eds.) Washington (DC): National Academies Press (US); 1996.

Stanford Medicine. (2019). *What Is Population Health?* Retrieved from http://med.stanford.edu/phs.html

Starfield, B. (1954). Primary care: Concept, evaluation, and policy. In M. S. Donaldson, K. D. Yordy, & K. N. Lohr et al., (eds.), *Primary care: America's health in a new era. Institute of medicine (US) committee on the*

future of primary care. Washington (DC): National Academies Press (US).

Statistics Canada. (2019). *Census profile 2016*. Retrieved from https://www12.statcan.gc.ca/census-recensement/2016/dp-pd/prof/index.cfm?Lang=E

Substance Abuse and Mental Health Services Administration. (2012). *The TEDS Report: A comparison of rural and urban substance abuse treatment admissions*. Rockville, MD: Substance Abuse and Mental Health Services Administration.

Tandon, A., Murray, C. J. L., Lauer, J. A., & Evans, D. B. (2000). Measuring overall health system performance for 191 countries [Global Programme on Evidence for Health Policy Discussion Paper No. 30]. Geneva, Switzerland: World Health Organization.

The Balance. (2018). *What are Standard and Poor's Credit Ratings?* Retrieved from https://www.thebalance.com/what-are-sandp-credit-ratings-and-scales-3305886

The Joint Committee on Taxation. (2017). Estimated revenue effects of modifications to the "Tax Cuts and Job Act," as reported by the Committee on Finance JCX-62-17. Retrieved from https://www.jct.gov/publications.html?func=startdown&id=5046

U.S. Department of Health & Human Services. (2015). Medical treatment in Hill-Burton funded healthcare facilities. Retrieved from https://www.hhs.gov/civil-rights/for-individuals/hill-burton/index.html

U.S. Department of Health and Human Services. Health Resources and Services Administration. The Office of Rural Health Policy. (2012). Office of Rural Health Policy Rural Guide to Health Professions Funding. *HRSA*, Retrieved from https://www.hrsa.gov/sites/default/files/ruralhealth/pdf/ruralhealthprofessionsguidance.pdf

U.S. Department of Labor, Bureau of Labor Statistics. (2018). Occupational employment and wages, May 2017. Retrieved from https://www.bls.gov/oes/2017/may/oes291123.htm

U.S. Public Health Service, Health Resources and Services Administration. (1996). Primary care: America's health in a new era. In Donaldson M. S., Yordy, K. D., Lohr K. N., & Vanselow, N. A. (eds.), *Institute of Medicine (US) Committee on the Future of Primary Care*. Washington (DC): National Academies Press (US).

United States Department of Agriculture. (2016). *Rural-urban commuting area codes*. Retrieved from https://www.ers.usda.gov/data-products/rural-urban-commuting-area-codes.aspx#.VCL_vufbYgA

United States Department of Agriculture USDA. (2018). *Opioid misuse in rural America*. Retrieved from https://www.usda.gov/topics/opioids

United States Department of Health & Human Services, National Center for Health Workforce Analysis. (2014). *Distribution of U.S. health care providers residing in rural and urban areas*. Retrieved from https://

www.ruralhealthinfo.org/assets/1275-5131/rural
-urban-workforce-distribution-nchwa-2014.pdf

United States Department of Health & Human Services. (2019). EMTALA Revisions to the State Operations Manual (SOM) Chapter 5 and Appendix V. *State Operations Provider Certification Centers for Medicare & Medicaid Services (CMS* (Pub. 100-07, p 12-17). Retrieved from https://www.cms.gov /Regulations-and-Guidance/Guidance/Transmittals /2019Downloads/R191SOMA.pdf

United States Department of Health and Human Services. (2015). *Medical treatment in Hill-Burton funded healthcare facilities.* Retrieved from https://www.hhs .gov/civil-rights/for-individuals/hill-burton/index .html

Weisman, J. S., Cohen, M. A., Reich, A. (2017). *Weakening the Affordable Care Act will boost hospitals' financial burden. STAT.* Retrieved from https://www.statnews .com/2017/10/11/affordable-care-act-hospitals/

Wells, R., Cody, M., Alpino, R., Van Dyne, M., Abbott, R. & King, N. (2017). *Physician assistants: Modernize laws to improve rural access.* Retrieved from https://www.ruralhealthweb.org/NRHA/media /Emerge_NRHA/Advocacy/Policy%20documents /04-09-18-NRHA-Policy-Physician-Assistants -Modernize-Laws-to-Improve-Rural-Access.pdf

Wilson, R. D., Lewis, S. A., & Murray, P. K. (2009). Trends in the rehabilitation therapist workforce in underserved areas: 1980–2000. *The Journal of Rural Health, 25*(1), 26–32. Retrieved from http://dx.doi .org/10.1111/j.1748-0361.2009.00195.x

World Health Organization, The World Bank. (2011). *World report on disability.* Geneva: World Health Organization. Retrieved from https://www.who.int /disabilities/world_report/2011/report.pdf?ua=1

World Health Organization. (1978). *Primary health care* [Report of the International Conference on the Primary Health Care]. Geneva: World Health Organization. Retrieved from http://apps.who.int/iris /bitstream/10665/39228/1/9241800011.pdf

Young, A. M., Havens, J. R., & Leukefeld, C. G. (2012). A comparison of rural and urban nonmedical prescription opioid users' lifetime and recent drug use. *American Journal of Drug and Alcohol Abuse, 38*(3), 220–227.

PART 3

Health Disparities in Rural Communities

CHAPTER 7

Cardiovascular Disease in Rural United States

Micah Zuhl, PhD
Maurice Tawil, MPH

LEARNING OBJECTIVES

At the end of this chapter, readers will be able to:

1. Discuss the prevalence of coronary heart disease, stroke, and heart failure in the United States.
2. Explain the pathophysiology of coronary heart disease, stroke, and heart failure.
3. Discuss the prevalence of cancers that are more prevalent in rural areas.
4. Discuss cardiovascular disease (CVD) disparities in the United States across geographic regions.
5. Discuss and contrast CVD disparities by gender in the United States.
6. Discuss and contrast racial/ethnic CVD disparities within rural and minority populations.
7. Explain the contributing factors to CVD disparities.
8. Discuss strategies to improve CVD health equity in rural regions of the United States.

KEY TERMS

Cardiovascular disease
Contributing factors
Coronary heart disease (CHD)
Health disparities
Heart failure
Interventions
Prevention
Stroke

CHAPTER OVERVIEW

This chapter explores the basic pathophysiology of cardiovascular diseases, including Coronary Artery Disease (CAD), Peripheral Artery Disease (PAD), **Stroke**, and **heart failure**. In addition, disparities among specific populations based on things such as regional difference, gender and ethnicity, as well as risk factors of these diseases are discussed. The chapter ends with a discussion on **prevention** and treatment for **cardiovascular disease**, providing details on where public health can have an impact on this global burden, and showing real examples of the impact certain groups have had on cardiovascular health. The chapter discusses all of these things while also encompassing differences between rural and urban populations. A common theme is that rural populations tend to have more difficulties with cardiovascular health for many different reasons, including socioeconomic status, access to care, inadequate treatment, insurance coverage, access to food, and recreational activities, and much more.

Introduction

CVD refers to disorders of the heart and blood vessels and remains the leading cause of death in the United States. Coronary artery disease (CAD), peripheral artery disease (PAD), stroke, heart arrhythmias, heart valve disorders, and heart failure are the most common types of CVDs. Early data from the late 1960s through the mid-1980s reported higher CVD-related death rates among those living in metropolitan compared with non-metropolitan locations in the United States (Ingram & Gillum, 1989). However, this pattern has shifted, and more current data (since the mid-1990s) shows that the prevalence of and death from heart diseases are considerably higher among Americans living in rural regions versus urban dwellers. For example, rates of CAD have been reported to be nearly 40% higher among those living in rural versus urban areas (O'Connor & Wellenius, 2012) and death rates from CAD were highest for both men and women in the nation's most rural counties (Meit et al., 2014). Similarly, in 2016, heart failure mortality rates were 18 deaths per 100,000 in metro areas across the United States compared with 24 per 100,000 in nonmetro regions (Towne Jr et al., 2019). In addition, rates of heart disease and mortality due to CVD are more prevalent in Southern rural regions compared with Northeast, Midwest, and Western regions; and, furthermore, the largest disparity existed between Southern rural and metro regions. Regarding gender disparities, heart disease deaths among men have been reported to be 18% higher in rural than urban areas across the United States and 20% higher among women. Heart disease mortality also differs among various ethnic groups who live in urban and rural regions of the United States. While mortality rates have declined since 1999 among both White and African American populations, age-adjusted death from heart disease remains higher in African American populations. Moreover, CVD-linked mortality is higher among African Americans compared with whites in all urban regions of the United States (Northeast, Midwest, West, South) (Kulshreshtha, Goyal, Dabhadkar, Veledar, & Vaccarino, 2014). The same disparity exists in rural regions except for the Northeast region of the United States. African Americans are also twice as likely to have a stroke and much more likely to die from the stroke than white Americans. Similarly, both Native Americans and Hispanic Americans also report higher rates of heart disease and also die earlier than white Americans.

It is well established that the prevalence of CVD and CVD-related death is more common among Americans living in rural regions, and that these **health disparities** are influenced by gender and ethnicity. Identifying the underlying causes that contribute to these differences will influence health policies and resource allocations, with the ultimate goal of advancing both CVD prevention and clinical care across all regions (both rural and urban) of the United States.

The purpose of this chapter is to identify cardiovascular disease pathophysiology; review prevalence of CVD disparities among urban and rural U.S. dwellers, along with gender and ethnic differences in CVD; discuss possible causes that contribute to heart disease; and, lastly, highlight strategies to improve CVD health equity through prevention and treatment.

Pathophysiology of Cardiovascular Diseases

Cardiovascular diseases include a category of disorders of the heart and circulatory systems of the body. Understanding CVD pathophysiology will assist policymakers and clinicians in developing appropriate therapies to treat disease and will also help identify prevention strategies. Some CVDs are much more prevalent than others in the United States, and for this reason, we will highlight the pathophysiology of coronary artery disease, peripheral artery disease, stroke, and heart failure.

Coronary Artery Disease

CAD is a result of plaque formations (blockage) in the coronary vessels of the heart and is the most common form of cardiovascular disease in the United States (Centers for Disease Control and Prevention (CDC)). It is also referred to as ischemic heart disease (IHD) or **coronary heart disease (CHD)**. The plaque substance develops from a complex atherosclerosis process that slowly builds in the arteries and eventually leads to reduced oxygen delivery to the heart. The disease may also manifest through a plaque rupture leading to occlusion of a coronary vessel, ultimately causing oxygen deprivation in heart tissue (i.e., myocardial infarction or heart attack). Patients commonly present with symptoms of angina (i.e., chest pain), shortness of breath, and/or radiating pain in the neck and shoulders.

Research within the past 15 years has shifted the understanding of atherosclerosis from a cholesterol storage process to what is now recognized as a chronic cascade of inflammatory events (Libby & Theroux, 2005). The inflammation develops from insult to the coronary vessel endothelial wall, which activates immune cell infiltration to the injured site, and promotes a cascade of inflammatory events, which causes a lesion, or plaque formation. Conditions such as hypertension, hyperglycemia, obesity, dyslipidemia, and cigarette smoking are all thought to cause damage to the arterial wall. The chronic state of these disorders enhances the continued progression of the atherosclerotic plaque. For example, someone who smokes two packs of cigarettes per day is consistently exposing their coronary vessels to damage, and the inflammatory events remain in a constant cycle. As the lesion progresses, the death of immune cells at the insult site (e.g., lipid-laden macrophages) can

lead to the development of a lipid rich necrotic core that is commonly associated with atherosclerosis. If the plaque ruptures, clotting factors will activate to prevent coronary vessel bleeding but will also occlude the vessel and cause a myocardial infarction. The plaque may also calcify and harden over time and may lead to the narrowing of the coronary vessel, which reduces oxygen delivery to the heart (ischemia).

Coronary artery disease is commonly treated through revascularization procedures such as coronary angioplasty combined with arterial stent placement, or coronary artery bypass graft. Patients are also prescribed numerous medications to prevent restenosis and to treat underlying causes such as hypertension, dyslipidemia, and diabetes.

Peripheral Artery Disease

PAD affects nearly 10 million Americans and has a similar underlying pathophysiology as CAD. The disease is mostly silent and symptoms typically emerge later in life among both men and women (>55 years of age). Atherosclerosis, or plaque formations, typically develops in the lower extremities, such as the thigh or calf muscles instead of the coronary vessels. Insufficient oxygen supply to the legs causes pain and occurs during walking activities and is alleviated upon rest. This type of pain is called intermittent claudication (IC), and the degree of pain along with tolerable walking distance assists with evaluating the seriousness of the blockages in the lower limbs (Criqui et al., 2016).

The pathophysiology of PAD is similar to coronary artery disease. Inflammatory events as a result of insult to peripheral arteries ignites the atherosclerosis process. The abdominal aorta, iliac, and femoral arteries are common sites for PAD lesions to form. In the early stages of the disease, the arteries will compensate by expanding (i.e., vasodilation) and oxygen delivery to tissue is sustained. The vessels lose the ability to properly vasodilate as the disease progresses, and the oxygen supply is greatly reduced. To compensate, PAD patients will shift blood flow to smaller parallel vessels, (collateral flow); however, symptoms (claudication) will appear once the smaller vessels reach their maximal oxygen delivery capacity (Zemaitis, Bah, Boll, & Dreyer, 2019). The risk factors that cause PAD are similar to CAD and include smoking, hypertension, diabetes, obesity, and dyslipidemia (Zemaitis et al., 2019). Due to the similarities with CAD, PAD patients are at a 70% risk for a cardiovascular event and an overall 80% increased risk of death than people without PAD (Grenon et al., 2014).

Stroke

A stroke is an abrupt decline in oxygen circulation to the brain, which causes neural ischemia, infarction, or intracranial hemorrhage. The interruption in blood flow results in a sudden onset of muscle weakness, numbness, paralysis, visions problems, and aphasia (loss of speech). For these reasons, stroke is responsible for reduced quality of life from both physical and mental disabilities and is also the third-leading cause of death in the United States. Nearly 800,000 Americans suffer a stroke each year, and it is estimated that someone has a stroke every 40 seconds (Benjamin et al., 2017).

The majority of strokes (~87%) are ischemic strokes and occur when oxygen delivery to the brain is blocked. Blood clots, or embolism, in the cerebrovascular vessels are a leading cause of ischemic strokes. The clot is thought to form from plaque rupture in the circulatory system, such as the heart or large arteries, and then travels to the brain and becomes lodged in a small vessel (American Stroke Association). A hemorrhagic stroke occurs less often and happens when a blood vessel in the brain ruptures. The blood surrounds neighboring tissue and causes an increase in cerebral pressure and cellular damage. In addition, a transient ischemic attack (TIA) is a short duration (<5 minutes) loss of brain oxygen delivery and is a warning sign

of a future stroke (Easton et al., 2009). Many people fail to recognize a TIA and it results in lack of treatment and increased susceptibility to future stroke. Similar to both CAD and PAD, the risk for stroke is increased among those who smoke, have high blood pressure and high cholesterol, and also those with diabetes (Benjamin et al., 2017). In addition, the risk for stroke is elevated among those with CAD and heart arrhythmias (e.g., atrial fibrillation). The treatment for stroke is highly dependent on recognizing symptoms and early access to medical care.

Heart Failure

Heart failure is a condition in which the heart is not capable of maintaining adequate cardiac output or blood supply to meet the metabolic needs of the body. There were approximately 6.2 million cases of heart failure in the United States reported between 2012 and 2106, and this number is expected to exceed 8 million by 2030 (Benjamin, Muntner, & Bittencourt, 2019).

The disease reduces the pumping ability of the left ventricle and can be a result of systolic or diastolic dysfunction. Systolic heart failure, or heart failure with reduced ejection fraction (HFrEF), is when the left ventricle is unable to contract and eject blood. Diastolic dysfunction is when the left ventricle does not fill properly and is defined as heart failure with preserved ejection fraction (HFpEF). It is estimated that 50% of heart failure patients suffer from HFpEF. Regardless of type, heart failure is primarily categorized by severity of symptoms (e.g., shortness of breath, fatigue, palpitations) during physical exertion (Dahlström, 2019).

HFrEF is diagnosed when left ventricular ejection fraction (LVEF) is less than 40%. LVEF is the ratio of blood ejected from the left ventricle in proportion to the volume filled. Healthy adults typically have LVEF values above 65% at rest. Loss of contractile function of the heart muscle is the primary cause of decline in LVEF observed in HFrEF, which is primarily attributed to myocardial ischemia and infarction. Damage to the contractile fibers of the heart reduces the ability of the heart to eject blood. The second leading contributor to HFrEF is uncontrolled hypertension, which forces the heart to contract against high arterial pressures and eventually leads to contractile dysfunction. Other factors that negatively affect myocardial contractile fibers are cardiotoxins from drugs used in chemotherapy, and viral infection (e.g., viral cardiomyopathy). It is important to realize that when the left ventricle is unable to eject blood effectively, the remaining blood in the heart will lead to elevated pressure in the lung, which will force fluid out of pulmonary capillaries. The excess fluid will cause pulmonary congestion and shortness of breath, which is a hallmark symptom of heart failure (Kemp & Conte, 2012).

Heart failure patients with HFpEF have normal LVEF but suffer from impaired filling of the heart (Pfeffer, Shah, & Borlaug, 2019). The left ventricle's inability to fill is caused by myocardial stiffness as a result of fibrosis, along with hypertrophied walls of the heart. Researchers have had a difficult time determining the major **contributing factors** that lead to development of fibrosis, but hypertension, obesity, coronary artery disease, atrial fibrillation, and female sex have all been linked (Lee et al., 2009).

Treating heart failure is complex and requires intensive medication regimens along with other therapies such as biventricular pacing, implanted cardioversion devices (ICD), and left ventricular assisted devices (LVAD). The progression of the disease will eventually lead to heart transplantation.

Cardiovascular Disease Disparities in the United States

It is established that CVD disparities exist in the United States (see **Figure 7-1**), and these inequities are apparent across geographic regions, gender, and ethnic groups. Furthermore, people living in rural regions of the United States are more likely to be diagnosed with CVD. This section will review the prevalence of CVD throughout the United States.

Regional Differences

Age-standardized rates of CVD disability adjusted life years (DALYs), which is the number of life years lost to CVD, decreased significantly in all states in the past 25 years, but there was wide regional variation in the amount of decline. For example, in a publication on CVD burden in the United States between 1990 and 2016, it was reported that it took 25 years for Southern states to achieve levels observed among the healthiest states. States, including Mississippi, West Virginia, Alabama, Arkansas, Louisiana, Tennessee, and Oklahoma are only now achieving the 1990 levels of CVD burden that higher ranked states had in 1990. These findings demonstrate that CVD burden has improved in regions that have the greatest prevalence, but disparities between states have not changed in the past 25 years.

Furthermore, adults living in rural households reported higher rates of cardiovascular disease and stroke than those in metro (more than one million residents) areas. As of 2015, according to the Rural Health Information Hub (RHIhub), metropolitan locations nationally averaged 56.6 deaths per 100,000 from heart disease whereas nonmetropolitan locations averaged 86.9 deaths per 100,000 from heart disease (Towne Jr et al., 2019). Persons living in rural areas also have higher rates of cardiovascular-linked hospitalizations, disabilities, and mortality than those living in urban areas (Jones, 2009). Possible causes for the CVD disparities in rural regions are limited access to treatment, heightened risk for CVD (e.g., obesity, inactivity, poor nutrition, hypertension, smoking), along with lower socioeconomic status. Each of these factors are discussed in Section 3. According to the CDC, in 2014, nearly 25,000 rural deaths

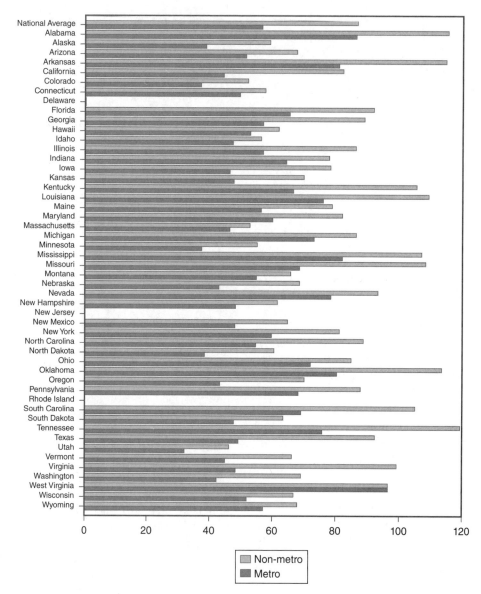

Figure 7-1 Comparison of Deaths from Heart Disease for Metro and Non-metro States.

Rural Health Information Hub.

from heart disease and 4,000 from stroke were considered to be preventable, which is higher than preventable death estimations among urban residents. Therefore, the implementation of strategies to improve overall health and treatment in rural regions will potentially prevent a large number of CVD-related deaths (García, 2019).

Regional and urban impacts on specific CVDs are more difficult to track. Rural populations tend to lack proper documentation of these cases, which makes direct comparisons of these populations difficult. In general, coronary artery disease death rates have been decreasing among Americans aged 35 to 84 over the previous decades. However, the death rate has declined faster in urban areas than in rural areas in all four regions of the United States, including the Northeast, Midwest, West, and South. This has resulted in rural areas having a higher CAD rate than urban areas, which is a trend that began roughly around 2007. Evidence also shows that the rural habitants are more highly afflicted with congestive heart failure, and heart failure patients hospitalized in less-populated regions are at higher risk of in-hospital death relative to patients living in large central metropolitan areas.

The data regarding stroke is quite compelling. For more than half a century, stroke mortality has been excessively high in the Southeast in an area known as the "stroke belt." According to the National Heart, Lung, and Blood Institute (NHLBI), the Stroke Belt consists of 11 states with the highest age-adjusted stroke mortality in the United States (National Heart & Institute, 1989). One interesting fact about this region is that the stroke belt also contains nearly half of the people in the United States who live in poverty. Additionally, the Appalachia region is heavily afflicted with high stroke rates (Wilson, Kratzke, & Hoxmeier, 2012). Researchers have failed to discover the exact underlying factors that cause stroke rates to be so much higher in these regions; however, there is an undeniably strong indication that stroke has severe effects in rural areas, specifically the rural South.

Within the Stroke Belt lies a sub-area called the "Stroke Buckle," which comprises a 153-county region in the coastal plains of North Carolina, South Carolina, and Georgia. This region has a stroke mortality rate substantially higher than the rest of the United States. The Stroke Buckle exhibits a stroke mortality rate roughly 1.3 to 1.5 times greater than the rest of the United States, and consistently has the highest stroke mortality in the United States (Shrira, Christenfeld, & Howard, 2008). There has even been evidence that visitors to this region increase their risk of stroke by up to 11% (Shrira et al., 2008). Additionally, according to CDC Data Trends & Maps, stroke appeared to affect the Southern region of the United States substantially more than the other regions as of 2017 (Mendy, Vargas, Payton, Sims, & Zhang, 2019).

Gender Differences

The cardiovascular disease burden in the United States is estimated to be twice as great for men as women in all states (Roth et al., 2018). While most types of cardiovascular disease (CAD, PAD, heart failure) are worse in men, it should be emphasized that risk factors (discussed in a later section) are actually very similar for both. Men tend to have heart attacks, or symptoms of heart disease at an earlier age (~65 years) compared with women (~72 years). Regardless, heart disease is linked to one of three deaths in both sexes, and more women than men have died from CVD in the United States since 1984, which is primarily because women generally live longer and have cardiac events in their later years. One explanation as to why younger women have less reported CVD is due to the protective benefits of the hormone estrogen (Lastra, Harbuz-Miller, Sowers, & Manrique, 2019). However, women tend to do worse than men after they have a cardiac-related event or experience symptoms of heart disease. Nearly 50% of women who have heart attacks will either die, develop heart failure, or experience a stroke within 5 years; compared with 36% among men. One reason may be that women often experience atypical CVD-related symptoms compared with men. For example, women report fatigue, dizziness, or nausea; while men commonly demonstrate more classical symptoms of chest pain and shortness of breath. The nontraditional symptoms lead to missed diagnoses of CVD. Another explanation of why women suffer worse outcomes after diagnosis is that women often receive suboptimal medical care for CVD. When women arrive at a hospital, treatments are often delayed or not available. Additionally, women are less likely to receive standard electrocardiogram (ECG) monitoring, be admitted to a coronary unit, and receive referrals for advance treatment (Canto et al., 2000; Canto et al., 1998; Garcia, Mulvagh, Bairey Merz, Buring, & Manson, 2016). Regarding stroke, women have a greater chance of having a stroke than men, and nearly 55,000 more women than men experience a stroke each year, which is attributed to a disproportionately larger number of older women having strokes as a result of longer life expectancy than men (Ennen & Beamon, 2012). One possible explanation is that women tend to experience more atrial fibrillation-related blood clots that travel to the brain and result in a stroke (Friberg, Scharling, Gadsbøll, Truelsen, & Jensen, 2004). Other potential links to higher stroke rates in women include oral contraceptives, hormone replacement therapy, and having many more frequent migraines (Reeves et al., 2008).

In comparison to urbanized regions of the United States, both men and women living in rural areas have higher rates of CVD-related mortality (Meit et al., 2014). Also, rural habitants fare worse after being diagnosed with heart disease. More specifically, men over the age of 20 years living in rural counties are 18% more likely to die from heart disease than men living in suburban areas. Similarly, rural women over the age of 20 have a 20% greater likelihood of dying from CVD than their urban counterparts. African American (AA) women living in rural regions have the highest mortality risk among women as a group (Taylor, Hughes, & Garrison, 2002). Rural regions such as Mississippi River Delta, southwest Oklahoma, and Northern Florida have some of the highest mortality rates for African American women in the country.

Ethnicity Differences

Since 1999, the death rates for cardiovascular disease have decreased for all racial and ethnic groups. As of 2017, nearly 11.5% of whites, 9.5% of non-Hispanic black adults, 7.5% of Hispanic adults, and 6.0% of non-Hispanic Asian adult Americans were being treated for some form of CVD (Wall et al., 2018). However, based on population, a disparity exists among various ethnic groups in the United States. For example, African Americans are 30% more likely to die from heart disease than Whites and have higher rates of myocardial infarction and heart failure (Wall et al., 2018). Stroke rates are two times higher among African Americans and cause higher morbidity and mortality rates, compared to whites (Gillum, 1999; Sharrief, Johnson, Abada, & Urrutia, 2016). Hispanic populations tend to have higher reported risk factors for CVD than whites and heart disease is the leading cause of death in this group (Rodriguez et al., 2014, AHA). Surprisingly, Hispanic populations have lower incidence and prevalence of most types of cardiovascular disease than non-Hispanic Whites and non-Hispanic Blacks, including but not limited to CAD, heart failure, stroke, and PAD (Balfour Jr, Ruiz, Talavera, Allison, & Rodriguez, 2016). This epidemiological phenomenon has confounded scientists and has been described as the Hispanic Paradox (Markides & Eschbach, 2005). More recent reports have come to the same conclusion with Hispanic Americans having lower rates of CVD despite greater CVD risk factors than non-Hispanics (Cortes-Bergoderi et al., 2013).

In addition, ethnic people living in rural regions of the United States experience higher rates of CVD compared with their urban counterparts. African Americans living in rural counties have higher rates of CVD risk factors such as hypertension, obesity, and diabetes compared with African Americans living in metro regions. This is notably apparent in the Southern rural states of the United States, including Louisiana, Mississippi, Alabama, South Carolina, and West Virginia (Appel, Harrell, & Deng, 2002). Additionally, Native Americans who live on rurally located reservation land have high rates of CVD risk factors, including prevalence of poor health, diabetes, physical inactivity, and poor diet, resulting in cardiovascular disease (Levin, Mayer-Davis, Ainsworth, Addy, & Wheeler, 2001). It should be noted; however, that for Native Americans/ Alaska Natives, and Asians/Pacific Islanders, there are substantially fewer data and results should be interpreted with caution, highlighting the common theme that minority groups are under-researched in the United States.

Barriers to CVD diagnosis and receiving lower-quality health care have been cited as reasons for ethnic groups CVD disparities in the rural United States (Mochari, Lee, Kligfield, & Mosca, 2006). This may explain why CVD rates are declining much slower in rural regions of the United States among African Americans and Hispanic Americans. Additionally, many CVD **interventions** are applied with one-size-fits-all approaches despite varying populations. Interventions tend to lack necessary adaptions for different communities, subcultures, and cultural competency for rural/urban and ethnic variations (Greenlund et al., 2004; Veeranna et al., 2013). Lower education levels are also a major contributing factor to CVD disparities between rural and urban regions (Logan, Guo, Dodd, Muller, & Riley, 2013). This is especially apparent for African American women living in rural counties who have lower educational attainment, as well as lower income than whites, higher BMI, and a much higher prevalence of CVD (Appel et al., 2002).

Contributing Factors to CVD Disparities

One major component that helps to explain the development of cardiovascular disease is CVD risk factor prevalence. Risk factors such as hypertension, obesity, tobacco smoking, diabetes, along with low levels of physical activity all help to predict a person's probability of developing heart disease. It is not surprising that U.S. regions with the highest rates of CVDs also report poor CVD risk factor rates. On a positive note, many of the CVD risk factors are modifiable, which indicates that with proper treatment the risk can be

alleviated. Unfortunately, another important factor that explains CVD disparities is limited access to medical treatment and healthcare coverage. In addition, socioeconomic factors such as lack of health-related education and income status contribute to CVD imbalances across the United States. Those with lower levels of education have higher incidents of mortality from CVD, and these same individuals receive markedly poorer healthcare services. This section will highlight CVD risk prevalence, healthcare access, and socioeconomic factors that contribute to the heart disease disparities between urban and rural regions of the United States.

Health-related Risk Factors

Hypertension is an elevation in arterial blood pressure. Untreated hypertension has a strong link to all forms of heart disease. Elevated pressure forces the heart muscle to pump harder, which puts considerable stress on the cardiovascular system. Guidelines for diagnosing hypertension were recently updated to reflect that normal systolic blood pressure (SBP) and diastolic blood pressure (DBP) are less than 120 mmHg and 80 mmHg, respectively (reported as 120/80 mmHg) (Whelton et al., 2018). Elevated blood pressure is 120–129/80 mmHg, stage 1 hypertension is 130–139/80–89 mmHg, and stage 2 hypertension is >140/>90 mmHg. Therefore, hypertension is diagnosed when BP exceeds 130/80 mmHg (Whelton et al., 2018). Treatment recommendations differ based on the patient's blood pressure classification. For example, someone with elevated blood pressure would be advised to change lifestyle habits such as engaging in physical exercise and dietary changes. Someone with stage 2 hypertension is advised to make lifestyle changes in addition to pharmacological therapy. Based on prevalence, hypertension is considered the most important modifiable risk factor for preventing cardiovascular disease (GBD global risk factor collaborators). Evidence suggests that hypertension accounts for 54% of all strokes and 47% of coronary artery disease and a 20 mmHg increase in SBP, and 10 mmHg increase in DBP doubles a person's risk of dying from heart disease (Lawes, Bennett, Feigin, & Rodgers, 2004). In addition, treating hypertension is paramount to preventing heart failure. For example, lowering SBP blood pressure from 139 to 136 mmHg was associated with a 13% reduction in the development of heart failure events among ~9,000 adults (Yusuf et al., 2000).

Shockingly, an estimated 46% of United States adults have hypertension or are being treated with an antihypertensive medication (Whelton et al., 2018). The prevalence of hypertension is slightly greater among men (48%) compared with women (43%). Rates are also higher among African Americans compared with whites, Asian Americans, and Hispanic Americans. Additionally, the rates of hypertension vary based on geographic locations. A significant higher prevalence of hypertension was reported in southern states compared with non-southern U.S. residents (Obisesan, Vargas, & Gillum, 2000). In fact, high rates of hypertension among African Americans living in the South have a strong link to stroke and heart disease mortality among the members of this group (Gillum, 1999). In 2016, Mississippi reported the highest number of life years lost to CVD in addition to the highest rates of hypertension per 100,000 residents. Louisiana, Alabama, and Tennessee followed closely in life years lost to CVD along with the corresponding link to hypertension. Conversely, Minnesota, Colorado, and Vermont had the lowest life years lost to CVD and have the lowest rates of hypertension in the United States (Roth et al., 2018). These data suggest that cardiovascular disease rates can be attenuated if efforts are made to diagnose hypertension earlier in life and then treat through encouraging lifestyle changes and medication compliance.

The influence of urbanization on hypertension rates in the United States is less clear. Estimates suggest that rural counties in America had a 0.2% higher rate of hypertension than populated counties (Harris et al., 2016). However, the U.S. Center for Disease Control and Prevention (CDC) recommended blood pressure screenings and treatment as a key initiative to preventing heart disease related death in rural regions (James et al., 2014).

Tobacco smoking rates have decreased substantially, but tobacco smoking still remains the leading cause of preventable death in the United States. The chemicals in cigarette smoke cause inflammation throughout the vascular system and notably effect the coronary and peripheral vessels (Siasos et al., 2014). Therefore, it is a major cause of coronary artery disease and peripheral artery disease. It has been reported that one of every four CVD-related deaths is linked to smoking. In addition, smoking increases the likelihood of developing 36 cardiovascular disease subtypes (Banks et al., 2019). However, within 5 years of quitting smoking, former smokers cut their risk for some CVDs to nearly the same levels as nonsmokers (Health & Services, 2010).

Similar to hypertension data, smoking rates are higher among African Americans (19%), compared with non-Hispanic white Americans (15%), and Hispanic Americans (10%). Also, the South (22%) and Midwest (22%) have the highest rates of smoking, and smoking in these regions is linked to coronary artery disease and stroke. In addition, 28% of residents living in rural counties who currently smoke compared with 18% in large metro regions of the United States. Moreover, smokers in rural regions are more likely to smoke 15 or more cigarettes per day. It has been reported that smoking as few as five cigarettes per day increases the likelihood of developing CVD, and the risk increases based on the number of cigarettes smoked per day (Control).

It is difficult to identify why smoking rates are substantially higher in the rural regions of the United States. One possible explanation is a lower level of completed education, which is inversely associated with smoking behavior. Those with a general education development (GED) certificate are nearly five times more likely to smoke than someone with an undergraduate degree. Another reason is due to lower household income among rural habitants. Twenty-one percent of Americans in the lowest household income bracket (<$35,000) currently smoke compared with 7% in the highest income brackets (>$100,000) (Control).

E-cigarettes, sometimes referred to as "vape pens," "e-cigs," or "mods" have grown in popularity in recent years. It produces an aerosol that contains nicotine, which is inhaled by the user. Researchers have been struggling to understand the other chemicals that are present in the aerosol mists primarily because so many types of products and delivery systems exist on the market. However, limited data suggest that cancer-causing agents, heavy metals, ultrafine particles, and chemicals are linked to serious lung disease (e.g., the flavoring agent diacetyl). Regardless, the U.S. Surgeon General cites e-cigarette use as one alternative to cigarette smoking. Similar to cigarette smoking trends, e-cigarette use in the United States is more prevalent in rural communities compared with urban areas (Mumford, Pearson, Villanti, & Evans, 2017). Part of the rationale is the emphasis placed on e-cigarettes as a replacement for cigarette smoking in some rural regions (Mumford et al., 2017). It is important to understand that despite efforts to market e-cigarettes as an alternative to cigarette smoking, the long-term health effects of e-cigarette use is not known. Therefore, the downstream impact on the development and progression of CVD among e-cigarette use may play a role in rural-urban CVD disparities.

Diabetes is a complex metabolic disease that results in elevated blood glucose. Type 2 diabetes (T2DM) is the common form and occurs when the body does not use insulin properly, which leads to chronic elevations in blood glucose. It develops as a result of poor lifestyle habits such as lack of physical exercise and unhealthy diets, along with obesity.

T2DM is a prime risk factor for developing CVD due to the vascular damage caused by hyperglycemia, and host of additional mechanisms (e.g., oxidative stress, inflammation) (Dokken, 2008). The prevalence of heart disease, and the risk of dying from a cardiac-related event among T2DM patients is eye opening. The American Heart Association (AMA) reported that adults with T2DM are two to four times more likely to die from heart disease than adults without diabetes.

The prevalence of diabetes throughout the United States helps to further explain the CVD disparities. Data suggest that rates of diabetes are 17% higher in rural areas than urban regions of the United States. Between 1999 and 2016, diabetes-related mortality decreased across urban regions of the United States. However, diabetes mortality remained unchanged in rural regions, especially in southern rural areas (Callaghan, Ferdinand, Akinlotan, Towne Jr, & Bolin, 2019). The strong link between diabetes and CVD helps to explain why heart disease is also more prevalent in rural regions of the United States.

Healthcare Coverage and Access

Lack of healthcare coverage among habitants of rural regions of the United States contributes to CVD disparity. It is estimated that nearly 10% of Americans living in rural areas do not have health insurance coverage, and that many of these people delay receiving health care due to the cost. Without coverage, people are more likely live with undiagnosed hypertension and diabetes, which dramatically increase risk for developing heart disease and dying from a cardiac event or a stroke. In addition, people tend to not fill and re-fill prescribed medications if they do not have prescription medication coverage. Further complicating rural habitants' health-related treatment is that many providers in rural regions do not accept charity insurance, or low-cost insurance that many rural residents receive coverage under. Also, recent research reported that health insurance premiums were higher in rural counties of the United States compared with urban counties (Barker et al., 2018).

A much larger factor in creating CVD health disparity is rural access to healthcare services. The largest barriers include transportation, distance to treatment centers, healthcare infrastructure, and climate. For example, public transportation services are commonly limited or unavailable in rural regions. In addition, it is common for rural residents to travel substantial distances to a provider's office, which results in disrupted or lack of care. Basic services such as pharmacy, routine check-ups, and physical rehabilitation are delayed as a result. This is especially apparent for rural habitants seeking cardiovascular and stroke services. Long travel times to see a cardiologist or delays in emergency treatment can lead to poorer outcomes and death.

Lack of rural healthcare services presents a major challenge for policymakers and public health workers. Recent hospital closures, and conversion of hospitals to emergency, or urgent care facilities limits access to specialty care such as cardiology. In addition, there is a large shortage of cardiologists nationwide, which has created a maldistribution favoring urban regions, which leaves primary care physicians to provide treatment in rural areas.

Socioeconomic Status

Socioeconomic status is a complex assessment of an individual's economic and social position compared with others. It is commonly composed of education (see **Figure 7-2**), income, and occupation. (Miner et al., 2014). It was recently reported that U.S. states with the lowest socioeconomic status also report the highest number of life years lost to cardiovascular disease (Roth et al., 2018). The states are all from the Southern regions of the United States and include: Mississippi, Louisiana, Arkansas, Alabama, West Virginia, and Kentucky. In addition, Southern states contain

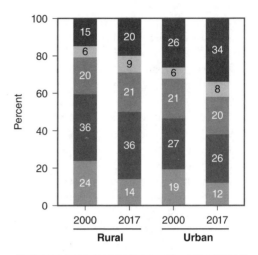

Note: Educational attainment for adults 25 and older. Urban and rural status is determined by Office of Management and Budget metropolitan and nonmetropolitan area definitions.

Figure 7-2 Socioeconomic Status—Educational Attainment in Rural Areas.

Rural Education. (n.d.). Retrieved from https://www.ers.usda.gov/topics/rural-economy-population/employment-education/rural-education/

nearly 50% of all rural habitants in the United States (Ratcliffe, Burd, Holder, & Fields, 2016). Conversely, the states with the highest socioeconomic status such as Massachusetts, Connecticut, and New Hampshire, also report low CVD-related life years lost. States in the Northeast region of the United States also contain the smallest number of rural residents (Ratcliffe et al., 2016). Therefore, it is easy to recognize that the low socioeconomic status of rural regions across the United States is highly linked to CVD disparities.

As previously stated, individuals with the lowest level of education and who are also in the lowest income range are more likely to smoke. Those who smoke also tend to have additional comorbidities such as hypertension, which increases the risk for cardiovascular disease. Additionally, people with a low socioeconomic status also have high rates of obesity and diabetes (Volaco, Cavalcanti, Filho, & Precoma, 2018). It is difficult to identify the reason, but it is likely linked to lack of education, poor lifestyle habits, along with limited access to health care. It is important to recognize that in many situations, it is a compilation of factors that contribute to the development of heart disease. Unfortunately, residents in rural regions of the United States are much more likely to have low socioeconomic status, along with more CVD risk factors, and limited access to health care. Combined, this helps to explain CVD disparities among Americans living in rural areas of the United States.

Prevention and Treatment for CVD

As discussed in previous sections, cardiovascular disease is a large burden across the United States due to a multitude of underlying factors. Unfortunately, rural regions of the United States experience higher rates of CVD, which is explained by socioeconomic status, lifestyle patterns, and various comorbidities, along with limited access to care (Moy et al., 2017; Shaw, 2016). Public health officials play a critical role in addressing both CVD prevention and treatment among rural residents in the United States. Technological initiatives such as upgrading information technology (IT) infrastructure and treating patients though telemedicine are contributing to this prevention. Other strategies include programs designed to increase access to cardiology physician specialists; development of recreational spaces to promote physical activity; and partnerships with communities and businesses to improve eating behaviors. The aim of this section is to discuss strategies to improve CVD health equity among those living in rural regions of the United States. In addition, several successful real-world examples will be highlighted.

Technological Initiatives

Health Information Technology (Health IT), which is the exchange of health information within an electronic format, plays a major role in hospital success. Health IT offers hospitals the ability to manage the storage and transfer of health information, provide medical treatment decision support from a care team, and assist with facilitating care from a distance. These health IT services have been shown to reduce medical errors, lower costs, and improve patient care, which create a larger problem for smaller, rural hospitals that have fewer resources to develop and maintain IT infrastructure (Association, 2007). One innovative way to address this issue is outsourcing rural hospital's health IT to larger, more technologically advanced hospitals in their regions (Reddy, Purao, & Kelly, 2008). Health IT outsourcing is the shift of responsibility for providing IT services to an external provider. These services include Electronic Health Records (EHR), IT advisory services, electronic data collection and real-time analysis, cybersecurity, and business intelligence and analytics. Rural hospitals have reported financial savings from sharing staff and access to expertise through health IT services that would otherwise not be accessible without outsourcing activities. In addition, health IT outsourcing has also been shown to shorten time required for clinicians working in rural hospitals to learn new technologies because the outsourcing hospital has resources to help guide them during the learning process (Reddy et al., 2008). Outsourcing health IT also has the potential to help alleviate the burden of specialty healthcare services being less abundant in rural regions (e.g., cardiology) by providing cheaper access to cardiologists, as well as providing better opportunity for management of chronic conditions to patients who can't travel to larger hospitals.

The use of telemedicine through mobile technologies is another key initiative to reduce barriers to cardiovascular treatment, and to prevent the development of CVD among those at high risk. Common treatments delivered through telemedicine services include: diagnosis of common medical problems, treatment recommendations, post-treatment checks, follow-up for chronic care, prescription fills, or any issue for patients incapable of leaving the home due to illness or weather conditions. Accumulating evidence of the efficacy of smartphone technologies for management and prevention of CVD has demonstrated promising results (Chow et al., 2015). One example is HeartBeat Connections (HBC) telemedicine program, which integrated with primary care for 333 residents of a rural community in Minnesota. The program used electronic health records (EHR) to screen, identify, and invite patients with metabolic syndrome or high Framingham Risk scores, aged 40–79 (without CVD or diabetes) to enroll. Nurse and dietitian-led telephonic coaching was provided, which focused on controlling CVD risk factors through medication compliance and diet. Results showed that those participants who completed more than four telephone meetings decreased their LDL by 16 mg/dL (Benson et al., 2014). Treatment through telemedicine services is also associated with a reduction in a host of important health outcomes among heart disease patients (Kruse, Soma, Pulluri, Nemali, & Brooks, 2017). Specifically, telemedicine services have improved self-management for heart failure patients, shortened hospital stays, and fewer emergency department visits. These impacts provided a substantial costs savings to both the healthcare system and costs for patients.

Another treatment successfully delivered through telemedicine technology is cardiac rehabilitation (CR). CR is a class I indication (strongly recommended) after heart surgery, for those with stable angina and PAD, along with chronic heart failure (Simon, Korn, Cho, & Raymond, 2018). It is comprehensive treatment centered on providing physical exercise combined with educational components to address CVD risk factors (e.g., smoking, diabetes, obesity, and psychosocial factors).

In traditional center-based CR programs, patients are asked to attend 36 exercise sessions over several months. Patient adherence has been a long-standing barrier to treatment among patients enrolled in traditional CR programs. A few reasons for lack of adherence include the CR program's geographic location, transportation services, and inconvenience (Ades et al., 2017; Jackson, Leclerc, Erskine, & Linden, 2005). There has been a recent surge of research exploring the benefits of home-based CR delivered through telemedicine services in an effort to improve adherence rates in CR (Ades et al., 2000; Thomas et al., 2019). Patients interact with a clinician through a smart device and receive their exercise programming and various education through a private server within the electronic medical record system. Data has shown that home-based CR is equally as effective as center-based CR for improving functional outcomes and quality-of-life measures among CVD patients at low risk for exercise-related events (Buckingham et al., 2016; Dalal, Zawada, Jolly, Moxham, & Taylor, 2010).

In summary, the advancement in technology has improved both infrastructure (IT enhancements), and delivery of treatment and prevention programs (telemedicine). It is likely that the continued advancement in technology will lead to improved CVD outcomes and lower prevalence among those living in rural America.

Access to Cardiology Care

Rural regions of the United States experience higher healthcare staff shortages than urban areas (National Agricultural Library). It is estimated that fewer than 10% of the country's physicians' practice in rural regions of the United States. Furthermore, specialty care physicians such as cardiologists are less likely to practice in rural regions for multiple reasons such as lower pay, lower job satisfaction, increased distance from metropolitan areas, and an overall decline in the number of trained cardiologists (Klein et al.,

2019; Laditka, Laditka, & Probst, 2009). An addition to these issues is that with the aging cardiology profession, as professionals get closer to retiring, they are less likely to be "on call" at hospitals in rural areas (Klein et al., 2019). The reduction in on-call services from cardiologists commonly results in additional strain on providers already working in rural hospitals.

One solution for cardiology shortages in rural locations is recruiting cardiologists to participate in rural outreach programs. An example of this has been reported from Iowa where 45% of the state's cardiologists agreed to consult rural residents through rural outreach (Gruca, Pyo, & Nelson, 2016). This effort reduced average driving time to the nearest cardiologists from 42.2 to 14.7 minutes for rural Iowans, and improved geographic access to office-based cardiology for more than 1 million Iowans (Gruca et al., 2016). Rural outreach programs are a short-term care approach and result in initial consultations for rural patients. In many situations, follow-up testing and reassessment of treatment strategies is required, which may lead to breakdown in therapy for rural patients. Therefore, outreach programs must be sustainable to provide a continuum of cardiology care for rural patients. Unfortunately, long-term solutions to the cardiology shortages in rural areas are difficult, and currently, there is not enough research to have a clear picture of successful programs. Additional efforts need to be made to recruit medical students to specialize in cardiology and offer them incentives to practice in rural regions or participate in rural outreach programs.

Recreational Space

The development of rural land for recreational purposes provides opportunity to promote physical activity. This can be achieved by creating outdoor hiking trails, bicycle paths, and exercise areas. In a cross-sectional study of rural youth in two Georgia counties, the odds of youth participating in physical activity increased by 20% when they had access to at least one physical activity area, and youth reporting access to multiple physical activity areas were twice as likely to be physically active than youth with no access (Shores, Moore, & Yin, 2010).

The National Recreation and Park Association (NRPA) Park Access initiative aims to address inequities in access to park and recreation spaces for rural regions of the United States. Since 2018, the NRPA has provided funds to six rural communities to improve access to parks, as well as improve the quality of their parks. Some ways in which these communities are improving their parks are by developing park and greenway plans, providing transportation opportunities to the parks, and engaging their communities during their park improvement processes (Acquino, 2019).

Evidence shows that improving parks and recreational areas while also providing active transportation to these locations can improve activity levels in rural communities. The financial cost to develop recreational spaces may hinder the ability of rural communities to invest in these types of initiatives. One option is to partner with the NRPA, which provides recommendations about converting spaces and assists with financial costs through granting opportunities. Check their website for more information (https://www.nrpa.org/). In addition, if rural communities are incapable of building new trails or developing recreational spaces, smaller investments in improving landscape of rural areas can have positive cardiovascular benefits. Interestingly, living in a neighborhood dense with trees, bushes, and other vegetation has been shown to reduce people's risk of having a heart attack, stroke, and other cardiovascular events regardless of these people undergoing physical activity (Yeager et al., 2020).

Another strategy is for rural communities to invest in community centers that provide exercise services along with educational programs (e.g., healthy eating, weight management) focused on heart health. This is commonly accomplished through partnerships with regional hospitals and not only creates a location for recreation and education but also for CVD treatment by providing clinical office space. Churches and other community-based organizations are also options for providing space for recreation and other educational programs. The benefits of a community program for improving CVD risk factors has been demonstrated among women living in rural regions of Montana and New York. In this study, a group of women participated in 48 classes across 24 weeks (2 classes/week) located at various community spaces. Classes included physical fitness, diet, weight loss, and other CVD risk education, along with stress management. In addition, the program also encouraged utilization of outdoor recreational spaces. The women who participated in the community program demonstrated improvements in dietary behavior and exercise activity compared with women who did not participate (Folta et al., 2019; Seguin-Fowler et al., 2020).

Access to Food

Rural communities have been negatively impacted by the evolving food environment in the United States over the past several decades. These changes have included an increase in the number of food establishments and an abundance of low nutritious food options, along with a shift toward more families having meals away from home (i.e., eating out) (Story et al., 2008, Ann Rev Public). These changes have been linked to the higher rates of obesity and heart disease in rural communities. Efforts are underway to increase access to nutritious foods for Americans living in rural regions (Ramirez, Diaz Rios, Valdez, Estrada, & Ruiz, 2017). For example, the Farmers Market Promotion Program (FMPP) funds projects that develop, coordinate, and expand direct producer-to-consumer

markets to help increase access to and availability of locally and regionally produced agricultural projects. One example was the Good Local Markets project in Texas during 2016. With nearly $250,000 in funding, the program team was able to improve access to food in rural regions surrounding Dallas, Texas. Funds were used to open food markets, strengthen the local nutrition assistance programs, develop new outreach and educational programs focused on eating local, and hosting regular events at the market to increase traffic. Another example is the *Produce on the Go* (POTG), which is a mobile farmer's market, designed to provide food access in a rural central California county. The community cited improved access to food with this mobile food service (Ramirez et al., 2017). The biggest challenge with food interventions in rural communities are the costs associated with sustaining access. Many interventions are reliant upon short-term grant funding (either federal or nonfederal) to support the initiatives. Other, possibly less costly strategies include increasing healthy menu options at restaurants, reducing portion sizes, and community programs that emphasize healthy grocery shopping.

Access to Healthcare Coverage

In rural populations, one of the biggest challenges with CVD treatment and prevention is access to care and affordable healthcare coverage. In 2010, the Affordable Care Act (ACA) was signed into law. It was designed to extend health insurance coverage to millions of uninsured Americans by expanding Medicaid eligibility, preventing companies from denying coverage due to pre-existing conditions, and qualifying lower-income families for extra savings on health insurance plans through premium tax credits and cost-sharing reductions. Following this act, the rates of uninsured rural Americans decreased by 8.5%

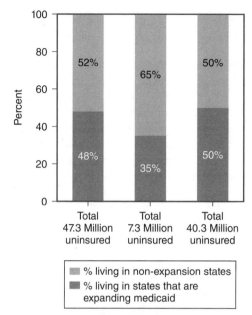

Note: "States expanding Medicaid" includes the 25 states and the District of Columbia expanding Medicaid as of March 1. "States not expanding" includes 25 states that are not expanding as of March 1, some of which may be considering expansion in the future.

Figure 7-3 Uninsured Individuals in Rural Areas Are Disproportionately Likely to Live in States that Are Not Expanding.

Retrieved from https://www.kff.org/uninsured/issue-brief/the-affordable-care-act-and-insurance-coverage-in-rural-areas/

(Benitez & Seiber, 2018). Despite the improvement in coverage, access to a regular source of medical care and doctor visitation did not improve (Benitez & Seiber, 2018). This may be explained by the high number of rural hospital closures since enacting the ACA, which has occurred mainly in states that decided not to adopt Medicaid expansion under the ACA (see **Figure 7-3**). Additionally, private insurers have not entered the rural marketplace, leaving little competition and higher priced insurance options sold in many rural areas.

With the enactment of the ACA in 2010, rural residents have had a mixture of benefits and hardships with insurance changes. The largest benefit of the ACA is that it slows the rise of healthcare costs, mainly because it provides insurance for millions and makes preventive care free (Hall, 2013). An additional major benefit of the ACA is that it requires all insurance plans to cover the 10 essential health benefits, one of which is treatment for chronic diseases such as CVDs. Children can remain on their parents' health insurance plans up to age 26, which has resulted in millions of previously uninsured young people being added since the enactment of the ACA (Sommers, 2012). Despite all of these improvements that came with the ACA, there have also been limitations to these benefits in rural locations. One example is that businesses with more than 50 employees must offer health insurance to their employees according to the ACA. However, many businesses in rural locations tend to be smaller and end up meeting the 50-employee mark less frequently. This results in many workers in rural locations not receiving the benefit of employer insurance.

Rural Health Clinics (RHCs) also play a major role in addressing health care in rural areas. In 1977, the rural health clinic certification program was started. This program aimed to boost rural provider availability for Medicare and Medicaid beneficiaries and is still present today. Certified providers are given clinic-specific, cost-based reimbursement for all services rendered to public payer patients, rather than having to accept a flat state (Medicaid) or federal (Medicare) payment rate. Certified clinics that can accept Medicaid offer appointments to Medicaid patients nearly 95% of the time, whereas rural clinics not certified by Medicaid offer appointments to these patients only 75% of the time (Richards, Saloner, Kenney, Rhodes, & Polsky, 2016). This program allows rural clinics to accept Medicaid patients without having to take on a financial burden for doing so and is a major way that the rural clinic has been able to contribute to treating and providing preventative care for rural populations.

Chapter Summary

While there is sometimes conflicting evidence for CVD disparities, there is no doubt that rural residents face unique challenges and risks for CVD that are not adequately addressed through current public health efforts. One of the many issues with current CVD initiatives is that they do not cater to the specific populations in which they are being implemented; many interventions could stand to benefit from added aspects of cultural competency. Additionally, there is not enough data for many subpopulations, such as American Indians/Alaska Natives and Asians/Pacific Islanders, and data for some topics dated. These issues reiterate the important role public health professionals play in collecting accurate and timely data of all population and subpopulation groups. Public health professionals must also strive to design and implement interventions that cater to the cultural aspects of the specific populations and/or communities with whom they are working.

Discussion Questions

1. Which cardiovascular disease discussed presents with leg pain during walking activities, which is alleviated upon rest?
2. What are the two main factors discussed that contribute to the development of heart failure with reduced ejection fraction?
3. Why does stroke lead to both physical and mental disabilities?
4. Which regions of the United States experience higher rates of CVD? (e.g., north, south, urban, rural, etc.)
5. Why do younger women generally have lower risk for cardiovascular events than men?
6. What are some possible explanations for why women tend to fare worse than men after experiencing a cardiac-related event?
7. Despite having higher risk factors for cardiovascular disease, which ethnic group tends to have lower prevalence of CVD?
8. What CVD risk factor is linked to 36 cardiovascular dieases?
9. What are the biggest challenges to healthcare access among rural residents in the United States?
10. What is the socioeconomic status and how does it affect CVD among rural residents in the United States?
11. What are some ways in which rural hospitals can utilize telemedicine to provide better care to patients?
12. What are some ways in which to mitigate physical inactivity, as well as poor access to food?

Student Activities and Worksheets are available inside the Navigate eBook, included with the printed text. Simply redeem the access code found at the front of the book at www.jblearning.com.

References

Acquino, M. Highlighting the "Power of Rural." *National Recreation and Park Association (NRPA)*. Retrieved from https://www.nrpa.org/blog/highlighting-the-power-of-rural/. Accessed July 6, 2020.

Ades, P. A., Keteyian, S. J., Wright, J. S., Hamm, L. F., Lui, K., Newlin, K., . . . Thomas, R. J. (2017). Increasing cardiac rehabilitation participation from 20% to 70%: A road map from the Million Hearts Cardiac

Rehabilitation Collaborative. *Mayo Clinic Proceedings, 92*(2), 234–242.

Ades, P. A., Pashkow, F. J., Fletcher, G., Pina, I. L., Zohman, L. R., & Nestor, J. R. (2000). A controlled trial of cardiac rehabilitation in the home setting using electrocardiographic and voice transtelephonic monitoring. *American Heart Journal, 139*(3), 543–548.

Appel, S. J., Harrell, J. S., & Deng, S. (2002). Racial and socioeconomic differences in risk factors for cardiovascular disease among Southern rural women. *Nursing Research, 51*(3), 140–147.

Association, A. H. (2007). Continued progress: Hospital use of information technology. *American Hospital Association: Washington DC.*

Balfour Jr, P. C., Ruiz, J. M., Talavera, G. A., Allison, M. A., & Rodriguez, C. J. (2016). Cardiovascular disease in Hispanics/Latinos in the United States. *Journal of Latina/o Psychology, 4*(2), 98–113.

Banks, E., Joshy, G., Korda, R. J., Stavreski, B., Soga, K., Egger, S., . . . Lopez, A. D. (2019). Tobacco smoking and risk of 36 cardiovascular disease subtypes: Fatal and non-fatal outcomes in a large prospective Australian study. *BMC Medicine, 17*(128). doi:10 .1186/s12916-019-1351-4

Benitez, J. A., & Seiber, E. E. (2018). US Health care reform and rural America: Results from the ACA's Medicaid expansions. *The Journal of Rural Health, 34*(2), 213–222. doi:10.1111/jrh.12284

Benjamin, E. J., Blaha, M. J., Chiuve, S. E., Cushman, M., Das, S. R., Deo, R., . . . Muntner, P. (2017). Heart disease and stroke statistics-2017 update: A report from the American Heart Association. *Circulation, 135*(10), e146–e603.

Benjamin, E. J., Muntner, P., Bittencourt, M. S., Callaway, C. W., Carson, A. P., Chamberlain, A. M., . . . Virni, S. S. (2019). Heart disease and stroke statistics-2019 update: A report from the American Heart Association. *Circulation, 139*(10), e56–e528.

Benson, G., Sidebottom, A., Sillah, A., Boucher, J., Knickelbine, T., & VanWormer, J. (2014). Primary cardiovascular disease prevention is leaving the office: Early results from the HeartBeat Connections integrated telemedicine program. *American College of Cardiology, 63*(12), 1219–154.

Buckingham, S., Taylor, R., Jolly, K., Zawada, A., Dean, S., Cowie, A., . . . Dalal, H. M. (2016). Home-based versus centre-based cardiac rehabilitation: Abridged Cochrane systematic review and meta-analysis. *Open Heart, 3*(2), e000463.

Callaghan, T., Ferdinand, A. O., Akinlotan, M. A., Towne Jr, S. D., & Bolin, J. (2020). The changing landscape of diabetes mortality in the United States across region and rurality, 1999–2016. *The Journal of Rural Health, 36*(3), 410–415.

Canto, J. G., Shlipak, M. G., Rogers, W. J., Malmgren, J. A., Frederick, P. D., Lambrew, C. T., . . . Kiefe, C. I. (2000). Prevalence, clinical characteristics, and mortality among patients with myocardial infarction presenting without chest pain. *JAMA, 283*(24), 3223–3229.

Canto, J. G., Taylor Jr, H. A., Rogers, W. J., Sanderson, B., Hilbe, J., & Barron, H. V. (1998). Presenting characteristics, treatment patterns, and clinical outcomes of non-black minorities in the National Registry of Myocardial Infarction 2. *The American Journal of Cardiology, 82*(9), 1013–1018.

Centers for Disease Control and Prevention (CDC). Health effects of cigarette smoking. Retrieved from https://www.cdc.gov/tobacco/data_statistics/fact _sheets/health_effects/effects_cig_smoking/index .htm#reduced-risks

Chow, C. K., Redfern, J., Hillis, G. S., Thakkar, J., Santo, K., Hackett, M. L., . . . Thiagalingam A. (2015). Effect of lifestyle-focused text messaging on risk factor modification in patients with coronary heart disease: A randomized clinical trial. *JAMA, 314*(12), 1255–1263.

Cortes-Bergoderi, M., Goel, K., Murad, M. H., Allison, T., Somers, V. K., Erwin, P. J., . . . Lopez-Jimenez, F. (2013). Cardiovascular mortality in Hispanics compared to non-Hispanic whites: A systematic review and meta-analysis of the Hispanic paradox. *European Journal of Internal Medicine, 24*(8), 791–799.

Criqui, M. H., Aboyans, V., Allison, M. A., Denenberg, J. O., Forbang, N., McDermott, M. M., . . . Wong, N. D. (2016). Peripheral artery disease and aortic disease. *Global Heart, 11*(3), 313–326.

Dahlström, U. (2019). Epidemiology of heart failure. In *Heart Failure* (pp. 3–36): Springer.

Dalal, H. M., Zawada, A., Jolly, K., Moxham, T., & Taylor, R. S. (2010). Home based versus centre based cardiac rehabilitation: Cochrane systematic review and meta-analysis. *The BMJ, 340*, b5631.

Department of Health and Human Services. (2010). How tobacco smoke causes disease: What it means to you. Atlanta: US Department of Health and Human Services, Centers for Disease Control and Prevention (CDC). *National Center for Chronic Disease Prevention and Health Promotion, Office on Smoking and Health.*

Dokken, B. B. (2008). The pathophysiology of cardiovascular disease and diabetes: Beyond blood pressure and lipids. *Diabetes Spectrum, 21*(3), 160–165.

Easton, J. D., Saver, J. L., Albers, G. W., Alberts, M. J., Chaturvedi, S., Feldmann, E., . . . Sacco, R. L. (2009). Definition and evaluation of transient ischemic attack: A scientific statement for healthcare professionals from the American Heart Association/ American Stroke Association Stroke Council; Council on Cardiovascular Surgery and Anesthesia; Council on Cardiovascular Radiology and Intervention; Council on Cardiovascular Nursing; and the Interdisciplinary

Council on Peripheral Vascular Disease: *The American Academy of Neurology affirms the value of this statement as an educational tool for neurologists. Stroke, 40*(6), 2276–2293.

Ennen, K. A., & Beamon, E. R. (2012). Women and stroke knowledge: Influence of age, race, residence location, and marital status. *Health Care for Women International, 33*(10), 922–942.

Folta, S. C., Paul, L., Nelson, M. E., Strogatz, D., Graham, M., Eldridge, G. D., . . . Seguin-Fowler, R. A. (2019). Changes in diet and physical activity resulting from the *Strong Hearts, Healthy Communities* randomized cardiovascular disease risk reduction multilevel intervention trial. *International Journal of Behavioral Nutrition and Physical Activity, 16*(1), 91.

Friberg, J., Scharling, H., Gadsbøll, N., Truelsen, T., & Jensen, G. B. (2004). Comparison of the impact of atrial fibrillation on the risk of stroke and cardiovascular death in women versus men (The Copenhagen City Heart Study). *The American Journal of Cardiology, 94*(7), 889–894.

Garcia, M., Mulvagh, S. L., Bairey Merz, C. N., Buring, J. E., & Manson, J. E. (2016). Cardiovascular disease in women: Clinical Perspectives. *Circulation Research, 118*(8), 1273–1293.

García, M. C., Rossen, Ł. M., Bastian, B., Faul, M., Dowling, N. F., Thomas, C. C., . . . Iademarco, M. F. (2019). Potentially excess deaths from the five leading causes of death in metropolitan and nonmetropolitan counties—United States, 2010–2017. *MMWR. Surveillance Summaries, 68*(10), 1–11.

Gillum, R. F. (1999). Risk factors for stroke in blacks: A critical review. *American Journal of Epidemiology, 150*(12), 1266–1274. doi:10.1093/oxfordjournals. aje.a009957

Greenlund, K. J., Keenan, N. L., Giles, W. H., Zheng, Z. J., Neff, L. J., Croft, J. B., & Mensah, G. A. (2004). Public recognition of major signs and symptoms of heart attack: Seventeen states and the US Virgin Islands, 2001. *American Heart Journal, 147*(6), 1010–1016.

Grenon, S. M., Chong, K., Alley, H., Nosova, E., Gasper, W., Hiramoto, J., . . . Owens, C. D. (2014). Walking disability in patients with peripheral artery disease is associated with arterial endothelial function. *Journal of Vascular Surgery, 59*(4), 1025–1034.

Gruca, T. S., Pyo, T. H., & Nelson, G. C. (2016). Providing cardiology care in rural areas through visiting consultant clinics. *Journal of the American Heart Association, 5*(7). doi:10.1161/jaha.115.002909

Hall, M. A. (2013). Evaluating the Affordable Care Act: The eye of the beholder. *HeinOnline, 51*, 1029.

Harris, J. K., Beatty, K., Leider, J., Knudson, A., Anderson, B. L., & Meit, M. (2016). The double disparity facing rural local health departments. *Annual Review of Public Health, 37*, 167–184.

Ingram, D. D., & Gillum, R. F. (1989). Regional and urbanization differentials in coronary heart disease mortality in the United States, 1968–1985. *Journal of Clinical Epidemiology, 42*(9), 857–868. doi:10.1016/0895-4356(89)90099-1

Jackson, L., Leclerc, J., Erskine, Y., & Linden, W. (2005). Getting the most out of cardiac rehabilitation: A review of referral and adherence predictors. *Heart, 91*(1), 10–14.

James, P. A., Oparil, S., Carter, B. L., Cushman, W. C., Dennison-Himmelfarb, C., Handler, J., . . . Ortiz, E. (2014). 2014 evidence-based guideline for the management of high blood pressure in adults: Report from the panel members appointed to the Eighth Joint National Committee (JNC 8). *JAMA, 311*(5), 507–520.

Jones, C. A. (2009). *Health status and health care access of farm and rural populations*: DIANE Publishing.

Kemp, C. D., & Conte, J. V. (2012). The pathophysiology of heart failure. *Cardiovascular Pathology, 21*(5), 365–371. doi:10.1016/j.carpath.2011.11.007

Klein, L. W., Rab, T., Anderson, H. V., Lotfi, A., Truesdell, A. G., Duffy, P. L., . . . Kleiman, N. S. (2019). The implications of acute clinical care responsibilities on the contemporary practice of interventional cardiology. *JACC: Cardiovascular Interventions, 12*(6), 595–599.

Kruse, C. S., Soma, M., Pulluri, D., Nemali, N. T., & Brooks, M. (2017). The effectiveness of telemedicine in the management of chronic heart disease–a systematic review. *JRSM Open, 8*(3), 2054270416681747. https://doi.org/10.1177/2054270416681747.

Kulshreshtha, A., Goyal, A., Dabhadkar, K., Veledar, E., & Vaccarino, V. (2014). Urban-rural differences in coronary heart disease mortality in the United States: 1999–2009. *Public Health Reports, 129*(1), 19–29.

Laditka, J. N., Laditka, S. B., & Probst, J. C. (2009). Health care access in rural areas: Evidence that hospitalization for ambulatory care-sensitive conditions in the United States may increase with the level of rurality. *Health & Place, 15*(3), 761–770. doi:10.1016/j.healthplace.2008.12.007

Lastra, G., Harbuz-Miller, I., Sowers, J. R., & Manrique, C. M. (2019). Estrogen receptor signaling and cardiovascular function. In *Sex Differences in Cardiovascular Physiology and Pathophysiology* (pp. 13–22): Academic Press.

Lawes, C. M., Bennett, D. A., Feigin, V. L., & Rodgers, A. (2004). Blood pressure and stroke: An overview of published reviews. *Stroke, 35*(3), 776–785.

Lee, D. S., Gona, P., Vasan, R. S., Larson, M. G., Benjamin, E. J., Wang, T. J., . . . Levy, D. (2009). Relation of disease pathogenesis and risk factors to heart failure with preserved or reduced ejection fraction: Insights from the National Heart, Lung, and Blood Institute's Framingham Heart Study. *Circulation, 119*(24), 3070–3077. doi:10.1161/circulationaha.108.815944

Levin, S., Mayer-Davis, E. J., Ainsworth, B. E., Addy, C. L., & Wheeler, F. C. (2001). Racial/ethnic health disparities in South Carolina and the role of rural locality and educational attainment. *Southern Medical Journal, 94*(7), 711.

Libby, P., & Theroux, P. (2005). Pathophysiology of coronary artery disease. *Circulation, 111*(25), 3481–3488.

Logan, H., Guo, Y., Dodd, V. J., Muller, K., & Riley, J. (2013). The burden of chronic diseases in a rural North Florida sample. *BMC Public Health, 13*(1), 906.

Markides, K. S., & Eschbach, K. (2005). Aging, migration, and mortality: Current status of research on the Hispanic paradox. *The Journals of Gerontology Series B, 60*(Special_Issue_2), S68–S75.

Meit, M., Knudson, A., Gilbert, T., Yu, A. T.-C., Tanenbaum, E., Ormson, E., . . . Popat, S. (2014). The 2014 update of the rural-urban chartbook. *RHRC Rural Health Research & Policy Centers.*

Mendy, V. L., Vargas, R., Payton, M., Sims, J. N., & Zhang, L. (2019). Trends in the stroke death rate among Mississippi adults, 2000–2016. *Preventing Chronic Disease, 16*, E21.

Mochari, H., Lee, J. R., Kligfield, P., & Mosca, L. (2006). Ethnic differences in barriers and referral to cardiac rehabilitation among women hospitalized with coronary heart disease. *Preventive Cardiology, 9*(1), 8–13.

Moy, E., Garcia, M. C., Bastian, B., Rossen, L. M., Ingram, D. D., Faul, M., . . . Iademarco, M. F. (2017). Leading causes of death in nonmetropolitan and metropolitan areas—United States, 1999–2014. *MMWR Surveillance Summaries, 66*(1), 1–8.

Mumford, E. A., Pearson, J. L., Villanti, A. C., & Evans, W. D. (2017). Nicotine and e-cigarette beliefs and policy support among US smokers and nonsmokers. *Tobacco Regulatory Science, 3*(3), 293–305.

National Agricultural Library. U.S. Department of Agriculture. Rural public health. Retrieved from https://www.nal.usda.gov/ric/rural-public-health

National Institutes of Health. (1989). Data fact sheet: The stroke belt: Stroke mortality by race and sex. *Hyattsville, MD: Dept of Health and Human Services.*

Obisesan, T. O., Vargas, C. M., & Gillum, R. F. (2000). Geographic variation in stroke risk in the United States: Region, urbanization, and hypertension in the Third National Health and Nutrition Examination Survey. *Stroke, 31*(1), 19–25.

O'Connor, A., & Wellenius, G. (2012). Rural-urban disparities in the prevalence of diabetes and coronary heart disease. *Public Health, 126*(10), 813–820. doi:10.1016/j.puhe.2012.05.029

Pfeffer, M. A., Shah, A. M., & Borlaug, B. A. (2019). Heart failure with preserved ejection fraction in perspective. *Circulation Research, 124*(11), 1598–1617. doi:10.1161/circresaha.119.313572

Ramirez, A. S., Diaz Rios, L. K., Valdez, Z., Estrada, E., & Ruiz, A. (2017). Bringing produce to the people: Implementing a social marketing food access intervention in rural food deserts. *Journal of Nutrition Education Behavior, 49*(2), 166–174.e161. doi:10.1016/j.jneb.2016.10.017

Ratcliffe, M., Burd, C., Holder, K., & Fields, A. (2016). Defining rural at the U.S. Census Bureau. *American Community Survey and Geography Brief, 1–8.*

Reddy, M. C., Purao, S., & Kelly, M. (2008). Developing IT infrastructure for rural hospitals: A case study of benefits and challenges of hospital-to-hospital partnerships. *Journal of the American Medical Informatics Association, 15*(4), 554–558.

Reeves, M. J., Bushnell, C. D., Howard, G., Gargano, J. W., Duncan, P. W., Lynch, G., . . . Lisabeth, L. (2008). Sex differences in stroke: Epidemiology, clinical presentation, medical care, and outcomes. *The Lancet Neurology, 7*(10), 915–926.

Richards, M. R., Saloner, B., Kenney, G. M., Rhodes, K. V., & Polsky, D. (2016). Availability of new Medicaid patient appointments and the role of rural health clinics. *Health services research, 51*(2), 570–591.

Roth, G. A., Johnson, C. O., Abate, K. H., Abd-Allah, F., Ahmed, M., Alam, K., . . . Murray, C. J. L. (2018). The Burden of Cardiovascular Diseases Among United States, 1990–2016. *JAMA Cardiology, 3*(5), 375–389. doi:10.1001/jamacardio.2018.0385

Seguin-Fowler, R. A., Strogatz, D., Graham, M. L., Eldridge, G. D., Marshall, G. A., Folta, S. C., . . . Paul, L. (2020). The Strong Hearts, Healthy Communities Program 2.0: An RCT Examining Effects on Simple 7. *American Journal of Preventive Medicine, 59*(1), 32–40.

Sharrief, A. Z., Johnson, B., Abada, S., & Urrutia, V. C. (2016). Stroke knowledge in African Americans: A narrative review. *Ethnicity & Disease, 26*(2), 255–262.

Shaw, K. M., Theis, K. A., Self-Brown, S., Roblin, D. W., & Barker, L. (2016). Chronic disease disparities by county economic status and metropolitan classification, Behavioral Risk Factor Surveillance System, 2013. *Preventing Chronic Disease, 13*, 160088.

Shores, K. A., Moore, J. B., & Yin, Z. (2010). An examination of triple jeopardy in rural youth physical activity participation. *The Journal of Rural Health, 26*(4), 352–360. doi:10.1111/j.1748-0361.2010.00301.x

Shrira, I., Christenfeld, N., & Howard, G. (2008). Exposure to the US Stroke Buckle as a risk factor for cerebrovascular mortality. *Neuroepidemiology, 30*(4), 229–233.

Siasos, G., Tsigkou, V., Kokkou, E., Oikonomou, E., Vavuranakis, M., Vlachopoulos, C., . . . Tousoulis, D. (2014). Smoking and atherosclerosis: Mechanisms of disease and new therapeutic approaches. *Current Medicinal Chemistry, 21*(34), 3936–3948. doi:10.2174/09298673213414101516153

Simon, M., Korn, K., Cho, L., & Raymond, C. (2018). Cardiac rehabilitation: A class 1 recommendation. *Cleveland Clinic Journal of Medicine, 85*(7), 551–558.

Sommers, B. D. (2012). Number of young adults gaining insurance due to the Affordable Care Act now tops 3 million. *ASPE Issue Brief.*

Story, M., Kaphingst, K. M., Robinson-O'Brien, R., & Glanz, K. 2008. Creating Healthy Food and Eating Environments: Policy and Environmental Approaches. *Annual Review of Public Health 29*, 253–272.

Taylor, H. A., Hughes, G. D., & Garrison, R. J. (2002). Cardiovascular disease among women residing in rural America: Epidemiology, explanations, and challenges. *American Journal of Public Health, 92*(4), 548–551.

Thomas, R. J., Beatty, A. L., Beckie, T. M., Brewer, L. C., Brown, T. M., Forman, D. E., . . . Whooley, M. A. (2019). Home-based cardiac rehabilitation: A scientific statement from the American Association of Cardiovascular and Pulmonary Rehabilitation, the American Heart Association, and the American College of Cardiology. *Journal of the American College of Cardiology, 74*(1), 133–153.

Towne Jr, S. D., Callaghan, T. H., Ferdinand, A. O., Akinlotan, M., Primm, K., & Bolin, J. (2019). Prevalence and mortality of heart disease and related conditions: Disparities affecting the South, Rural areas, and American Indian and Alaska Natives. *Policy Brief.*

Veeranna, V., Zalawadiya, S. K., Niraj, A., Kumar, A., Ference, B., & Afonso, L. (2013). Association of novel biomarkers with future cardiovascular events is influenced by ethnicity: Results from a multi-ethnic cohort. *International Journal of Cardiology, 166*(2), 487–493.

Volaco, A., Cavalcanti, A. M., Filho, R. P., & Précoma, D. B. (2018). Socioeconomic status: The missing link between obesity and Diabetes Mellitus? *Current Diabetes Reviews, 14*(4), 321–326. doi:10.2174 /1573399813666170621123227

Wall, H. K., Ritchey, M. D., Gillespie, C., Omura, J. D., Jamal, A., & George, M. G. (2018). Vital signs: Prevalence of key cardiovascular disease risk factors for million hearts 2022—United States, 2011–2016. *MMWR Morbidity and Mortality Weekly Report, 67*(35), 983–991. doi:10.15585 /mmwr.mm6735a4

Whelton, P. K., Carey, R. M., Aronow, W. S., Casey, D. E., Collins, K. J., Himmelfarb, C. D., . . . Jones, D. W. (2018). 2017 ACC/AHA/AAPA/ABC/ACPM /AGS/APhA/ASH/ASPC/NMA/PCNA guideline for the prevention, detection, evaluation, and management of high blood pressure in adults: A report of the American College of Cardiology/American Heart Association Task Force on Clinical Practice Guidelines. *Journal of the American College of Cardiology, 71*(19), e127–e248.

Wilson, S. L., Kratzke, C., & Hoxmeier, J. (2012). Predictors of access to healthcare: What matters to rural Appalachians? *Global Journal of Health Science, 4*(6), 23–35.

Winters-Miner, L. A., Bolding, P. S., Hilbe, J. M., Goldstein, M., Hill, T., Nisbet, R., . . . Miner, G. D. (2015). *Practical predictive analytics and decisioning systems for medicine: Informatics accuracy and cost-effectiveness for healthcare administration and delivery including medical research*: Academic Press.

Yeager, R., Riggs, D. W., DeJarnett, N., Srivastava, S., Lorkiewicz, P., Xie, Z., . . . Bhatnagar, A. (2020). Association between residential greenness and exposure to volatile organic compounds. *Science of The Total Environment, 707*, 135435.

Yusuf, S., Sleight, P., Pogue, J., Bosch, J., Davies, R., & Dagenais, G. (1999). Effects of an angiotensin-converting-enzyme inhibitor, ramipril, on cardiovascular events in high-risk patients. *The New England Journal of Medicine, 342*(3), 145–153. doi:10.1056 /nejm200001203420301

Zemaitis, M. R., Bah, F., Boll, J. M., & Dreyer, M. A. (2019). Peripheral Arterial Disease.

CHAPTER 8

Obesity, Type 2 Diabetes, and Physical Activity

Rachael Nelson, PhD
Naveen Sharma, PhD

LEARNING OBJECTIVES

At the end of this chapter, the readers will be able to:

1. Describe the prevalence of obesity and type 2 diabetes in rural U.S. communities.
2. Identify how behavioral, socioeconomic, and environmental factors may contribute to obesity and other chronic health issues in rural settings.
3. Discuss how physical activity can mitigate obesity-related health concerns, including type 2 diabetes.
4. Recognize the unique barriers to achieving healthy lifestyles in rural settings.

KEY TERMS

Adiposity
Body mass index
Exercise
Insulin resistance

CHAPTER OVERVIEW

Obesity, clinically defined by a **body mass index (BMI)** greater than 30 kg/m² as shown in **Table 8-1** and characterized by an excess accumulation of body fat, is arguably the greatest epidemic impacting the health and well-being of individuals and communities worldwide. Obesity is associated with numerous negative health outcomes, including increased risk of cardiovascular disease, hypertension, certain types of cancer, cognitive impairment, and type 2 diabetes mellitus (T2DM) (Apovian, 2016; L. Dye, Boyle, Champ, & Lawton, 2017; Lega & Lipscombe, 2020).

Globally, nowhere is obesity more pronounced than the United States, where greater than 40% of all American adults are now classified as obese (Hales, Carroll, Fryar, & Odgen, 2020). Intriguingly, it is well reported that the prevalence of obesity in rural areas is significantly greater than that of urban areas (Befort, Nazir, & Perri, 2012; Chea & Kim, 2020; S. A. Cohen, Cook, Kelley, Foutz, & Sando, 2017; S. A. Cohen, Greaney, & Sabik, 2018; Hill, You, & Zoellner, 2014; Lundeen et al., 2018; Wen, Fan, Kowaleski-Jones, & Wan, 2018), contributing to a further disparity in health outcomes among these populations. The causes of obesity are complex and multifactorial, however, poor dietary habits contributing to excess calorie consumption and increased

Table 8-1 Obesity Defined by BMI

Body mass index classifications	
BMI value (kg/m²)	Classification
<18.5	Underweight
18.5–24.9	Normal Weight
25.0–29.9	Overweight
30.0–34.9	Class I Obesity
35.0–39.9	Class II Obesity
≥40.0	Class III Obesity

Data from the National Institutes of Health.

sedentary behavior are often cited as the main reasons for the tremendous increase in obesity in the United States (Katzmarzyk et al., 2019; Matthews et al., 2008; Mozaffarian, 2016; Murray et al., 2013; Sisson et al., 2009). The goal of this chapter is to highlight aspects of U.S. rural communities that have not only led to the observed increase in overall obesity prevalence in recent decades but also importantly underscore potential reasons for rural-urban disparities in obesity rates. Consequently, we will further delve into the impact of obesity on pathogenesis of T2DM and discuss how engagement in regular physical activity is vital to reducing health disparities in rural communities.

Obesity: Prevalence and Etiology

Data from several sources indicate that the prevalence of obesity in rural areas is greater than that in urban areas in the United States. Self-reported data from 10,032 participants of the 2003–2008 National Health and Nutrition Examination Survey (NHANES) indicated that obesity prevalence was 41% in rural communities compared with only 32% in urban areas (Wen et al., 2018). Using measured, rather than self-reported, data acquired from the 2005–2008 NHANES data set, obesity prevalence was 40% among rural versus 34% in

urban adults (Befort et al., 2012). Findings from the 2016 Behavioral Risk Factor Surveillance Survey (BRFSS) also indicated that obesity prevalence was higher in adults from rural counties (34%) compared with those living in metropolitan counties (29%) (Lundeen et al., 2018). Potential reasons for higher rural obesity prevalence rates have been proposed but remain unclear. It has been suggested that this discrepancy between rural and urban areas is related to both individual as well as community-based factors (Bennett, Probst, & Pumkam, 2011; Wen et al., 2018). To that point, the etiology of obesity is multifactorial and can be influenced by a combination of behavioral (e.g., physical activity and dietary habits), socioeconomic, environmental, and genetic influences (Albuquerque, Nobrega, Manco, & Padez, 2017; Bilal, Auchincloss, & Diez-Roux, 2018; Giskes, van Lenthe, Avendano-Pabon, & Brug, 2011; Katzmarzyk et al., 2019; Mozaffarian, 2016; Nicolaidis, 2019; Volaco, Cavalcanti, Filho, & Precoma, 2018; Wende et al., 2020). Collectively, these factors contribute to an imbalance between energy intake (dietary calories) and energy expenditure (i.e., basal metabolic rate, activity thermogenesis, and dietary effect of feeding), favoring greater energy intake than expenditure and ultimately resulting in weight gain leading to obesity. Therefore, a rural setting is likely associated with a unique set of challenges influencing dietary behaviors and physical activity contributing to weight gain and obesity.

It is important to highlight potentially meaningful limitations to using BMI only as diagnostic criteria for obesity. One such limitation of BMI is that it does not distinguish between fat mass and lean mass in the calculation of body mass. Since lean mass (including muscle) has a higher density than fat mass (adipose tissue), an individual who has a higher percentage of muscle can be characterized as overweight or obese, despite their lack of **adiposity**. Furthermore, a basic assumption of BMI is that among adults, weight gain is associated with primarily gaining fat mass while weight loss is primarily associated with losing primarily fat mass. However, there are various populations where these assumptions are false including older adults who can experience sarcopenia (i.e., muscle wasting) as they lose weight with age (Wannamethee & Atkins, 2015) and athletes who gain muscle mass from regular strength/resistance training. Additionally, although racial/ethnic disparities exist between BMI and adiposity, BMI classification categories are uniform regardless of race/ethnicity (Rush et al., 2007).

Rural Disparities in Sociodemographic Factors Related to Obesity

According to the US Census Bureau, less than 20% of the U.S. population lives in nonurban or rural areas (Ratcliffe, 2016). Within this rural population, established markers of socioeconomic status have been identified regularly as different from urban populations, partially contributing to obesity and health discrepancies between these communities. Data from the 2015 American Community Survey revealed that the median household income in rural households was about 3.5% lower than urban households ($54,296 versus $52,386) (Survey, 2016). Data from the 1999–2006 NHANES survey revealed that a higher percentage of rural households fall below the federal poverty levels compared with urban households (Trivedi et al., 2015).

Educational access and achievement are often positively associated with upward social mobility and future earning potential (Baum, Kurose, & McPherson, 2013; Haveman & Smeeding, 2006). There is evidence that educational attainment is often lower in residents of rural areas. More specifically, while the proportion of residents achieving a high school diploma (or equivalent) is higher in rural versus urban communities (36 vs. 26%), only 20% of rural residents complete a bachelor's degree (or higher) compared with 34% among urban residents (*Rural education at a glance,*

2017). Other characteristics, including region of country, sex, and racial/ethnic background may also be used to reveal unique trends associated with urban and racial disparities. However, there are consistent and significant trends when age is considered a factor. Households with householders ages 45 to 64 had a higher median household income in urban areas than rural areas by about 6.9% ($66,399 versus $62,169). Similarly, for those households with a householder age 65 and over, those in urban areas had a higher median household income than those in rural areas by about 4.9% ($39,202 versus $37,310) (Survey, 2016). As obesity prevalence is more pronounced in older populations compared with younger ones (Hales, Fryar, Carroll, Freedman, & Ogden, 2018), it suggests that fewer economic resources contribute to age-associated obesity, particularly in a rural setting.

Dietary Patterns in Rural Environments Contributing to Obesity

The U.S. Dietary Guidelines generated by the federal government is a tool designed for policymakers and health professionals to aid the American public into making healthful nutritional choices. The current 2015–2020 Dietary Guidelines for Americans comprises five overarching guidelines, including: 1) consuming a variety of vegetables, 2) consuming nutrient-dense foods, 3) limiting calories from added sugar, saturated fat, and sodium, 4) shifting to healthier food and beverages choices, and 5) supporting healthier eating patterns in general (*Dietary guidelines for Americans, 2015 — 2020,* 2015). Adherence to these recommendations is intended to provide its followers with a healthy lifestyle, thereby reducing the risk of chronic diseases, such as obesity. Implementation of these guidelines is clearly a challenge for policymakers and health experts in the United States based on the current expanding prevalence of obesity (Hales et al., 2018). Moreover, these guidelines are even more difficult to successfully implement in rural communities based on the increased prevalence of obesity in these regions. Rural environments are often synonymous to food deserts, areas with limited accessibility to nutritionally dense foods (Bennett et al., 2011; Hansen, Umstattd Meyer, Lenardson, & Hartley, 2015; Lenardson, Hansen, & Hartley, 2015; Powell, Slater, Mirtcheva, Bao, & Chaloupka, 2007; Valdez, Ramirez, Estrada, Grassi, & Nathan, 2016; Walker, Keane, & Burke, 2010; Yousefian, Leighton, Fox, & Hartley, 2011). Consequently, these areas cultivate unhealthy dietary patterns, including overconsumed, low–nutrient-dense foods characterized by added sugars, saturated fats, and sodium (Befort et al., 2012; Bove & Olson, 2006; Champagne et al., 2004; S. A. Cohen et al., 2018; Trivedi et al., 2015). Approximately 95% of rural adults exceed the dietary guidelines for saturated fat and sodium intake, while 70% do not meet dietary guidelines for fruit, vegetables, and whole grain intake (Savoca et al., 2009). Collectively, higher intake of added sugar, sodium, and saturated fat contribute to obesity and other chronic diseases, including cardiovascular disease and T2DM (Lega & Lipscombe, 2020; Mozaffarian, 2016).

Regardless of the macronutrient source (e.g., carbohydrate, fat, or protein), total caloric intake impacts weight gain. In the United States, average calorie intake has increased due to several factors, including the increased prevalence of cheap processed food, larger portion sizes, and the amount of calories consumed away from home (Afshin et al., 2017; An, 2016; Casagrande & Cowie, 2017; Duffey & Popkin, 2011, 2013; Finkelstein, Strombotne, Zhen, & Epstein, 2014; McCrory, Harbaugh, Appeadu, & Roberts, 2019; B. T. Nguyen & Powell, 2014; Poti, Duffey, & Popkin, 2014; Powell, Chriqui, Khan, Wada, & Chaloupka, 2013; Powell et al., 2007; Todd, 2017). In summation, over the last several decades (i.e., from the 1970s onwards), daily calorie intake has risen from an estimated 2,016 kcal/day to 2,390 kcals/day, providing an average surplus

of over 300 kcal/day (Bentley, 2017). Over this same time period, there has been a parallel rise prevalence of obesity (Gordon-Larsen, The, & Adair, 2010). Intriguingly, in some reports, daily caloric intake has been reported to be similar between residents of rural and urban communities (Befort et al., 2012; Champagne et al., 2004; Trivedi et al., 2015). Therefore, while overconsumption of calories and unhealthy eating patterns are undoubtedly contributing to obesity and poor health outcomes, diet alone is not the sole reason for these health disparities between rural and urban populations.

Sedentary Behavior in Rural Communities Contributing to Obesity

Current **exercise** guidelines recommend accumulating 150–300 minutes of moderate, 75–150 minutes of vigorous, or an equivalent combination of physical activity, each week for health retention and promotion (*Physical Activity Guidelines for Americans*, 2008). These guidelines also recommend engaging regular strength and flexibility training, which are important for fall prevention and other quality-of-life measures like muscular endurance and stamina (Hart, 2019; Schmid et al., 2018). These guidelines are intended to counteract the decades-long decline in physical activity levels of Americans (Brownson, Boehmer, & Luke, 2005). Despite the known health benefits of regular exercise, a nationally representative sample of U.S. adults estimates that only 19% of rural-community residents meet current exercise guidelines compared with 25% of adults in urban communities (Whitfield et al., 2019). However, those data are self-reported and objective measures of physical activity behavior using accelerometers suggest that a much lower proportion of U.S. adults meet exercise guidelines at closer to 10% among women (Troiano et al., 2008). No physical activity during leisure time was reported in 38.8% of rural individuals compared with 31.8% of urban individuals

(Trivedi et al., 2015). Furthermore, data obtained from NHANES have revealed that when rural residents are physically active, they generally spend more time engaged in low-intensity household physical activity but less time in high-intensity physical activity than their urban counterparts (Fan, Wen, & Kowaleski-Jones, 2014).

It is well established that physical activity trends in rural environments are impacted by the quality and accessibility of where that physical activity is likely to occur, including recreational areas, the workplace, and school (Boehmer, Lovegreen, Haire-Joshu, & Brownson, 2006; Kasehagen, Busacker, Kane, & Rohan, 2012; Kelly et al., 2014; Lo et al., 2017; Perry et al., 2015; Seguin, Lo, Sriram, Connor, & Totta, 2017; Watson, Harris, Carlson, Dorn, & Fulton, 2016). The Rural Active Living Assessment (RALA) tool was developed to evaluate the physical activity environment of rural communities (Yousefian et al., 2010). Studies utilizing the RALA tool have generally described less than ideal physical activity infrastructure, including parks, playgrounds, and sidewalks, in rural communities across the U.S. (Hege, Christiana, Battista, & Parkhurst, 2017; Perry et al., 2015; Robinson et al., 2014; Thomson, Goodman, & Landry, 2019). Therefore, it is commonplace to find suboptimal facilities and opportunities to perform physical activities in rural areas. Despite rural communities acknowledging value in recreational infrastructure for health promotion as well as community aesthetics, costs are often cited as a limitation for the inability to improve or develop these spaces (Chrisman, Nothwehr, Yang, & Oleson, 2015; Cohen et al., 2015; Gunn, Lee, Geelhoed, Shiell, & Giles-Corti, 2014; Kirby, Levesque, Wabano, & Robertson-Wilson, 2007; Knell et al., 2019; Lal et al., 2019; Olsen, 2013).

A persistent labor trend suggests that Americans are spending more time in their daily jobs than previously. Globally, it has been documented that weight gain is associated with long working hours (Virtanen et al., 2019). Obesity is also more prevalent as time on the job increases throughout the week for American workers (Luckhaupt, Cohen, Li, & Calvert, 2014). Those working ≥40 hours/weekly had about 1.4 times greater odds of becoming obese than those who work <40 hours/weekly (Doerrmann, Oancea, & Selya, 2020). With the advancement of labor-saving technology, Americans who are performing less physical activity are, therefore, expending fewer calories in the workplace, potentially contributing to obesity and decreasing overall health and fitness. This is evident in rural communities where agricultural jobs are common and have been greatly impacted by technology. NHANES 1999–2004 shows that employees in the agricultural sector, including farm operators, forestry, and fishing occupations had a higher percentage of workers with lower cardiovascular fitness (Lewis et al., 2011). Additionally, activity levels at work impact leisure activity levels. In a study involving 26,334 women in the United States, low occupational activity was associated with lower leisure-time physical activity (Ekenga, Parks, Wilson, & Sandler, 2015). Considered together, these finding suggest that recent work trends that have reduced or replaced traditional occupations in rural areas may limit expenditure of calories thus promoting an obesogenic environment.

T2DM—Definition, Prevalence, and Etiology

While obesity contributes to a number of chronic diseases (e.g., cardiovascular disease, hypertension, nonalcoholic fatty liver disease), it is the number one risk factor for the development of T2DM (Barnes, 2011; Colditz, Willett, Rotnitzky, & Manson, 1995). T2DM is a metabolic disease characterized by **insulin resistance** accompanied by progressive beta-cell death. Approximately 10% of the U.S. population has been diagnosed (see **Table 8-2**

Exhibit 8-1 Genetics and Epigenetics of Obesity

Obesity has a great component of heritability based on human research, particularly on the strength of pioneering twin and adoption studies (Afshin et al., 2017; Goodarzi, 2018; Silventoinen, Rokholm, Kaprio, & Sorensen, 2010; Singh, Kumar, & Mahalingam, 2017; Young, Graff, Fernandez-Rhodes, & North, 2018). However, there is abundant complexity in how genetics influences obesity. Genetics has been demonstrated to impact several aspects related to weight gain and adipose tissue accumulation, including food-seeking behavior, metabolic rate, lipid storage, penchant for physical activity, among numerous other factors related to physiology and behavior (Gulyaeva, Dempersmier, & Sul, 2019; Lin, Eaton, Manson, & Liu, 2017; O'Rahilly & Farooqi, 2006; Wardle & Cooke, 2008). Though single gene mutations can be associated with an obese phenotype, it is probable that obesity is due to multiple genes (polygenic) contributing sequentially or simultaneously to a microenvironment primed for increased fat storage and weight gain (Farooqi, 2008; Hinney & Hebebrand, 2008). Although it is feasible that genetic changes or mutations can be responsible for obesity, this may not be a practical explanation for the great surge in obesity prevalence in humans over the past few decades. Consequently, epigenetics has become a burgeoning field for scientists to explain the heritability of obesity (Lopomo, Burgio, & Migliore, 2016). Epigenetics is defined as the study of heritable phenotype changes that do not involve alterations in the DNA (Berger, Kouzarides, Shiekhattar, & Shilatifard, 2009; Dupont, Armant, & Brenner, 2009; Jaenisch & Bird, 2003). Environmental factors are widely assumed to impact phenotype; however, some can functionally change the genome of a cell without changing the DNA sequence. Notably, poor or inadequate maternal nutrition can lead to increased DNA methylation or histone modification, which are epigenetic mechanisms associated with metabolic disorders, including obesity and T2DM (Ling & Ronn, 2019; Parrillo et al., 2019; Rees, Hay, Brown, Antipatis, & Palmer, 2000; Stel & Legler, 2015). Endocrine disrupting chemicals (EDCs) have been demonstrated to have an obesogenic impact through an epigenetic mechanism altering cellular nuclear receptors that can lead to adipogenesis (Maradonna & Carnevali, 2018; Ozgyin, Erdos, Bojcsuk, & Balint, 2015). Still a burgeoning field, an epigenetic-based mechanism for obesity might provide future insight into potential therapeutics for obesity and/or its comorbidities.

for diagnostic criteria) with T2DM, and approximately 1 in 3 adults have prediabetes (*National Diabetes Statitics Report, 2020*). Notably, higher rates of obesity in rural communities are accompanied by higher rates of T2DM (*National Diabetes Statitics Report*, 2020; Trivedi et al., 2015). The prevalence of T2DM is 17% higher in rural communities than in urban areas (Bolin et al., 2015; Brown-Guion, Youngerman, Hernandez-Tejada, Dismuke, & Egede, 2013; O'Brien & Denham, 2008). Although the exact mechanisms by which obesity results in insulin resistance and beta-cell death have not been completely elucidated, contributing factors, including increased lipolysis rate (the breakdown of stored fat)

Table 8-2 Clinical Diagnosis of Type 2 Diabetes

Diagnostic Test	Normal	Prediabetes	Type 2 diabetes
Fasting plasma glucose (FPG)	<100 mg/dL	100–125 mg/dL	≥126 mg/dL
Oral glucose tolerance test (OGTT)	<140 mg/dL	140–199 mg/dL	≥200 mg/dL
Hemoglobin A1C (HbA1C)	<5.7%	≥5.7–≤6.4%	>6.5%

Data from the American Diabetes Association.

and a chronic state of low-grade inflammation are more often observed in obese adults (Arner, 2002; Ferrannini, 1995; Goossens, 2017).

The fasting plasma glucose (FPG) test instantly determines blood sugar levels after an 8 hour fast, typically from a finger-prick sample read on a glucometer. An oral glucose tolerance test (OGTT) follows an 8 hour fast and checks your blood sugar levels 2 hours after drinking a standard 8 oz. glucose solution (75g). The HbA1C test is a blood test that provides information of average blood sugar levels over the three previous 3 months and is based on the attachment of glucose to hemoglobin found in red blood cells.

Relationship Between Obesity and T2DM

As previously stated, obesity is a major independent risk factor for T2DM, as the vast majority of people afflicted with T2DM are either overweight or obese (Eckel et al., 2011). Glucose metabolism is regulated by a number of hormones but is largely dependent on the hormone insulin. In nondiabetics, following a meal when blood glucose levels rise, specialized cells in the pancreas, referred to as beta-cells, are stimulated to release insulin. Once released into the blood, insulin promotes glucose absorption into various tissues and organs, most notably skeletal muscle and to a lesser extent the liver and adipose tissue. In healthy, nondiabetic adults, 80% of glucose in each meal is absorbed and stored in skeletal muscle (Defronzo, 2009). However, skeletal muscle glucose uptake is reduced by approximately 40% in T2DM patients who are "insulin resistant" (DeFronzo, Gunnarsson, Bjorkman, Olsson, & Wahren, 1985). Therefore, glucose that would normally be stored in skeletal muscle remains in the blood, contributing to hyperglycemia. The exact mechanism by which obesity contributes to insulin resistance remains unknown. However, two characteristics of obesity, including ectopic lipid accumulation (when lipid accumulation is in an abnormal place or position) and chronic, low-grade inflammation have been highlighted as two potential mediators of insulin resistance.

One way in which obesity contributes to insulin resistance is by disrupting normal lipid storage and release from adipose tissue. When we eat lipid, it is stored in adipose tissue. Conversely, when we are not eating (e.g., at night while sleeping) and during physical activity/exercise, lipid is released from adipose tissue and used for energy production. Importantly, these periods when lipid is released from adipose tissue are temporary and the lipids are almost immediately used (rather than accumulating in the body). However, lipid release is even higher among obese compared with nonobese adults (Horowitz et al., 1999). Additionally, the extra lipid released from adipose tissue is not immediately used but rather accumulates throughout the body, contributing to ectopic lipid accumulation. One of the places where these lipids accumulate is in skeletal muscle. In fact, obese adults have approximately 20% more lipid stored in their skeletal muscle than their nonobese counterparts (Amati et al., 2011). Importantly, accumulation of lipid within skeletal muscle has been shown to directly impair key steps involved in insulin-stimulated glucose uptake (Itani, Ruderman, Schmieder, & Boden, 2002; Ussher et al., 2010).

Obesity also contributes to insulin resistance by promoting a state of low-grade chronic inflammation. Once thought of as simply a storage depot for excess nutrients, it is now understood that adipose tissue can also act as an important paracrine and endocrine organ, secreting inflammatory proteins known to influence insulin resistance (Itoh, Suganami, Hachiya, & Ogawa, 2011; Olefsky & Glass, 2010). The regulation and release of inflammatory proteins from adipose tissue is not completely understood. However, hypertrophy of adipocytes (fat cells), as observed in obesity, induces secretion of proinflammatory proteins (Itoh et al., 2011). Similar to lipid accumulating in skeletal muscle, proinflammatory proteins secreted from adipose tissue are also

---

Exhibit 8-2 Why Don't All T2DM Patients Need to Take Insulin?

As T2DM progresses, it can be accompanied by progressive beta-cell dysfunction (i.e., an inadequate ability to secrete insulin from the pancreas in response to elevated blood glucose levels), ultimately resulting in exogenous insulin therapy. This explains why some T2DM patients are only on oral medications (e.g., biguanides, sulfonylureas) while other patients take insulin in addition or oral agents for glycemic control. Beta-cell dysfunction is detectable early in the diagnosis of T2DM and gets progressively worse over time (Kahn, 2003). In fact, beta-cell dysfunction has even been observed prior to the onset of T2DM in first-degree relatives diagnosed with T2DM, suggesting a genetic component (Knowles, Landchild, Fujimoto, & Kahn, 2002). However, no gene or set of genes has been identified as causing beta-cell dysfunction and thus diabetes. Conversely, an abundance of research exists identifying lipotoxicity and inflammation causing beta-cell dysfunction (Lupi et al., 2002; Oprescu et al., 2007; Prentki, Joly, El-Assaad, & Roduit, 2002). More specifically, when lipid and proinflammatory cytokines accumulate in pancreatic beta-cells (as observed in obesity), it results in beta-cell death. However, this process takes time. Consequently, initiation of insulin therapy is typically observed 10–15 years after the initial diabetes diagnosis (Nathan, 2002). Additionally, it is possible to preserve beta-cell function with medication (e.g., thiazolidinedione), regular exercise, and dietary changes aimed at improving glycemic control (Cerf, 2013). Therefore, with appropriate lifestyle changes and medication compliance, it is possible for some T2DM patients to avoid insulin therapy completely.

---

directly linked to impaired insulin stimulated glucose uptake (Wei et al., 2008).

Additional Health Consequences Associated with T2DM

Unfortunately, T2DM has been associated with or is known to contribute to the progression of numerous other debilitating conditions, including the main cause of death globally, cardiovascular disease (Balakumar, Maung, & Jagadeesh, 2016; Collins et al., 2017). Also, individuals with T2DM often have an increased prevalence of hypertension and associated vascular and microvascular disease (Colberg et al., 2010; Cryer, Horani, & DiPette, 2016; Lamacchia & Sorrentino, 2020; Sasaki et al., 2020; Strain & Paldanius, 2018). Concomitantly, this leads to elevated levels of adult blindness, nontraumatic limb amputation, and renal failure (Braunwald, 2019; Flaxman et al., 2017; Thorud, Plemmons, Buckley, Shibuya, & Jupiter, 2016). Moreover, insulin resistance is thought to be a major contributor to the development of dyslipidemia (Bjornstad & Eckel, 2018; Franssen, Monajemi, Stroes, &

Kastelein, 2011; Jornayvaz, Samuel, & Shulman, 2010; Ormazabal et al., 2018; Wu & Parhofer, 2014), which is associated with several other pathologies, including atherosclerosis, nonalcoholic fatty liver disease, and metabolic syndrome (Akhtar, Iqbal, Vazquez-Montesino, Dennis, & Ahmed, 2019; Gaggini et al., 2013; Grundy, 2016). In addition, the impact of T2DM and insulin resistance is implicated in brain disorders and cognitive impairments (Moheet, Mangia, & Seaquist, 2015; Nguyen, Ta, Nguyen, Le, & Vo, 2020; Sharma et al., 2020; Zilliox, Chadrasekaran, Kwan, & Russell, 2016). With T2DM contributing to numerous conditions and complications, it is imperative that its root source, poor nutrition and sedentary behavior, be seriously treated at various levels of society.

Physical Activity— Benefits, and Barriers

With higher prevalence of obesity and T2DM in rural communities, it is important to identify effective interventions to reduce these health disparities. Importantly, regular physical activity/exercise can improve glycemic control as well as reduce cardiovascular disease risk even in the absence of weight loss (Despres, 2015; Kadoglou et al., 2012; Martinez-Gomez et al., 2019; Neeland, Poirier, & Despres, 2018). However, in addition to the aforementioned environmental and socioeconomic burdens limiting physical activity in rural communities, individual perceptions of physical activity and exercise may be another barrier to overcome in an effort to improve rural health.

Health Benefits of a Physically Active Lifestyle

Regular exercise is recommended for individuals with T2DM to not only reduce cardiovascular disease risk factors like hypertension, dyslipidemia, and inflammation, but also to aid in the maintenance of blood glucose levels, also known as glycemic control (Amanat, Ghahri, Dianatinasab, Fararouei, & Dianatinasab, 2020; Kirwan, Sacks, & Nieuwoudt, 2017; Knudsen & Pedersen, 2015; Mann, Beedie, & Jimenez, 2014; Park, Kim, & Lee, 2020; Pedersen, 2017; Pedersen & Saltin, 2015; Rijal et al., 2019; Sharman, La Gerche, & Coombes, 2015; Sylow, Kleinert, Richter, & Jensen, 2017; Teich, Zaharieva, & Riddell, 2019; Wang & Xu, 2017). Exercise can improve glycemic control by reducing insulin resistance, the underlying cause of T2DM. In healthy, nondiabetic individuals, insulin stimulates glucose uptake into insulin sensitive tissues (e.g., skeletal muscle, adipose tissue, liver), in a process referred to as "insulin-mediated glucose uptake." However, among T2DM patients, insulin-mediated glucose uptake is reduced by upwards of 40% (Abdul-Ghani & DeFronzo, 2010; DeFronzo & Ferrannini, 1991; Stanford & Goodyear, 2014). Importantly, just a single session of exercise has been shown to improve insulin-mediated glucose uptake in T2DM in patients (Braun, Zimmermann, & Kretchmer, 1995; Devlin, Hirshman, Horton, & Horton, 1987; Newsom, Everett, Hinko, & Horowitz, 2013; Oguri, Adachi, Ohno, Oshima, & Kurabayashi, 2009) as well as those at increased risk of developing T2DM (Devlin & Horton, 1985; Nelson & Horowitz, 2014). Additionally, glycemic control has also been shown to occur independent of insulin in skeletal muscle, due to increased muscle contraction (Borghouts & Keizer, 2000; Buresh, 2014; Hawley, 2004; Hayashi, Wojtaszewski, & Goodyear, 1997; Stanford & Goodyear, 2014; Sylow et al., 2017; Wiernsperger, 2005). Taken together, this underscores the importance of performing physical activity and regular exercise for individuals with or at risk for T2DM. Consequently, in addition to performing regular exercise, it important to avoid prolonged periods of sedentary behavior, including sitting, which can further one's risk for T2DM (Asvold, Midthjell, Krokstad, Rangul, & Bauman, 2017; Bailey, Hewson, Champion, & Sayegh, 2019; Biswas et al., 2015; Chau et al., 2013; Dempsey et al., 2016; Duvivier et al., 2017; Wilmot et al., 2012). Finally, there is also evidence to suggest that regular exercise can increase pancreatic beta-cell insulin secretion in T2DM patients (Bloem & Chang, 2008). Collectively, these data underscore the importance of promoting a physically active lifestyle for individuals with T2DM.

While exercise can aid in glycemic control, exercise can also cause and/or exacerbate complications associated with T2DM, including hypoglycemia (i.e., low blood glucose) and ketoacidosis (i.e., accumulation of blood ketones accompanied by a drop in blood pH). Therefore, certain precautions should be considered when diabetic patients exercise. First, as previously discussed, exercise causes skeletal muscle to absorb glucose. Importantly, glucose absorption into skeletal muscle is directly proportional to exercise intensity (Rose & Richter, 2005). Unfortunately, this can stimulate further production of ketones intensifying ketoacidosis. Additionally, it is common for T2DM patients to be on one or more glucose-lowering medications. Unfortunately, when exercise is paired with glucose-lowering medications, specifically insulin or a medication that promotes insulin secretion (e.g., GLP-1 receptor agonists) can cause or worsen hypoglycemia. Despite these concerns, with proper blood glucose monitoring, complications related to hypoglycemia and ketoacidosis can be avoided.

Perceived Barriers/ Motivators to Physical Activity in Rural Communities

Engaging rural community members in physical activity/exercise in rural communities comes with its own unique set of challenges that must be overcome in order to promote health (Aronson & Oman, 2004; Boehm et al., 2013; Bopp, Wilcox, Oberrecht, Kammermann, & McElmurray, 2004; Dye & Wilcox, 2006; Walia & Leipert, 2012; Wilcox, Bopp, Oberrecht, Kammermann, & McElmurray, 2003; Wilcox, Oberrecht, Bopp, Kammermann, & McElmurray, 2005). For example, men in rural areas believe that they get "enough exercise at work"; therefore, they do not feel the need to exercise in a nonwork setting (Gavarkovs, Burke, & Petrella, 2017). In addition, survey responses such as "I'm too tired" and "I don't have enough time" are frequent explanations for lack of participation in formal exercise. On the contrary, rural men report a desire to be healthier and support from family/friends promotes exercise, suggesting that if more opportunities for physical activity were presented, they would exercise more (Gavarkovs et al., 2017). Women in rural communities report a different set of barriers and motivators to a physically active lifestyle compared with their male counterparts. Specifically, lack of motivation, tiredness, and cold-weather-related problems are perceived barriers to physical activity among rural women (Cadmus-Bertram, Gorzelitz,

Dorn, & Malecki, 2019). Notably, women in rural communities are interested in particular physical activities, specifically walking, yoga, and strength training (Cadmus-Bertram et al., 2019). Collectively, this suggests that in addition to providing appropriate infrastructure, individual perceived barriers to physical activity/exercise should also be considered for promoting physically active lifestyles in rural communities. Furthermore, interventions to promote a physically active lifestyle should also be aimed at capitalizing on individual motivators, including support systems and modality of exercise.

Chapter Summary

Obesity prevalence has been consistently reported as higher in rural (34-41%) versus urban (29–34%) communities. While the causes of obesity are complex and multifactorial, poor dietary habits contributing to excess calorie consumption and increased sedentary behavior are the main reasons for the tremendous rise in U.S. obesity rates. Notably, limited accessibility of nutritionally dense foods and decreased levels of physical activity are common among residents in rural communities. Additionally, meaningful sociodemographic and environmental differences in rural versus urban communities have supported sedentary behavior contributing to weight gain and ultimately obesity. Consequently, the higher prevalence of obesity in rural U.S. communities has led to several rural-urban health disparities, including a higher prevalence of T2DM. Importantly, engagement in healthy behaviors, including regular physical activity is vital to reducing health disparities in rural communities. However, community infrastructure as well as individual perceptions of barriers and motivators to engagement in a physically active lifestyle must be considered when developing interventions aimed at U.S. rural health promotion and disease prevention.

Discussion Questions

1. What are some of the rates and causes of obesity in the United States, and what are some specific concerns for rural America?
2. Which factors may contribute to obesity and other chronic health issues in rural settings?
3. How can physical activity mitigate obesity-related health concerns, including type 2 diabetes?
4. As a rural health educator, what do you believe are unique barriers to achieving healthy lifestyles in your service area?

Student Activities and Worksheets are available inside the Navigate eBook, included with the printed text. Simply redeem the access code found at the front of the book at www.jblearning.com.

References

Abdul-Ghani, M. A., & DeFronzo, R. A. (2010). Pathogenesis of insulin resistance in skeletal muscle. *BioMed Research International, 2010*, 476279. http://dx.doi.org/10.1155/2010/476279

Afshin, A., Peñalvo, J. L., Del Gobbo, L., Silva, J., Michaelson, M., O'Flaherty, M., . . . Mozaffarian, D. (2017). The prospective impact of food pricing on improving dietary consumption: A systematic review and meta-analysis. *PLoS One, 12*(3), e0172277. http://dx.doi.org/10.1371/journal.pone.0172277

Akhtar, D. H., Iqbal, U., Vazquez-Montesino, L. M., Dennis, B. B., & Ahmed, A. (2019). Pathogenesis of insulin resistance and atherogenic dyslipidemia in nonalcoholic fatty liver disease. *Journal of Clinical Translational Hepatology, 7*(4), 362–370. http://dx.doi.org/10.14218/JCTH.2019.00028

Albuquerque, D., Nóbrega, C., Manco, L., & Padez, C. (2017). The contribution of genetics and environment to obesity. *British Medical Bulletin, 123*(1), 159–173. http://dx.doi.org/10.1093/bmb/ldx022

Amanat, S., Ghahri, S., Dianatinasab, A., Fararouei, M., & Dianatinasab, M. (2020). Exercise and type 2 Diabetes. *Physical Exercise for Human Health, 1228*, 91–105. http://dx.doi.org/10.1007/978-981-15-1792-1_6

Amati, F., Dube, J. J., Alvarez-Carnero, E., Edreira, M. M., Chomentowski, P., Coen, P. M., . . . Goodpaster, B. H. (2011). Skeletal muscle triglycerides, diacylglycerols, and ceramides in insulin resistance: Another paradox in endurance-trained athletes? *Diabetes, 60*(10), 2588–2597. http://dx.doi.org/10.2337/db10-1221

An, R. (2016). Fast-food and full-service restaurant consumption and daily energy and nutrient intakes in US adults. *European Journal of Clinical Nutrition, 70*(1), 97–103. http://dx.doi.org/10.1038/ejcn.2015.104

Apovian, C. M. (2016). Obesity: Definition, comorbidities, causes, and burden. *American Journal of Managed Care, 22*(7 Suppl), s176–185.

Arner, P. (2002). Insulin resistance in type 2 diabetes: Role of fatty acids. *Diabetes Metabolism Research and Reviews, 18*(Suppl 2), S5–S9. http://dx.doi.org/10.1002/dmrr.254

Aronson, R. E., & Oman, R. F. (2004). Views on exercise and physical activity among rural-dwelling senior citizens. *The Journal of Rural Health, 20*(1), 76–79. http://dx.doi.org/10.1111/j.1748-0361.2004.tb00010.x

Åsvold, B. O., Midthjell, K., Krokstad, S., Rangul, V., & Bauman, A. (2017). Prolonged sitting may increase diabetes risk in physically inactive individuals: An 11 year follow-up of the HUNT Study, Norway. *Diabetologia, 60*(5), 830–835. http://dx.doi.org/10.1007/s00125-016-4193-z

Bailey, D. P., Hewson, D. J., Champion, R. B., & Sayegh, S. M. (2019). Sitting time and risk of cardiovascular disease and diabetes: A systematic review and meta-analysis. *American Journal of Preventive Medicine, 57*(3), 408–416. http://dx.doi.org/10.1016/j.amepre.2019.04.015

Balakumar, P., Maung, U. K., & Jagadeesh, G. (2016). Prevalence and prevention of cardiovascular disease and diabetes mellitus. *Pharmacological Research, 113*(Pt A), 600–609. http://dx.doi.org/10.1016/j.phrs.2016.09.040

Barnes, A. S. (2011). The epidemic of obesity and diabetes: Trends and treatments. *Texas Heart Institute Journal, 38*(2), 142–144.

Baum, S., Kurose, C., & McPherson, M. (2013). An overview of American higher education. *The Future of Children, 23*(1), 17–39. http://dx.doi.org/10.1353/foc.2013.0008

Befort, C. A., Nazir, N., & Perri, M. G. (2012). Prevalence of obesity among adults from rural and urban areas of the United States: Findings from NHANES (2005-2008). *The Journal of Rural Health, 28*(4), 392–397. http://dx.doi.org/10.1111/j.1748-0361.2012.00411.x

Bennett, K. J., Probst, J. C., & Pumkam, C. (2011). Obesity among working age adults: The role of county-level persistent poverty in rural disparities. *Health & Place, 17*(5), 1174–1181. http://dx.doi.org/10.1016/j.health place.2011.05.012

Bentley, J. (2017). *U.S. trends in food availability and a dietary assessment of loss-adjusted food availability, 1970-2014* (166). Retrieved from https://www.ers .usda.gov/webdocs/publications/82220/eib-166 .pdf?v=42762%20

Berger, S. L., Kouzarides, T., Shiekhattar, R., & Shilatifard, A. (2009). An operational definition of epigenetics. *Genes & Development, 23*(7), 781–783. http://dx.doi .org/10.1101/gad.1787609

Bilal, U., Auchincloss, A. H., & Diez-Roux, A. V. (2018). Neighborhood environments and diabetes risk and control. *Current Diabetes Reports, 18*(62). http://dx .doi.org/10.1007/s11892-018-1032-2

Biswas, A., Oh, P. I., Faulkner, G. E., Bajaj, R. R., Silver, M. A., Mitchell, M. S., & Alter, D. A. (2015). Sedentary time and its association with risk for disease incidence, mortality, and hospitalization in adults: A systematic review and meta-analysis. *Annals of Internal Medicine, 162*(2), 123–132. http://dx.doi .org/10.7326/M14-1651

Bjornstad, P., & Eckel, R. H. (2018). Pathogenesis of lipid disorders in insulin resistance: A brief review. *Current Diabetes Reports, 18*(127). http://dx.doi.org/10.1007 /s11892-018-1101-6

Bloem, C. J., & Chang, A. M. (2008). Short-term exercise improves beta-cell function and insulin resistance in older people with impaired glucose tolerance. *The Journal of Clinical Endocrinology & Metabolism, 93*(2), 387–392. http://dx.doi.org/10.1210/jc.2007 -1734

Boehm, J., Franklin, R. C., Newitt, R., McFarlane, K., Grant, T., & Kurkowski, B. (2013). Barriers and motivators to exercise for older adults: A focus on those living in rural and remote areas of Australia. *The Australian Journal of Rural Health, 21*(3), 141–149. http://dx.doi.org/10.1111/ajr.12032

Boehmer, T. K., Lovegreen, S. L., Haire-Joshu, D., & Brownson, R. C. (2006). What constitutes an obesogenic environment in rural communities? *American Journal of Health Promotion, 20*(6), 411–421. http:// dx.doi.org/10.4278/0890-1171-20.6.411

Bolin, J. N., Bellamy, G. R., Ferdinand, A. O., Vuong, A. M., Kash, B. A., Schulze, A., & Helduser, J. W. (2015). Rural Healthy People 2020: New decade, same challenges. *The Journal of Rural Health, 31*(3), 326–333. http://dx.doi.org/10.1111/jrh.12116

Bopp, M., Wilcox, S., Oberrecht, L., Kammermann, S., & McElmurray, C. T. (2004). Correlates of strength training in older rural African American and Caucasian women. *Women & Health, 40*(1), 1–20. doi:10.1300 /J013v40n01_01

Borghouts, L. B., & Keizer, H. A. (2000). Exercise and insulin sensitivity: A review. *International Journal of Sports Medicine, 21*(1), 1–12. doi:10.1055/s-2000-8847

Bove, C. F., & Olson, C. M. (2006). Obesity in low-income rural women: Qualitative insights about physical activity and eating patterns. *Women & Health, 44*(1), 57–78. doi:10.1300/J013v44n01_04

Braun, B., Zimmermann, M. B., & Kretchmer, N. (1995). Effects of exercise intensity on insulin sensitivity in women with non-insulin-dependent diabetes mellitus. *Journal of Applied Physiology (1995), 78*(1), 300–306. doi:10.1152/jappl.1995.78.1.300

Braunwald, E. (2019). Diabetes, heart failure, and renal dysfunction: The vicious circles. *Progress in Cardiovascular Diseases, 62*(4), 298–302. doi:10.1016/j.pcad .2019.07.003

Brown-Guion, S. Y., Youngerman, S. M., Hernandez-Tejada, M. A., Dismuke, C. E., & Egede, L. E. (2013). Racial/ethnic, regional, and rural/urban differences in receipt of diabetes education. *The Diabetes Educator, 39*(3), 327–334. doi:10.1177/0145721713480002

Brownson, R. C., Boehmer, T. K., & Luke, D. A. (2005). Declining rates of physical activity in the United States: What are the contributors? *Annual Review of Public Health, 26*, 421–443. doi:10.1146/annurev .publhealth.26.021304.144437

Buresh, R. (2014). Exercise and glucose control. *The Journal of Sports Medicine and Physical Fitness, 54*(4), 373–382.

Cadmus-Bertram, L. A., Gorzelitz, J. S., Dorn, D. C., & Malecki, K. M. C. (2019). Understanding the physical activity needs and interests of inactive and active rural women: A cross-sectional study of barriers, opportunities, and intervention preferences. *Journal of Behavioral Medicine.* doi:10.1007/s10865-019-00070-z

Casagrande, S. S., & Cowie, C. C. (2017). Trends in dietary intake among adults with type 2 diabetes: NHANES 1988–2012. *Journal of Human Nutrition and Dietetics, 30*(4), 479–489. doi:10.1111/jhn.12443

Cerf, M. E. (2013). Beta cell dysfunction and insulin resistance. *Frontiers in Endocrinology, 4*, 37. doi:10.3389 /fendo.2013.00037

Champagne, C. M., Bogle, M. L., McGee, B. B., Yadrick, K., Allen, H. R., Kramer, T. R., . . . Lower Mississippi Delta Nutrition Intervention Research, I. (2004). Dietary intake in the lower Mississippi delta region: Results from the foods of our Delta Study. *Journal of the American Dietetic Association, 104*(2), 199–207. doi:10.1016/j.jada.2003.11.011

Chau, J. Y., Grunseit, A. C., Chey, T., Stamatakis, E., Brown, W. J., Matthews, C. E., . . . van der Ploeg, H. P. (2013). Daily sitting time and all-cause mortality: A meta-analysis. *PLoS One, 8*(11), e80000. doi:10.1371 /journal.pone.0080000

Chea, H., & Kim, H. (2020). Examining spatial disparities of obesity: Residential segregation and the urban-rural divide. *The Professional Geographer, 72*(2), 206–218. doi:10.1080/00330124.2019.1676800

Chrisman, M., Nothwehr, F., Yang, G., & Oleson, J. (2015). Environmental influences on physical activity in rural Midwestern adults: A qualitative approach. *Health Promotion Practice, 16*(1), 142–148. doi:10.1177/1524839914524958

Cohen, D. A., Han, B., Isacoff, J., Shulaker, B., Williamson, S., Marsh, T., . . . Bhatia, R. (2015). Impact of park renovations on park use and park-based physical activity. *Journal of Physical Activity and Health, 12*(2), 289–295. doi:10.1123/jpah.2013-0165

Cohen, S. A., Cook, S. K., Kelley, L., Foutz, J. D., & Sando, T. A. (2017). A closer look at rural-urban health disparities: Associations between obesity and rurality vary by geospatial and sociodemographic factors. *The Journal of Rural Health, 33*(2), 167–179. doi:10.1111/jrh.12207

Cohen, S. A., Greaney, M. L., & Sabik, N. J. (2018). Assessment of dietary patterns, physical activity and obesity from a national survey: Rural-urban health disparities in older adults. *PLoS One, 13*(12), e0208268. doi:10.1371/journal.pone.0208268

Colberg, S. R., Sigal, R. J., Fernhall, B., Regensteiner, J. G., Blissmer, B. J., Rubin, R. R., . . . Braun, B. (2010). Exercise and type 2 diabetes: The American College of Sports Medicine and the American Diabetes Association: Joint position statement. *Diabetes Care, 33*(12), e147–167. doi:10.2337/dc10-9990

Colditz, G. A., Willett, W. C., Rotnitzky, A., & Manson, J. E. (1995). Weight gain as a risk factor for clinical diabetes mellitus in women. *Annals of Internal Medicine, 122*(7), 481–486. doi:10.7326/0003-4819-122-7-199504010-00001

Collins, D. R., Tompson, A. C., Onakpoya, I. J., Roberts, N., Ward, A. M., & Heneghan, C. J. (2017). Global cardiovascular risk assessment in the primary prevention of cardiovascular disease in adults: Systematic review of systematic reviews. *BMJ Open, 7*(3), e013650. doi:10.1136/bmjopen-2016-013650

Cryer, M. J., Horani, T., & DiPette, D. J. (2016). Diabetes and hypertension: A comparative review of current guidelines. *Journal of Clinical Hypertension (Greenwich), 18*(2), 95–100. doi:10.1111/jch.12638

Defronzo, R. A. (2009). Banting Lecture. From the triumvirate to the ominous octet: A new paradigm for the treatment of type 2 diabetes mellitus. *Diabetes, 58*(4), 773–795. doi:10.2337/db09-9028

DeFronzo, R. A., & Ferrannini, E. (1991). Insulin resistance. A multifaceted syndrome responsible for NIDDM, obesity, hypertension, dyslipidemia, and atherosclerotic cardiovascular disease. *Diabetes Care, 14*(3), 173–194. doi:10.2337/diacare.14.3.173

DeFronzo, R. A., Gunnarsson, R., Björkman, O., Olsson, M., & Wahren, J. (1985). Effects of insulin on peripheral and splanchnic glucose metabolism in noninsulin-dependent (type II) diabetes mellitus. *Journal of Clinical Investigation, 76*(1), 149–155. doi:10.1172/JCI111938

Dempsey, P. C., Larsen, R. N., Sethi, P., Sacre, J. W., Straznicky, N. E., Cohen, N. D., . . . Dunstan, D. W. (2016). Benefits for type 2 diabetes of interrupting prolonged sitting with brief bouts of light walking or simple resistance activities. *Diabetes Care, 39*(6), 964–972. doi:10.2337/dc15-2336

Despres, J. P. (2015). Obesity and cardiovascular disease: Weight loss is not the only target. *Canadian Journal of Cardiology, 31*(2), 216–222. doi:10.1016/j.cjca.2014.12.009

Devlin, J. T., Hirshman, M., Horton, E. D., & Horton, E. S. (1987). Enhanced peripheral and splanchnic insulin sensitivity in NIDDM men after single bout of exercise. *Diabetes, 36*(4), 434–439. doi:10.2337/diab.36.4.434

Devlin, J. T., & Horton, E. S. – (1985). Effects of prior high-intensity exercise on glucose metabolism in normal and insulin-resistant men. *Diabetes, 34*(10), 973–979. doi:10.2337/diab.34.10.973

Dietary guidelines for Americans, 2015–2020. (2015). Retrieved from https://www.dietaryguidelines.gov/sites/default/files/2019-05/2015-2020_Dietary_Guidelines.pdf

Doerrmann, C., Oancea, S. C., & Selya, A. (2020). The Association between hours spent at work and obesity status: Results from NHANES 2015 to 2016. *American Journal of Health Promotion, 34*(4), 359–365. doi:10.1177/0890117119897189

Duffey, K. J., & Popkin, B. M. (2011). Energy density, portion size, and eating occasions: Contributions to increased energy intake in the United States, 1977–2006. *PLoS Med, 8*(6), e1001050. doi:10.1371/journal.pmed.1001050

Duffey, K. J., & Popkin, B. M. (2013). Causes of increased energy intake among children in the U.S., 1977–2010. *American Journal of Preventive Medicine, 44*(2), e1–e8. doi:10.1016/j.amepre.2012.10.011

Dupont, C., Armant, D. R., & Brenner, C. A. (2009). Epigenetics: Definition, mechanisms and clinical perspective. *Seminars in Reproductive Medicine, 27*(5), 351–357. doi:10.1055/s-0029-1237423

Duvivier, B. M., Schaper, N. C., Hesselink, M. K., van Kan, L., Stienen, N., Winkens, B., . . . Savelberg, H. H. (2017). Breaking sitting with light activities vs structured exercise: A randomised crossover study demonstrating benefits for glycaemic control and insulin sensitivity in type 2 diabetes. *Diabetologia, 60*(3), 490–498. doi:10.1007/s00125-016-4161-7

Dye, C. J., & Wilcox, S. (2006). Beliefs of low-income and rural older women regarding physical activity: You have to want to make your life better. *Women & Health, 43*(1), 115–134. doi:10.1300/J013v43n01_07

Dye, L., Boyle, N. B., Champ, C., & Lawton, C. (2017). The relationship between obesity and cognitive health and decline. *Proceedings of the Nutrition Society, 76*(4), 443–454. doi:10.1017/S0029665117002014

Eckel, R. H., Kahn, S. E., Ferrannini, E., Goldfine, A. B., Nathan, D. M., Schwartz, M. W., . . . Smith, S. R. (2011). Obesity and type 2 diabetes: What can be unified and what needs to be individualized? *The Journal of Clinical Endocrinology & Metabolism, 96*(6), 1654–1663. doi:10.1210/jc.2011-0585

Ekenga, C. C., Parks, C. G., Wilson, L. E., & Sandler, D. P. (2015). Leisure-time physical activity in relation to occupational physical activity among women. *Preventive Medicine, 74*, 93–96. doi:10.1016/j.ypmed .2015.03.003

Fan, J. X., Wen, M., & Kowaleski-Jones, L. (2014). Rural-urban differences in objective and subjective measures of physical activity: Findings from the National Health and Nutrition Examination Survey (NHANES) 2003-2006. *Preventing Chronic Disease, 11*, E141. doi:10.5888/pcd11.140189

Farooqi, I. S. (2008). Monogenic human obesity. *Frontiers in Hormonal Research, 36*, 1–11. doi:10.1159 /000115333

Ferrannini, E. (1995). Physiological and metabolic consequences of obesity. *Metabolism, 44*(9 Suppl 3), 15–17. doi:10.1016/0026-0495(95)90313-5

Finkelstein, E. A., Strombotne, K. L., Zhen, C., & Epstein, L. H. (2014). Food prices and obesity: A review. *Advances in Nutrition, 5*(6), 818–821. doi:10.3945/an.114.007088

Flaxman, S. R., Bourne, R. R. A., Resnikoff, S., Ackland, P., Braithwaite, T., Cicinelli, M. V., . . . Vision Loss Expert Group of the Global Burden of Disease, S. (2017). Global causes of blindness and distance vision impairment 1990-2020: A systematic review and meta-analysis. *Lancet Global Health, 5*(12), e1221–e1234. doi:10.1016/S2214-109X(17)30393-5

Franssen, R., Monajemi, H., Stroes, E. S., & Kastelein, J. J. (2011). Obesity and dyslipidemia. *Medical Clinics of North America, 95*(5), 893–902. doi: S0025-7125(11)00061-7 [pii]10.1016/j.mcna.2011 .06.003

Gaggini, M., Morelli, M., Buzzigoli, E., DeFronzo, R. A., Bugianesi, E., & Gastaldelli, A. (2013). Non-alcoholic fatty liver disease (NAFLD) and its connection with insulin resistance, dyslipidemia, atherosclerosis and coronary heart disease. *Nutrients, 5*(5), 1544–1560. doi:10.3390/nu5051544

Gavarkovs, A. G., Burke, S. M., & Petrella, R. J. (2017). The physical activity-related barriers and facilitators perceived by men living in rural communities. *American Journal of Men's Health, 11*(4), 1130–1132. doi:10.1177/1557988315598368

Giskes, K., van Lenthe, F., Avendano-Pabon, M., & Brug, J. (2011). A systematic review of environmental factors and obesogenic dietary intakes among adults: Are we getting closer to understanding obesogenic environments? *Obesity Reviews, 12*(5), e95–e106. doi:10.1111/j.1467-789X.2010.00769.x

Goodarzi, M. O. (2018). Genetics of obesity: What genetic association studies have taught us about the biology of obesity and its complications. *Lancet Diabetes Endocrinol, 6*(3), 223–236. doi:10.1016/S2213-8587 (17)30200-0

Goossens, G. H. (2017). The Metabolic phenotype in obesity: Fat mass, body fat distribution, and adipose tissue function. *Obesity Facts, 10*(3), 207–215. doi:10.1159/000471488

Gordon-Larsen, P., The, N. S., & Adair, L. S. (2010). Longitudinal trends in obesity in the United States from adolescence to the third decade of life. *Obesity (Silver Spring), 18*(9), 1801–1804. doi:10.1038 /oby.2009.451

Grundy, S. M. (2016). Metabolic syndrome update. *Trends in Cardiovascular Medicine, 26*(4), 364–373. doi:10.1016/j.tcm.2015.10.004

Gulyaeva, O., Dempersmier, J., & Sul, H. S. (2019). Genetic and epigenetic control of adipose development. *Biochimica Biophysica Acta (BBA) - Molecular Cell Biology of Lipids, 1864*(1), 3–12. doi:10.1016/j .bbalip.2018.04.016

Gunn, L. D., Lee, Y., Geelhoed, E., Shiell, A., & Giles-Corti, B. (2014). The cost-effectiveness of installing sidewalks to increase levels of transport-walking and health. *Preventive Medicine, 67*, 322–329. doi:10 .1016/j.ypmed.2014.07.041

Hales, C. M., Carroll, M. D., Fryar, C. D., & Odgen, C. L. (2020). Prevalence of obesity and severe obesity among adults: United States, 2017 – 2018. *NCHS Data Brief* (360).

Hales, C. M., Fryar, C. D., Carroll, M. D., Freedman, D. S., & Ogden, C. L. (2018). Trends in obesity and severe obesity prevalence in us youth and adults by sex and age, 2007–2008 to 2015–2016. *JAMA, 319*(16), 1723–1725. doi:10.1001/jama.2018.3060

Hansen, A. Y., Umstattd Meyer, M. R., Lenardson, J. D., & Hartley, D. (2015). Built environments and active living in rural and remote areas: A review of the literature. *Current Obesity Reports, 4*(4), 484–493. doi:10.1007/s13679-015-0180-9

Hart, P. D. (2019). Grip strength and health-related quality of life in U.S. adult males. *Journal of Lifestyle Medicine, 9*(2), 102–110. doi:10.15280/jlm.2019 .9.2.102

Haveman, R., & Smeeding, T. (2006). The role of higher education in social mobility. *The Future of Children, 16*(2), 125–150. doi:10.1353/foc.2006.0015

Hawley, J. A. (2004). Exercise as a therapeutic intervention for the prevention and treatment of insulin resistance. *Diabetes Metabolism Research and Reviews, 20*(5), 383–393. doi:10.1002/dmrr.505

Hayashi, T., Wojtaszewski, J. F., & Goodyear, L. J. (1997). Exercise regulation of glucose transport in skeletal muscle. *American Journal of Physiology, 273*(6), E1039–E1051. doi:10.1152/ajpendo.1997.273.6.E1039

Hege, A., Christiana, R. W., Battista, R., & Parkhurst, H. (2017). Active living in rural Appalachia: Using the rural active living assessment (RALA) tools to explore environmental barriers. *Preventive Medicine Reports, 8*, 261–266. doi:10.1016/j.pmedr.2017.11.007

Hill, J. L., You, W., & Zoellner, J. M. (2014). Disparities in obesity among rural and urban residents in a health disparate region. *BMC Public Health, 14*, 1051. doi:10.1186/1471-2458-14-1051

Hinney, A., & Hebebrand, J. (2008). Polygenic obesity in humans. *Obesity Facts, 1*(1), 35–42. doi:10.1159/000113935

Horowitz, J. F., Coppack, S. W., Paramore, D., Cryer, P. E., Zhao, G., & Klein, S. (1999). Effect of short-term fasting on lipid kinetics in lean and obese women. *American Journal of Physiology, 276*(2), E278–E284. doi:10.1152/ajpendo.1999.276.2.E278

Itani, S. I., Ruderman, N. B., Schmieder, F., & Boden, G. (2002). Lipid-induced insulin resistance in human muscle is associated with changes in diacylglycerol, protein kinase C, and IkappaB-alpha. *Diabetes, 51*(7), 2005–2011. doi:10.2337/diabetes.51.7.2005

Itoh, M., Suganami, T., Hachiya, R., & Ogawa, Y. (2011). Adipose tissue remodeling as homeostatic inflammation. *International Journal of Inflammation, 2011*, 720926. doi:10.4061/2011/720926

Jaenisch, R., & Bird, A. (2003). Epigenetic regulation of gene expression: How the genome integrates intrinsic and environmental signals. *Nature Genetics, 33 Suppl*, 245–254. doi:10.1038/ng1089

Jornayvaz, F. R., Samuel, V. T., & Shulman, G. I. (2010). The role of muscle insulin resistance in the pathogenesis of atherogenic dyslipidemia and nonalcoholic fatty liver disease associated with the metabolic syndrome. *Annual Reviews of Nutrition, 30*, 273–290. doi:10.1146/annurev.nutr.012809.104726

Kadoglou, N. P., Vrabas, I. S., Kapelouzou, A., Lampropoulos, S., Sailer, N., Kostakis, A., . . . Angelopoulou, N. (2012). The impact of aerobic exercise training on novel adipokines, apelin and ghrelin, in patients with type 2 diabetes. *Medical Science Monitor, 18*(5), CR290295. doi:10.12659/msm.882734

Kahn, S. E. (2003). The relative contributions of insulin resistance and beta-cell dysfunction to the pathophysiology of Type 2 diabetes. *Diabetologia, 46*(1), 3–19. doi:10.1007/s00125-002-1009-0

Kasehagen, L., Busacker, A., Kane, D., & Rohan, A. (2012). Associations between neighborhood characteristics and physical activity among youth within rural-urban commuting areas in the US. *Maternal and Child Health Journal, (16 Suppl 2)*, 258–267. doi:10.1007/s10995-012-1188-3

Katzmarzyk, P. T., Powell, K. E., Jakicic, J. M., Troiano, R. P., Piercy, K., Tennant, B., & Physical Activity Guidelines Advisory, C. (2019). Sedentary behavior and health: Update from the 2018 Physical Activity Guidelines Advisory Committee. *Medical & Science in Sports & Exercise, 51*(6), 1227–1241. doi:10.1249/MSS.0000000000001935

Kelly, C., Wilson, J. S., Schootman, M., Clennin, M., Baker, E. A., & Miller, D. K. (2014). The built environment predicts observed physical activity. *Frontiers in Public Health, 2*, 52. doi:10.3389/fpubh.2014.00052

Kirby, A. M., Levesque, L., Wabano, V., & Robertson-Wilson, J. (2007). Perceived community environment and physical activity involvement in a northern-rural Aboriginal community. *International Journal of Behavioral Nutrition and Physical Activity, 4*, 63. doi:10.1186/1479-5868-4-63

Kirwan, J. P., Sacks, J., & Nieuwoudt, S. (2017). The essential role of exercise in the management of type 2 diabetes. *Cleveland Clinic Journal of Medicine, 84*(7 Suppl 1), S15–S21. doi:10.3949/ccjm.84.s1.03

Knell, G., Brown, H. S., Gabriel, K. P., Durand, C. P., Shuval, K., Salvo, D., & Kohl, H. W., 3rd. (2019). Cost-effectiveness of improvements to the built environment intended to increase physical activity. *Journal of Physical Activity and Health, 16*(5), 308–317. doi:10.1123/jpah.2018-0329

Knowles, N. G., Landchild, M. A., Fujimoto, W. Y., & Kahn, S. E. (2002). Insulin and amylin release are both diminished in first-degree relatives of subjects with type 2 diabetes. *Diabetes Care, 25*(2), 292–297. doi:10.2337/diacare.25.2.292

Knudsen, S. H., & Pedersen, B. K. (2015). Targeting inflammation through a physical active lifestyle and pharmaceuticals for the treatment of type 2 diabetes. *Current Diabetes Reports, 15*(10), 82. doi:10.1007/s11892-015-0642-1

Lal, A., Moodie, M., Abbott, G., Carver, A., Salmon, J., Giles-Corti, B., . . . Veitch, J. (2019). The impact of a park refurbishment in a low socioeconomic area on physical activity: A cost-effectiveness study. *International Journal of Behavioral Nutrition and Physical Activity, 16*(1), 26. doi:10.1186/s12966-019-0786-5

Lamacchia, O., & Sorrentino, M. R. (2020). Diabetes mellitus, arterial stiffness and cardiovascular disease: Clinical implications and the influence of SGLT2i. *Current Vascular Pharmacology*. doi:10.2174/1570161118666200317150359

Lega, I. C., & Lipscombe, L. L. (2020). Review: Diabetes, obesity, and cancer-pathophysiology and clinical implications. *Endocrine Reviews, 41*(1). doi:10.1210/endrev/bnz014

Lenardson, J. D., Hansen, A. Y., & Hartley, D. (2015). Rural and remote food environments and obesity. *Current Obesity Reports, 4*(1), 46–53. doi:10.1007/s13679-014-0136-5

Lewis, J. E., Clark, J. D., 3rd, LeBlanc, W. G., Fleming, L. E., Caban-Martinez, A. J., Arheart, K. L., . . . Lee, D. J.

(2011). Cardiovascular fitness levels among American workers. *Journal of Occupational and Environmental Medicine, 53*(10), 1115—1121. doi:10.1097/JOM .0b013e31822cfe8e

Lin, X., Eaton, C. B., Manson, J. E., & Liu, S. (2017). The Genetics of Physical Activity. *Current Cardiology Reports, 19*(119). doi:10.1007/s11886-017-0938-7

Ling, C., & Rönn, T. (2019). Epigenetics in human obesity and type 2 diabetes. *Cell Metabolism, 29*(5), 1028–1044. doi:10.1016/j.cmet.2019.03.009

Lo, B. K., Morgan, E. H., Folta, S. C., Graham, M. L., Paul, L. C., Nelson, M. E., . . . Seguin, R. A. (2017). Environmental influences on physical activity among rural adults in montana, United States: Views from built environment audits, resident focus groups, and key informant interviews. *International Journal of Environmental Research and Public Health, 14*(10). doi:10.3390/ijerph14101173

Lopomo, A., Burgio, E., & Migliore, L. (2016). Epigenetics of Obesity. *Progress in Molecular Biology and Translational Science, 140,* 151–184. doi:10.1016/bs.pmbts .2016.02.002

Luckhaupt, S. E., Cohen, M. A., Li, J., & Calvert, G. M. (2014). Prevalence of obesity among U.S. workers and associations with occupational factors. *American Journal of Preventive Medicine, 46*(3), 237–248. doi:10 .1016/j.amepre.2013.11.002

Lundeen, E. A., Park, S., Pan, L., O'Toole, T., Matthews, K., & Blanck, H. M. (2018). Obesity Prevalence Among Adults Living in Metropolitan and Nonmetropolitan Counties - United States, 2016. *MMWR Morbidity and Mortality Weekly Report, 67*(23), 653–658. doi:10.15585/mmwr.mm6723a1

Lupi, R., Dotta, F., Marselli, L., Del Guerra, S., Masini, M., Santangelo, C., . . . Marchetti, P. (2002). Prolonged exposure to free fatty acids has cytostatic and pro-apoptotic effects on human pancreatic islets: Evidence that beta-cell death is caspase mediated, partially dependent on ceramide pathway, and Bcl-2 regulated. *Diabetes, 51*(5), 1437–1442. doi:10.2337 /diabetes.51.5.1437

Mann, S., Beedie, C., & Jimenez, A. (2014). Differential effects of aerobic exercise, resistance training and combined exercise modalities on cholesterol and the lipid profile: Review, synthesis and recommendations. *Sports Medicine, 44*(2), 211–221. doi:10.1007 /s40279-013-0110-5

Maradonna, F., & Carnevali, O. (2018). Lipid metabolism alteration by endocrine disruptors in animal models: An overview. *Frontiers in Endocrinology (Lausanne), 9,* 654. doi:10.3389/fendo.2018.00654

Martinez-Gomez, D., Lavie, C. J., Hamer, M., Cabanas-Sanchez, V., Garcia-Esquinas, E., Pareja-Galeano, H., . . . Rodriguez-Artalejo, F. (2019). Physical activity without weight loss reduces the development of cardiovascular disease risk factors—a prospective

cohort study of more than one hundred thousand adults. *Progress in Cardiovascular Diseases, 62*(6), 522–530. doi:10.1016/j.pcad.2019.11.010

Matthews, C. E., Chen, K. Y., Freedson, P. S., Buchowski, M. S., Beech, B. M., Pate, R. R., & Troiano, R. P. (2008). Amount of time spent in sedentary behaviors in the United States, 2003–2004. *American Journal of Epidemiology, 167*(7), 875–881. doi:10.1093/aje /kwm390

McCrory, M. A., Harbaugh, A. G., Appeadu, S., & Roberts, S. B. (2019). Fast-Food offerings in the United States in 1986, 1991, and 2016 show large increases in food variety, portion size, dietary energy, and selected micronutrients. *Journal of the Academy of Nutrition and Dietetics, 119*(6), 923–933. doi:10.1016/j .jand.2018.12.004

Moheet, A., Mangia, S., & Seaquist, E. R. (2015). Impact of diabetes on cognitive function and brain structure. *Annals of the New York Academy of Sciences, 1353,* 60–71. doi:10.1111/nyas.12807

Mozaffarian, D. (2016). Dietary and policy priorities for cardiovascular disease, diabetes, and obesity: A comprehensive review. *Circulation, 133*(2), 187–225. doi:10.1161/CIRCULATIONAHA.115.018585

Murray, C. J., Atkinson, C., Bhalla, K., Birbeck, G., Burstein, R., Chou, D., . . . Collaborators, U. S. B. o. D. (2013). The state of US health, 1990–2010: Burden of diseases, injuries, and risk factors. *JAMA, 310*(6), 591–608. doi:10.1001/jama.2013.13805

Nathan, D. M. (2002). Clinical practice. Initial management of glycemia in type 2 diabetes mellitus. *The New England Journal of Medicine, 347*(17), 1342–1349. doi:10.1056/NEJMcp021106

National Diabetes Statitics Report. (2020). Retrieved from https://www.diabetesresearch.org/file/national -diabetes-statistics-report-2020.pdf

Neeland, I. J., Poirier, P., & Despres, J. P. (2018). Cardiovascular and metabolic heterogeneity of obesity: Clinical challenges and implications for management. *Circulation, 137*(13), 1391–1406. doi:10.1161 /CIRCULATIONAHA.117.029617

Nelson, R. K., & Horowitz, J. F. (2014). Acute exercise ameliorates differences in insulin resistance between physically active and sedentary overweight adults. *Applied Physiology, Nutrition, and Metabolism, 39*(7), 811–818. doi:10.1139/apnm-2013-0525

Newsom, S. A., Everett, A. C., Hinko, A., & Horowitz, J. F. (2013). A single session of low-intensity exercise is sufficient to enhance insulin sensitivity into the next day in obese adults. *Diabetes Care, 36*(9), 2516–2522. doi:10.2337/dc12-2606

Nguyen, B. T., & Powell, L. M. (2014). The impact of restaurant consumption among US adults: Effects on energy and nutrient intakes. *Public Health Nutrition, 17*(11), 2445–2452. doi:10.1017 /S1368980014001153

Nguyen, T. T., Ta, Q. T. H., Nguyen, T. T. D., Le, T. T., & Vo, V. G. (2020). Role of insulin resistance in the Alzheimer's disease progression. *Neurochemical Research, 45*, 1481–1491. doi:10.1007/s11064-020-03031-0

Nicolaidis, S. (2019). Environment and obesity. *Metabolism, 100S*, 153942. doi:10.1016/j.metabol.2019.07.006

O'Brien, T., & Denham, S. A. (2008). Diabetes care and education in rural regions. *The Diabetes Educator, 34*(2), 334–347. doi:10.1177/0145721708316318

O'Rahilly, S., & Farooqi, I. S. (2006). Genetics of obesity. *Philosophical Transactions of the Royal Society of London Biological Sciences, 361*(1471), 1095–1105. doi:10.1098/rstb.2006.1850

Oguri, M., Adachi, H., Ohno, T., Oshima, S., & Kurabayashi, M. (2009). Effect of a single bout of moderate exercise on glucose uptake in type 2 diabetes mellitus. *Journal of Cardiology, 53*(1), 8–14. doi:10.1016/j.jjcc.2008.07.014

Olefsky, J. M., & Glass, C. K. (2010). Macrophages, inflammation, and insulin resistance. *Annual Review of Physiology, 72*, 219–246. doi:10.1146/annurev-physiol-021909-135846

Olsen, J. M. (2013). An integrative review of literature on the determinants of physical activity among rural women. *Public Health Nursing, 30*(4), 288–311. doi:10.1111/phn.12023

Oprescu, A. I., Bikopoulos, G., Naassan, A., Allister, E. M., Tang, C., Park, E., . . . Giacca, A. (2007). Free fatty acid-induced reduction in glucose-stimulated insulin secretion: Evidence for a role of oxidative stress in vitro and in vivo. *Diabetes, 56*(12), 2927–2937. doi:10.2337/db07-0075

Ormazabal, V., Nair, S., Elfeky, O., Aguayo, C., Salomon, C., & Zuniga, F. A. (2018). Association between insulin resistance and the development of cardiovascular disease. *Cardiovascular Diabetology, 17*(1), 122. doi:10.1186/s12933-018-0762-4

Ozgyin, L., Erdos, E., Bojcsuk, D., & Balint, B. L. (2015). Nuclear receptors in transgenerational epigenetic inheritance. *Progress in Biophysics and Molecular Biology, 118*(1–2), 34–43. doi:10.1016/j.pbiomolbio.2015.02.012

Park, S., Kim, J., & Lee, J. (2020). Effects of exercise intervention on adults with both hypertension and type 2 diabetes mellitus: A systematic review and meta-analysis. *Journal of Cardiovascular Nursing.* [ePub ahead of print] doi:10.1097/JCN.0000000000000651

Parrillo, L., Spinelli, R., Nicolo, A., Longo, M., Mirra, P., Raciti, G. A., . . . Beguinot, F. (2019). Nutritional factors, DNA methylation, and risk of type 2 diabetes and obesity: Perspectives and challenges. *International Journal of Molecular Science, 20*(12). doi:10.3390/ijms20122983

Pedersen, B. K. (2017). Anti-inflammatory effects of exercise: Role in diabetes and cardiovascular disease. *European Journal of Clinical Investigation, 47*(8), 600–611. doi:10.1111/eci.12781

Pedersen, B. K., & Saltin, B. (2015). Exercise as medicine—evidence for prescribing exercise as therapy in 26 different chronic diseases. *Scandinavian Journal of Medicine &Science in Sports, 25*(Suppl 3), 1–72. doi:10.1111/sms.12581

Perry, C. K., Nagel, C., Ko, L. K., Duggan, C., Linde, S., Rodriguez, E. A., & Thompson, B. (2015). Active living environment assessments in four rural Latino communities. *Preventive Medicine Reports, 2*, 818–823. doi:10.1016/j.pmedr.2015.09.001

Physical Activity Guidelines for Americans. (2008). Retrieved from https://health.gov/sites/default/files/2019-09/Physical_Activity_Guidelines_2nd_edition.pdf

Poti, J. M., Duffey, K. J., & Popkin, B. M. (2014). The association of fast food consumption with poor dietary outcomes and obesity among children: Is it the fast food or the remainder of the diet? *American Journal of Clinical Nutrition, 99*(1), 162–171. doi:10.3945/ajcn.113.071928

Powell, L. M., Chriqui, J. F., Khan, T., Wada, R., & Chaloupka, F. J. (2013). Assessing the potential effectiveness of food and beverage taxes and subsidies for improving public health: A systematic review of prices, demand and body weight outcomes. *Obesity Review, 14*(2), 110–128. doi:10.1111/obr.12002

Powell, L. M., Slater, S., Mirtcheva, D., Bao, Y., & Chaloupka, F. J. (2007). Food store availability and neighborhood characteristics in the United States. *Preventive Medicine, 44*(3), 189–195. doi:10.1016/j.ypmed.2006.08.008

Prentki, M., Joly, E., El-Assaad, W., & Roduit, R. (2002). Malonyl-CoA signaling, lipid partitioning, and glucolipotoxicity: Role in beta-cell adaptation and failure in the etiology of diabetes. *Diabetes, 51*(Suppl 3), S405–S413. doi:10.2337/diabetes.51.2007.s405

Ratcliffe, M., Burd, C., Holder, K., and Fields, A. (2016). *Defining rural at the U.S. Census Bureau.* Retrieved from https://www.census.gov/content/dam/Census/library/publications/2016/acs/acsgeo-1.pdf

Rees, W. D., Hay, S. M., Brown, D. S., Antipatis, C., & Palmer, R. M. (2000). Maternal protein deficiency causes hypermethylation of DNA in the livers of rat fetuses. *The Journal of Nutrition, 130*(7), 1821–1826. doi:10.1093/jn/130.7.1821

Rijal, A., Nielsen, E. E., Hemmingsen, B., Neupane, D., Gaede, P. H., Olsen, M. H., & Jakobsen, J. C. (2019). Adding exercise to usual care in patients with hypertension, type 2 diabetes mellitus and/or cardiovascular disease: A protocol for a systematic review with meta-analysis and trial sequential analysis. *Systematic Reviews, 8*(1), 330. doi:10.1186/s13643-019-1233-z

Robinson, J. C., Carson, T. L., Johnson, E. R., Hardy, C. M., Shikany, J. M., Green, E., . . . Baskin, M. L. (2014). Assessing environmental support for better health: Active living opportunity audits in rural communities in the southern United States. *Preventive Medicine,* *66,* 28–33. doi:10.1016/j.ypmed.2014.05.021

Rose, A. J., & Richter, E. A. (2005). Skeletal muscle glucose uptake during exercise: How is it regulated? *Physiology (Bethesda), 20,* 260–270. doi:10.1152/physiol.00012.2005

Rural education at a glance. (2017). Retrieved from https://www.ers.usda.gov/webdocs/publications/83078/eib-171.pdf?v=0

Rush, E. C., Goedecke, J. H., Jennings, C., Micklesfield, L., Dugas, L., Lambert, E. V., & Plank, L. D. (2007). BMI, fat and muscle differences in urban women of five ethnicities from two countries. *International Journal of Obesity (London), 31*(8), 1232–1239. doi:10.1038/sj.ijo.0803576

Sasaki, H., Kawamura, N., Dyck, P. J., Dyck, P. J. B., Kihara, M., & Low, P. A. (2020). Spectrum of diabetic neuropathies. *Diabetology International, 11*(2), 87–96. doi:10.1007/s13340-019-00424-7

Savoca, M. R., Arcury, T. A., Leng, X., Bell, R. A., Chen, H., Anderson, A., . . . Quandt, S. A. (2009). The diet quality of rural older adults in the South as measured by healthy eating index-2005 varies by ethnicity. *Journal of the American Dietetic Association, 109*(12), 2063–2067. doi:10.1016/j.jada.2009.09.005

Schmid, A. A., Atler, K. E., Malcolm, M. P., Grimm, L. A., Klinedinst, T. C., Marchant, D. R., . . . Portz, J. D. (2018). Yoga improves quality of life and fall risk-factors in a sample of people with chronic pain and Type 2 Diabetes. *Complementary Therapies in Clinical Practice, 31,* 369–373. doi:10.1016/j.ctcp.2018.01.003

Seguin, R. A., Lo, B. K., Sriram, U., Connor, L. M., & Totta, A. (2017). Development and testing of a community audit tool to assess rural built environments: Inventories for community health assessment in rural towns. *Preventive Medicine Reports, 7,* 169–175. doi:10.1016/j.pmedr.2017.06.008

Sharma, G., Parihar, A., Talaiya, T., Dubey, K., Porwal, B., & Parihar, M. S. (2020). Cognitive impairments in type 2 diabetes, risk factors and preventive strategies. *Journal of Basic and Clinical Physiology and Pharmacology, 31*(2), 1–14. doi:10.1515/jbcpp-2019-0105

Sharman, J. E., La Gerche, A., & Coombes, J. S. (2015). Exercise and cardiovascular risk in patients with hypertension. *American Journal of Hypertension, 28*(2), 147–158. doi:10.1093/ajh/hpu191

Silventoinen, K., Rokholm, B., Kaprio, J., & Sorensen, T. I. (2010). The genetic and environmental influences on childhood obesity: A systematic review of twin and adoption studies. *International Journal of Obesity (London), 34*(1), 29–40. doi:10.1038/ijo.2009.177

Singh, R. K., Kumar, P., & Mahalingam, K. (2017). Molecular genetics of human obesity: A comprehensive review. *Comptes Rendus Biologies, 340*(2), 87–108. doi:10.1016/j.crvi.2016.11.007

Sisson, S. B., Church, T. S., Martin, C. K., Tudor-Locke, C., Smith, S. R., Bouchard, C., . . . Katzmarzyk, P. T. (2009). Profiles of sedentary behavior in children and adolescents: The US National Health and Nutrition Examination Survey, 2001–2006. *International Journal of Pediatric Obesity, 4*(4), 353–359. doi:10.3109/17477160902934777

Stanford, K. I., & Goodyear, L. J. (2014). Exercise and type 2 diabetes: Molecular mechanisms regulating glucose uptake in skeletal muscle. *Advances in Physiology Education, 38*(4), 308–314. doi:10.1152/advan.00080.2014

Stel, J., & Legler, J. (2015). The role of epigenetics in the latent effects of early life exposure to obesogenic endocrine disrupting chemicals. *Endocrinology, 156*(10), 3466–3472. doi:10.1210/en.2015-1434

Strain, W. D., & Paldanius, P. M. (2018). Diabetes, cardiovascular disease and the microcirculation. *Cardiovascular Diabetology, 17*(1), 57. doi:10.1186/s12933-018-0703-2

Sylow, L., Kleinert, M., Richter, E. A., & Jensen, T. E. (2017). Exercise-stimulated glucose uptake — regulation and implications for glycaemic control. *Nature Reviews Endocrinology, 13*(3), 133–148. doi:10.1038/nrendo.2016.162

Teich, T., Zaharieva, D. P., & Riddell, M. C. (2019). Advances in exercise, physical activity, and Diabetes Mellitus. *Diabetes Technology & Therapeutics, 21*(S1), S112–S122. doi:10.1089/dia.2019.2509

Thomson, J. L., Goodman, M. H., & Landry, A. S. (2019). Assessment of town and park characteristics related to physical activity in the lower Mississippi delta. *Preventing Chronic Disease, 16,* E35. doi:10.5888/pcd16.180410

Thorud, J. C., Plemmons, B., Buckley, C. J., Shibuya, N., & Jupiter, D. C. (2016). Mortality after nontraumatic major amputation among patients with diabetes and peripheral vascular disease: A systematic review. *Journal of Foot and Ankle Surgery, 55*(3), 591–599. doi:10.1053/j.jfas.2016.01.012

Todd, J. E. (2017). Changes in consumption of food away from home and intakes of energy and other nutrients among US working-age adults, 2005–2014. *Public Health Nutrition, 20*(18), 3238–3246. doi:10.1017/S1368980017002403

Trivedi, T., Liu, J., Probst, J., Merchant, A., Jhones, S., & Martin, A. B. (2015). Obesity and obesity-related behaviors among rural and urban adults in the USA. *Rural and Remote Health, 15*(4), 3267.

Troiano, R. P., Berrigan, D., Dodd, K. W., Masse, L. C., Tilert, T., & McDowell, M. (2008). Physical activity in the United States measured by accelerometer. *Medicine & Science in Sports & Exercise, 40*(1), 181–188. doi:10.1249/mss.0b013e31815a51b3

United States Census Bureau. (2016). *New Census Data Show Differences Between Urban and Rural Populations.* Retrieved from https://www.census.gov/newsroom/press-releases/2016/cb16-210.html

Ussher, J. R., Koves, T. R., Cadete, V. J., Zhang, L., Jaswal, J. S., Swyrd, S. J., . . . Lopaschuk, G. D. (2010). Inhibition of de novo ceramide synthesis reverses diet-induced insulin resistance and enhances whole-body oxygen consumption. *Diabetes, 59*(10), 2453–2464. doi:10.2337/db09-1293

Valdez, Z., Ramirez, A. S., Estrada, E., Grassi, K., & Nathan, S. (2016). Community perspectives on access to and availability of healthy food in rural, low-resource, Latino communities. *Preventing Chronic Disease, 13*, E170. doi:10.5888/pcd13.160250

Virtanen, M., Jokela, M., Lallukka, T., Magnusson Hanson, L., Pentti, J., Nyberg, S. T., . . . Kivimaki, M. (2019). Long working hours and change in body weight: Analysis of individual-participant data from 19 cohort studies. *International Journal of Obesity, 44*, 1368–1375. doi:10.1038/s41366-019-0480-3

Volaco, A., Cavalcanti, A. M., Filho, R. P., & Precoma, D. B. (2018). Socioeconomic status: The missing link between obesity and Diabetes Mellitus? *Current Diabetes Review, 14*(4), 321–326. doi:10.2174/1573399813666170621123227

Walia, S., & Leipert, B. (2012). Perceived facilitators and barriers to physical activity for rural youth: An exploratory study using photovoice. *Rural and Remote Health, 12*, 1842.

Walker, R. E., Keane, C. R., & Burke, J. G. (2010). Disparities and access to healthy food in the United States: A review of food deserts literature. *Health & Place, 16*(5), 876–884. doi:10.1016/j.healthplace.2010.04.013

Wang, Y., & Xu, D. (2017). Effects of aerobic exercise on lipids and lipoproteins. *Lipids in Health & Disease, 16*(1), 132. doi:10.1186/s12944-017-0515-5

Wannamethee, S. G., & Atkins, J. L. (2015). Muscle loss and obesity: The health implications of sarcopenia and sarcopenic obesity. *Proceedings of the Nutrition Society, 74*(4), 405–412. doi:10.1017/S002966511500169X

Wardle, J., & Cooke, L. (2008). Genetic and environmental determinants of children's food preferences. *British Journal of Nutrition, 99*(Suppl 1), S15–S21. doi:10.1017/S000711450889246X

Watson, K. B., Harris, C. D., Carlson, S. A., Dorn, J. M., & Fulton, J. E. (2016). Disparities in adolescents' residence in neighborhoods supportive of physical activity — United States, 2011–2012. *MMWR Morbidity and Mortality Weekly Report, 65*(23), 598–601. doi:10.15585/mmwr.mm6523a2

Wei, Y., Chen, K., Whaley-Connell, A. T., Stump, C. S., Ibdah, J. A., & Sowers, J. R. (2008). Skeletal muscle insulin resistance: Role of inflammatory cytokines and reactive oxygen species. *American Journal of Physiology Regulatory, Integrative and Comparative Physiology, 294*(3), R673–R680. doi:10.1152/ajpregu.00561.2007

Wen, M., Fan, J. X., Kowaleski-Jones, L., & Wan, N. (2018). Rural-urban disparities in obesity prevalence among working age adults in the United States: Exploring the mechanisms. *American Journal of Health Promotion, 32*(2), 400–408. doi:10.1177/0890117116689488

Wende, M. E., Stowe, E. W., Eberth, J. M., McLain, A. C., Liese, A. D., Breneman, C. B., . . . Kaczynski, A. T. (2020). Spatial clustering patterns and regional variations for food and physical activity environments across the United States. *International Journal of Environmental Health Research*, 1–15. doi:10.1080/09603123.2020.1713304

Whitfield, G. P., Carlson, S. A., Ussery, E. N., Fulton, J. E., Galuska, D. A., & Petersen, R. (2019). Trends in meeting physical activity guidelines among urban and rural dwelling adults - United States, 2008–2017. *MMWR Morbidity and Mortality Weekly Report, 68*(23), 513–518. doi:10.15585/mmwr.mm6823a1

Wiernsperger, N. F. (2005). Is non-insulin dependent glucose uptake a therapeutic alternative? Part 1: physiology, mechanisms and role of non insulin-dependent glucose uptake in type 2 diabetes. *Diabetes & Metabolism, 31*(5), 415–426. doi:10.1016/s1262-3636(07)70212-4

Wilcox, S., Bopp, M., Oberrecht, L., Kammermann, S. K., & McElmurray, C. T. (2003). Psychosocial and perceived environmental correlates of physical activity in rural and older African American and white women. *The Journals of Gerontology Series B, 58*(6), P329–P337. doi:10.1093/geronb/58.6.p329

Wilcox, S., Oberrecht, L., Bopp, M., Kammermann, S. K., & McElmurray, C. T. (2005). A qualitative study of exercise in older African American and white women in rural South Carolina: Perceptions, barriers, and motivations. *Journal of Women & Aging, 17*(1–2), 37–53. doi:10.1300/J074v17n01_04

Wilmot, E. G., Edwardson, C. L., Achana, F. A., Davies, M. J., Gorely, T., Gray, L. J., . . . Biddle, S. J. (2012). Sedentary time in adults and the association with diabetes, cardiovascular disease and death: Systematic review and meta-analysis. *Diabetologia, 55*(11), 2895–2905. doi:10.1007/s00125-012-2677-z

Wu, L., & Parhofer, K. G. (2014). Diabetic dyslipidemia. *Metabolism, 63*(12), 1469–1479. doi:10.1016/j.metabol.2014.08.010

Young, K. L., Graff, M., Fernandez-Rhodes, L., & North, K. E. (2018). Genetics of obesity in diverse populations. *Current Diabetes Reports, 18*(12), 145. doi:10.1007/s11892-018-1107-0

Yousefian, A., Hennessy, E., Umstattd, M. R., Economos, C. D., Hallam, J. S., Hyatt, R. R., & Hartley, D. (2010). Development of the rural active living assessment tools: Measuring rural environments. *Preventive Medicine, 50* (Suppl 1), S86–S92. doi:10.1016/j.ypmed.2009.08.018

Yousefian, A., Leighton, A., Fox, K., & Hartley, D. (2011). Understanding the rural food environment—perspectives of low-income parents. *Rural & Remote Health, 11*(2), 1–11.

Zilliox, L. A., Chadrasekaran, K., Kwan, J. Y., & Russell, J. W. (2016). Diabetes and cognitive impairment. *Current Diabetes Reports, 16*(9), 87. doi:10.1007/s11892-016-0775-x

CHAPTER 9

Nutrition, Food Desert, and Weight Status

Roschelle Heuberger, PhD, RD

LEARNING OBJECTIVES

At the end of this chapter, readers will be able to:

1. Define and describe the principle components of the macro, micro, trace nutrients, and their recommended intakes and relationships to overall health.
2. Define and describe the principle components of the electrolytes and water and their recommended intakes and relationships to overall health.
3. Outline and categorize the nutritional concepts pertinent to the life stages.
4. Describe and classify major food and drug/alcohol interactions.
5. Explain terminology related to food deserts, surveillance, and the built environment.
6. Categorize and explain levels of weight status and their assessment; relationship to health and stratification by gender, age, socioeconomics; and other demographic factors.
7. Describe and analyze the relationships between nutrient density and energy balance, with its concomitant associations with geographic locale, comorbid conditions, life stage and access to nutritious foods, health care, and health literacy.

KEY TERMS

Anthropometry
Atherosclerosis
Body composition
Built environment
Dysbiosis
Energetics
Food desert
Food insecurity
High Density Lipoprotein (HDL)
Low Density Lipoprotein (LDL)
Macronutrients
Malnutrition
Microbiome
Micronutrients
Morbidity
Nutrient density
Surveillance

CHAPTER OVERVIEW

Nutrition is the basis of life. You cannot live without food and water. Dietary habits interact with the genome to dictate what your health will look like in the future. Patterns of intake are solidified in early life and can be difficult to change as you age. The availability of nutritious foods is limited in certain parts of the country, for a variety of reasons. Geography interacts

Table 9-1 Metric Equivalents

Volume		Weight	
1 liter	1,000 milliliters	1 gram	1,000 milligrams
0.95 liter	1 quart	1 gram	0.04 ounce
1 milliliter	0.03 fluid ounces	1 ounce	28.35 grams
240 milliliter	1 cup	1 kilogram	2.2 pounds
Energy		Length	
1 kilocalorie	1,000 calories	100 centimeters	1 meter
Water	0 kcals/gram	2.54 centimeters	1 inch
Carbohydrates	4 kcal/gram	Energy	
Protein	4 kcal/gram	Vitamins	0 kcals/gram
Fat	9 kcals/gram	Minerals	0 kcals/gram
Alcohol	7 kcals/gram	Fiber	0 kcals/gram

with demand, culture, habit, sociodemographics, and many other factors to dictate what and how people eat. Rural persons are at a disadvantage with respect to the food supply and subsequently there are disparities in nutrition-related **morbidity** and mortality.

Nutrition

Introduction

Nutrients are the building blocks of the body. **Malnutrition** is "bad" nutrition, or too much or too little of important nutrients. Each nutrient can have a deficiency or a toxicity syndrome. There are nutrients that must be obtained from the diet, as the body is unable to synthesize them from other substrates. These nutrients are called "essential." There are also "conditionally essential" nutrients, or those that should be obtained from the diet, because it is too difficult to make them or because their precursors are in short supply. In the United States, malnutrition often presents as obesity from too many empty calories. Empty calories do not have vitamins, minerals, trace elements

or protein, thus they do not contribute to any essential category and do nothing for nutritional status. Malnutrition has strong risks for chronic disease. Combined with other factors, it increases morbidity, mortality, healthcare costs, and decreases quality of life. **Table 9-1** outlines measures that are used to determine important nutritional parameters.

Macronutrients

Carbohydrates provide energy and are used as building blocks. There are many types of carbohydrates, some better than others, in terms of overall health status. There are simple sugars, refined sugars, starches, complex carbohydrates, and fibers. Glucose is a simple sugar, but it is the preferred energy source for muscles and the brain. Refined sugars are carbohydrates, but they should not be consumed in excess. An example of a refined sugar is sucrose (table sugar). Fibers are also carbohydrates, but they are not digestible or used for energy; however, they are very important to overall health. Fibers feed the desirable bacteria in the gut. The gut contains many strains of bacteria whose metabolism interacts with the host to either promote or degrade health. These are called the microbiota; and as a whole, constitute the **microbiome**. If unfavorable bacteria colonize the microbiome, it is called dysbiosis.

Dysbiosis has been linked to almost every chronic disease and its progression. Examples of fibers are the oligosaccharides, soluble and insoluble fibers, such as oats and bran. Starches and sugars can be broken down into glucose for energy or converted to fat if there is an excess. Carbohydrates like starch and sugar stimulate the release of insulin, which allows nutrients to enter the cells. Abnormal insulin levels and/or cellular response to insulin is the basis of diabetes, which is currently an enormous public health problem. Obesity increases the risk for type 2 diabetes (T2DM). This is especially true when there is increased deposition of fat in the center of the body, also known as central obesity or visceral adiposity. This type of obesity is related to the development of metabolic syndrome. The characteristics of metabolic syndrome are outlined in **Table 9-2**. Metabolic syndrome increases the risks for heart disease, diabetes, stroke, gout, and other chronic diseases.

Protein is a macronutrient that is used for building muscle, cell components, and blood cells. In general, Americans get much more protein than they need. Excess protein is hard on kidneys and liver, because it needs to be converted to fat. In order to do that, the body needs extra water and the processing of the ammonia left behind is inefficient. Excess protein has also been linked to bone loss, cancer and other chronic diseases. Protein needs are based on age, gender, stage of life, periods of growth, pregnancy, lactation, and older age. Elite athletes do need higher levels of protein, but it is rare that their needs are not met by the average U.S. diet. Protein can be found in dairy, eggs, beans, grains, vegetables, fish, and meats. Egg whites are the highest protein source and do not contain cholesterol or fat. Proteins are absorbed and metabolized differently based on their source. That is why rice and beans are combined in many cultures; the combination presents a complete array of protein components (amino acids).

Fats, also known as triglycerides or lipids, are needed in small quantities. There are many types of fats. Saturated fats are associated with chronic disease. A saturated fat can be described as being solid at room temperature.

Table 9-2 Metabolic Syndrome

Characteristics	National Cholesterol Education Program (U.S.)	International Diabetes Foundation (Global)
Obesity	Visceral Obesity	Visceral Obesity
High Blood Sugar	Fasting Blood Glucose >100 mg/dl	Fasting Blood Glucose >100 mg/dl
Abnormal Blood Triglycerides (fats)	Triglycerides >150 mg/dl	Triglycerides >150 mg/dl
Low Good Cholesterol (HDL)	HDL <40 mg/dl men, <50 mg/dl women	HDL <40 mg/dl men, <50 mg/dl women
Hypertension (Blood Pressure)	130 mmHg systolic or >85 mg Hg diastolic	130 mmHg systolic or >85 mg Hg diastolic
Requirements for Diagnosis	Any of three criteria above	Obesity (general) plus two of the criteria above

Saturated fats are present in many products, either naturally or by processing. Coconut oil, lard, shortening, cream, and full-fat products are high in saturated fats. Trans fats occur naturally in food but are added by processing in products ranging from baked goods to salty snacks and spreads. Recent regulations have forced manufacturers to disclose the amount of trans fats contained in a product, if the serving contains more than half a gram. Trans fats are associated with chronic diseases as well. Monounsaturated and polyunsaturated fats are liquid at room temperature, and although they should still be eaten in moderation, they still have better risk profiles. Another example of fats with heart-healthy profiles are the omega-3 fatty acids. Examples of fats in foods that are associated with health benefits include olive oil, fatty fish like salmon, and flaxseeds. Erroneously, people believe that cholesterol is a fat. Cholesterol is a sterol and is found exclusively in animal products. Cholesterol should be limited, particularly in those who have a predisposition to heart disease and metabolic syndrome. Fast food, highly processed foods and fatty snacks like chips, and doughnuts are very high in saturated fat, trans fats, calories, sodium, and cholesterol.

Rural residents are at significantly greater risk for poor nutrition and nutrition-related chronic disease (Cohen et al., 2013). Cardiovascular disease is the number one cause of mortality in the United States and rural women are particularly at risk due to behavioral and metabolic factors, which include unhealthy diet (Kelli et al., 2019). Khare et al., (2014) implemented a community-based intervention for rural women, with modest increases in vegetable intake and a decrease in total cholesterol. However, cholesterol level decrements were not maintained at one year (Khare et al., 2014). Similarly, Wang et al., (2019) found that while community-based interventions for cardiovascular disease were cost-effective, they resulted in modest improvements in risk profile of rural participants. It has been established that costs for healthy foods are greater

and access is more limited for rural residents (Carlson & Frazão, 2014). Because diet quality is inherently tied to the development of metabolic syndrome and chronic disease, several federal, state, and local initiatives have been launched to improve risk profiles for rural persons in the United States (Flynt & Daepp, 2015).

Micronutrients

The **micronutrients** or "small" nutrients are essential for the human body to function properly. While it is not common to see gross deficiencies in the United States, even subtle deficiencies accumulate over time to confer disease. The micronutrients encompass vitamins, minerals, and trace elements. Each has an absolute requirement, especially during periods of growth and development. These vary by age, life stage, gender, and genetics. The recommendations are based on studies that add a safety factor of two standard deviations from the means found to be adequate for persons of a given age, gender, etc. Therefore, these recommendations are sufficient for 95% of healthy people in the U.S. population (See **Figure 9-1**). Global recommendations differ slightly from those established by the United States; they are often lower because of scarcity of resources in impoverished nations. **Table 9-3** outlines the micronutrients needed for function. There are also guidelines for the highest acceptable intakes. These guidelines are to prevent toxicity from supplementation. Toxicity levels are difficult to achieve without using vitamin-mineral preparations available at stores. Specific Dietary Recommendations for Intake for Americans from the Institute of Medicine can be found at https://www.nal.usda.gov/fnic/dietary-reference-intakes.

Rural dwelling families are vulnerable to deficiencies in micronutrients because of their lower socioeconomic status, less access to large grocery stores, which have better availability of healthy foods, fruits and vegetables, and proximity to convenience stores

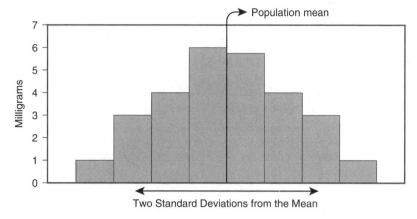

Figure 9-1 Dietary Recommendations for Nutrients for Populations.

Table 9-3 Micronutrients

Vitamins Water Soluble Vitamins	Minerals Electrolytes	Trace Elements Minor Elements*
Thiamin (vitamin B1)	Sodium	Sulfur
Riboflavin (vitamin B2)	Chloride	Boron
Niacin (vitamin B3)	Potassium	Nickel
Biotin	Phosphorus	Vanadium
Pantothenic Acid	Magnesium	Bromine
Pyridoxine (vitamin B6)		Cobalt
Folate	**Major Minerals**	
Cyanocobalamin (vitamin B12)	Calcium	**Phytochemicals**
Vitamin C	Iron	Carotenoids
Choline	Zinc	Flavinoids
	Iodine	Isoflavones
Fat Soluble Vitamins	Selenium	Sterols
Vitamin A (retinol)	Copper	Stanols
Vitamin D (cholecalciferol)	Manganese	Indoles
Vitamin E (tocopherol)	Fluoride	Phenolics
Vitamin K (phylloquinone)	Chromium	Isothiocyanates
	Molybdenum	Terpenes

*No requirements but necessary for functionality.
**No requirements, but known to have health benefits.

and fast food establishments known for their micronutrient poor selections (Larson et al., 2017; Wang et al., 2016). In a survey based on the Rural Healthy People 2010 guidelines, nearly 1,000 respondents ranked nutrition as their number two concern, and the top 10 included several concerns related to diet quality and disease (Bolin et al., 2015). The food access and availability environments are a strong determinant of health outcomes. In an analysis of the food environment and age-adjusted mortality, Ahern et al., (2011) found that distinct differences exist between urban and rural dwelling persons.

Because the intake of healthy fruits, vegetables, low-fat protein, and whole grains are often established at an early age, research into the rural family's home food environment has been undertaken. It is clear that poverty, rural residence, minority status and availability of foods in the home are essential for establishing lifelong micronutrient adequacy for children (Amuta et al., 2015). In order to improve the **nutrient density** of diets in rural settings, the consensus of the research community is that broad-based partnerships, infrastructure, and environmental and policy interventions must be undertaken (Barnidge et al., 2013).

Fluids and Electrolytes

There is an absolute requirement for the intake of fluids. Water is essential for regulating body temperature and allows normal metabolism to occur. Fluid needs increase during periods of growth, pregnancy, and lactation and in older age. Older adults are particularly vulnerable to dehydration. Heat and cold both increase fluid needs, as does physical activity, alcohol intake, drug use, and body weight. Beverages containing caffeine, non-nutritive sweeteners, and certain additives do not replace water in terms of functionality. Caffeine, high sugar load, and certain artificial sweeteners act as diuretics, as do other drugs and alcohol. A diuretic causes increased water excretion. Dehydration can be life threatening. Water levels in the body are

linked to the presence of electrolytes. Electrolytes are minerals that cause water to diffuse through membranes. Sodium, for example, causes water to be retained. Sodium chloride, or table salt, has a marked impact on where body water accumulates. Body water accumulation in the blood vessels increases blood pressure. Therefore, salt intake needs to be monitored for people who have hypertension (high blood pressure), or other vascular diseases, such as heart failure or kidney disease.

Electrolytes have another important function, and that is to act as buffers. The body must be kept at neutral pH, not too acidic or basic. Too much in either direction can cause life-threatening illness. Phosphorus is another electrolyte, which can be very high in the diets of soda consumers. Phosphorus levels must be kept in control for people with a predisposition to kidney disease. Too much phosphorus causes an imbalance of electrolytes. Potassium is another important electrolyte. Potassium is essential for normal signaling to the heart, muscles, and other vital organs. Potassium is high in fruits and vegetables. Higher levels of potassium intake are associated with better overall health profiles and decreased risk of metabolic syndrome.

Sodium and sugar intake are very high in people who consume processed foods. Pre-packaged, convenience, fast foods, and items such as snacks, soda, and canned goods contribute significantly to poor diet quality. These items are generally more available in underserved communities, such as in African American rural inhabitants. These communities also have a higher predisposition, both genetically and socioeconomically, for chronic disease (Taber et al., 2016; Robinson et al., 2014). Since prices are higher for healthful foods, and access is limited for poorer persons, there have been trials of corner store transformation. Increasing the healthy foods and providing nutrition education and recipes for low-cost preparation has resulted in increases in diet quality for residents in the vicinity of the rural corner store (Rushakoff et al., 2017;

Jilcott et al., 2017). In addition, influencing availability and access to nutritious foods also increases people's positive perceptions of their diet and health (Walker et al., 2014). It should also be noted that since poor diet affects oral health, which is directly tied to chronic disease outcomes, the policy implications of availability and access are critical to the overall health of rural America (Heuberger, 2011; Huang et al., 2012).

Life Stages

There are many life stages. These are outlined in **Table 9-4**. Although it is no longer acceptable to collapse older age and oldest old due to the heterogeneity of the two groups, for the purposes of nutritional recommendations, the differences have not been clearly delineated. The same holds true for early adulthood, adulthood, and late middle age. The research combines all three into "adulthood." In addition, there are differences in nutritional needs between males and females beginning in late childhood and ending prior to the oldest old classification. Prior to age nine years and after 85 years, the recommendations are the same between males and females for **macronutrients**, micronutrients, fluids, electrolytes, trace minerals, and other ancillary compounds.

Periods of rapid growth increase nutritional needs dramatically. All of the nutrients are required at higher levels adjusted for body weight, length, head circumference (infants), and body weight, height, and physical activity. Nutrient needs level off in adulthood, but then increase again for older adults. Aging decreases the body's ability to absorb, transport, metabolize, and utilize nutrients. Aging also decreases the need for calories as metabolism slows down. Excess calorie consumption leads to increased problems among older adults, because physical function has already declined.

Childhood obesity is a global public health problem. There is evidence that nutrition during pregnancy influences the risk of being obese in childhood. Childhood obesity is related to obesity in adulthood. It becomes more difficult to lose weight as one gets older. Childhood obesity is related to early onset chronic disease. Diseases such as T2D, hypertension, and cardiovascular risk factors, like high **low-density lipoprotein (LDL)** cholesterol, low **high-density lipoprotein (HDL)** cholesterol, **atherosclerosis**, and metabolic syndrome are now seen at much earlier ages. This equates to increased morbidity and mortality early in life.

Rural dwellers are more likely to be obese. **Surveillance** data from the government has

Table 9-4 Life Stage Delineations by Year

Life Stage	Years	Life Stage	Years
Early infancy	0–0.5	Pregnancy	>18
Late infancy	0.5–1.0	Lactation	>18
Early childhood	1–3	Early adulthood	18–24
Middle childhood	4–8	Adulthood	25–49
Late Childhood	9–13	Late middle age	50–69
Adolescence	14–18	Older age	70–85
Adolescent pregnancy	<18	Oldest old	>85
Adolescent lactation	<18		

shown that obesity and chronic diseases related to obesity are greater in all stages of life among rural inhabitants in the United States and globally. Rural obesity incidence is the primary driver for the global obesity and chronic disease epidemics (Befort et al., 2012; Bixby et al., 2019; Alkon & Agyeman, 2011). While these relationships exist in all races and socioeconomic classes of rural inhabitants, there is a predilection for higher morbidity and mortality among those of minority and low socioeconomic status who are rural residents. The most vulnerable are older adults and children, who have less control over what foods are available to them (Li et al., 2015; Mejia de Grubb et al., 2017; Peters et al., 2016).

Food-Drug Interactions

Many different drugs interact with nutrients. Alcohol, while classified as a drug, its intake is technically a nutritional issue. Alcohol has calories, 7 kcals/gram, more than either protein or carbohydrate. Alcoholic beverages contain few, if any, micronutrients. Alcohol has empty calories. Alcohol serving sizes can be found in **Table 9-5**. According to the National Institute on Alcohol Abuse and Alcoholism (NIAAA), drinking five or more alcoholic drinks in one sitting is considered binge drinking. That means that if a Zombie or Long Island Iced Tea is consumed, each having five shots of alcohol, one drink is considered binge drinking. It also means that 600+ calories are consumed in one drink. Heavy drinking is defined as consuming three drinks for women and four drinks for men on any given day (https://www.niaaa.nih.gov/overview -alcohol-consumption). There is a belief that because red wine is healthful due to its phytochemical constituents, it is reasonable to engage in heavy wine drinking. This is a fallacy. While wine does have phytochemicals, the ethanol content has the same deleterious effects on the liver and gastrointestinal tract. It is also true that an individual's genomic makeup determines how rapidly he or she

Table 9-5 Alcohol Serving Sizes, Caloric Values

Alcohol Type— Serving in Fluid Ounces (U.S.)	% Ethanol by Volume	Caloric Value
Standard Beer— 12 fl. oz.	5%	~100 kcals
Standard Wine— 5 fl. oz.	12%	~100 kcals
Standard Wine Cooler—10 fl. oz.	7%	~100 kcals
Standard Distilled—1.5 fl. oz. at 80 proof*	40%	~100 kcals

*Distilled spirits include alcoholic beverages such as vodka, whiskey, gin, rum, and tequila, which have considerable variability in alcohol content, resulting in large variances in serving size and caloric value.

metabolizes alcohol and how quickly the detrimental effects occur. The Dietary Guidelines for Americans specifically state that if an adult drinks alcohol, he or she should do so in moderation. Moderation is defined as one drink for women and two for men. Alcohol drinking significantly negatively impacts children and adolescents, predisposing them to addiction and nutritional deficit.

Pregnant and breastfeeding women should not consume alcohol. Fetal Alcohol Syndrome, Fetal Alcohol Spectrum Disorder, Alcohol-Related Neurodevelopmental Disorder, and Alcohol-Related Birth Defects are life-long disabilities, with huge costs to both the healthcare system and society at large. It is a fallacy that consistent wine drinking does not affect the fetus. The extent of the damage to the developing embryo depends on a variety of factors. Maternal nutritional status is diminished by alcohol and drugs of abuse, and the needs are far higher in terms of both macro and micro-nutrition during pregnancy (Sebastiani et al., 2018).

Very specific enzymes in the liver metabolize alcohol, and its degradation takes precedence over the metabolism of any other nutritional component. This is due to the body being wired to eliminate ethanol (drinking alcohol) before any other substrate. As a result, all nutrients and their trafficking are put on hold until the ethanol is detoxified. This is the basis for determining Blood Alcohol Levels (BALs), since there is a maximum rate by which detoxification by hepatocytes (liver cells) can occur. The ethanol is converted to acetaldehyde, which is toxic to cells and must be immediately converted to acetate, which is then routed to conversion into either energy or fat. Because the conversion of ethanol to fat is more likely, the fatty acids reside in the liver and build up until fatty streaks become apparent.

Consistent drinking leads to a fatty infiltrate-mediated inflammation, called alcoholic hepatitis, which can quickly cause scar tissue formation around the buildup of pockets of fat, thus destroying the surrounding tissue. Once the progression to cirrhosis of the liver occurs, through consistent heavy alcohol intake, the damage is irreversible. The liver is responsible for the vast majority of the metabolism of nutrients, in addition to acting as a reservoir for important minerals, vitamins, trace elements, and proteins. Cirrhosis causes life threatening nutritional issues, which are very difficult to remediate. Alcohol also causes irritation to the stomach and esophagus. Heavy drinking can lead to ruptures in the esophagus, making swallowing extremely painful and dangerous. Stomach inflammation is also a consequence, as is gout, visceral obesity, metabolic disorder, and pancreatitis.

Almost every drug of abuse is associated with nutritional consequences. Addiction is usually associated with poor food choices, diversion of resources away from nutritious food purchases, and alterations in liver function, the major organ of detoxification. **Figure 9-2** shows some common choices that users of drugs of abuse make which contribute to poor oral health and nutritional inadequacy (Morio, 2008).

Tips from the Field

Exhibit 9-1 Health Professional Expert Advice

Even if fresh fruits and vegetables are not available, due to season, geography, or other factors, the nutrients needed can be obtained by buying frozen fruits and vegetables. Canned is not a good choice, unless the product specifies that there is no added sugar, salt, high fructose corn syrup, preservatives, or other non-nutritive ingredients. These low-sodium, low-sugar products are usually more expensive. To preserve the nutrients in frozen vegetables, briefly microwave or steam on the stovetop. For frozen fruits, just defrosting the package is sufficient. The recommendation is to eat five or more servings of fruits and vegetables per day. Serving sizes will vary on the product. It is advisable to read the package labels, but the rule of thumb is one cup equals a serving. Adding sugar and salt at the table decreases the nutrient density of foods and should be avoided. Most people lose their sweet tooth or salt preference by abstaining from high-sugar and salty products for a period of approximately three months. After that, taste buds begin to sense the true flavors in foods, making added salt, sugar, and fat unnecessary. Increasing consumption of nutrient-dense foods such as fruits and vegetables, whole grains, and lean proteins, not only aids in weight control but increases the body's ability to counteract chronic diseases. Extensive food preparation knowledge is not necessary to cook nutritiously at home. The greater the amount of raw fruits and vegetables consumed, the fewer the calories and the greater the fiber, potassium, and mineral content of the meal.

Tips from the Dietitian

Exhibit 9-2 Sample Meal Plan

Breakfast

1 cup oatmeal (no sugar added), 1 cup defrosted berries or a banana
1 cup apple or orange juice (no sugar or artificial sweeteners)
1 cup decaffeinated coffee or tea
1 cup skim milk (splash for oatmeal, coffee/tea)

Lunch

1 cup raw carrots, 1 tablespoon ranch dressing
1 cup raw celery (combine with peanut butter and raisins for ants on a log)
3 Tablespoons Peanut Butter, ½ cup raisins
1 apple, 1 serving string cheese
2 cups water

Dinner

½ cup lettuce or other raw leafy greens, 1 cup tomato, ½ cup cucumber
¼ cup sunflower seeds hulled, ¼ cup grated cheese, 2 tablespoons salad dressing
1 chicken breast baked, roasted, or boiled, seasoned with pepper, spices to taste
1 baked potato with 1 teaspoon butter, 1 tablespoon sour cream or yogurt
1 cup peas boiled
1 cup pineapple chunks in their own juice
2 cups water

Snack

2 cups air popped popcorn
1 tablespoon butter
2 cups water

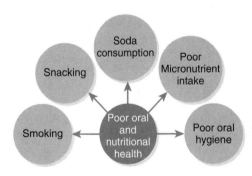

Figure 9-2 Contributions to Poor Oral Health and Nutritional Inadequacy in Users of Drugs of Abuse.

Data from Morio, K. A., Marshall, T. A., Qian, F., & Morgan, T. A. (2008). Comparing diet, oral hygiene and caries status of adult methamphetamine users and nonusers: A pilot study. *The Journal of the American Dental Association, 139*(2), 171-176. doi:10.14219/jada.archive.2008.0133.

Several drugs of abuse have very specific nutritional consequences. An example is opioid-induced constipation. Opioids decrease gut motility, slowing the movement of the intestines to the point where normal elimination is no longer possible. The constipation is so severe that it must be treated as a separate medical issue. The nutritional consequences of this syndrome can be quite severe, and in many cases, irreparable. Another example is methamphetamine. Because it is a stimulant, the nutrients move through the gut at a rate too rapid for proper absorption. There are many other drugs with addictive potential that interfere with nutritional competency. Significant increases in mortality are seen in older adults who have difficulty metabolizing exogenous compounds. Older persons also have difficulty maintaining nutritional adequacy. In addition, older adults are more predisposed to falls and fractures, so that alcohol and drug use complicates the diagnostic picture (Tevik et al., 2019).

Food Desert

Definition

Rural residency is associated with what has been termed "Food Deserts." A **food desert** is defined as a geographic locale characterized by limited access to affordable and nutritious foods. Rural residents make up approximately 20% of the U.S. population. Rural residency is defined by the U.S. Census Bureau as all population, housing, and territory not included in an urbanized area or urban cluster. Urbanization and urban clusters are more dense, large populations in a built-up, close-proximity environment. Rural areas are becoming increasingly more attractive to older persons and there is migration of Baby Boomers to areas with fewer residents. This is a very different trend than in previous decades, where migration out of rural jurisdiction was common due to lack of employment opportunities, fewer resources, and decreased numbers of farming families. For those persons who are established in rural residency, generally have lower levels of education and health literacy, more poverty and greater prevalence of chronic disease. There have been numerous studies tying the latter to geographic areas of food deserts (Jiao et al., 2012).

In addition, roughly 16% of rural residents are food insecure. **Food insecurity** is defined as the state of being without reliable access to a sufficient quantity of affordable, nutritious food. It is estimated that 6% of the rural population must travel between 10 and 20 miles to the nearest supermarket. Supermarkets, particularly the largest ones, have a better selection and lower pricing for nutritious foods. This is especially the case for fruits, vegetables, and whole grain products (Colman, 2018).

Geographic Classification

The Census Bureau and the Economic Research Service (ERS) have defined geographic areas of low food access, the new nonpejorative term for "food desert." The criteria include distance to the nearest supermarket and the percentage of low-income inhabitants according to census tracts. Additional criteria have been applied, including the ability to walk to a supermarket, take

public transportation and the actual comparative costs of nutritious foods across supermarket chains and types. The ERS has an interactive map of food accessibility, found at: https://www.ers.usda.gov/data-products/food-access-research-atlas/go-to-the-atlas/. Several organizations have started to use GIS mapping to identify areas of low income, low access, and low availability to characterize geographical areas requiring intervention. (McEntee, 2009; Alviola, 2013; LeClair & Aksan, 2014).

The "Let's Move" Initiative, included addressing the inequity faced by poorer persons in the United States with regard to healthy food access. The Food, Conservation and Energy Act of 2008 led by the U.S. Department of Agriculture provisioned for researching food distribution and the elimination of food deserts. The bill had three agencies coming together to subsidize healthy eating in food access deprived-communities. The U.S. Department of Agriculture (USDA), the Department of Health and Human Services (DHHS), and the Department of the Treasury (USDT) received a budget of $50 million to promote the development of healthy food access points in food deserts. The preliminary outcome was the use of both population characteristics and store access characteristics to define areas that would benefit most from subsidies (Ver Ploeg et al., 2015). The four area indicators used as food access measures can be found in **Table 9-6**. In a review of 31 available, large studies on food access issues in the United States, Walker et al., (2010) summarized the following results:

- Poor persons travel further to access the same resources and have less access to large chain stores. There is increased accessibility to small convenience stores.
- Areas in which there were a high percentage of African Americans had less access to grocery stores. Supermarkets were much further away and there was a sixfold greater increase in the number of fast-food establishments.

Table 9-6 Indicators used for Subsidizing Healthy Food Access in Food Deserts. Food Research and Action Center https://frac.org/

Individual Level	Store Location	Households without Vehicles
Residence Location	Type	Distance >0.5 miles from supermarkets
Resources—Income	Size	
Resources—Transportation	Prices	Survey question to individuals about whether getting to the store is difficult
Socio-demographics	Competition	
Education		
Disability	Store Attributes	Low income areas where residents are more than one mile from a supermarket
Perceived access	Square footage	
Area level	Store counts	
Population density		Low-income areas where the square footage of supermarkets/per capita are relatively low compared with other low-income areas
Poverty rate	Average prices	
Percentage without vehicles	Ratio of healthy to unhealthy food	
Percentage of minorities		
Percentage of older adults		

Data from Ver Ploeg, M., Dutko, P., & Breneman, V. (2015). Measuring food access and food deserts for policy purposes. *Applied Economic Perspectives and Policy, 37*(2), 205–225. doi:10.1093/aepp/ppu035

- Disadvantaged areas have greater rates of obesity and chronic disease.
- Easy access to large grocery stores was correlated with higher intakes of fresh fruits and vegetables.
- Poor areas have higher food prices, 30% fewer grocery stores, 50% fewer supermarkets, and less healthy food availability.
- Access to full-service restaurants, carry out meals, and healthy options equates to greater income and fewer fast food sources for area residents.

Convenience stores are known for having higher prices and food selections that are high in salt, sugar, trans and saturated fats, empty calories, and few healthy options. There have been trials of reworking policies to increase the healthful selections in the convenience

stores located in food deserts. There have also been attempts to establish healthy food access through mobile markets, farmer's markets, ethnic grocery stores, schools, work sites, community centers, and faith-based institutions in low income, rural areas. All of these approaches have been shown to increase diet quality if sustained over time (Hsaio et al., 2019; Belansky et al., 2009; Kato & McKinney, 2015; Block & Subramanian, 2015; Khojasteh & Raja, 2017; Campbell et al., 2017; Cornish et al., 2016, Escoffrey et al., 2011; Freedman et al., 2016). Community partnership and local policies that aid in implementation are essential for the success of these programs long term. An example is the Healthy2Go initiative in the Cumberland food desert of Appalachian Kentucky, where poverty, obesity, and chronic disease risks were identified as being exceptionally high. Convenience store owners were assisted with developing more healthful selection areas in their stores and were given education regarding nutrition and easy-to-use cookbooks for inexpensive meal preparation. In the one-year follow-up, trends toward better food environments and eating habits of residents were noted, particularly with children eating more vegetables (Rushakoff et al., 2017).

Socioeconomic Implications

Hunger is defined as the physical pain caused by a lack of food that starts food-seeking behavior. Hunger is a consequence of food insecurity and food insufficiency. There are approximately 50 million Americans who go hungry, a third of whom are children. The poverty line for a single adult is $12,500 per year. **Table 9-7** outlines poverty lines for households in the contiguous states; the rates for Hawaii and Alaska are higher. Unhealthy foods may be more accessible and less costly than fresh fruits and vegetables, such that food insecurity goes hand in hand with obesity. There are tools used to determine the level of food security in households, and they are available in long and short forms, Spanish, and self-report. The long form from the USDA can be found in **Table 9-8**. Several federal and state programs subsidize nutritious food for persons near or below the poverty line. In addition, there are nutrition programs for older adults, women, infants, and children, Native Americans, disaster victims, veterans, disabled, and homeless people. **Table 9-9** outlines some of the requirements and benefits of some of these programs (Whitley, 2013; Zenk et al., 2017).

The 2018 provisions for the Farm Bill have altered the state's plan requirements so that federal monies given to the contiguous 48 states to run nutrition programs can be used with greater flexibility. Changes to the Supplemental Nutrition Assistance Program

Table 9-7 Health and Human Services Poverty Guidelines for 2020

| 2020 Poverty Guidelines for the 48 Contiguous States and the District of Columbia ||
Persons in Family/ Household	Poverty Guideline
For families/households with more than eight persons, add $4,480 for each additional person.	
1	$12,760
2	$17,240
3	$21,720
4	$26,200
5	$30,680
6	$35,160
7	$39,640
8	$44,120

U.S. Department of Health & Human Services. Retrieved from https://aspe.hhs.gov/poverty-guidelines

(SNAP) were recommended to address food deserts in rural areas. Allowing these benefits to be extended to farmer's market purchases, mobile markets, and community sites were implemented to increase the intake of fresh fruits and vegetables among SNAP recipients while assisting local farmers and distributors. This was also done with the Women, Infants, and Children (WIC) Nutrition Program and the Title III Older Americans Act Senior Nutrition Programs. Electronic Benefit Cards (EBT), formerly known as Food Stamps, and Vouchers for nutrient dense items in the WIC packages and coupons for the senior nutrition programs were extended to local Farmer's and Mobile Markets. There is evidence that these changes have improved nutritionally dense food access and intake for those qualifying for benefits (Wu et al., 2017; Andrews et al., 2013; Bales, 2011; Chang et al., 2015; Fitzpatrick et al., 2016).

Table 9-8 Questions Used to Identify Food Insecurity in U.S. Households. Long Form for Households with Children

The following questions pertain to the past 12 months. Two or fewer positive responses = food secure. Three to seven positive responses = food insecure. Eight or more positive responses = very low food security (hunger).

1. Did you worry whether food would run out before you got money to buy more?

2. Did you find that the food that you bought just did not last and you did not have money to buy more?

3. Were you unable to afford to eat balanced meals?

4. Did you or other adults in your household ever cut the size of your meals or skip meals because there was not enough food?

5. Did this happen in three or more months of the previous year?

6. Did you ever eat less than you felt you should because there wasn't enough money for food?

7. Were you ever hungry but did not eat because you couldn't afford enough food?

8. Did you lose weight because you did not have money for food?

9. Did you or other adults in your household ever not eat for a whole day because you ran out of money to buy food?

10. Did this happen in three or more months during the previous year?

11. Did you rely on only a few kinds of low-cost foods to feed your children because you were running out of money to buy food?

12. Were you unable to feed your children a balanced meal because you could not afford it?

13. Were your children not eating enough because you couldn't afford enough food?

14. Did you ever cut the size of your children's meals because there was not enough money for food?

15. Were your children ever hungry but you just couldn't afford more food?

16. Did your children ever skip a meal because there wasn't enough money for food?

17. Did this happen three or more months in the previous year?

18. Did your children ever not eat for a whole day because there was not enough money for food?

United States Department of Agriculture Economic Research Service. Retrieved from https://www.ers.usda.gov/topics/food-nutrition-assistance/food -security-in-the-us/survey-tools/

Sovereign Native Nations have also been shown to live on reservations that have become food deserts. The native foodways that served these peoples over time have largely been lost, replaced by fast food, convenience items, and alcohol. Obesity, T2DM, alcoholism, metabolic disease, and malnutrition are common. Native Americans have jurisdiction over their public health policies, and they also have a different branch of government at the federal level in charge of subsidies and nutrition assistance. The Food Commodities Programs and the Food Distribution Program on Indian Reservations (FDPIR) are examples. The funds are

Table 9-9 Federal and State Nutrition Program Requirements for Benefits

SNAP—Supplemental Nutrition Assistance Program		WIC—Women, Infants, Children		Senior Nutrition Services		Child Nutrition and Education Services	
Must apply in the state of residence	Child support deduction	Income requirement	WIC-Eligible foods, Farmers Market:	Congregate meals program	60 or older	School Lunch	Daycare worker education
Household Requirement	Employment Training	Child <5 years	Legumes, Juice, Eggs, Peanut Butter	Nutrition Education/counseling	No strict income requirements	School breakfast	Snack provision
Resource limitations	Citizenship requirements	Infants- and/or	Cereal, milk, yogurt/cheese	Home delivered meals	Limited slots—preference given:	After school meals	Milk provision
Vehicle limitation	Tax Filing requirement	Pregnancy and/or	Fruit/vegetables	Provide one hot meal with 1/3 DRI	Low income	Childcare meals	1/3 DRI provision
Income requirement	Exemption: child, senior	Lactation and/or	Whole wheat products	Nutrition screening	Minority	Day program meals	<130% Poverty line
Shelter cost deduction	Exemption pregnant women, disabled	Education/training requirement/work requirement	Infant cereal, formula, baby food	Nutrition assessment	Rural	Teacher nutrition education	Eligible foods
Dependent care deduction	Food purchase restrictions	Resource limitation	Fish/tofu/soy beverages	Home health aide/services	Risk of institutionalization	Child nutrition education	School district audit

managed by Indian Tribal Organizations (ITO) or local agencies of state government. There are 276 tribes, 102 ITOs, and three state/local agencies receiving benefits in the United States. Changes to the foods available through these programs have sought to increase foods that had been utilized in native foodways tailored to tribes. Data have shown that increasing the awareness of native foodways and increasing access to ancient foods, fresh foods, and spices improves many facets of native health (Hodge & Nandy, 2011). It is important to understand that Native American views on health and nutrition are highly heterogeneous, dependent on geographic locale and custom, and any changes made must come from within the tribe as opposed to being mandated from outsiders.

There are also National Food Recovery Programs and a network of over 200 food banks across the United States. Locally, there are faith-based and nonfaith-based community programs, with food pantries, soup kitchens, and food drives designed to aid the hungry. **Table 9-10** outlines parameters for food recovery and local efforts. Use of these programs has been shown to improve access, intake, nutritional status, and selection of nutrient-dense

items (Vaterlaus et al., 2018). There are many barriers to using these resources. Pride, shame, low literacy, or lack of knowledge of the resources are all significant barriers. An example is that some programs have complicated applications and require that the applicant submit records and paperwork that would be difficult for a low-literacy person to complete (Wang et al., 2014; Guest et al., 2015).

Built Environment and Factors Affecting Nutritional Status

The **built environment** is defined as those places where people live, work, and play. This is a very broad definition, which encompasses many different components to consider in terms of the food desert, nutrition, and health. There have been studies that looked at the availability of places where people could engage in physical activity, which is known to improve nutritional status secondarily, and decrease health risks overall. In addition, there have been studies showing how walking proximity to a place where healthy fresh food could be accessed is a key determinant of whether there is access to nutrient-dense diets

---

Table 9-10 Food Systems for Feeding Hungry Persons

Food drive—nonperishable donated items with no check for "use by" date or dented cans

Food pantry—nonperishable items, dry goods (cereals, rice, pasta) with oversight

Soup kitchen—prepared foods, usually hot, cooked and served on the premises

Food bank—Food collection agencies that distribute products to organizations that feed the hungry

Food recovery systems: collection of wholesome food with a distribution mechanism

Field gleaning—Collecting crops from fields that were left over

Gleaning—collecting food from retailers

Salvage—collection of perishable foodstuff from wholesalers, markets

Prepared food rescue—Collection of cooked or prepared food from commercial kitchens

Nonperishable food rescue—collection of canned, processed, or otherwise shelf-stable products from large distributors, wholesalers, markets, or vendors

in the home of rural impoverished persons. Points of purchase farther than a half mile walking distance is a barrier. The latter may be tied to the lack of a reliable mechanism of transportation or insufficient funds to buy fuel and maintain an existing vehicle (Botchwey et al., 2015; Li et al., 2015). A proposed solution has been to test the feasibility of mobile markets that park in a different place each day in areas where there is no supermarket and no access to fresh foods. Mobile markets face challenges—dissemination of their schedules; inability of target populations needing the resource; inability of participants to reach the designated market location; inability of the buyer to use government benefits like coupons, vouchers, or EBT cards and obstacles like weather, roads, or physical barriers. Implementation of mobile market services over time has been shown to be beneficial to nutritional status of mobile market participants (Hsiao et al., 2019; Robinson et al., 2014; Rodriguez & Grahame, 2016).

Nutritional Surveillance

Surveillance programs are defined according to the World Health Organization (www.WHO.org), as the "continuous, systematic collection, analysis and interpretation of nutrition and health-related data needed for the planning, implementation, and evaluation of public health nutrition practice." Several such programs have been used to obtain data on the subsets of persons who were food insecure, rural, and lived within a food desert, in an effort to construct suitable public health policies. The National Health and Nutrition Examination Surveys (NHANES) have been conducted every few years using stratified, weighted, extrapolated, randomly sampled, population surveys. The data collected includes physical testing, laboratory analyses and questionnaires regarding food intake, income, socio-demographics, **anthropometry** and long-form food frequencies corrected for seasonality. There has also been a systematic

collection of data from the Behavioral Risk Factor Surveillance System (BRFSS) and the subset of questions regarding fruit and vegetable intake, using self-reported data in addition to direct interview protocols. The primary drawback for using surveillance data is that it often fails to capture the most vulnerable persons, because they are migrants, homeless, not listed, or fall below the age of 18, among other reasons (Wright et al., 2016, Walker et al., 2010; Smith et al., 2013; Semple & Giguere, 2018; Loo, 2014; Kongats et al., 2019).

The surveillance data is used to map areas of nutritional deficit and overlay geographic features and community resources. The USDA and the Agricultural Research Division maintain databases of the nutritional content of foods and nutritional status information on survey respondents or NHANES participants that are open to researchers at any institution who wish to use them (https://www.nal.usda.gov/ks). Another surveillance activity is the Healthy People Initiative, which is characterized as the nations' goals and objectives for public health improvements for the nation, based on surveys done throughout the United States. It should be noted that not all the goals and objectives for Healthy People 2000 were met, and the current cycle of Healthy People 2010 faced similar challenges. It is anticipated that this next cycle of recommendations for 2020 will continue to face obstacles in terms of meeting stated goals and objectives. The mission statement, goals, and objectives of the Healthy People Initiative for 2020 can be found at https://www.cdc.gov/dhdsp/hp2020.htm.

There are also regional surveillance efforts, which are funded by the National Institutes of Health Area Agencies and undertaken by researchers at academic or nonprofit institutions. Nutritional epidemiologists nationwide analyze these data and a variety of nutrition and health outcomes for specific rural populations, such as those with HIV. Worldwide, many countries engage in surveillance for the same purposes. Most countries, developing or not, maintain records of the population's unique nutritional and health concerns. Several global agencies exist for monitoring nutritional surveillance, such as the WHO, United Nations Taskforces, UNICEF, CARE, Bill and Melinda Gates Foundation, along with many others (Kalichman et al., 2014; Popkin, 2019).

NHANES and BRFSS data have shown that there are specific areas of concern for rural residents, particularly in food deserts. Primary concerns include obesity and concomitant metabolic syndrome; healthcare disparities, food access inequality and disproportionately adverse health outcomes, and mortality rates among residents. African American rural residents in underserved, impoverished communities fare worse than their other minority counterparts. The number of rural older adults is higher than it has ever been and will continue to increase as the graying of the nation continues. Older African American rural residents are much more disadvantaged and require additional resources. Of note, data have shown that obesity rates in rural older

adults are very high and fresh fruit and vegetable consumption is very low (Chai et al., 2018; Chang et al., 2015; Chasekwa et al., 2018; Baernholdt et al., 2012; Cohen et al., 2018).

Nutritional Outcomes and Comorbid Conditions

Food insecurity, poverty, geographic isolation, and poor access to healthy foods is associated with obesity. Older age, minority status, and household size are all correlated with obesity and health disparity. Rural inhabitants are significantly more at risk for obesity and its complications. Food deserts are associated with greater rates of obesity, morbidity and mortality. Therefore, when the combination of rural locale, food desert, and unfavorable socioeconomic and nutritional profiles intersect, the relative risk for malnutrition increases disproportionately. Malnutrition increases the risk for morbidity, and in turn, mortality. Malnutrition, or "bad nutrition" goes hand

---

Tips from the Nutritionist

Exhibit 9-3 Health Professional Expert Advice

There is considerable evidence that kitchen gardens teach children about nutrition and improve micronutrient status in poorer people. Growing fruits and vegetables in a rural setting is not only less expensive, it improves access to healthy food and improves life-long dietary quality and food habits. Starting a kitchen garden from seed is an economically sound practice. Community gardens can also be very beneficial, if there is not enough tillable land in close proximity to the home. Starting tomatoes, cucumbers, herbs, squashes, and other fruits and vegetables from seed in early spring can take place indoors in paper cups. When all frost warnings have passed, planting a garden outside can be a family activity. Children can assist in thinning the plants, weeding, watering, and supporting the young plants as they grow. They can learn about how plants flower and then produce edible components. Eating just-picked produce is a key component in getting young children to enjoy eating vegetables and understanding where food actually comes from. They can also learn about plant diseases, bugs, and beneficial gardening practices such as planting certain flowers to keep away pests. An example is planting inexpensive marigolds along the perimeter of the garden plot. Once the fruits and vegetables start to ripen, children can learn about picking, washing, storing, and preservation. Learning how to pickle, can, and freeze for winter months is a practical skill. These are all excellent learning activities for the entire family. There are also opportunities to learn about conservancy, organic growing, fertilizing practices, and different varieties of cultivars for every plant. There are also seed programs, which supply seeds at low or no cost, or provide heirloom varieties that are not grown commercially and are generally inaccessible to the ordinary consumer.

in hand with obesity and the intersection of the food-health milieu. Complex patterns of interaction occur because nutrition, genetics and health are inextricably tied (Firth, 2012; Kegler et al., 2008; Lebel et al., 2016).

Interventions at any level, individual, local, regional, national, or global must address many specific components. Often, intercession for population subsegments must be tailored and supported from within for sustained impact. Longitudinal assessment of the impact of any intervention must be very long term and must inform policy and procedure at each level of implementation. Changes with regard to nutrition occur slowly over time and health outcomes can only be assessed in the distant future. Funding from outside sources must remain available to ensure viability of positive outcomes. These may include the federal, state, and local government; community organizations; non-profit organizations and research groups, as well as global NGOs and agencies. (Dubowitz et al., 2013; Beaulac et al., 2009; Carnahan et al., 2016)

Weight Status

Epidemiology and Surveillance

Rural obesity rates are climbing, and this phenomenon is thought to be driving the global obesity epidemic. The usual cut points for adult underweight are BMI <18 kg/m². Overweight is classified as a BMI >25–29.9, obesity is 30–39.9, and morbid or Grade 3 obesity is >40 kg/m². Children are characterized by percentiles on growth charts, based on age, weight, length (height), and head circumference (for infants). The WHO growth charts for girls and boys, including those for infants can be found at https://www.who.int/childgrowth /standards/chart_catalogue/en/. The WHO Growth chart interpretation guidelines can be found at https://www.who.int/childgrowth /en/. The CDC also has growth charts specific to the United States. These charts can be found at https://www.cdc.gov/growthcharts /clinical_charts.htm along with standards for interpretation. Those CDC charts used for participants of WIC are also included in their clinical chart section. Childhood obesity calculators and BMI by age charts are also available from the CDC along with tutorials at https://www.cdc.gov/obesity/childhood /defining.html. It should be noted that there are more specific situations in children that complicate screening for obesity. There are periods of catch-up growth for premature infants, and stages of childhood in which there are growth trajectories that need to be adjusted prior to the calculation of percentile. Generally, greater than the 95th percentile on the growth charts is considered obese.

Older adults have more leniency in cutoff points, and overweight is usually classified starting at >29.9 kg/m² and obesity at >34.9 kg/m². It is generally recognized that older people with a BMI equal to 20 or less, are at significant risk for morbidity and mortality, so much so that weight losses of 10% of body weight in a period of six months or fewer is considered a top criterion for malnutrition screening. The older adult group of 65 years or older is so diverse and heterogeneous in their state of health that it is not appropriate to treat the group based on chronological age, but rather by physical attribute.

Surveillance has shown that the obesity epidemic is affecting rural inhabitants disproportionately. Analyses of the NHANES data, representing 138 million Americans, showed that adults in rural areas were 1.2 times as likely to be obese and have metabolic syndrome. This has also been shown in regional and local-level investigations (Hill et al., 2014; Robinson et al., 2014, Dean & Sharkey, 2011; Kegler et al., 2008; Spurrier et al., 2018). In adults, this finding was significantly associated with the following:

- Age (older)
- Race (African American)

- Physical activity (less than 10,000 steps per day)
- Leisure activity (less leisure activities)
- Screen time (more hours of television, phone, computer, video games)
- Fruits and vegetable consumption (less servings)
- Fiber intake (fewer sources)
- Sweetened beverage consumption (more soda, sweetened drinks)
- Saturated and Trans Fat (higher intakes)
- Skipping breakfast (more times per week)

In children, analyses of the NHANES data showed that rural children were 33% more likely to become obese than their urban counterparts. Overweight among children has more than tripled since the 1960s. The incidence increases are alarming, but the severity of obesity is even more so. The number of T2D cases among children and teens has risen dramatically, such that 76% of newly diagnosed T2D in Native Americans are teenagers. This has also been shown in other national, regional, and local surveillance data (Moore et al., 2008; Nanney et al., 2013; Dennison et al., 2008; King & Ling, 2015; Li et al., 2015; Lu et al., 2019). Rural childhood obesity and metabolic syndrome is significantly associated with:

- Low income
- Parents with less education
- Parents who were obese
- Parents who were not physically active
- Parents who were food insecure
- Race (African American, Hispanic)
- Sex (Female)
- Degree of rurality (most rural at highest risk)
- Less physical activity
- Fewer leisure activities (sports teams, lessons, etc.)
- More hours of screen time
- More time spent indoors
- Minimal intake of fruits and vegetables
- Increased consumption of sweetened beverages

- Increased consumption of fat, all types, all sources
- Limited access to dietitians
- Less access to counseling
- Less access to healthcare providers and resources

In older adults, surveillance data report rural inhabitants are more likely to be obese and sedentary than older urban people. It has also been noted that this population has poorer health outcomes due to chronic disease burden. This may be due in part to decreased access to healthcare services. In an analysis of the BRFSS data, Cohen et al., (2018) found that among 153 thousand respondents aged 65 years or older, African Americans were less likely to have had a check-up within the past year, geographic locale was associated with self-perception of health and with actualization of healthy behaviors (Lohman et al., 2019; Baernholdt et al., 2012; Bales, 2011; Cohen et al., 2018; Heuberger, 2011; Huang et al., 2012; Sylvie et al., 2013). Vieira et al., found that in NHANES data, those older people receiving home delivered or congregate meals through Title III Older Americans Act, were more food insecure and less functionally abled (2017). Rural obesity in older people has been linked to the following characteristics:

- Inequitable social conditions across the lifespan
- Increased susceptibility to environmental exposures
- Lower income
- Poor infrastructure
- Family dynamics and caring systems
- Barriers to accessing services
- Poorer overall perception of health
- Less social interaction, poorer social functioning
- Dependence on built environment characteristics (public transportation, proximity to senior centers)
- Less physical activity
- Race (African American)

- Sex (Female)
- Lower intake of vegetables
- Less education
- Less opportunity
- Poorer functional status
- Greater food insecurity
- More chronic disease

Energy Balance

Energy balance is an equation where the number of calories taken in must equal the number of calories expended. There are several components of energy expenditure. The greatest percentage is for Basal Metabolic Rate (BMR). Basal metabolism is related to age, gender, size, muscle mass, brown adipocyte numbers, and the cost of maintaining cellular processes. The BMR for women, older age, sedentary, obese, short stature, metabolically unstressed individuals is going to be lower than their counterparts. The greater the amount of muscle and the larger the organ sizes of the body, the greater the BMR and Resting Metabolic Rate (RMR) or the cost of being at rest for cellular processes, breathing, heartbeat, gastrointestinal motility, and other autonomic activities. This cost increases when physical activity is added, meaning more calories will be burned and more muscle mass will be active and accrued over time. In addition, there is a cost to the thermic effect of food (TEF). This accounts for less than 10% of the total costs of RMR. The TEF is related to the intake of food and the **energetics** of digestion, absorption, transport, metabolism, utilization, detoxification, and excretion. Starvation decreases the overall costs of total energy expenditure.

Skipping meals has a disproportionate effect on slowing of metabolism and decreasing energy utilization. Loss of muscle mass also has a disproportionate effect on energy expenditure. During starvation, the body catabolizes its own muscle to use for needed proteins involved in cellular processes. Inactivity, starvation, aging, and increased fat deposits have a cumulative effect on metabolism. Over time, these can permanently decrease the number of calories a person needs on a daily basis. One pound of fat is equal to 3,500 kcals. To lose one pound, someone would need to burn 3,500 kcals or spend five hours jumping rope at a relatively fast pace, or four hours cycling uphill, or three hours running a seven-minute mile. It is easier to cut 3,500 kcals from the diet than it is to lose the pound through vigorous activity.

Cutting 500 calories per day, by eating low-calorie foods and cutting out sweets, soda, fats, fast foods, snack type foods, and processed foods is a far better option for healthy weight loss when combined with incremental increases in activity that promote the formation of muscle mass, like weight training and cumulative cardiovascular exercise like walking or taking the stairs. It has also been shown that screen time decreases metabolic rate, to levels lower than sleeping. That is because during sleep there are many involuntary muscle movements, particularly during the REM cycle, while there are far fewer when sitting watching television, for example. Screen time has been significantly shown to increase BMI.

Body Composition

Not all body shapes and sizes are equal in terms of their associations with chronic disease. The gynoid, or "pear" shape is associated with a decreased risk of metabolic syndrome. The android, or "apple" shape is the opposite. The deposition of fat in the central or visceral area of the body is least favorable in terms of disease risk. This equates to a higher waist circumference (WC), and waist to hip ratio (WHR) (measure of the waist divided by the measure of the hips). A WHR greater than one is unhealthy, less than one is preferable. Cutoffs exist from epidemiological data as to what WC confers health benefit or risk. Table 9-10 shows the procedure and cutoffs for WC in males and females. A visual representation of

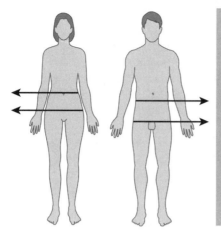

Using a tape measure, wrap the tape snugly at the end of an exhaled breath at the two points indicated to the left.

For the waist, locate the top of the hipbone and the top of the iliac crest and make sure the tape is parallel to the floor.

For the hip measurement, find the greatest circumference around the buttocks and hips.

Record the measures three times and take the average for each, the waist and the hip. Divide one by the other to get a waist to hip ratio.

Figure 9-3 Procedure for Measuring Waist Circumference and Waist-to-Hip Ratio in Males and Females.

how to measure WC and WHR can be found in **Figure 9-3**. There are a variety of ways to determine the amount of body fat relative to muscle mass. An examination with Dual X-Ray Absorptiometry (DEXA) can give highly accurate percentages of fat, lean, and bone mass. Using a DEXA to measure fracture risk is commonplace, whole **body composition** analyses is not. There are portable DEXA machines that are used for surveillance but are still too costly to use for determination of mass of adipocytes and muscle for all respondents (Slack et al., 2014; Smith, 2013).

Life Stages

Different levels of adiposity are found in males versus females and through different stages of life. Females generally have more body fat than men, older adults have more than younger people. A concern is a phenomenon called sarcopenic obesity, usually associated with older people but now is being seen in young children and teens. This is the condition in which there is such poor muscle mass quantity and quality, that the individual is essentially disabled, despite being very obese (See **Table 9-11**). This is a condition of malnutrition coupled with

Table 9-11 Waist Circumference Cutoffs for Males and Females Based on U.S. Surveillance, Relative to Normal Weight and Circumference Risk for Morbidity

	Obesity Class	Women >88 cm or 35 Inches	Men >102 cm or 40 Inches
Overweight		Moderate	Moderate
Obese	I	High	High
	II	Very High	Very High
Morbid Obesity	III	Extremely High	Extremely High

U.S. Department of Health & Human Services. Classification of Overweight and Obesity by BMI, Waist Circumference, and Associated Disease Risks. Retrieved from https://www.nhlbi.nih.gov/health/educational/lose_wt/BMI/bmi_dis

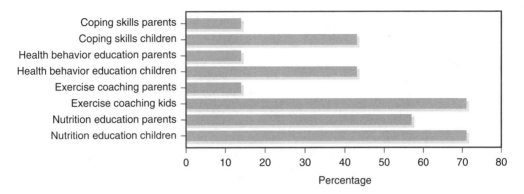

Figure 9-4 Micro-level Approaches to Stem Obesity in Youth.

sedentary behavior (Thomsen et al., 2016; Yousefian et al., 2011).

Several different strategies have been used to combat sedentary behavior and obesity, particularly in rural children. Public health measures should address inequality in "education," "policy," "place," and "access" (Fox & Heaton, 2012; King & Ling, 2015; Moore et al., 2008). Guidance for practitioners and policymakers include a variety of approaches. **Figures 9-4** and **9-5** depict some considerations for addressing the underlying systemic issues that drive this epidemic among youth (Kim-Godwin & McMurry, 2012; Frost & Porterfield, 2012; Boelens et al., 2019; Greder et al., 2017; Howlett et al., 2016; Berry et al., 2018; Karpyn et al., 2012). There are interventions that can be done at the individual

level or at the "micro" level and then there are those that are aimed at organizations or government. The latter include policies, procedures, legislation, taxation, and other "macro" level approaches. Both need to be used for effective, sustained change.

Health Status

Obesity is related to the rise in T2D. Strom et al., (2011) found that rural residents were less likely to receive diabetes education, despite the incidence of T2D increasing by 11% in this population. Diabetes self-care involves scheduling regular visits to a health professional, footcare, eye exams, blood glucose, and glycosylated hemoglobin testing and vaccinations against pneumonia and

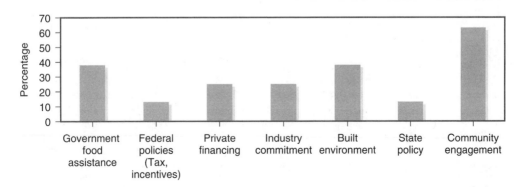

Figure 9-5 Macro-level Approaches to Stem Obesity in Youth.

influenza. Characteristics associated with higher T2D were the least population-dense, larger minority populations, less education, lower income, and declining housing value. The fewer supermarkets and more fast food and convenience stores, the higher the diabetes prevalence. A similar relationship is seen in other morbidities, such as heart failure. Living in a food desert is associated with increased disease and repeat hospitalizations. It should also be noted that poorer, sicker people are more susceptible to marketing of nutritionally supplemented foods, which may be too costly to warrant their purchase versus healthful food preparation in the home from available basic ingredients (Strom et al., 2011; Haynes-Maslow & Leone, 2017; Liese, 2018; Morris et al., 2019; Wanyama, 2019).

Drug Use and Comorbidity

Poorer nutritional health has been well established with regard to substance abusers. In opioid-dependent persons, Richardson and Wiest (2015) found that nutritional risk is associated with a decreased treatment retention rate. Methadone treatment for opioid-dependent persons was associated with a substantial, clinically significant weight gain that led to obesity. Substance abuse is also found to be highly associated with food insecurity. Comorbid mood disorders increase the strength of these relationships (Richardson & Wiest, 2015; Fenn et al., 2015; Sigmon & Fenn, 2015; Karen et al., 2018; Davison et al., 2016). It is well established that substance abuse and mood disorders are often comorbid.

Applications from the Experts

Exhibit 9-4 Health Professional Expert Advice

Changing behaviors is difficult, even when there is access and resources for healthy food options, environmental constructs that allow greater physical activity and the income to spend on getting help with making good choices. There are several ways to go about making better choices and being healthier. The methods that often work best are those that incorporate very small steps and a long period practicing each little increment before trying to make another tiny change.

An example might be that someone wants to lose weight. We know that decreasing the calories and increasing the physical activity results in weight losses. We also know that cutting calories makes people feel hungry and deprived and it doesn't behoove long-term weight loss maintenance. A strategy for decreasing calories while increasing the perception of fullness is to increase the amount of the fiber in the diet. Fruits and vegetables, whole grains, and beans/legumes are high in fiber. Substituting a serving of fresh fruit for a dessert every other day could be a first step. Using vegetables, like baby carrots or celery as a snack between meals, can be a second small step. Switching to whole grain bread, pasta, or brown rice could be a third step. Replacing soda with seltzer plus a squeeze of lemon, lime, or orange could be a fourth step, and so on. Over time, these small incremental, practiced steps build into the decrement of enough calories to lose weight slowly but surely.

The same can be said for increasing physical activity. Parking further away from where you need to go will force you to walk there and then walk back. A second step might be to take the stairs and not use the elevator. A third step might be to get a pedometer and chart how many steps you make during a day, and then add a few more each day. A fourth might be to get up and walk around your workplace every few hours if you sit at a desk, and so on. Over time, these steps accumulate to increase the amount of physical activity you get each day. The coupling of increased physical expenditure and decreased caloric intake over time results in weight loss and behavior change. Small successes lead to a better outlook and then support sustained efforts to make healthier choices, without feeling overwhelmed, discouraged or tiresome.

Environmental, Socioeconomic, and Other Factors

Increased obesity and metabolic syndrome risks have been established for rural dwelling persons. Interventions targeted at this population must incorporate culturally sensitive, cost-effective, transportation-friendly approaches. Several studies have investigated using healthcare self-management through educational opportunities, health coaching, and remote sensing technologies. Access to health care can also be provided through community centers, faith-based organizations, and the workplace. Direct care can be achieved for rural home-bound persons through mobile providers and the use of telemedicine.

Telemedicine, or telehealth, allows rural residents access to providers who can remotely evaluate, diagnose, and treat patients using technological advancements at a much lower cost and without requirements for patient transportation. Home health, or the provision of health care by mobile providers, allows the use of nutritional intervention and improvements in patient care for rural persons home-bound either through disability, geographic isolation, lack of transportation, or low resources. An example would be a single parent unable to find or afford child care so they can seek medical attention at a distance (Meit & Knudson, 2017; Haldane et al., 2019; Horning et al., 2018; Myers et al., 2015).

Geographical Considerations

The costs of having a balanced diet for rural inhabitants is higher in food deserts. Obesity rates are correlated with living within a food desert. There has been speculation that the USDA Thrifty Food Plan, which outlines how to achieve nutrients sufficiently on a low-cost budget for those receiving nutrition supplemental benefits does not work for many rural families. This is due in part to the costs of transportation to places where these basic foods can be purchased. The costs of transportation are high and not included in federal budgeting procedures for poor persons receiving benefits. Dimensions for cost and food security involve proximity when assessing fresh fruit and vegetable consumption, not just purchasing power or "direct costs." Another dimension not figured into the Thrifty Food Plan calculations is time. The most vulnerable persons who do not have vehicles must rely on other people's schedules for rides, or must combine walking with public transport to shop at a cost-conscious market. Researchers have assessed the influence of community adaptations to low access, poor proximity, lack of time, and resources (childcare, time off work to shop, flexible schedule), and found that the use of existing infrastructure, such as schools, zoning, municipal buildings to disseminate information, transportation, volunteer assistance, and childcare are all useful tools. Another solution has been to deploy the local food system to bridge the gaps in nutrient-dense food access. Entrepreneurial foodways include farmer's markets, kitchen gardens, community-supported agriculture, farm-to-institution programs (farm to fork), and food hubs, either mobile or stationary. In addition, combining private emergency food assistance with local food systems and entrepreneurial foodways can overcome gross deficiencies in communities that are impoverished, obese, and rural. While a "patchwork" approach to geography, policy, and food insecurity is not ideal, until a more unified approach is implemented, these methods provide respite for nutritionally underserved communities (Hilbert et al., 2014; Michimi & Wimberly, 2010; Strome et al., 2016; Hallet & McDermott, 2011; Dolstad et al., 2016; Sitaker et al., 2014; Pine & Bennett, 2014; Nguyen, 2017; McEntee & Naumova, 2012; Miller et al., 2016).

Conclusion

Rural, low-income persons are more likely to be obese, have chronic diseases, live in a food desert, and be food insecure. Food deserts dictate household food environments and impact nutritional adequacy. Rural households have less access to healthy foods, such as fruits and vegetables and whole grain products at low cost and poorer persons may not be able to use their nutrition supplemental benefits to improve their diets, due to poor proximity to a supermarket and/or other obstacles. Large supermarkets have better selections at lower cost compared with convenience stores. There is more access to unhealthy fast food establishments in low income, rural areas, where the educational attainment is lower. Models of nutritious food access have identified economics, service delivery, spatial-temporal, social, and personal dimensions that affect intake. Minorities are at greater disadvantage in terms of nutritional adequacy and food security. The latter impacts BMI. Parents are key in the process of food acquisition, processing and feeding, and low-income parents may not have the ability to make healthy choices, or even to put enough food on the table. Interventions for improving access and increasing the quality of the foods that rural persons eat should include cultural sensitivity. Tailored strategies to improve access, like subsidizing healthier choices in the local stores and using community infrastructure to provide education, access, and policies is important for success. Industry commitment to providing better food choices, using mobile food access points, farmers' markets, and food banks or pantries are essential. Sustainable changes involving the local food system do work but require assurance that implementation will be supported locally and federally or privately funded. Concerted efforts to stem the obesity and metabolic syndrome epidemics in rural areas is needed to decrease the escalating fiscal, health, and social costs being incurred. (Liese, 2014; Strome et al., 2016; Kyureghian & Nayga, 2013; Hubley, 2011; Freedman et al., 2013; Ro & Osborn, 2018; Macnell, 2011; Walker et al., 2012; Ken, 2014; Mader & Busse, 2011; Singleton et al., 2017).

Chapter Summary

Nutrition is the basis of life. Malnutrition is either a deficit or excess of nutrients. Rural persons are at risk for nutritional inadequacies, which result in disease. Obesity is a state of malnourishment and is associated with Metabolic Syndrome, which has T2D, cardiovascular disease, and other conditions under its umbrella. Rates of obesity among rural persons, particularly low income, poorly educated minorities, is escalating. Rural African Americans fare worst across all ages and regions. Subgroups within rural tracts are also at heightened risk for malnutrition, notably those that are food insecure. Food insecurity is related to several factors in addition to income. There are special populations that are notably food insecure, such as those who struggle with substance abuse and comorbid mental health issues.

Food deserts are areas that do not have access to healthy food choices. Rural areas often have more limited access to large supermarkets that have healthier foods at lower costs. Rural areas have more small convenience stores. Fast food, which is generally worse in terms of nutrient density, is also more accessible in poor rural areas. Programs that subsidize low-income person's purchasing power may not be effective in increasing the access to fruits and vegetables or healthy choices in general. Some groups, although subsidized, such as Native Americans, still exhibit alarming increases in obesity and comorbid disease rates. Surveillance of the nutritional landscape of rural areas has overwhelmingly shown that poor nutrition is rampant. Policy, intervention, and cultural competency are required to address this epidemic.

Discussion Questions

1. Discuss the contributions of specific nutrients to nutritional status and the development of obesity and comorbid conditions, such as metabolic syndrome.
2. Analyze the differences between different life-stage requirements for nutrients.
3. Describe the components of body composition and the manifestation of fat accumulation in the central region.
4. Discuss how surveillance measures nutrition and obesity. Which measures are useful and which are not? Explain your answers.
5. Discuss the phenomenon of dysbiosis and its relationship to disease.
6. Describe food and drug interactions and concomitant effects on overall nutritional status and health. Which groups exhibit the most serious consequences of these interactions? Explain your answer.
7. Define the following: food desert, food insecurity, food access points, built environment, disproportionate disadvantage, subsidies, poverty line, supplemental nutrition assistance, commodities, foodways, food recovery, surveillance, and longitudinal intervention. Using all of the words above explain how they intertwine and how there are relationships between each of them that can be used to comprehensively characterize rural nutrition challenges.
8. Describe how obesity is measured; what risks are commonplace for obese, rural residents; what variables are correlated with increased rates of rural obesity; and how life stage affects these relationships.
9. Explain how each of the following might be used to address nutritional problems related to rural residence: farmer's markets, mobile food access points, telehealth, community food drives, food pantries, food recovery, faith-based organizations, home visits, rideshares, health coaching, nutrition education, cooking classes, local food systems, cultural sensitivity, infrastructure improvements, private subsidies, industry commitments, kitchen gardens, incremental behavior change, and child care/school based programming.

Additional Reading

1. James, C. V., Moonesinghe, R., Wilson-Frederick, S. M., Hall, J. E., Penman-Aguilar, A., & Bouye, K. (2017). Racial /ethnic health disparities among rural adults — United States, 2012–2015. *MMWR Surveillance Summary,* 66(23), 1–9.
2. Hardin-Fanning, F., & Rayens, M. K. (2015). Food cost disparities in rural communities. *Health Promotion Practice, 16*(3), 383–391. doi:10.1177/1524839914554454
3. Rural Health Information Hub. (2019). *Rural hunger and access to healthy food.* https://www.ruralhealthinfo.org/topics /food-and-hunger.
4. Gregory C., A., &, A. Coleman-Jensen. (2017). Food insecurity, chronic disease, and health among working-age adults. *U.S. Department of Agriculture, ERR 235,* 1–31.
5. Rural Health Information Hub. (2020). *Rural food access toolkit.* https://www .ruralhealthinfo.org/toolkits/food-access

Student Activities and Worksheets are available inside the Navigate eBook, included with the printed text. Simply redeem the access code found at the front of the book at www.jblearning.com.

References

Ahern, M., Brown, C., & Dukas, S. (2011). A national study of the association between food environments and county-level health outcomes. *The Journal of Rural Health, 27*(4), 367–379. doi:10.1111/j.1748-0361.2011.00378.x

Alkon, A. H., & Agyeman, J. (Eds.). (2011). *Cultivating food justice: Race, class, and sustainability*. Cambridge, MA: The MIT Press.

Alviola, P. A., Nayga, R. M., & Thomsen, M. (2013). Food deserts and childhood obesity. *Applied Economic Perspectives and Policy, 35*(1), 106–124. doi:10.1093/aepp/pps035

Alviola, P. A., Nayga, R. M., Thomsen, M. R., & Wang, Z. (2013). Determinants of food deserts. *American Journal of Agricultural Economics, 95*(5), 1259–1265. doi:10.1093/ajae/aat029

Amuta, A. O., Jacobs, W., Idoko, E. E., Barry, A. E., & McKyer, E. L. J. (2015). Influence of the home food environment on children's fruit and vegetable consumption: A study of rural low-income families. *Health Promotion Practice, 16*(5), 689–698. doi:10.1177/1524839915589733

Andrews, M., Bhatta, R., & Ploeg, M. V. (2013). An alternative to developing stores in food deserts: Can changes in SNAP benefits make a difference? *Applied Economic Perspectives and Policy, 35*(1), 150–170. doi:10.1093/aepp/pps042

Baernholdt, M., Yan, G., Hinton, I., Rose, K., & Mattos, M. (2012). Quality of life in rural and urban adults 65 years and older: Findings from the national health and nutrition examination survey. *The Journal of Rural Health, 28*(4), 339–347. doi:10.1111/j.1748-0361.2011.00403.x

Bales, C. W. (2011). Paradise lost? Rural life and nutritional well being in the 21st century. *Journal of Nutrition in Gerontology and Geriatrics, 30*(3), 201–203. doi:10.1080/21551197.2011.597648

Barnidge, E. K., Radvanyi, C., Duggan, K., Motton, F., Wiggs, I., Baker, E. A., & Brownson, R. C. (2013). Understanding and addressing barriers to implementation of environmental and policy interventions to support physical activity and healthy eating in rural communities. *The Journal of Rural Health, 29*(1), 97–105. doi:10.1111/j.1748-0361.2012.00431.x

Beaulac, J., Kristjansson, E., & Cummins, S. (2009). A systematic review of food deserts, 1966-2007. *Preventing Chronic Disease, 6*(3), A105.

Befort, C. A., Nazir, N., & Perri, M. G. (2012). Prevalence of obesity among adults from rural and urban areas of the United States: Findings from NHANES (2005-2008). *Journal of Rural Health, 28*(4), 392–397. doi:10.1111/j.1748-0361.2012.00411.x

Belansky, E. S., Cutforth, N., Delong, E., Ross, C., Scarbro, S., Gilbert, L., . . . Marshall, J. A. (2009). Early impact of the federally mandated local wellness policy on physical activity in rural, low-income elementary schools in Colorado. *Journal of Public Health Policy, 30*(S1), S141–S160. doi:10.1057/jphp.2008.50

Berry, D. C., McMurray, R. G., Schwartz, T. A., & Adatorwovor, R. (2018). Benefits for African American and white low-income 7–10-year-old children and their parents taught together in a community-based weight management program in the rural southeastern United States. *BMC Public Health, 18*(1), 1107. doi:10.1186/s12889-018-6006-4

Block, J. P., & Subramanian, S. V. (2015). Moving beyond "food deserts": Reorienting United States policies to reduce disparities in diet quality. *PLoS Medicine, 12*(12), e1001914. doi:10.1371/journal.pmed.1001914

Boelens, M., Windhorst, D., Jonkman, H., Hosman, C., Raat, H., & Jansen, W. (2019). Evaluation of the promising neighbourhoods community program to reduce health inequalities in youth: A protocol of a mixed-methods study. *BMC Public Health, 19*(1), 555. doi:10.1186/s12889-019-6901-3

Bolin, J. N., Bellamy, G. R., Ferdinand, A. O., Vuong, A. M., Kash, B. A., Schulze, A., & Helduser, J. W. (2015). Rural healthy people 2020: New decade, same challenges. *The Journal of Rural Health, 31*(3), 326–333. doi:10.1111/jrh.12116

Botchwey, N. D., Falkenstein, R., Levin, J., Fisher, T., & Trowbridge, M. (2015). The built environment and *actual causes of death*: Promoting an ecological approach to planning and public health. *Journal of Planning Literature, 30*(3), 261–281. doi:10.1177/0885412214561337

Campbell, E. A., Shapiro, M. J., Welsh, C., Bleich, S. N., Cobb, L. K., & Gittelsohn, J. (2017). Healthy food availability among food sources in rural Maryland counties. *Journal of Hunger & Environmental Nutrition, 12*(3), 328–341. doi:10.1080/19320248.2017.1315328

Carlson, A., & Frazão, E. (2014). Food costs, diet quality and energy balance in the United States. *Physiology & Behavior, 134*, 20–31. doi:10.1016/j.physbeh.2014.03.001

Carnahan, L. R., Zimmermann, K., & Peacock, N. R. (2016). What rural women want the public health community to know about access to healthful food: A qualitative study, 2011. *Preventing Chronic Disease, 13*, E57. doi:10.5888/pcd13.150583

Chai, W., Fan, J. X., & Wen, M. (2018). Association of individual and neighborhood factors with home food availability: Evidence from the national health and nutrition examination survey. *Journal of the Academy of Nutrition and Dietetics, 118*(5), 815–823. doi:10.1016/j.jand.2017.11.009

Chang, K., Zastrow, M., Zdorovtsov, C., Quast, R., Skjonsberg, L., & Stluka, S. (2015). Do SNAP and

WIC programs encourage more fruit and vegetable intake? A household survey in the Northern Great Plains. *Journal of Family and Economic Issues, 36*(4), 477–490. doi:10.1007/s10834-014-9412-5

Chasekwa, B., Maluccio, J. A., Ntozini, R., Moulton, L. H., Wu, F., Smith, L. E., . . . The SHINE Trial Team. (2018). Measuring wealth in rural communities: Lessons from the sanitation, hygiene, infant nutrition efficacy (SHINE) trial. *PLoS ONE, 13*(6), 1–19. doi:10.1371/journal.pone.0199393

Chen, D., Jaenicke, E., & Volpe, R. (2016). Food environments and obesity: Household diet expenditure versus food deserts. *American Journal of Public Health, 106*(5), 881–888. doi:10.2105/AJPH.2016.303048

Cohen, S. A., Greaney, M. L., & Sabik, N. J. (2018). Assessment of dietary patterns, physical activity and obesity from a national survey: Rural-urban health disparities in older adults. *PLoS ONE, 13*(12), e0208268. doi:10.1371/journal.pone.0208268

Colman, A. (2018). Addressing health disparities in rural America. *Parks & Recreation, 53*(10), 42–44.

Cornish, D., Askelson, N., & Golembiewski, E. (2016). "Reforms looked really good on paper": Rural food service responses to the healthy, Hunger-Free Kids Act of 2010. *The Journal of School Health, 86*(2), 113–120. doi:10.1111/josh.12356

Crow, R., Lohman, M., Titus, A., Cook, S., Bruce, M. L., McKenzie, S., . . . Batsis, J. A. (2019). Association of obesity with frailty in older adults: NHANES 1999–2004. *Journal of Nutrition, Health & Aging, 23*(2), 138–144.

Davison, K., Gondara, L., & Holloway, C. (2016). Relationships between previous 12-month and lifetime illicit substance use and food insecurity in British Columbia. *Journal of Nutrition Education and Behavior, 48*(7S), S91–S92. doi:10.1016/j.jneb.2016.04.242

Davison, K. M., Holloway, C., Gondara, L., & Hatcher, A. S. (2018). Independent associations and effect modification between lifetime substance use and recent mood disorder diagnosis with household food insecurity. *PLoS ONE, 13*(1), e0191072. doi:10.1371/journal.pone.0191072

Dean, W. R., & Sharkey, J. R. (2011). Food insecurity, social capital and perceived personal disparity in a predominantly rural region of Texas: An individual-level analysis. *Social Science & Medicine, 72*(9), 1454–1462. doi:10.1016/j.socscimed.2011.03.015

Dennison, D. A., Yin, Z., Kibbe, D., Burns, S., & Trowbridge, F. (2008). Training health care professionals to manage overweight adolescents: Experience in rural Georgia communities. *The Journal of Rural Health, 24*(1), 55–59. doi:10.1111/j.1748-0361.2008.00137.x

Dolstad, H. A., Woodward, A. R., Green, C. L., & McSpirit, S. J. (2016). Interest in nutrition and local food systems among food-insecure households in an Appalachian community. *Journal of Hunger & Environmental Nutrition, 11*(3), 340–353. doi:10.1080/19320248.2016.1146191

Dubowitz, T., Ghosh-Dastidar, M., Collins, R. L., & Escarce, J. J. (2013). Food policy research: We need better measurement, better study designs, and reasonable and measured actions based on the available evidence. *Obesity, 21*(1), 5–6. doi:10.1002/oby.20035

Escoffery, C., Kegler, M. C., Alcantara, I., Wilson, M., & Glanz, K. (2011). A qualitative examination of the role of small, rural worksites in obesity prevention. *Preventing Chronic Disease, 8*(4), A75.

Fenn, J. M., Laurent, J. S., & Sigmon, S. C. (2015). Increases in body mass index following initiation of methadone treatment. *Journal of Substance Abuse Treatment, 51*, 59–63. doi:10.1016/j.jsat.2014.10.007

Firth, J. (2012). Healthy choices and heavy burdens: Race, citizenship and gender in the 'obesity epidemic.' *Journal of International Women's Studies, 13*(2), 33–50.

Fitzpatrick, K., Greenhalgh-Stanley, N., & Ver Ploeg, M. (2016). The impact of food deserts on food insufficiency and SNAP participation among the elderly. *American Journal of Agricultural Economics, 98*(1), 19–40. doi:10.1093/ajae/aav044

Flynt, A., & Daepp, M. I. G. (2015). Diet-related chronic disease in the northeastern United States: A model-based clustering approach. *International Journal of Health Geographics, 14*(25). doi:10.1186/s12942-015-0017-5

Fox, K., & Heaton, T. B. (2012). Child nutritional status by rural/urban residence: A cross-national analysis. *The Journal of Rural Health, 28*(4), 380–391. doi:10.1111/j.1748-0361.2012.00408.x

Freedman, D. A., Blake, C. E., & Liese, A. D. (2013). Developing a multicomponent model of nutritious food access and related implications for community and policy practice. *Journal of Community Practice, 21*(4), 379–409. doi:10.1080/10705422.2013.842197

Freedman, D. A., Vaudrin, N., Schneider, C., Trapl, E., Ohri-Vachaspati, P., Taggart, M., . . . Flocke, S. (2016). Systematic review of factors influencing farmers' market use overall and among low-income populations. *Journal of the Academy of Nutrition and Dietetics, 116*(7), 1136–1155. doi:10.1016/j.jand.2016.02.010

Frost, D., & Porterfield, S. (2012). Health promotion guidance for a rural community. *The Journal for Nurse Practitioners, 8*(9), 712–716. doi:10.1016/j.nurpra.2012.04.011

Gamba, R., Schuchter, J., Rutt, C., & Seto, E. (2015). Measuring the food environment and its effects on obesity in the United States: A systematic review of methods and results. *Journal of Community Health, 40*(3), 464–475. doi:10.1007/s10900-014-9958-z

Greder, K., Peng, C., Doudna, K. D., & Sarver, S. L. (2017). Role of family stressors on rural low-income children's behaviors. *Child & Youth Care Forum, 46*(5), 703–720. doi:10.1007/s10566-017-9401-6

Guest, M. A., Freedman, D., Alia, K. A., Brandt, H. M., & Friedman, D. B. (2015). Dissemination of an electronic manual to build capacity for implementing farmers' markets with community health centers. *Clinical and Translational Science, 8*(5), 484–489. doi:10.1111/cts.12318

Haldane, V., Chuah, F. L. H., Srivastava, A., Singh, S. R., Koh, G. C. H., Seng, C. K., & Legido-Quigley, H. (2019). Community participation in health services development, implementation, and evaluation: A systematic review of empowerment, health, community, and process outcomes. *PLoS ONE, 14*(5), e0216112. doi:10.1371/journal.pone.0216112

Hallett, L. F., & McDermott, D. (2011). Quantifying the extent and cost of food deserts in Lawrence, Kansas, USA. *Applied Geography, 31*(4), 1210–1215. doi:10.1016/j.apgeog.2010.09.006

Haynes-Maslow, L., & Leone, L. A. (2017). Examining the relationship between the food environment and adult diabetes prevalence by county economic and racial composition: An ecological study. *BMC Public Health, 17*, 648. doi:10.1186/s12889-017-4658-0

Heuberger, R. (2011). Impact of housing type on nutritional status and oral health of rural older adults residing in the Midwestern United States. *Seniors Housing & Care Journal, 19*(1), 49–63.

Hilbert, N., Evans-Cowley, J., Reece, J., Rogers, C., Ake, W., & Hoy, C. (2014). Mapping the cost of a balanced diet, as a function of travel time and food price. *Journal of Agriculture, Food Systems, and Community Development, 5*(1), 105–127. doi:10.5304/jafscd.2014.051.010

Hill, J. L., You, W., & Zoellner, J. M. (2014). Disparities in obesity among rural and urban residents in a health disparate region. *BMC Public Health, 14*(1). doi:10.1186/1471-2458-14-1051

Hodge, F. S., & Nandy, K. (2011). Predictors of wellness and American Indians. *Journal of Health Care for the Poor and Underserved, 22*(3), 791–803. doi:10.1353/hpu.2011.0093

Hollinger, D. L. (Ed.). (2018). Sites in review. *Journal of the Academy of Nutrition and Dietetics, 118*(11), 2201. https://doi.org/10.1016/j.jand.2018.08.162

Horning, M., Olsen, J., Lell, S., Thorson, D., & Monsen, K. (2018). Description of public health nursing nutrition assessment and interventions for home-visited women. *Public Health Nursing, 35*(4), 317–326. doi:10.1111/phn.12410

Howlett, E., Davis, C., & Burton, S. (2016). From food desert to food oasis: The potential influence of food retailers on childhood obesity rates. *Journal of Business Ethics, 139*(2), 215–224. doi:10.1007/s10551-015-2605-5

Hsiao, B. S., Sibeko, L., & Troy, L. M. (2019). A systematic review of mobile produce markets: Facilitators and barriers to use, and associations with reported fruit and vegetable intake. *Journal of the Academy of Nutrition and Dietetics, 119*(1), 76–97. doi:10.1016/j.jand.2018.02.022

Huang, D. L., Rosenberg, D. E., Simonovich, S. D., & Belza, B. (2012). Food access patterns and barriers among midlife and older adults with mobility disabilities. *Journal of Aging Research*, 2012, 231489. doi:10.1155/2012/231489

Hubley, T. A. (2011). Assessing the proximity of healthy food options and food deserts in a rural area in Maine. *Applied Geography, 31*(4), 1224–1231. doi:10.1016/j.apgeog.2010.09.004

Jiao, J., Moudon, A., Ulmer, J., Hurvitz, P., & Drewnowski, A. (2012). How to identify food deserts: Measuring physical and economic access to supermarkets in King County, Washington. *American Journal of Public Health, 102*(10), e32–e39.

Jilcott Pitts, S. B., Wu, Q., Truesdale, K. P., Laska, M. N., Grinchak, T., McGuirt, J. T., . . . Ammerman, A. S. (2017). Baseline assessment of a healthy corner store initiative: Associations between food store environments, shopping patterns, customer purchases, and dietary intake in eastern North Carolina. *International Journal of Environmental Research and Public Health, 14*(10), e1189. doi:10.3390/ijerph14101189

Kalichman, S., Hernandez, D., Cherry, C., Kalichman, M. O., Washington, C., & Grebler, T. (2014). Food insecurity and other poverty indicators among people living with HIV/AIDS: Effects on treatment and health outcomes. *Journal of Community Health, 39*(6), 1133–1139. doi:10.1007/s10900-014-9868-0

Karpyn, A., Young, C., & Weiss, S. (2012). Reestablishing healthy food retail: Changing the landscape of food deserts. *Childhood Obesity, 8*(1), 28–30. doi:10.1089/chi.2011.0113

Kato, Y., & McKinney, L. (2015). Bringing food desert residents to an alternative food market: A semi-experimental study of impediments to food access. *Agriculture and Human Values, 32*(2), 215–227. doi:10.1007/s10460-014-9541-3

Kegler, M. C., Escoffery, C., Alcantara, I., Ballard, D., & Glanz, K. (2008). A qualitative examination of home and neighborhood environments for obesity prevention in rural adults. *International Journal of Behavioral Nutrition and Physical Activity, 5*(65). doi:10.1186/1479-5868-5-65

Kelli, H. M., Kim, J. H., Samman Tahhan, A. S., Liu, C., Ko, Y. A., Hammadah, M., . . . Quyyumi, A. A. (2019). Living in food deserts and adverse cardiovascular outcomes in patients with cardiovascular disease. *Journal of the American Heart Association, 8*(4), e010694. doi:10.1161/JAHA.118.010694

Ken, I. (2014). Profit in the food desert: Walmart stakes its claim. *Theory in Action, 7*(4), 13–32. doi:10.3798/tia.1937-0237.14025

Khare, M. M., Koch, A., Zimmermann, K., Moehring, P. A., & Geller, S. E. (2014). Heart smart for women: A community-based lifestyle change intervention to reduce cardiovascular risk in rural women. *The Journal of Rural Health, 30*(4), 359–368. doi:10.1111/jrh.12066

Khojasteh, M., & Raja, S. (2017). Agents of change: How immigrant-run ethnic food retailers improve food environments. *Journal of Hunger & Environmental Nutrition, 12*(3), 299–327. doi:10.1080/19320248.2015.1112759

Kim-Godwin, Y., & McMurry, M. J. (2012). Perspectives of nurse practitioners on health care needs among Latino children and families in the rural southeastern United States: A pilot study. *Journal of Pediatric Health Care, 26*(6), 409–417. doi:10.1016/j.pedhc.2011.02.013

King, K. M., & Ling, J. (2015). Results of a 3-year, nutrition and physical activity intervention for children in rural, low-socioeconomic status elementary schools. *Health Education Research, 30*(4), 647–659. doi:10.1093/her/cyv029

Kongats, K., McGetrick, J. A., Raine, K. D., & Voyer, C. (2019). Assessing general public and policy influencer support for healthy public policies to promote healthy eating at the population level in two Canadian provinces. *Public Health Nutrition, 22*(8), 1492–1502. doi:10.1017/S1368980018004068

Kyureghian, G., & Nayga, R. M. (2013). Food store access, availability, and choice when purchasing fruits and vegetables. *American Journal of Agricultural Economics, 95*(5), 1280–1286. doi:10.1093/ajae/aat043

Larson, K. L., Mullaney, M., Mwangi, E., Xiong, D., & Ziegler, F. (2017). Access to healthy foods in rural Minnesota: A pilot analysis of corner stores. *American Journal of Health Studies, 32*(3), 144–148.

Lebel, A., Noreau, D., Tremblay, L., Oberlé, C., Girard-Gadreau, M., Duguay, M., & Block, J. P. (2016). Identifying rural food deserts: Methodological considerations for food environment interventions. *Canadian Journal of Public Health, 107*(Suppl 1), eS21–eS26. doi:10.17269/CJPH.107.5353

LeClair, M. S., & Aksan, A. (2014). Redefining the food desert: Combining GIS with direct observation to measure food access. *Agriculture and Human Values, 31*(4), 537–547. doi:10.1007/s10460-014-9501-y

Li, Y., Kidd, T., Lindshield, E., Adhikari, K., Muturi, N., Kattelmann, K., & Zies, S. (2015). Analyses of the built environment and perceptions related to nutritious foods in rural low-income ethnic communities in Kansas. *Journal of the Academy of Nutrition and Dietetics, 115*(9), A83. doi:10.1016/j.jand.2015.06.300

Liese, A. D., Hibbert, J. D., Ma, X., Bell, B. A., & Battersby, S. E. (2014). Where are the food deserts? An evaluation of policy-relevant measures of community food access in South Carolina. *Journal of Hunger & Environmental Nutrition, 9*(1), 16–32. doi:10.1080/19320248.2013.873009

Liese, A. D., Lamichhane, A. P., Garzia, S. C. A., Puett, R. C., Porter, D. E., Dabelea D., . . . Liu, L. (2018). Neighborhood characteristics, food deserts, rurality, and type 2 diabetes in youth: Findings from a case-control study. *Health and Place, 50*, 81–88. doi:10.1016/j.healthplace.2018.01.004

Loo, C. (2014). Towards a more participative definition of food justice. *Journal of Agricultural and Environmental Ethics, 27*(5), 787–809. doi:10.1007/s10806-014-9490-2

Lu, C., Huang, G., & Corpeleijn, E. (2019). Environmental correlates of sedentary time and physical activity in preschool children living in a relatively rural setting in the Netherlands: A cross-sectional analysis of the GECKO Drenthe cohort. *BMJ Open, 9*(5), e027468. doi:10.1136/bmjopen-2018-027468

Macnell, L. (2011). A geo-ethnographic analysis of low-income rural and urban women's food shopping behaviors. *Appetite, 128*, 311–320. doi:10.1016/j.appet.2018.05.147

Mader, E., & Busse, H. (2011). Hungry in the heartland: Using community food systems as a strategy to reduce rural food deserts. *Journal of Hunger & Environmental Nutrition, 6*(1), 45–53. doi:10.1080/19320248.2011.549377

Maguire, J. S. (2016). Introduction: Looking at food practices and taste across the class divide. *Food, Culture & Society, 19*(1), 11–18. doi:10.1080/15528014.2016.1144995

McEntee, J. (2009). Highlighting food inadequacies: Does the food desert metaphor help this cause? *British Food Journal, 111*(4), 349-363. doi:10.1108/00070700910951498

McEntee, J., & Naumova, E. (2012). Building capacity between the private emergency food system and the local food movement: Working toward food justice and sovereignty in the global north. *Journal of Agriculture, Food Systems, and Community Development, 3*(1), 235–253.

Meit, M., & Knudson, A. (2017). Leveraging interest to decrease rural health disparities in the United States. *American Journal of Public Health, 107*(10), 1563–1564. doi:10.2105/AJPH.2017.304025

Mejia de Grubb, M. C., Levine, R. S., & Zoorob, R. J. (2017). Diet and obesity issues in the underserved. *Primary Care: Clinics in Office Practice, 44*(1), 127–140. doi:10.1016/j.pop.2016.09.014

Michimi, A., & Wimberly, M. (2010). Associations of supermarket accessibility with obesity and fruit and vegetable consumption in the conterminous United States. *International Journal of Health Geographics, 9*(1), 49. doi:10.1186/1476-072X-9-49

Miller, W. C., Rogalla, D., Spencer, D., Zia, N., Griffith, B. N., & Heinsberg, H. B. (2016). Community adaptations to an impending food desert in rural Appalachia, USA. *Rural and Remote Health, 16*(4), 3901, 1–12.

Moore, J. B., Davis, C. L., Baxter, S. D., Lewis, R. D., & Yin, Z. (2008). Physical activity, metabolic syndrome, and overweight in rural youth. *The Journal of Rural Health, 24*(2), 136–142. doi:10.1111/j.1748-0361.200800144.x

Morio, K. A., Marshall, T. A., Qian, F., & Morgan, T. A. (2008). Comparing diet, oral hygiene and caries status of adult methamphetamine users and non-users: A pilot study. *The Journal of the American Dental Association, 139*(2), 171–176. doi:10.14219/jada.archive.2008.0133

Morris, A. A., McAllister, P., Grant, A., Geng, S., Kelli, H. M., Kalogeropoulos, A., . . . Butler, J. (2019). Relation of living in a "food desert" to recurrent hospitalizations in patients with heart failure. *The American Journal of Cardiology, 123*(2), 291–296. doi:10.1016/j.amjcard.2018.10.004

Myers, C., Slack, T., Martin, C., Broyles, S., & Heymsfield, S. (2015). Regional disparities in obesity prevalence in the United States: A spatial regime analysis. *Obesity, 23*(2), 481–487. doi:10.1002/oby.20963

Nanney, M. S., Davey, C. S., & Kubik, M. Y. (2013). Rural disparities in the distribution of policies that support healthy eating in US secondary schools. *Journal of the Academy of Nutrition and Dietetics, 113*(8), 1062–1068. doi:10.1016/j.jand.2013.04.021

National Institute on Alcohol Abuse and Alcoholism. Rethinking drinking: Alcohol and your health. https://www.rethinkingdrinking.niaaa.nih.gov/how-much-is-too-much/what-counts-as-a-drink/whats-a-standard-drink.aspx

NCD Risk Factor Collaboration (NCD-RisC). (2019). Rising rural body-mass index is the main driver of the global obesity epidemic in adults. *Nature, 569*(7755), 260–264. doi:10.1038/s41586-019-1171-x

Nguyen, L. T. (2017). Would you like tax exemptions with that? How food exemptions under state sales tax are not reaching lower income communities in food deserts. *Journal of Gender, Race and Justice, 20*(1), 187–207.

Peters, P., Gold, A., Abbott, A., Contreras, D., Keim, A., Oscarson, R., . . . Mobley, A. R. (2016). A quasi-experimental study to mobilize rural low-income communities to assess and improve the ecological environment to prevent childhood obesity. *BMC Public Health, 16*(376). doi:10.1186/s12889-016-3047-4

Pine, A., & Bennett, J. (2014). Food access and food deserts: The diverse methods that residents of a neighborhood in Duluth, Minnesota use to provision themselves. *Community Development, 45*(4), 317–336. doi:10.1080/15575330.2014.930501

Popkin, B. (2019). Rural areas drive the global weight gain. *Nature, 569*(7755), 200–201. doi:10.1038/d41586-019-01182-x

Richardson, R., & Wiest, K. (2015). A preliminary study examining nutritional risk factors, body mass index,

and treatment retention in opioid-dependent patients. *The Journal of Behavioral Health Services & Research, 42*(3), 401–408. doi:10.1007/s11414-013-9371-x

Ro, A., & Osborn, B. (2018). Exploring dietary factors in the food insecurity and obesity relationship among Latinos in California. *Journal of Health Care for the Poor and Underserved, 29*(3), 1108–1122. doi:10.1353/hpu.2018.0082

Robinson, J. C., Carson, T. L., Johnson, E. R., Hardy, C. M., Shikany, J. M., Green, E., . . . Baskin, M. L. (2014). Assessing environmental support for better health: Active living opportunity audits in rural communities in the southern United States. *Preventive Medicine, 66*, 28–33. doi:10.1016/j.ypmed.2014.05.021

Robinson, J., Weissman, E., Adair, S., Potteiger, M., & Villanueva, J. (2016). An oasis in the desert? The benefits and constraints of mobile markets operating in Syracuse, New York food deserts. *Agriculture and Human Values, 33*(4), 877–893. doi:10.1007/s10460-016-9680-9

Rodriguez, R. M., & Grahame, K. M. (2016). Understanding food access in a rural community: An ecological perspective. *Food, Culture & Society, 19*(1), 171–194. doi:10.1080/15528014.2016.1145010

Rushakoff, J. A., Zoughbie, D. E., Bui, N., Devito, K., Makarechi, L., & Kubo, H. (2017). Evaluation of Healthy2Go: A country store transformation project to improve the food environment and consumer choices in Appalachian Kentucky. *Preventive Medicine Reports, 7*, 187–192. doi:10.1016/j.pmedr.2017.06.009

Salinas, J., Abdelbary, B., Klaas, K., Tapia, B., & Sexton, K. (2014). Socioeconomic context and the food landscape in Texas: Results from hotspot analysis and border/non-border comparison of unhealthy food environments. *International Journal of Environmental Research and Public Health, 11*(6), 5640–5650. doi:10.3390/ijerph110605640

Santorelli, M., & Okeke, J. (2017). Evaluating community measures of healthy food access. *Journal of Community Health, 42*(5), 991–997. doi:10.1007/s10900-017-0346-3

Schafft, K., Jensen, E., & Hinrichs, C. (2009). Food deserts and overweight schoolchildren: Evidence from Pennsylvania. *Rural Sociology, 74*(2), 153–177. doi:10.1111/j.1549-0831.2009.tb00387.x

Sebastiani, G., Borrás-Novell, C., Casanova, M. A., Tutusaus, M. P., Martínez, S. F., Roig, M. D. G., & García-Algar, O. (2018). The effects of alcohol and drugs of abuse on maternal nutritional profile during pregnancy. *Nutrients, 10*(8), 1008. doi:10.3390/nu10081008

Semple, H., & Giguere, A. (2018). The evolution of food deserts in a small midwestern city: The case of Ypsilanti, Michigan: 1970 to 2010. *Journal of Planning Education and Research, 38*(3), 359–370. doi:10.1177/0739456X17702222

Sigmon, S. C., & Fenn, J. (2015). Examining the association between methadone maintenance treatment and body mass index. *Drug and Alcohol Dependence, 146*, e99. doi:10.1016/j.drugalcdep.2014.09.637

Singleton, C., Li, Y., Duran, A., Zenk, S., Odoms-Young, A., & Powell, L. (2017). Food and beverage availability in small food stores located in healthy food financing initiative eligible communities. *International Journal of Environmental Research and Public Health, 14*(10), e1242. doi:10.3390/ijerph14101242

Sitaker, M., Kolodinsky, J., Pitts, S. J., & Seguin, R. (2014). Do entrepreneurial food systems innovations impact rural economies and health? Evidence and gaps. *American Journal of Entrepreneurship, 7*(2), 3–16.

Slack, T., Myers, C., Martin, C., & Heymsfield, S. (2014). The geographic concentration of US adult obesity prevalence and associated social, economic, and environmental factors. *Obesity, 22*(3), 868–874. doi:10.1002/oby.20502

Smart, M. J. (2018). Walkability, transit, and body mass index: A panel approach. *Journal of Transport & Health, 8*, 193–201. doi:10.1016/j.jth.2017.12.012

Smith, D., Miles-Richardson, S., Dill, L., & Archie-Booker, E. (2013). Interventions to improve access to fresh food in vulnerable communities: A review of the literature. *International Journal on Disability and Human Development, 12*(4), 409–417. doi:10.1515/ijdhd-2013-0203

Spurrier, A. E., Suttle, C., Matheson, L., & Baker-Watson, A. (2018). The effects of a health promotion program on rural, West Virginia adults. *Family and Community Health, 41*(2), 95–104. doi:10.1097/FCH.0000000000000179

Strom, J. L., Lynch, C. P., & Egede, L. E. (2011). Rural/urban variations in diabetes self-care and quality of care in a national sample of US adults with diabetes. *The Diabetes Educator, 37*(2), 254–262. doi:10.1177/0145721710394875

Strome, S., Johns, T., Scicchitano, M. J., & Shelnutt, K. (2016). Elements of access: The effects of food outlet proximity, transportation, and realized access on fresh fruit and vegetable consumption in food deserts. *International Quarterly of Community Health Education, 37*(1), 61–70. doi:10.1177/0272684X16685252

Sylvie, A., Jiang, Q., & Cohen, N. (2013). Identification of environmental supports for healthy eating in older adults. *Journal of Nutrition in Gerontology and Geriatrics, 32*(2), 161–174. doi:10.1080/21551197.2013.779621

Taber, D., Chriqui, J., Quinn, C., Rimkus, L., & Chaloupka, F. (2016). Cross-sector analysis of socioeconomic, racial/ethnic, and urban/rural disparities in food policy enactment in the United States. *Health & Place, 42*, 47–53. doi:10.1016/j.healthplace.2016.08.006

Tevik, K., Selbæk, G., Engedal, K., Seim, A., Krokstad, S., & Helvik, A. S. (2019). Mortality in older adults with frequent alcohol consumption and use of drugs with addiction potential – The Nord Trøndelag Health Study 2006-2008 (HUNT3), Norway, a population-based study. *PLoS ONE, 14*(4), e0214813. doi:10.1371/journal.pone.0214813

Thomsen, M. R., Nayga, R. M., Alviola, P. A., & Rouse, H. L. (2016). The effect of food deserts on the body mass index of elementary school children. *American Journal of Agricultural Economics, 98*(1), 1–18. doi:10.1093/ajae/aav039

Vaterlaus, J. M., Cottle, N. M., Patten, E. V., & Gibbons, R. (2018). Understanding customers: The jobs to be done theory applied in the context of a rural food pantry. *Journal of the Academy of Nutrition and Dietetics, 118*(10), 1895–1902. doi:10.1016/j.jand.2018.02.011

Ver Ploeg, M., Dutko, P., & Breneman, V. (2015). Measuring food access and food deserts for policy purposes. *Applied Economic Perspectives and Policy, 37*(2), 205–225. doi:10.1093/aepp/ppu035

Vieira, E. R., Vaccaro, J. A., Zarini, G. G., & Huffman, F. G. (2017). Health indicators of US older adults who received or did not receive meals funded by the Older Americans Act. *Journal of Aging Research*, 2160819. https://doi.org/10.1155/2017/2160819

Walker, J. O. Y., & Cunningham, G. B. (2014). The influence of perceived access to healthy food and physical activity on the subjective health of African Americans in rural communities. *American Journal of Health Studies, 29*(2), 165.

Walker, R. E., Block, J., & Kawachi, I. (2012). Do residents of food deserts express different food buying preferences compared to residents of food oases? A mixed-methods analysis. *International Journal of Behavioral Nutrition and Physical Activity, 9*(1), 41. doi:10.1186/1479-5868-9-41

Walker, R. E., Butler, J., Kriska, A., Keane, C., Fryer, C. S., & Burke, J. G. (2010). How does food security impact residents of a food desert and a food oasis? *Journal of Hunger & Environmental Nutrition, 5*(4), 454–470. doi:10.1080/19320248.2010.530549

Walker, R. E., Fryer, C. S., Butler, J., Keane, C. R., Kriska, A., & Burke, J. G. (2011). Factors influencing food buying practices in residents of a low-income food desert and a low-income food oasis. *Journal of Mixed Methods Research, 5*(3), 247–267. doi:10.1177/1558689811412971

Walker, R. E., Keane, C. R., & Burke, J. G. (2010). Disparities and access to healthy food in the United States: A review of food deserts literature. *Health and Place, 16*(5), 876–884. doi:10.1016/j.healthplace.2010.04.013

Wang, H., Kenkel, D., Graham, M., Paul, L., Folta, S., Nelson, M., . . . Seguin, R. A. (2019). Cost-effectiveness of a community-based cardiovascular disease prevention intervention in medically underserved rural areas. *BMC Health Services Research, 19*(1), 315. doi:10.1186/s12913-019-4117-y

Wang, H., Qiu, F., & Swallow, B. (2014). Can community gardens and farmers' markets relieve food desert problems? A study of Edmonton, Canada. *Applied Geography, 55,* 127–137. doi:10.1016/j.apgeog.2014.09.010

Wang, H., Tao, L., Qiu, F., & Lu, W. (2016). The role of socio-economic status and spatial effects on fresh food access: Two case studies in Canada. *Applied Geography, 67,* 27–38. doi:10.1016/j.apgeog.2015.12.002

Wanyama, R., Gödecke, T., Jager, M., & Qaim, M. (2019). Poor consumers' preferences for nutritionally enhanced foods. *British Food Journal, 121*(3), 755–770. doi:10.1108/BFJ-09-2018-0622

Whitley, S. (2013). Changing times in rural America: Food assistance and food insecurity in food deserts. *Journal of Family Social Work, 16*(1), 36–52. doi:10.1080/10522158.2012.736080

Wright, J., Donley, A., Gualtieri, M., & Strickhouser, S. (2016). Food deserts: What is the problem? What is the solution?. *Society, 53*(2), 171–181. doi:10.1007/s12115-016-9993-8

Wu, Q., Saitone, T., & Sexton, R. (2017). Food access, food deserts, and the Women, Infants, and Children program. *Journal of Agricultural and Resource Economics, 42*(3), 310–328.

Yousefian, A., Leighton, A., Fox, K., & Hartley, D. (2011). Understanding the rural food environment-perspectives of low-income parents. *Rural and Remote Health, 11*(2), 1631.

Zenk, S., Tarlov, E., Wing, C., Matthews, S., Jones, K., Tong, H., & Powell, L. M. (2017). Geographic accessibility of food outlets not associated with body mass index change among veterans, 2009–14. *Health Affairs, 36*(8), 1433–1442. doi:10.1377/hlthaff.2017.0122

CHAPTER 10

Maternal and Child Health in Rural Areas

Shayesteh Jahanfar, PhD
Fathima Wakeel, PhD, MPH

LEARNING OBJECTIVES

At the end of this chapter, the readers will be able to:

1. Name the division of the Centers for Disease Control and Prevention (CDC) that provides leadership in the promotion of women's and infant health.
2. Cite approximately what percentage of women in the United States live in rural areas.
3. List factors related to maternal mortality in rural areas.
4. Describe key components of the school health programs.
5. List the advantages of family planning practices.
6. Name the most common forms of sexually transmitted infections (STIs).

KEY TERMS

Contraception
Diaphragm
Hormonal contraception
Infant mortality
Low birth weight
Maternal morbidity
Maternal mortality
Non hormonal contraceptives
Prenatal care
Preterm Birth
Sexually transmitted infection
Unintended pregnancy

CHAPTER OVERVIEW

The health of women and children is a vital part of the right to health, incorporating reproductive and maternal health (prenatal and postnatal), and child health care. The CDC's Division of Reproductive Health provides leadership in the promotion of women's and infants' health before, during, and after pregnancy. The major task of this division is to reduce disease and death among mothers and babies, with special attention to reducing racial and ethnic differences in health in these populations. Women living in rural areas are among the most vulnerable populations due to lack of access to health care as well as disparity issues.

In this chapter, we present the most important concepts under the umbrella of maternal child health, with a focus on rural health. First, we will provide a description of the foundational lens through which maternal and child health has been largely conceptualized in the past two decades—the life course approach. In this section, we will discuss the five guiding principles of the life course approach as well as three temporal concepts related to one's development over the life course. Second, we describe the epidemiology of maternal health.

This section describes major health disparities among women living in rural areas, points to disparity in terms of access to health care, and divides the reasons for such disparities into a "patient" factor and a "delivery of care" factor. The section ends with a description of various public health programs that are introduced to improve access to services across the United States.

The third section of this chapter explores issues related to maternal and infant health. The prevalence of and major reasons for maternal and **infant mortality** are discussed. Utilizing prenatal care services has been noted as the best way to reduce both maternal and infant mortality. Prenatal care visits and types of screening and monitoring of maternal and fetal health are described. Next, barriers to prenatal care are presented. Finally, a short history of public health programs in the United States is given.

Fourth, children's health is discussed, with an emphasis on the differential health outcomes that rural children experience, potential determinants of these disparities, and evidence-based initiatives to address these disparities.

The fifth section of the chapter encompasses adolescent reproductive health, with a discussion on salient reproductive health issues among rural adolescents as well as evidence-based initiatives to address these issues.

The sixth section covers nutrition in pregnancy and lactation with a description of the nutritional requirements of these stages and challenges that rural pregnant women may face in terms of meeting these requirements.

Seventh, family planning is discussed, with a focus on accessibility and acceptability. The two major categories of contraception, permanent and temporary, are defined and briefly explained. Public health programs disseminating contraception across the United States are discussed.

The eighth and final section of this chapter is dedicated to sexually transmitted diseases. The prevalence of such infectious diseases

during pregnancy and barriers to prevention are discussed briefly.

Life Course Approach to Maternal and Child Health

Before delving into salient maternal and health issues in rural areas, it is important to better understand the conceptual underpinnings of this field. Toward the end of the twentieth century, health researchers and practitioners began to acknowledge that disparities in maternal and child health are likely due to upstream determinants of health that extend beyond issues related to access to and delivery of care. The Life Course Health Development (LCHD) framework proposed that health is the culmination of and interaction between multiple determinants (biological, genetic, behavioral, social, and economic) that evolve during one's life span; furthermore, this theory emphasizes that both risk and protective exposures can shape a person's health during the life course (Halfon and Hochstein, 2002).

The life course approach comprises five guiding principles, including life-span development, timing, human agency, linked lives, and historical time and place (Elder et al., 1998). Life-span development involves the idea that one's health must be viewed as a life-long process that is impacted by exposures through the entire life span. For example, low infant birthweight has been linked to a greater risk of chronic diseases later in life (Rasmussen et al., 2001). The principle of timing proposes that a person's health is not only dependent on what happens to us but also when these events occur as well as the order in which events occur. For example, childbearing may differentially impact a woman's potential educational attainment based on when it occurs. Furthermore, the concept of human agency emphasizes that individuals do have control over their own decisions, which ultimately impacts their health outcomes as well. On the other hand, the principle of linked lives also recognizes that individuals exist in social networks, which can have significant risky or protective influences over one's health decisions and outcomes. For example, research has shown that children who are exposed to intimate partner violence in their families may be more likely to experience negative mental and behavioral health outcomes (McTavish, et al., 2016). Finally, the concept of historical time and place points to the notion that one's health can also be greatly impacted by the broader historical context. For example, during wartime, women and children may experience unique stressors that inevitably impact their long-term health outcomes.

In addition to these guiding principles, there are three temporal concepts related to one's development over the life course—trajectories, transitions, and turning points. A trajectory is a type of long-term pattern that defines a substantial portion of one's life, such as health, education, work, and relationship trajectories (Elder, et al., 2003; George et al., 2003). On the other hand, transitions occur over a short time frame, are embedded within a trajectory, and typically entail a change in one's status or role (Elder, et al., 2003). For example, the onset of parenthood may be a transition that occurs in a relationship trajectory. Lastly, a transition can sometimes be a turning point as well if it results in significant changes in one's views or behavior (Cappeliez, et al., 2008). For example, pregnancy may be a turning point that propels some women to quit smoking. Tying in the five guiding principles of the life course approach with these three temporal concepts, it is important to note that the influences of risky and protective factors accumulate over one's various trajectories and that there are sensitive and critical times (i.e., transitions and turning points) in which these impacts may be especially salient.

Epidemiology of Maternal Health in Rural Areas

Rural America represents 75% of the national landmass and is home to 22.8% of U.S. women aged 18 and older, with substantial variance in the ethnic and racial composition of this population (American Academy of Obstetricians and Gynecologist, 2014).

The word "rural" is defined differently by different authors. Since the definition is used to determine eligibility for federal and state programs, as well as for implementing laws and comparing research findings and data, it is important to define this word correctly. The different definitions of the word "rural" can be found in Chapter 1 of this textbook.

There are major health disparities between rural and urban areas. Women in rural America experience higher rates of adverse health conditions compared with their urban counterparts. These conditions include, but are not limited to, mortality due to cerebrovascular diseases, ischemic heart diseases (Jukic et al., 2007), suicide, unintentional injuries, motor vehicle accidents, and morbidities such as cervical cancer, poor health in general, obesity, as well as high-risk behaviors such as higher rates of smoking and alcohol consumption compared with women living in urban areas.

Apart from higher risks of health outcomes, access to health care is complicated for rural women. Such complications are due to either patient factors or delivery of care.

Patient Factors

Residents of rural areas are more likely to be poor, lack health insurance, or rely extensively on Medicaid and Medicare. Women often must travel longer distances to receive care or to access a variety of reproductive health care or more general healthcare services (medical, dental, and mental health specialty services; Hart et al., 2005). In about half of all rural areas across the United States, the average travel time from the nearest hospital is estimated at around 30 minutes' drive, if the patient has the means to travel. Within a 60-minute drive, the proportion increases to 87.6% in rural townships and 78.7% in the most remote areas (Finley et al., 2013). Apart from distance, the other factor impacting rural women's access to care is the cost. During 2008–2010, 18.6% of rural women reported that they had delayed or not received medical care due to cost and more than 23% reported having no health insurance coverage (National Center for Health Statistics, 2013).

One of the most important indicators of reproductive health is the frequency of very low birth weight (VLBW), defined as birth weight lower than 1,500 grams. Based on this indicator, nine of the 12 states ranked high for having VLBW in rural populations. That exceeds one-third of the state population (US Census Bureau, 2010; Health Resources and Services Administration, 2017). What makes this statistic more relevant to the concept of access to care is that VLBW infants are more likely to be born in areas that are more distant from a subspecialty hospital. This translates into inadequate prenatal care, which in turn leads to an increase in the likelihood of delivery in a lower level-facility (Gould et al., 1999; Samuelson et al., 2002). Reports also reveal that prenatal care initiation in the first trimester was lower for pregnancies in more rural areas compared with suburban areas (Agency for Healthcare Research and Quality, 2013). In 2008, rural women experienced slightly higher rates of hospitalization with complications during pregnancy than women living in large metropolitan and medium to small metropolitan areas (Romano et al., 2003).

Although VLBW is more frequent in rural areas, with respect to adverse birth outcomes, a study found that women living in the two most rural communities in Pennsylvania experienced risks of **low birth weight (LBW)** and preterm birth similar to those identified for women living in urban areas, even after adjusting for maternal characteristics such as age, gestational age, and number of prenatal visits (Hillemeier et al., 2007).

Another relevant indicator of reproductive health is access of rural women to reproductive health services between 15–45 years of age, when women are sexually active. Women in rural areas were less likely to report having had access to such services in the past year than women living in metropolitan areas (National Center for Health Statistics, 2012). For example, 35% of rural women reported a lack of access to female sterilization, compared with 24% of women living in central metropolitan areas and 25% in fringe metropolitan (25%) areas (Jones et al., 2012). A study in Colorado suggested that women between the ages of 11 and 44 years living in small towns or rural areas indicated less use of contraceptive methods and, therefore, were more likely to have had an **unintended pregnancy** than women in more urban areas (Jones et al., 2012).

Delivery of Care

There is a potential decrease in the rural, health-related workforce. This will contribute to poor care delivery, which may have a detrimental effect on health outcomes of rural women. Data show that in 2008, only 6.4% of obstetrician–gynecologists practiced in rural areas (American College of Obstetricians and Gynecologists, 2014). By 2010, approximately half of the 3,143 US counties lacked an obstetrician–gynecologist. This means that over 10 million rural women (or 8.2% of all-American women) did not have access to a specialized reproductive healthcare professional. These disparities exist in all states but are most prevalent in the central and mountain west states. The ratio of obstetrician–gynecologists per 10,000 women is highest in metropolitan areas and decreases in less populated and rural counties (Rayburn et al., 2012). The same pattern is observable for general practitioners. In some rural areas, family physicians provide most of the obstetric care in the absence of a specialist. Even under such circumstances, the provision of obstetric services by general practitioners is declining, with only 19.2% providing deliveries (American Academy of Family Physicians, 2010). Although an increasing proportion of women are choosing obstetrics and family practice as their field of specialty, fewer female clinicians choose to practice in rural areas compared with their male counterparts (Rayburn et al., 2012; Emmons et al., 2006).

Moreover, the range of available obstetric and gynecologic health services is limited in many nonmetropolitan areas. For instance, vaginal deliveries after cesarean section (VBAC) are performed less often in rural areas. Considerable decreases in the availability of VBAC services were reported for rural areas in Colorado, Montana, Oregon, and Wisconsin from 1999 through 2005 (Roberts et al., 2007). This is because facilities such as theatre rooms and anesthesiologists should be accessible in such cases, a luxury limited to tertiary healthcare centers such as referral hospitals. Hence, if a complication develops during VBAC, because tertiary centers aren't available in rural areas, women can't be referred to them.

Another example of a service lacking in rural areas is access to abortion services. In 2008, no such services were provided for 35% of reproductive-age women. Obstetrician–gynecologists who practiced in rural areas were 6.5% less likely to perform abortions than their urban colleagues (17.0 %; Stulberg et al., 2011). This meant that rural women seeking abortions had to travel substantially greater distances than women living in metropolitan areas. A report in 2008 suggests that 31% of rural women traveled more than 100 miles and an additional 42.9% traveled between 50 miles and 100 miles to get an abortion, compared with 3.8% and 7%, respectively, for their nonrural counterparts (Jones, 2013).

The lack of access to publicly funded contraceptive services and supplies has also been studied. Among the 14 states ranked the highest on the percentage of women aged 13–44 years in need of such services, nine have rural populations surpassing 33% of the state population (U.S. Census Bureau, 2010). Another study revealed that less than half of the agencies providing publicly funded family planning services reported having clinic sites located in rural areas (Frost et al., 2013). A lack of access to pharmacy or health clinics has also been reported in Colorado, where almost 3/4 of the counties are considered rural (Prevention First Colorado, 2017); in these situations, filling initial or refill prescriptions for contraceptives is not possible. Which types of contraception are available in rural areas is also not clear and neither is whether barrier methods such as condoms are accessible. This can have a detrimental health effect on those who may be exposed to HIV/AIDS through their partners. Moreover, there is a lack of crucial data on the current, over-the-counter availability of emergency contraception in rural pharmacies in the United States.

Public Health Programs to Improve Services

A variety of programs has been implemented to address the difficulties in providing care to rural women. Such programs are funded by a range of state and federal programs and academic institutions. For instance, in Wyoming, out-of-state healthcare providers and facilities in addition to state Medicaid providers were permitted to provide care for pregnant women or infants, allowing the state to compensate transport to and care and delivery in an out-of-state subspecialty hospital when medically required (Wyoming Department of Health, 2014). Another example was the development of the Regional Maternal & Child Health Program in the University of Texas Medical Branch in Galveston's Department of Obstetrics and Gynecology. The program was originally developed to assist geographically underserved women and children in multiple off-site clinics. This program addressed transportation needs and adopted culturally relevant services and the use of electronic medical records to facilitate continuity of care. The program is far reaching and provided housing facilities, referred to Regional Perinatal Care facilities, for high-risk women to ease their access to regional center when hospitalization is not required (Lowery et al., 2007).

Maternal and Infant Health

Two important indicators of the general health and well-being of a society are maternal and infant mortality. We will discuss these two in depth.

Maternal Mortality

Rates of **maternal morbidity** and mortality are rising in the United States. Currently, 700 women die every year in the United States as a result of pregnancy or delivery complications (Center for Disease Control, Division of Reproductive Health, 2019).

Historically, in the United States, the risk of death to mothers was substantial at the beginning of the 20th century. **Maternal mortality**, however, has been markedly reduced since then. Nevertheless, the United States still has the highest rate of maternal mortality in the developed world. Maternal mortality refers to the death of a woman during pregnancy or up to a year after pregnancy has terminated. Maternal mortality due to accidental causes is not counted in this statistic. The maternal death rate averaged 9.1 maternal deaths per 100,000 live births from 1979 to 1986. However, it rose quickly to 14 per 100,000 in 2000 and also increased between 2000 and 2014, from 14 to 21.5 maternal deaths per 100,000 live births, at a time when 157 of 183 countries in a World Health Organization (WHO, 2019) study reported decreases in maternal mortality. Among 31 countries in the Organization for Economic Cooperation and Development

(2019) reporting maternal mortality data in 2014, the United States ranked 30th, ahead of only Mexico and more than three times higher than Canada and the United Kingdom. There is a long way to go to reach zero maternal mortality.

The major reasons for maternal mortality are postpartum hemorrhage, high blood pressure, obstructed labor, preexisting complications, infections, and complications of abortion. If a proper number of prenatal care visits (at least eight visits during 40 weeks of gestation) is provided, maternal mortality can be reduced dramatically. Types of prenatal care visits include serial surveillance, risk assessment, health education, and psychosocial support.

In general, access to obstetric services may be hampered by affordability, availability, and acceptability barriers. Services may be unequally distributed, with differences between socioeconomic groups and geographic areas being most important. Rural women face the greatest barriers, including the lengthiest travel times, highest costs associated with delivery, and lowest levels of service acceptability, compared with urban residents.

In the United States, a major reason for maternal mortality in rural areas is disparity. Rural America, which represents 75% of the national mainland land mass and is home to 22.8% of U.S. women, suffers from substantial variance in ethnic and racial disparity. The lack of data on rural America is one major setback to planning and improving prenatal care.

Second, as described earlier, rural residents are spread over a large geographic area; hence, rural women are less likely to receive preventive health services or any screening during pregnancy or in the postpartum period. Data show that about half of rural women live within a 30 minutes' drive to a hospital with perinatal services. Some rural areas such as Wyoming do not have any care centers for pregnant women. Many smaller hospitals (Kozhimannil et al., 2018) are under threat of being shut down due to financial instability or lack of medical personnel in the communities. According to the American College of Obstetricians and Gynecologists (Academy of Obstetricians and Gynecologist, 2014), 49% of the nation's counties lack an obstetrician–gynecologist. This leaves over 10 million women in the United States with no obstetric service.

Third, apart from the lack of perinatal care services, societal, maternal, and structural barriers play a major role in access to prenatal care (Phillippi et al., 2009). A systematic review of women's perceptions of access to prenatal care identified several societal and maternal barriers to prenatal care, such as fear of medical procedures or disclosing the pregnancy to others, depression, and a belief that prenatal care is unnecessary. Structural barriers include long wait times, the location and hours of the clinic, the language and attitude of the clinic staff and provider, the cost of services, and a lack of child-friendly facilities.

An analysis of Minnesota Pregnancy Risk Assessment Monitoring System (PRAMS) data from 2009–2010 suggested that approximately one in every 10 mothers in rural Minnesota reported that they did not receive prenatal care as early in their pregnancy as they wanted. Barriers reported by this group included not having enough money or insurance to pay for the visit; not knowing they were pregnant; and physicians or health plans not starting prenatal care as early as the mother wanted. They also noted that the initial prenatal appointments were not scheduled due to lack of personnel. Moreover, mothers from rural Minnesota were less likely to report that their clinician discussed topics such as smoking, alcohol use, illegal drug use, HIV screening, physical abuse, or seat belt use during the prenatal care visit (Centers for Disease Control and Prevention, 2015).

Fourth, non-Hispanic Black women are at highest risk for adverse health outcomes compared with women of other races/ethnicities. A recent review of the literature revealed the relationship between prenatal care utilization, social determinants of health, and racial disparities in maternal outcomes (Hillemeier et al., 2007). Black women are also more likely to be late to prenatal care or be inadequate users of prenatal care. Maternal mortality among Black Americans is more likely to occur in younger, less-educated, and unmarried women (National Center for Health Statistics, 2012).

According to a Cochrane systematic review (Till et al., 2015) there is no strong evidence as to how incentivizing women would improve prenatal health visits (giving cash, vouchers, coupons or products not generally offered to women as a standard part of prenatal care). Pregnant women receiving incentives were no more likely to initiate prenatal care (risk ratio (RR) 1.04, 95% confidence interval (CI) 0.78 to 1.38, one study, and 104 pregnancies). However, women receiving incentives were more likely to attend prenatal visits on a frequent basis (RR 1.18, 95% CI 1.01 to 1.38, one study, 606 pregnancies), and to obtain adequate prenatal care as defined by the number of "procedures," such as testing blood sugar or blood pressure, vaccinations, and counseling about breastfeeding and birth control (mean difference (MD) 5.84, 95% CI 1.88 to 9.80, one study, 892 pregnancies).

Infant Mortality

Infant mortality, the death of an infant before his or her first birthday, is measured by the number of infant deaths per 1,000 live births. In 2017, the infant mortality rate in the United States was 5.8 deaths per 1,000 live births (Jones et al., 2012). Major causes of infant death are birth defects, **preterm birth**, maternal pregnancy complications, sudden infant death syndrome, and injuries (mostly suffocation). A preterm birth is when a baby is born sooner than at 37 weeks of pregnancy. A preterm baby lacks growth and development of essential organs such as the brain, liver, and lungs. Most infants who die are both very premature and have very low birth weight. From

2007 to 2014, preterm birth in the United States was in decline, but the CDC reports (2019) indicate that it rose in 2016. Preterm birth affected approximately one of every 10 infants born in the United States. Higher rates of preterm birth are found among African American women (14%) compared with white women (9%). Low birth weight, a birth weight of less than 2,500 grams, is associated with preterm birth and is an indicator of infant mortality and morbidity. In the United States, the rate of low birth weight was 8.2% in 2008. The rate has slowly but steadily increased over the last two decades.

Prenatal Care

Prenatal care is a type of preventive care with the goal of providing regular check-ups that allow obstetricians–gynecologists or midwives to detect, treat, and prevent potential health problems throughout the course of the pregnancy, while also promoting healthy lifestyles that benefit both mother and child. Prenatal care covers areas such as prenatal nutrition, breastfeeding, lifestyle changes, injury and illness prevention, and methods to monitor potentially dangerous health conditions. During prenatal visits, medical professionals will inform the mother about the birthing process and the basic skills for taking care of a newborn. Each prenatal visit is dedicated to examination such as physical and pelvic exams, lab work, and ultrasound measurements. Ultrasounds are used to measure fetus growth, heartbeats, and movement, as well as to identify physically abnormalities. Regular check-ups allow clinicians to assess changes to the mother's blood pressure, weight, uterus size, protein supplies from urine samples, and various diseases such as diabetes through screening tests. The frequency of prenatal care visits varies depending on maternal complications. More frequent visits are warranted for women older than 35 years or in the case of a high-risk pregnancy, with the number and types of extra visits depending on individual risk factors. The optimal number of prenatal visits is 8 to 11 visits for a pregnant woman of low risk. However, many American expectant mothers living in rural areas do not visit a clinician as often as they are supposed to. Black women are at disproportionate risk for this outcome. PRAMS data (2015) indicates that Black and Hispanic women who die of pregnancy-related causes are more likely than White women to have initiated prenatal care in the second and third trimesters, rather than in the first trimester. Apart from late presentation, poor adherence to prenatal care visits is observed among Black American women. Inadequate prenatal care is associated with risk factors such as smoking, alcohol consumption, insufficient weight gain, precipitous labor, and no breastfeeding (Jonas et al., 2012).

Public Health Programs to Improve Services

The involvement of the federal government in maternal child health began in 1935, when the Social Security Act Title IV&V raised concerns over maternal child health during the Great Depression era. In 1943, the Emergency Maternity and Infant Care Program addressed the needs of maternal child health following the onset of World War II. Medicare was enacted in 1965, leading to the launch of programs such as *The Healthy Start*, which is administered by the MCH Bureau. Fifteen urban and rural communities were selected annually to receive funds to facilitate community-driven approaches to infant mortality. Beginning in 1984, Medicaid provided coverage to single pregnant women. In 1987, Medicaid expansions improved the uptake of prenatal care in low-income populations at risk for disparities. These programs have had long-term success in providing better health for infants.

One program still running, which supports infants in the United States is the "Women, Infants and Children (WIC)" program. This program provides nutrition education, breastfeeding education and support, referrals, and food. Home visits by nurses and community health workers give pregnant women and families, especially those at risk, the required resources and skills to raise children who are physically, socially, and emotionally healthy and ready to learn. Home visit programs have been shown to improve prenatal care utilization (American College of Obstetricians and Gynecologists, 2014). Another program, titled "Administration for Children and Families (ACF)," is responsible for promoting the economic and social well-being of children, families, individuals, and communities with leadership and resources for compassionate, effective delivery of human services. Other programs that support the growth and development of children include the Child & Adult Care Food Program (CACFP), Fresh Fruit & Vegetable Program (FFVP), National School Lunch Program (NSLP), School Breakfast Program (SBP), and Summer Food Service Program (SFSP).

Children's Health

Childhood encompasses two primary stages in the life course—the toddler and school-age years. These stages are characterized by accelerated physical, social, emotional, language, and cognitive development that lay the foundation for an individual's long-term health and well-being. Children in rural areas experience unique challenges that may lead to suboptimal health outcomes that extend to adolescence and adulthood. In this section, we will discuss differential health outcomes that rural children experience, potential determinants of these disparities, and evidence-based initiatives to address these disparities.

Differential Health Outcomes among Rural Children

Compared with urban children, children in rural areas are more likely to experience certain chronic conditions, including obesity/ overweight, oral health problems, and adverse childhood experiences (ACEs). Based on data from the U.S. Department of Health and Human Services (USDHHS) Maternal and Child Health Bureau (2015), children living in rural areas have a higher prevalence (approximately 35-38%) of overweight and obesity than their urban counterparts (30%); furthermore, in rural areas, non-Hispanic Black and Hispanic children are even more likely than White children to be obese or overweight. Related to obesity, rural families are more likely to reside in food deserts (i.e., areas characterized by lack of access to affordable, fresh, and nutritious foods) and experience food insecurity (Sharkey et al., 2009; Gregory and Coleman-Jensen, 2017). Obesity, overweight, and food insecurity have long-lasting implications for one's health over the life course as they have been strongly linked to chronic diseases, including heart disease, type 2 diabetes, hypertension, and kidney disease (National Institute of Diabetes and Digestive and Kidney Diseases, 2015; Gregory and Coleman-Jensen, 2017).

Furthermore, children in rural regions are more likely to experience poor oral health than their urban counterparts (Institute of Medicine and National Research Council, 2011). Data from the National Survey of Children's Health suggest that rural children are less likely to receive preventative dental care and are also less likely to have "excellent" or "very good" teeth, based on parental reporting; minority rural children lag behind White rural children on these statistics as well (Martin, et al., 2017). Additionally, although the fluoridation of water has been a major Public Health achievement to protect against dental caries, rural residents are less likely to access sufficiently fluoridated water, either through private wells or through the public water supply, and are, therefore, vulnerable to tooth decay (Hendryx, et al., 2012).

Additionally, children in rural areas have been shown to experience more adverse childhood experiences (ACEs). ACEs are defined as chronic stressors or trauma that occur during childhood and have both short- and long-term impacts on one's health (National Advisory Committee on Rural Health and Health Services, 2018). Based on data from the 2011–2012 National Survey on Children's Health, almost 29% of rural children experienced two or more ACEs compared with 21% of urban children (USDHHS, 2015). A seminal study by the Centers for Disease Control and Prevention (CDC) and Kaiser Permanente (Felitti, et al., 1998) identified 10 ACEs, including physical, emotional, and sexual abuse; physical and emotional neglect; and household dysfunction (i.e., mental illness, incarcerated relative, mother who is a victim of violence, divorce, and substance abuse). This study also discovered that children who experience four or more of these ACEs are significantly more likely to engage in negative health behaviors (e.g., substance abuse, lack of physical activity) and have impaired long-term physical and mental health (e.g., obesity, depression, ischemic heart disease, **sexually transmitted infections**).

Determinants of Children's Health in Rural Areas

Overarching social determinants of children's health in rural areas include poverty, inadequate access to health care and health services, and housing and water concerns. Data from the U.S. Department of Agriculture indicates that 28% of rural counties have persistent child poverty (i.e., at least 20% of children living in poverty), compared with only 13% of urban counties (Parker, 2015). Similarly, rural children are more likely to live in low socioeconomic status families; overall, 19% of rural counties are considered low education (i.e., at least 20% of residents aged 25–64 have less than a high school education) compared with 9% of urban counties, and 36% of rural counties are low employment (i.e., less than 65% of residents aged 21–64 are employed) compared with 16% of urban counties (Parker, 2015). Furthermore, it should be noted that race/ ethnicity is an added layer to consider in the spectrum of poverty in the United States— two-thirds of minority children, including African American, Hispanic, and American Indian/Alaska Native children, live in concentrated poverty, compared with one-third of White children (Gabe, 2015). Poverty in rural children has been strongly associated with a wide range of negative outcomes, including poor academic progress and achievement; physical health; behavioral, social, and emotional problems; mental health disorders; developmental delays; obesity; and the onset of chronic diseases (e.g., heart and lung diseases) later in life (Pascoe, et al., 2016).

Another salient social determinant of health among rural children is adequate access to health care and health services. While rural and urban children are likely to have similar insurance rates, rural children are more likely to be covered by Medicaid (USDHHS, 2015). Importantly, this coverage does not always include dental care services, thereby placing rural children at greater risk for oral health problems (Liu, et al., 2007). Rural areas are also more likely to contain an insufficient number of healthcare providers and be designated as "health professional shortage areas" (HPSAs), which are determined by a person-to-provider ratio, percentage of population living below 100% of the federal poverty level, and travel time to the nearest source of care (Doescher, et al., 2009; Health Resources Services Administration, 2019). Hence, as rural areas lack an adequate primary care and dental health workforce, rural children are less likely to receive necessary preventative services and experience a greater risk of unmet medical need (Doescher, et al., 2009; Mertz, 2009; USDHHS, 2015; Clark, et al., 2001). Furthermore, when compared with urban settings, rural areas have significantly fewer mental healthcare providers; physical, occupational, and speech therapists; and medical social workers; thus placing rural children with special healthcare and mental health needs at even greater risk for negative outcomes (Roots and Li, 2013; Daniels, et al., 2007). Therefore, due to a lack of a usual source of care, rural families are significantly more likely to use emergency departments for nonemergency situations (Diedhiou, et al., 2010; Huffman, et al., 2012). Additionally, in terms of unmet medical need, rural children face a higher risk of dying from unintentional injuries, such as motor vehicle injuries, due to the greater distance first responders need to travel to address the injury, the longer distance to the nearest healthcare facility, and the dearth of trauma-related medical expertise in rural areas (Garcia, et al., 2017).

Unsafe housing conditions and water supply are also critical social determinants of health in rural areas, especially for children, as these environmental exposures may substantially alter their health trajectories early in life. A report from the Housing Assistance Council (2012) revealed that certain rural, poverty-stricken communities, such as residents of Appalachia, the Mississippi Delta, Native American regions, and the U.S.-Mexico border areas, are more likely to experience low-quality or lack of plumbing and wastewater systems, unsafe heating and cooling processes, lack of home safety devices (i.e., smoke alarms, carbon monoxide detectors), mold, and lead-based paint and water pipes. These types of housing conditions have been linked to long-term health problems, such as respiratory infections, asthma, lead poisoning, and injuries (Krieger and Higgins, 2002). Further, many rural families often rely on a water supply, such as well water or water systems, that are contaminated by a variety of hazards (e.g., waste from mines, pesticides, manure, landfills, road salt, etc.), that is not covered by the Safe Water Drinking Act (Environmental Protection Agency, 2015). Exposure to unsafe water has been associated with gastrointestinal infections, cancers, liver, kidney, and intestinal deterioration, and reproductive health problems later in life (Environmental Protection Agency, 2018).

Interventions to Address Children's Health in Rural Areas

Various types of interventions, including early childhood development and education programs, coordinated school health programs, and school-based food programs, have been instrumental in improving children's health in rural settings. The Head Start program, which is funded by the U.S. Department of Health and Human Services, promotes early learning, family well-being, and importantly, health services (e.g., health and development screenings, healthy meals, and oral health and mental health services) to low-income children from birth to five years old (USDHHS, 2019). It has been determined that in a 10-state sample, there are 48 rural counties that would otherwise not contain a child care center without the Head Start program and that there are Heart Start programs in 86% of rural counties in the U.S. (Malik and Schochet, 2018). Furthermore, coordinated school health programs comprise eight key components, including health services; health education; biophysical and psychosocial environments; psychological, counseling, and social services; physical education; nutrition services; employee health promotion and integrated family and community involvement; and may help compensate for the various challenges that rural children face in accessing adequate healthcare services in resource-poor areas (Kolbe, 2005; Cornwell, et al., 2007). Additionally, a variety of school-based food programs, including reduced and free lunch and after school meals for low-income students as well as universal breakfast, farm to school programs (which expose students to locally grown fresh fruits and vegetables), backpack school programs (which provide students with nonperishable foods to take home during the weekend or long breaks), and summer meals (which are typically free or low-cost lunches provided during the summer months) for all students, have been implemented to combat food insecurity and obesity among rural children (Rural Health Information Hub, 2019).

Adolescent Reproductive Health

The risk and protective factors that children experience accumulate and accompany them into adolescence, a period characterized by rapid physical, social, and psychological growth beginning after the onset of puberty and ending in early adulthood (i.e., the teenage years). In this section, we will briefly discuss reproductive health issues among rural adolescents as well as evidence-based initiatives to address these issues.

Leading Reproductive Health Issues among Rural Adolescents

In rural areas, two salient issues that adolescents face in terms of reproductive health are teenage pregnancy, which is further elaborated upon in the "Family Planning" section below; and sexually transmitted infections (STIs). It has been found that STI rates, specifically rates of gonorrhea, chlamydia, and syphilis, have generally increased among adolescents in the U.S. (Centers for Disease Control and Prevention (CDC), 2017), but they have also experienced particularly high increases in some rural regions (Pinto, et al., 2017; Gesink, et al., 2013). For example, one study found that there was an increase in gonorrhea or chlamydia rates in eight of 12 rural Pennsylvania counties between 2004 and 2014 (Pinto, et al., 2017). Another important trend is that although the vaccination rates for human papillomavirus (HPV), which is the most common STI in the United States, have increased nationally, the percentage of rural adolescents who received the first dose of HPV vaccine in 2017 was 11 percentage points lower than among their urban counterparts (Centers for Disease Control and Prevention, 2018).

In addition to the social determinants of health that adolescents face in rural areas, including poverty and inadequate access to health care and health services (i.e., access to contraception and STI screening services), social stigma and fears about lack of confidentiality are significant barriers that likely prevent rural adolescents from seeking reproductive health care to prevent pregnancy and STIs. Rural communities often comprise small towns, in which residents have a significant reduced ability to maintain confidentiality when seeking reproductive health care, such as contraception and STI screening and treatment services (Garside, et al., 2002). Furthermore, as certain rural areas, such as the rural southern United States, have more conservative and religion-based social norms surrounding reproductive health, perceived societal stigma among rural adolescents may hinder them from attempting to access more controversial types of reproductive healthcare services, such as abortion, contraception (specifically emergency contraception), and screening for STIs (Shellenberg and Tsui, 2012; Lichtenstein, et al., 2005; Pew Research Center, 2013).

Interventions to Improve Adolescent Reproductive Health in Rural Areas

Two key types of interventions that have been used to improve rural adolescent reproductive health are school-based programs and digital media. School-based programs aim to provide integrated health services to adolescents in the school setting, thereby circumventing potential challenges to accessing care, such as transportation (Rural Health Information Hub, 2019). Various forms of school-based service programs include school-linked services, school-based health centers, and Whole School, Whole Community, Whole Child (WSCC) (Rural Health Information Hub, 2019). School-linked services connect students and families to community health organizations to access services through referrals, mobile health units, family resource centers, etc. (Levy & Shepardson, 1992). Similarly, school-based health centers offer students and their families a wide array of services, including, but not limited to, preventative screenings (e.g. dental, vision, and hearing), primary health care, mental and behavioral health care, substance abuse counseling, and nutrition education (Health Resources Services Administration, 2017). Finally, the WSCC, which is very similar to coordinated school health programs, is a holistic, student-centered framework developed by the Centers for Disease Control and Prevention (CDC) that focuses on 10 components, including physical education and physical activity, nutrition environment and services, health education, social and emotional school climate, physical environment, health services, counseling, psychological and social services, employee wellness, community involvement, and family engagement (Centers for Disease Control and Prevention (CDC), 2019).

In addition to school-based programs, the use of digital media, such as the Internet, social networking sites, and text messaging, has emerged as a promising strategy to improve adolescent reproductive health (Guse, et al., 2012). In rural areas, where barriers such as lack of transportation and distance often hinder individuals from accessing health information as well as healthcare services, communication via digital media can be particularly beneficial. For example, in one study that examined the impact of a computer-based intervention on pregnancy and STI risk among rural tenth-graders, the intervention group experienced statistically significant increases in knowledge, condom negotiation skills, abstinence attitudes, and situational self-efficacy as well as delayed initiation of sex for students who were "sexually naïve" at the beginning of the intervention (Roberto, et al., 2007). The use of digital media also likely helps maintain confidentiality and enables rural adolescents access reproductive health information and services with less fear of encountering social stigma; however, this strategy does necessitate a stable Internet connection, which may be problematic for some rural residents.

Nutrition in Pregnancy and Lactation

A significant critical period in the lives of women is pregnancy. As the physiological demands of pregnancy and the metabolic demands of the growing fetus can be extremely taxing, women's nutritional needs are especially high during the prenatal period. Poor maternal nutrition during pregnancy has been linked to increased maternal and infant mortality, intrauterine growth retardation of the fetus, congenital anomalies and low birthweight among infants, and increased risk of chronic disease for the child later in life (Kramer, 1987; Kramer, 2003; Kanaka-Gantabein, 2010; Barker, 1998). In order to help achieve a healthy pregnancy and baby, women are recommended to consume an additional 300 kcal per day during pregnancy as well as the necessary micronutrients, such as folic acid and iron, before and during pregnancy (Food and Nutrition Board, 1998; Kominiarek and Rajan, 2016). Furthermore, it is recommended that breastfeeding mothers consume an additional 500 kcal and an additional 25 grams of protein per day compared with nonpregnant mothers (American Academy of Pediatrics and American College of Obstetricians and Gynecologists, 2012; Kominiarek and Rajan, 2016). Increased micronutrient intake, especially vitamins A and E, is also required during lactation and thus breastfeeding women are urged to continue taking the prenatal multivitamin after pregnancy (Otten, et al., 2006).

Rural women experience unique challenges related to nutrition during pregnancy and lactation. Many rural areas are characterized by food deserts and, therefore, lack ready access to affordable and fresh foods. For example, American Indian communities, especially those residents who reside in rural settings, tend to have high food insecurity rates, with a rate as high as 28% in the Northern Plains region (Kaufman, et al., 2014; Jernigan, et al., 2017). Additionally, although there is a gap in the literature regarding potential differences in knowledge of preconception, prenatal, and lactation requirements among rural versus urban pregnant women in the United States, rural pregnant women may be less likely than their urban counterparts to have knowledge about these nutritional requirements due to the inadequate access to health information and services characterized by many rural settings.

Family Planning

Family planning was globally accepted as a human right at the 1994 International Conference on Population and Development. Subsequently, universal access to reproductive health was included as a fundamental piece of the United Nations' Millennium Development Goals. Family planning was also identified to eradicate extreme poverty and hunger, achieve universal primary education, promote gender equality, empower women, and ensure environmental sustainability (Rayburn et al., 2012).

Accessibility

Access to contraceptives has saved the lives of millions of women worldwide, assisted in decreasing uncontrolled population growth, helped numerous families break the cycle of poverty, and transformed the lives of hundreds of millions more. Use of contraceptives has proven to be effective in reducing the number of unplanned pregnancies, increasing birth intervals and providing the ability for families to plan when and how many children they would like to bear, which has eventually led to a decrease in the average family size (American Academy of Family Physicians, 2013).

Contraception use in rural areas in America has not been optimal due to a lack of access to reproductive health services by sexually active women. Moreover, rural America is changing, yet much of the existing research on rural reproductive health and contraceptive use dates to the 1990s. A 2006 survey of women of reproductive age in Colorado suggested that women in rural areas plan less for contraceptive use and were more likely to have had unwanted pregnancies than their counterparts living in metropolitan areas (Emmons et al., 2006). An unintended pregnancy is one that was either mistimed or unwanted. If a woman did not want to become pregnant at the time the pregnancy occurred but did want to become pregnant at some point in the future, the pregnancy is considered mistimed. If a woman did not want to become pregnant then or at any time in the future, the pregnancy is considered unwanted. A more recent study in Michigan estimated that postpartum use of contraceptives in rural areas is low compared with urban areas, and the types of contraceptives used are more permanent types such as sterilization or long-acting reversible contraception, rather than condoms or pills. This study analyzed phase 5 of (2004–2008) of the Michigan Pregnancy Risk Assessment Monitoring System survey among 6,468 women. Contraceptive methods used by women in this study included sterilization (14.4%), long-acting reversible contraception (6.7%), hormonal methods (37.3%), condoms or no method (38.4%), and abstinence (3.2%).

Lack of access to health care can be a major reason for poor utilization of contraception in rural areas. Hence, unintended pregnancies may occur more often in rural areas than urban areas. Moreover, unintended pregnancies often involve a more vulnerable population: adolescents. According to the National Campaign to Prevent Teen and Unplanned Pregnancy (NCPTUP, 2010), the teenage birth rate is nearly one-third higher in rural areas of the United States (42.9) than it is in urban areas (32.6) of the country, and teen pregnancy rates have been much slower to decline in rural counties over the past decade. Teen girls living in rural counties account for 20% of teen births, although they only account for 16% of the adolescent population. This increase in teen rate is higher for rural Hispanic teens (71.7%) compared with those from the same ethnicity living in urban areas (51%).

Factors contributing to teenage pregnancy can be categorized into direct and indirect factors. Direct factors include sexual activities and use of contraceptives. In a survey by NCPTUP, rural teenage girls were more likely to say they had ever had sex (55%) compared with their counterparts in urban areas (40%). Moreover, based on data from NCPTUP, 41% of rural teenage girls had been sexually active in the three months preceding the survey compared with 29% of urban teens. Rural teen girls are also significantly less likely to have used a contraceptive method in their first sexual encounter (71% to 81%). The method of contraceptive used, however, is like that of the urban teen population: condom use is 27% in rural areas compared with 17% in urban areas, and both hormonal and condom use are estimated at 72% (urban) and 53% (rural) in the first sexual encounter.

Indirect factors contributing to the prevalence of contraceptive use are acceptability, availability, and affordability of contraception. Moreover, confidentiality issues and stigmatization may limit teen access to badly needed health services in rural areas. A study in Midwestern public universities across the United States (n=388) identified more barriers to accessing contraception in rural areas, and those who experienced more barriers were less likely to obtain contraceptives while in high school (Roberts et al., 2007). The study concludes that pregnancy prevention programs should take these barriers into account when developing future interventions. Apart from sex education, improving access to health care and building close relationships between pregnancy prevention programs and the community can positively impact the usage of family planning methods. In addition, computer-based interventions, peer educators, school-based programs, and educating parents and care providers may remove some of the barriers.

Acceptability

Despite the mass availability of evidence-based research demonstrating the critical value of contraception for families and society, it remains a debated topic in many political landscapes for a wide array of social, cultural, and religious reasons. Our American population is extremely diverse and, as a result, there are a wide range of religious or cultural beliefs that shape an individual's willingness to use contraceptives. The religious influence over politics in the United States has become so significant that political leaders utilize their religious beliefs in political debates; as a result, many Americans vote based on the shared religious beliefs expressed by political leaders. Christianity is the most practiced religion in American society today, with over 70% of the population reporting affiliation with this religion. Hence, many of the fundamental values of policymakers are shaped by their Christian doctrine. Because of this, a strong political backlash against contraceptives has resulted (Stulberg et al., 2011).

Even though America, as a developed country, has a strong health service infrastructure, we still suffer from higher rates of unintended pregnancies than other comparable industrialized countries. The reason for these high rates is probably due to policies preferring abstinence, which result from the religious influence on American policy. A good example of the influence of political will based on religious beliefs about family planning occurred in 2017, when the elected federal or state administration issued a regulatory relief to combat the contraceptive coverage mandate issued under the Affordable Care Act. This act makes it possible for employers to reject certain coverage requirements, including coverage of contraceptives, on religious grounds. There have also been budgetary cuts for governmentally funded family planning programs such as those provided under Title X of the Public Health Service Act (Stulberg et al., 2011). These services prevented 1.9 million unintended pregnancies in 2014 alone. The absence of funding for such important programs would be damaging to the health and well-being of American women and children nationwide (Jones et al., 2013).

Other barriers to contraception relate to high levels of social disadvantage that delay access to the existing infrastructure for a large portion of women living in rural America (SmithBattle et al., 2012). As a result of the barriers that rural women face in impoverished and minority groups in the United States, the highest rates of unintended pregnancy in the United States are noted among women who are young, unmarried, have a low income, or are members of a racial or ethnic minority and live in rural areas (Institute of Medicine, 1995). This has created a striking disparity in the frequency of unwanted pregnancy rates among socioeconomically disadvantaged women. As a result, nearly 20 million women of reproductive age in America are left with an unmet need for publicly funded contraceptive services; a large portion of them live in rural areas (Jonas et al., 2013).

Unwanted pregnancy poses various health burdens on women. Children have better outcomes if born to mothers who are not at the extremes of childbearing age (younger than 18 years or older than 35), if births are spaced at least two years apart, and if children are born at low birth order. Women who get pregnant intentionally are more likely to seek prenatal care, use less alcohol, or smoke less. The product of such pregnancies tends to be normal pregnancies with fewer complications. Higher rates of low birth weight and preterm births are expected as a major complication of unwanted pregnancy, and women are four times more likely to be abused during such pregnancies.

What Is Contraception?

Contraception, also known as birth control, is the deliberate use of artificial methods or other techniques to prevent pregnancy. It is important to understand the successes, failures, indications, and complications of various contraceptive methods. No one family planning method is entirely satisfactory for all women or for all circumstances. In this section, we will focus on these concepts.

The current and future focus of contraceptive research and development has expanded to include male methods. The major methods of family planning can be divided into two main categories:

1. Permanent methods
2. Temporary methods

Permanent Methods

These include either tubal ligation or vasectomy. Tubal ligation refers to a surgical procedure that permanently blocks or cuts the fallopian tube, a part of the female internal reproductive system attached to the uterus, to prevent passage of an ovum from the ovary to the uterus or to prevent the passage of a formed egg. Vasectomy, the blockage/cutting of the vas deferens (male tubes in scrotum that carry sperm), is also a surgical procedure but a much easier one that does not require full anesthesia. Both methods have small failure rates (0.5% for female sterilization and 0.15% for male sterilization) and are, therefore, considered to be the most effective methods of family planning.

Temporary Methods

Such methods *are inclusive of nonhormonal and hormonal methods.*

Non Hormonal Methods

Non hormonal contraceptives have fewer or no side effects compared with hormonal contraceptives but are considered less reliable.

Male and female condoms are called barrier methods; they physically or chemically block sperm from reaching an egg and provide barriers against direct skin-to-skin contact. Such blocks between partners have the benefit of protection against STIs. Male condoms are made of thin layers of rubber, latex, plastic, or animal membrane that are rolled over an erect penis. The condom prevents semen from entering the woman's vagina. These have a higher failure rate than sterilization (18%) but are easy to use and prevent STIs. Female condoms are harder to wear and less effective (failure rate: 21%) and are also more expensive and less widely available.

A **diaphragm**, another barrier method, is a soft silicone cup with a flexible outer ring. The cup should be inserted into the vagina to completely cover the cervix. Usually, a fitting by a clinician is necessary prior to use. A gel containing spermicide, a sperm-killing substance, is applied to the diaphragm beforehand to decrease the possibility of pregnancy. The diaphragm is inserted into the vagina before having a sexual encounter and must be left in place for at least six hours afterwards. Diaphragms are reliable if they are used correctly.

Another type of nonhormonal method is a copper intrauterine device (IUD). These contraceptives are inserted into the uterus by a clinician. Copper interferes with sperm by reducing its motility, prevents fertilization, and prevents implantation of the egg in the lining of the uterus. IUDs can stay in place for up to 5 years. The possible side effects include heavier periods and pelvic infections.

The natural method (calendar method) is used to determine when a woman ovulates, hence is fertile, based on her body temperature in the morning, as well as on her vaginal discharge. Such methods have a high failure rate—up to 24%—and are not very reliable. These also require a lot of determination and discipline in order to be effective. Another natural method is withdrawal, before the man's penis ejaculates. This method has a high failure rate (22%) mainly because millions of sperm can live in one drop of semen and only a few drops are enough to cause pregnancy. However, those who have religious considerations will use such methods or choose abstinence to avoid unwanted pregnancies.

Hormonal contraception includes pills (failure rate 9%), vaginal rings (failure rate 9%), hormonal IUDs (failure rate of 0.2 to 0.8%), injectable (failure rate 6%) or patches (failure rate 9%). All of these methods contain a combination of hormones, namely estrogen and progesterone, to stop ovulation or interfere with sperm motility and function. Pills are either sequential or combined and are taken for 21 to 22 days per cycle. A female has a menstrual period in the week when she does not take the pill. Mini pills or progesterone pills only are used during the breastfeeding period or when women cannot tolerate the effect of estrogen (e.g., nausea and bloating, headache) or have contraindications for the use of such hormones (e.g., coagulation diseases). Hormonal IUDs release levonorgestrel, a hormone that prevents implantation of any fertilized eggs. Vaginal rings also contain a combination of hormones that are absorbed via the vaginal wall. These rings are fitted by a clinician and should be taken out for cleaning in case of discharge or during menstrual cycles. Patches are placed on the body's surface and release a combination of estrogen and progesterone. Patches are more expensive and should be changed weekly for three weeks of the menstrual cycle.

Public Health Programs Disseminating Contraception

The Title X National Family Planning Program, originally founded in 1970, is the only publicly funded program in the United States. This program provides subsidized family planning and related preventative services to teens and low-income adults. The services funded by Title X are available at about

4,000 sites across the nation, including public health departments and community health agencies, family planning agencies, and additional nonprofit agencies. Of those who utilized services provided by Title X in 2016, 43% were uninsured and 37% had public insurance. The Affordable Care Act increased access to contraceptive methods and services such as patient education and contraceptive counseling at no cost to the individual. Both private insurance and Medicaid expansion are needed to fully cover methods approved by the U.S. Food and Drug Administration (FDA). The FDA recognizes 18 different contraceptive methods, including permanent (i.e., tubal ligation and vasectomy), and temporary contraception (e.g., IUDs, oral contraceptive pills, patches, shots, and condoms).

The Affordable Care Act, signed into law in 2010, is another political measure assisting in increasing access to contraceptives for American women. This law mandates that all health insurance plans provide coverage of prescription contraceptives without cost sharing for patients' preventative care. Implementation of this mandate of the Affordable Care Act resulted in a 19% decline in the number of women in need of publicly funded contraceptive services who had no public or private insurance in 2011, just one year following the enactment of the mandate.

Sexually Transmitted Infections

Sexually transmitted infections (STIs) are defined as venereal diseases that are passed from one person to another via sexual contact through vaginal intercourse, oral sex, and anal sex. Examples of STIs are chlamydia, syphilis, trichomoniasis, gonorrhea, herpes simplex virus, human papilloma virus, hepatitis B, and human immunodeficiency virus. All of these diseases are nationally reportable conditions.

Pregnant women are vulnerable to the consequences of STIs. A CDC report suggests that the most common types of STIs are chlamydia and gonorrhea, both of which have been on the rise during the last few years (11% for chlamydia over the last four years and 33.4% for gonorrhea—141.8 cases per 100,000—in recent years; Frost, 2012).

Social barriers to STI prevention and control efforts as well as individual-level risky behaviors contribute to infectious disease prevalence. The adverse effect of STIs on pregnancy outcomes include premature delivery, premature rupture of the membranes, low birth weight, and stillbirth. Untreated maternal infection can also affect the infant, causing conjunctivitis, other eye infections, and pneumonia. Mother-to-child transmission of congenital syphilis has been reported to be on the rise since 2013; in 2017, it was reported to be around 23.3 cases per 100,000 live births, the highest rate in two decades. If left untreated, syphilis may lead to fetal death, preterm birth, and congenital infection, which in turn can result in both physical and mental developmental disabilities. Most cases of congenital syphilis are preventable if women are screened for syphilis during prenatal care visits and treated early during prenatal care (Prevention First Colorado, 2017).

Infection with the trichomonas vaginalis parasite is also associated with adverse health outcomes such as preterm birth and symptomatic vaginitis. According to the 2016 National Disease and Therapeutic Index, the number of initial visits for Trichomonas vaginalis infection in 2015 was 139,000. The National Health and Nutrition Examination Survey (NHANES) report for 2001–2004 reported the highest prevalence of infection among non-Hispanic Blacks, at 13.3%.

Public Health Programs

The best way to prevent STIs is to use condoms. If used correctly, condoms can dramatically reduce the risk of STI infection. However, it should be noted that the most effective way to prevent STIs is to abstain from sexual activity or stay faithful to a lifelong partner. The types of interventions discussed in the literature to prevent STIs include individually focused interventions, community-focused interventions, health communication interventions, policy-focused interventions, and behavioral intervention programs. A few examples of successful programs in the United States that were able to reduce STI infection among high-risk populations, including pregnant mothers, are:

Wear One Campaign. A condom distribution program that provides local businesses with free condoms and education on STI services, including testing and treatment. Anyone can pick up a Wear One condom bag for free, whenever the business is open.

Project Respect. In this program, public STI clinic patients who underwent a series of counseling sessions based on the Health Belief Model were significantly more likely to adopt protective behaviors and were less likely to acquire new STDs at six months of follow-up compared with those who received only informational messages.

Women in Group Support (WINGS). Community women at high risk for STIs improved condom use and communication skills through a small group intervention and were able to increase protected sex at three months of follow-up compared with a control group.

AIDS Evaluation of Street Outreach Projects (AESOP). For injection drug users and youth in high-risk situations, contact with street outreach programs was a predictor of having a condom at post-enhancement interviews, and having a condom at these interviews was a strong predictor of condom use with partners.

Chapter Summary

Women in rural areas face many challenges when it comes to health care. This chapter presented the life course approach to maternal and child health and the three temporal concepts related to personal development. The epidemiology of maternal health care described the major health disparities among women living in rural areas. A short history of public health in the United States is also explored. Other areas include children's health and adolescent reproductive health nutritional needs during pregnancy. The chapter concludes with family planning access and acceptability also describing contraception methods. Sexually transmitted infection prevalence during pregnancy and barriers to prevention end the unit.

Discussion Questions

1. Apply at least three of the five life course approach principles to discuss the one salient children's health issue in rural areas and its impact over the life course.
2. Discuss some of the significant barriers that hinder rural adolescents' access to reproductive health care. What are some approaches to address these barriers?
3. Discuss some of the challenges that rural women encounter in terms of accessing adequate nutrition during pregnancy and lactation.
4. Name family planning types and discuss the method briefly.
5. What is the definition of maternal mortality and what is the rate of maternal mortality in the state in which you are living?
6. Discuss some of the challenges that rural women are facing in terms of access to prenatal clinics during pregnancy?
7. Name various public health programs that improve access to services across the United States.
8. Briefly discuss issues pertaining to maternal and infant health.

References

Agency for Healthcare Research and Quality. (2013). *2012 National healthcare disparities report. AHRQ Publication No. 13-0003.* Rockville (MD): AHRQ.

American Academy of Family Physicians. (2010). *Cesarean delivery in family medicine. Position paper.* Leawood (KS): AAFP. Retrieved from https://www.aafp.org/about/policies/all/cesarean-delivery.html

American Academy of Obstetricians and Gynecologists. (2014). Committee Opinion No. 586: Health disparities in rural women. *Obstetrics & Gynecology, 123*(2 Pt 1), 384–388. Retrieved from https://doi.org/10.1097/01.AOG.0000443278.06393.d6

American Academy of Obstetrician and Gynecologists. (2015). *Access to contraception committee on health care for underserved women.* Retrieved from https://www.acog.org/-/media/Committee-Opinions/Committee-on-Health-Care-for-Underserved-Women/co615.pdf?dmc=1&ts=20171016T1854058857

American Academy of Pediatrics and the American College of Obstetricians and Gynecologists. (2012). *Guidelines for perinatal care.* Washington, DC: National Academies Press.

American College of Obstetricians and Gynecologists. (2014). *Health disparities in rural women.* Retrieved from https://www.acog.org/clinical/clinical-guidance/committee-opinion/articles/2014/02/health-disparities-in-rural-women

Barker, D. J. P. (1998). *Mothers, babies and health in later life* (2nd ed.). Edinburgh: Churchill Livingstone.

Bekemeier, B., Grembowski, D., Yang, Y. R., & Herting, J. R. (2012). Local public health delivery of maternal child health services: Are specific activities associated with reductions in black–white mortality disparities? *Maternal and Child Health Journal, 16*(3), 615–623. Retrieved from https://doi.org/10.1007/s10995-011-0794-9

Cappeliez, P., Beaupré, M., & Robitaille, A. (2008). Characteristics and impact of life turning points for older adults. *Ageing International, 32,* 54–64. 10.1007/s12126-008-9005-4

Centers for Disease Control and Prevention (CDC). (2015). *CDC—Minnesota: PRAMS data to inform policies and planning for improved rural birth outcomes—PRAMS—Reproductive health.* Retrieved from https://www.cdc.gov/prams/state-success-stories/Minnesota.html

Centers for Disease Control and Prevention (CDC). (2017). *Sexually transmitted diseases (STDs): Adolescents and young adults.* Retrieved from https://www.cdc.gov/std/life-stages-populations/adolescents-youngadults.htm.

Centers for Disease Control and Prevention (CDC). (2018). *CDC healthy schools: Whole school, whole community, whole child (WSCC).* Retrieved from https://www.cdc.gov/healthyschools/wscc/index.htm

Centers for Disease Control and Prevention (CDC). (2019). *Rural health: Vaccination in rural communities.* Retrieved from https://www.cdc.gov/ruralhealth/vaccines/

Centers for Disease Control and Prevention (CDC). Division of Reproductive Health. (2016). *Infant Mortality, Maternal and Infant Health, Reproductive Health, CDC.* Retrieved from http://www.cdc.gov/reproductivehealth/maternalinfanthealth/infantmortality.htm

Centers for Disease Control and Prevention (CDC), Division of Reproductive Health. (2019). *Reproductive health.* Retrieved from https://www.cdc.gov/reproductivehealth/index.html

Centers for Disease Control and Prevention (CDC). (2017). *STDs in Women and Infants.* Retrieved from https://www.cdc.gov/std/stats18/slides/STD-SurvRpt-2018-WOMEN-and-INFANTS_F.pptx

Clark, S. J., Savitz, L. A., & Randolph, R. K. (2001). Rural children's health. *Western Journal of Medicine, 174*(2), 142–147. doi:10.1136/ewjm.174.2.142

Cornwell, L., Hawley, S. R., & St. Romain, T. (2007). Implementation of a coordinated school health program in a rural, low-income community. *Journal of School Health, 77*(9), 601–606.

Creanga, A. A., Berg, C. J., Ko, J. Y., Farr, S. L., Tong, V. T., Bruce, F. C., & . . . Callaghan, W. M. (2014). Maternal mortality and morbidity in the United States: Where are we now? *Journal of Women's Health, 23*(1), 3–9. Retrieved from https://doi.org/10.1089/jwh.2013.4617

Daniels, Z. M., Vanleit, B. J., Skipper, B. J., Sanders, M. L., & Rhyne, R. L. (2007). Factors in recruiting and retaining health professionals for rural practice. *Journal of Rural Health, 23*(1), 62–71.

Department of Health and Human Services National Institute of Diabetes and Digestive and Kidney Diseases. (2015). *Health risks of being overweight.* Retrieved from https://www.niddk.nih.gov/health-information/weight-management/health-risks-overweight.

Diedhiou, A., Probst, J. C., Hardin, J. W, Martin, A. B., & Xirasagar, S. (2010). Relationship between presence of a reported medical home and emergency department use among children with asthma. *Medical Care Research and Review, 67*(4), 450–75.

Doescher, M. P., Keppel, G. A., Skillman, S. M., & Rosenblatt, R. A. (2009). *The crisis in rural dentistry.* Seattle, Washington: WWAMI Rural Health Research Center. Retrieved from http://depts.washington.edu/uwrhrc/uploads/Rural_Dentists_PB_2009.pdf/

Elder, G. H. Jr. (1998). *The life course and human development*. In R.M. Lerner (Ed.). *Volume 1: Theories of Human Development: Contemporary Perspectives in William Damon (editor-in-chief), The Handbook of Child Psychology* (5th ed.). New York: Wiley.

Elder, G. H., Johnson, M. K., & Crosnoe, R. (2003). The emergence and development of life course theory. In J. T. Mortimer & M. J. Shanahan (Eds.), *Handbook of the life course. Handbooks of sociology and social research*. Springer, Boston, MA.

Emmons, S. L., Nichols, M., Schulkin, J., James, K. E., & Cain, J. M. (2006). The influence of physician gender on practice satisfaction among obstetrician gynecologists. *American Journal of Obstetrics and Gynecology, 194*(6), 1728–1738.

Environmental Protection Agency (EPA). (2015). *Getting up to speed: Ground water contamination*. Retrieved from https://www.epa.gov/sites/production/files/2015-08/documents/mgwc-gwc1.pdf

Environmental Protection Agency (EPA). (2018). *Potential well water contaminants and their impacts*. Retrieved from https://www.epa.gov/privatewells/potential-well-water-contaminants-and-their-impacts

Felitti, V. J., Anda, R. F., Nordenberg, D., Williamson, D. F., Spitz, A. M., Edwards, V., & Koss, M. P. (1998). Relationship of childhood abuse and household dysfunction to many of the leading causes of death in adults: The Adverse Childhood Experiences (ACE) Study. *American Journal of Preventive Medicine, 14*(4), 245–258.

Finley, C., & Stewart, A. (2013). *Working with rural teens: Adolescent reproductive health in rural America*. Paper presented at the Third Annual Teen Pregnancy Prevention Grantee Conference, National Harbor, MD.

Food and Nutrition Board. (1998). *Dietary reference intakes: Thiamin, riboflavin, niacin, vitamin B_6, folate, vitamin B_{12}, pantothenic acid, biotin, and choline*. Washington, D.C.: National Academy Press.

Fowler, C., Gable, J., Wang, J., & Lasater, B. (2017). *Family planning annual report: 2016 National summary*. RTI International. Retrieved from https://www.hhs.gov/opa/sites/default/files/title-x-fpar-2016-national.pdf

Frost, J. J., Jerman, J., & Sonfield, A. (2012). *Health information technology and publicly funded family planning agencies: Readiness, use and challenges*. New York (NY): Guttmacher Institute. Retrieved from http://www.guttmacher.org/pubs/Health-IT.pdf.

Frost, J. J., Zolna, M. R., & Frohwirth, L. (2013). *Contraceptive needs and services, 2010*. Guttmacher Institute. Retrieved from https://www.guttmacher.org/report/contraceptive-needs-and-services-2010

Gabe, T. (2015). *Poverty in the United States: 2013. Congressional Research Service Report to Congress*. Washington, DC: Congressional Research Service.

Garcia, M. C., Faul, M., Massetti, G, Thomas, C. C., Hong, Y., Bauer, U. E., . . . Iademarco, M. F. (2017). Reducing potentially excess deaths from the five leading causes of death in the rural United States. *Morbidity and Mortality Weekly Report— Surveillance Summaries, 66*(2), 1–7.

Garside, R., Ayres, R., Owen, M., Pearson, V. A. H., & Roizen, J. (2002). Anonymity and confidentiality: Rural teenagers' concerns when accessing sexual health services. *BMJ Sexual & Reproductive Health, 28*, 23–26.

George, L. K. (2003). Life course research. In J. T. Mortimer & M. J. Shanahan (Eds.), *Handbook of the Life Course. Handbooks of Sociology and Social Research*. Springer, Boston, MA.

Gesink, D., Sullivan, A. B., Norwood, T., Serre, M. L., & Miller, W.C. (2013). Does core area theory apply to STIs in rural environments? *Sexually Transmitted Diseases, 40*(1), 32–40.

Gould, J. B., Sarnoff, R., Liu, H., Bell, D. R., & Chavez, G. (1999). Very low birth weight births at non-NICU hospitals: The role of sociodemographic, perinatal, and geographic factors. *Journal of Perinatology, 19*(3), 197–205.

Gregory, C. A. & Coleman-Jensen, A. (2017). *Food insecurity, chronic disease, and health among working-age adults*. ERR-235. U.S. Department of Agriculture, Economic Research Service.

Guse, K., Levine, D., Martins, S., Lira, A., Gaarde, J., Westmorland, W., & Gilliam, M. (2012). Interventions using new digital media to improve adolescent sexual health: A systematic review. *Journal of Adolescent Health, 51*(6), 535–543.

Halfon, N., & Hochstein, M. (2002). Life course health development: An integrated framework for developing health, policy, and research. *The Milbank Quarterly, 80*(3), 433–479. doi:10.1111/1468-0009.00019

Hart, L. G., Larson, E. H., Lishner, D. M. (2005). Rural definitions for health policy and research. *American Journal of Public Health, 95*(7), 1149–1155.

Health Resources & Services Administration. (2017). *School-based health centers*. Retrieved from https://www.hrsa.gov/our-stories/school-health-centers/index.html

Health Resources & Services Administration. (2019). *Health professional shortage area (HPSA) application scoring process*. Retrieved from htpps://bhw.hrsa.gov/shortage-designation/hpsa-process.

Hendryx, M., Weiner, R. C., & Gurka, M. (2011). *Water fluoridation and dental health indicators in rural and urban areas of the United States*. West Virginia Rural Health Research Center. Retrieved from https://www.ruralhealthresearch.org/mirror/4/473/2011_fluoridation_final_report.pdf

Hillemeier, M. M., Weisman, C. S., Chase, G. A., & Dyer, A.-M. (2007). Individual and community predictors of preterm birth and low birthweight along the rural-urban continuum in central Pennsylvania. *The Journal of Rural Health, 23*(1), 42–48. Retrieved from https://doi.org/10.1111/j.1748-0361.2006.00066.x

Housing Assistance Council. (2012). *Taking stock: Rural people, poverty, and housing in the 21st century.* Retrieved from http://www.ruralhome.org/storage/documents/ts2010/ts_full_report.pdf

Huffman, L. C., Wang, N. E., Saynina, O., Wren, F. J., Wise, P. H., & Horwitz, S. M. (2012). Predictors of hospitalization after an emergency department visit for California youths with psychiatric disorders. *Psychiatry Services, 63*(9), 896–905.

Institute of Medicine. (1995). *1995 Report.* Washington, DC: The National Academies Press.

Institute of Medicine and National Research Council. (2011). *Improving access to oral health care for vulnerable and underserved populations.* Washington, DC: The National Academies Press.

Issel, L. M., Forrestal, S. G., Slaughter, J., Wiencrot, A., & Handler, A. (2011). A review of prenatal home-visiting effectiveness for improving birth outcomes. *Journal of Obstetric, Gynecologic, and Neonatal Nursing, 40*(2), 157–165. Retrieved from https://doi.org/10.1111/j.1552-6909.2011.01219.x

Jernigan, V. B. B., Huyser, K. R., Valdes, J., Simonds, V. W. (2017). Food insecurity among American Indians and Alaska Natives: A national profile using the current population survey—food security supplement. *Journal of Hunger & Environmental Nutrition, 12*(1), 1–10.

Jones, J., Mosher, W., & Daniels, K. (2012). Current contraceptive use in the United States, 2006–2010, and changes in patterns of use since 1995. *National Health Statistics Report, 60,* 1–25. Retrieved from https://pubmed.ncbi.nlm.nih.gov/24988814/

Jones, R. K., & Jerman, J. (2013). How far did US women travel for abortion services in 2008? *Journal of Women's Health (2002), 22*(8), 706–713. Retrieved from https://doi.org/10.1089/jwh.2013.4283

Jukic, A. M., Weinberg, C. R., Baird, D. D., & Wilcox, A. J. (2007) Lifestyle and reproductive factors associated with follicular phase length. *Journal of Women's Health, 16*(9), 1340–1347.

Kanaka-Gantenbein, C. (2010). Fetal origins of adult diabetes. *Annals of the New York Academy of Sciences, 1205*(1), 99–105.

Kaufman, P., Dicken, C., & Williams, R. (2014). *Measuring access to healthful, affordable food in American Indian and Alaska Native tribal areas.* Washington (DC): US Department of Agriculture. Bulletin Number 131. Retrieved from 10.22004/ag.econ.262120

Kolbe, L. J. (2005). A framework for school health programs in the 21st century. *Journal of School Health, 75*(6), 226–228.

Kominiarek, M. A., & Rajan, P. (2016). Nutrition recommendations in pregnancy and lactation. *The Medical Clinics of North America, 100*(6), 1199–1215. Retrieved from doi:10.1016/j.mcna.2016.06.004

Kozhimannil, K. B., Hung, P., Henning-Smith, C., Casey, M. M., & Prasad, S. (2018). Association between loss of hospital-based obstetric services and birth outcomes in rural counties in the United States. *Journal of the American Medical Association, 319*(12), 1239–1247.

Kramer, M. S. (1987). Determinants of low birth weight: Methodological assessment and meta-analysis. *Bulletin of the World Health Organization, 65*(5), 663–737.

Kramer, M. S. (2003). The epidemiology of adverse pregnancy outcomes: An overview. *The Journal of Nutrition, 133*(5 Suppl 2), 1592S–1596S.

Krieger, J., & Higgins, D. L. (2002). Housing and health: Time again for public health action. *American Journal of Public Health, 92*(5), 758–768. Retrieved from doi:10.2105/ajph.92.5.758

Levy, J. E. & Shepardson, W. (1992). A look at current school-linked service efforts. *The Future of Children, 2*(1), 44–55.

Lichtenstein, B., Hook, E. W., & Sharma, A. K. (2005). Public tolerance, private pain: Stigma and sexually transmitted infections in the American Deep South. *Culture, Health & Sexuality, 7*(1), 43–57.

Liu, J., Probst, J. C., Martin, A. B., Wang, J. Y., & Salinas, C. F. (2007). Disparities in dental insurance coverage and dental care among US children. The national survey of children's health. *Pediatrics, 119*(Suppl 1), S12–S21.

Lowery, C., Bronstein, J., McGhee, J., Ott, R., Reece, E. A., & Mays, G. P. (2007). ANGELS and University of Arkansas for medical sciences paradigm for distant obstetrical care delivery. *American Journal of Obstetrics and Gynecology, 196*(6), 534.e1–534.e9.

Malik, R. & Schochet, L. (2018). *A compass for families: Head Start in rural America.* Retrieved from https://www.americanprogress.org/issues/early-childhood/reports/2018/04/10/448741/a-compass-for-families/

Probst, J. C., and Jones, K. M. (2017). *Chartbook: Trends in Rural Children's Oral Health and Access to Care.* Columbia, SC: South Carolina Rural Health Research Center.

McTavish, J. R., MacGregor, J. C., Wathen, C. N., & MacMillan, H. L. (2016). Children's exposure to intimate partner violence: An overview. *International Review of Psychiatry, 28*(5), 504–518.

Mertz, E. & Mouradian, W. E. (2009). Addressing children's oral health in the new millennium: Trends in the dental workforce. *Academic Pediatrics, 9*(6), 433–439.

Michigan Department of Health and Human Services. (n.d.). Michigan pregnancy risk assessment monitoring system. Retrieved from https://www.michigan.gov/mdhhs/0,5885,7-339-73971_4911_21428---,00.html

National Campaign to Prevent Teen and Unplanned Pregnancy. (2010). *Why it Matters.* Washington, DC:

National Campaign to Prevent Teen and Unplanned Pregnancy. [Online]. Retrieved from https://powerto decide.org/what-we-do/information/why-it-matters

National Center for Health Statistics. (2012). *Health, United States, 2012: With special feature on emergency care*. Hyattsville (MD): NCHS. [Internet]. Retrieved from http://www.cdc.gov/nchs/data/hus/hus12.pdf

Organization for Economic Cooperation and Development. (2020). *OECD health statistics 2020 definitions, sources and methods*. Retrieved from http://www.oecd.org/els/health-systems/health-data.htm

Otten, J. J., Pitzi, H. J., Meyers, L. D., (Eds.). (2006). *Dietary reference intakes. The essential guide to nutrient requirements*. Washington, DC: National Academies Press.

Parker T. (2015). *Updated ERS County Economic Types Show a Changing Rural Landscape*. United States Department of Agriculture Economic Research Service. Retrieved from Retrieved from https://www.ers.usda.gov/amber-waves/2015/december/updated-ers-county-economic-types-show-a-changing-rural-landscape

Pascoe, J. M., Wood, D. L., Duffee, J. H., & Kuo, A. (2016). Mediators and adverse effects of child poverty in the United States. *Pediatrics, 137*(4), e20160340. doi:10.1542/peds.2016-0340

Pew Research Center. (2013). *Widening regional divide over abortion laws*. Washington, D.C.: Pew Research Center.

Phillippi, J. C. (2009). Women's perceptions of access to prenatal care in the United States: A literature review. *Journal of Midwifery & Women's Health, 54*(3), 219–225. Retrieved from https://doi.org/10.1016/j.jmwh.2009.01.002

Pinto, C. N., Dorn, L. D., Chinchilli, V. M., Du, P., & Chi, G. (2017). Rural counties chlamydia and gonorrhea rates in Pennsylvania among adolescents and young adults. *Annals of Epidemiology, 27*(9), 606–610.

Prevention First Colorado. (2017). Allow advanced practice nurses with prescriptive authority to distribute and administer prescription contraceptives. In Planning, protection, prevention: Reducing unintended pregnancy in Colorado. Denver, CO: PFC.

Rasmussen, K. M. (2001). The "fetal origins" hypothesis: Challenges and opportunities for maternal and child nutrition. *Annual Review of Nutrition, 21*, 73–95.

Rayburn, W. F., Klagholz, J. C., Murray-Krezan, C., Dowell, L. E., & Strunk, A. L. (2012) Distribution of American congress of obstetricians and gynecologists fellows and junior fellows in practice in the United States. *Obstetrics & Gynecology, 119*(5), 1017–1022.

Roberto, A. J., Zimmerman, R. S., Carlyle, K. E., & Abner, E. L. (2007). A computer-based approach to preventing pregnancy, STD, and HIV in rural adolescents. *Journal of Health Communication: International Perspectives, 12*(1), 53–76.

Roberts, R. G., Deutchman, M., King, V. J., Fryer, G. E., & Miyoshi, T. J. (2007). Changing policies on vaginal birth after cesarean: Impact on access. *Birth (Berkeley, Calif.), 34*(4), 316–322. Retrieved from https://doi.org/10.1111/j.1523-536X.2007.00190.x

Romano, P. S., Geppert, J. J., Davies, S., Miller, M. R., Elixhauser, A, & McDonald, K. M. (2003). A national profile of patient safety in U.S. hospitals. *Health Affairs, 22*(2). Retrieved from https://doi.org/10.1377/hlthaff.22.2.154

Roots, R. K., & Li, L. C. (2013). Recruitment and retention of occupational therapists and physiotherapists in rural regions: A meta-synthesis. *BMC Health Services Research, 13*(59).

Rural Health Information Hub. (2019). *School-based models*. Retrieved from Retrieved from https://www.ruralhealthinfo.org/toolkits/food-access/2/school-based-models.

Samuelson, J. L., Buehler, J. W., Norris, D., & Sadek, R. (2002). Maternal characteristics associated with place of delivery and neonatal mortality rates among very-low-birthweight infants, Georgia. *Paediatric Perinatal Epidemiology, 16*(4), 305–313.

Sharkey, J. R. (2009). Measuring potential access to food stores and food-service places in rural areas in the U.S. *American Journal of Preventive Medicine, 36*(4), s151–s155. doi:10.1016/j.amepre.2009.01.004

Shellenberg, K. M. & Tsui, A. O. (2012). Correlates of perceived and internalized stigma among abortion patients in the USA: An exploration by race and hispanic ethnicity. *International Journal of Gynaecology & Obstetrics, 118*(S2), S152–S159.

SmithBattle, L. (2012). Moving policies upstream to mitigate the social determinants of early childbearing. *Public Health Nursing, 29*(5), 444–454. Retrieved from http://online.library.wiley.com/doi/10.1111/j.1525-1446.2012.01017.x/full

Stulberg, D. B., Dude, A. M., Dahlquist, I., & Curlin, F. A. (2011). Abortion provision among practicing obstetrician–gynecologists. *Obstetrics & Gynecology, 118*(3), 609–614.

The National Academies of Sciences, Engineering, Medicine. (2011). *Clinical preventive services for women: Closing the gaps*. Washington, DC: The National Academies Press. Retrieved from http://www.nap.edu/catalog.php?record_id=13181.

Till, S. R., Everetts, D., & Haas, D. M. (2015). Incentives for increasing prenatal care use by women in order to improve maternal and neonatal outcomes. *Cochrane Systematic Review,* (12), CD009916. PMID: 26671418. Retrieved from: https://www.cochranelibrary.com/cdsr/doi/10.1002/14651858.CD009916.pub2/full

U.S. Census Bureau. (2010). *Table P2: Urban and rural*. Washington, DC: U.S. Census Bureau.

U.S. Department of Health and Human Services. (2019). *Head start programs*. Retrieved from https://www.acf.hhs.gov/ohs/about/head-start.

U.S. Department of Health and Human Services Health Resources and Services Administration Maternal and Child Health Bureau. (2015). *The health and well-being of children in rural areas: A portrait of the nation, 2011-2012.* Rockville, Maryland: U.S. Department of Health and Human Services.

U.S. Department of Health and Human Services National Advisory Committee on Rural Health and Human Services. (2018). *Exploring the rural context for adverse childhood experiences (ACEs).* Retrieved from https://www.hrsa.gov/sites/default/files/hrsa/advisory-committees/rural/publications/Rural-Context-for-ACEs-August2018.pdf

Wyoming Department of Health. *State narrative for Wyoming: Application for 2014 annual report for 2012.* Maternal and Child Health Services Title V Block Grant. Cheyenne (WY): Wyoming Department of Health; 2013. Retrieved from http://www.health.wyo.gov/Medi

CHAPTER 11

Oral Health in Rural Areas

Livingstone Aduse-Poku, MPH
Joseph N. Inungu, MD, DrPH, MPH

LEARNING OBJECTIVES

At the end of this chapter, readers will be able to:

1. Explain the importance of a healthy and well-functioning dentition to the general health of individuals.
2. Understand the nature of oral health disparities in rural populations and how it imparts the general health of these populations.
3. Gain knowledge on the current approaches to mitigate oral health disparities and how these approaches can be adopted within individual communities.
4. Describe Medicaid coverage of dental health benefits and how it affects oral health in rural populations.
5. Appreciate public health efforts used to improve oral health in rural communities.

KEY TERMS

Dental therapists
Disparities
Fluoridation
Medicaid
Oral health
Sealants

CHAPTER OVERVIEW

Brief Anatomy of the Oral/Buccal Cavity

The term oral refers to the mouth, which is comprised of the teeth, gums, tongue, lips, salivary glands, the masticatory muscles, jaws, temporomandibular joints, hard and soft palate, skeletal nerves, and the mucosal lining of the mouth and the throat (Battle, 2009). The health of the teeth and surrounding craniofacial structures is central to general health and well-being. The teeth are the hardest substances in the body. **Figure 11-1** (Hoffman, 2018) depicts a healthy tooth cut in half lengthways showing the layers of the tooth and its internal structure. The tooth is made of two sections: The crown: the upper part of the tooth and the root: the distal section of the tooth that is below the gum. The neck is the region of the tooth at the gum line between the root and the crown.

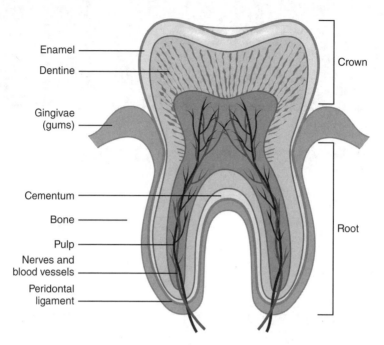

Enamel
Dentine
Gingivae (gums)
Cementum
Bone
Pulp
Nerves and blood vessels
Peridontal ligament
Crown
Root

Figure 11-1 Internal Structure of a Healthy Tooth.

The Crown

The crown is made of two layers: the enamel and the dentin. The enamel is the hard outer layer of the crown. It is the hardest substance of the body, yet it can decay if not properly cared for. The dentin is a layer of mineralized tissue just below the enamel. It extends from the crown down through the neck. Dentine is sensitive. It contains tiny tubules throughout its structure that connect with the central nerve of the tooth within the pulp.

Root

Although some teeth have only one root, such as incisors and canines, others have four roots such as molars and premolars. The root has two important layers: The dentine of the root is covered with a thin layer, which is not as hard as the enamel but with a similar hardness to the bone. It is called cementum. This membrane bonds the root of the tooth to the bone of the jaw. If the cementum becomes exposed to the oral cavity through gingival recession, this surface can become very sensitive to temperature changes in the mouth (hot and cold).

The pulp is the central chamber of the tooth where all of the nerves and blood vessels that supply the tooth are housed. The pulp is divided into two areas: the pulp chamber, located in the crown of the tooth; and the pulp canals, which are located in the root(s) of the tooth. If the pulp area becomes exposed to decay, a bacterial infection can occur and may require root canal therapy in order to save the tooth.

Background

Rural areas cover 97% of the nation's land but contain 19.3% of the American population (American Community Survey, 2015). Over the next decade, the migration of the retired baby boomers will further increase the population in nonmetropolitan areas (Economic Research Service, 2009). The rural population aged 55–75 is expected to increase by 30% between 2010 and 2020 if baby boomers follow past migration

Table 11-1 HRSA's FY18 Third-Quarter Report on Dental Health Professional Shortage Areas

Rural/Nonrural Designation	Number of Designations	Percentage of All Designations	Population of Designated HPSAs	Dental Practitioners Needed to Remove Designations
Rural	3,494	59.03%	20,582,142	3,533
Nonrural	2,047	34.58%	29,333,095	5,101
Partially rural	374	6.32%	13,385,082	2,225
Unknown	4	0.07%	38,762	7

From National Advisory Committee on Rural Health and Human Services, Retrieved from https://www.hrsa.gov/sites/default/files/hrsa/advisory-committees/rural/publications/2018-Oral-Health-Policy-Brief.pdf

patterns (Cromartie & Nelson, 2009). With the general improvement in health systems in the United States, older members of the population are living longer; most are retaining their own teeth and as a result will need dental care later in life than was the case some generations ago (Skillman et al., 2010). Also, older rural residents have less-favorable dental indicators and have a lower rate of dental insurance coverage than urban residents (Vargas, Yellowitz, & Hayes, 2003).

The Designated Health Professional Shortage Area (HPSA) Statistics report in 2018 showed that there was a total of 5,899 (**Table 11-1**) dental HPSAs nationally, 65% of which are located in rural and partially rural areas, accounting for approximately 40 million people. This means that of the nation's 60 million rural residents, 66.6% of them lack access to dental care. This is a clear indication of the need for proper attention to be given to **oral health** in the United States, especially in rural communities.

Magnitude of the Problem in the United States

Two major oral diseases are common in the United States: dental caries (caused by action of acids on the enamel surface) and periodontal disease (a pathological inflammatory condition of the gum and bone surrounding the teeth).

The oral cavity acts as more than just the window to conditions that are not visible to the naked eye; it is an integral part of the body and if poorly cared for, can lead to various health complications (Musgrove, 2018). One typical case that gained national attention was the death of Deamonte Driver, a child who died from a tooth infection when the bacteria traveled into the brain. According to the Institute of Medicine, (2011), approximately 7,500 people of 30,000 annual cases die of pharyngeal cancer. Poor oral health may inhibit an individual's ability to speak, smile, taste, touch, and effectively convey emotions (Kamer, 2008).

Oral infections such as periodontitis may increase the risk of preterm or low birthweight deliveries (Offenbacher et al., 2001). A study done by Lopez, Smith & Gutierrez in 2005, revealed that women with periodontal disease were between 3.7 to 7 times more likely than those who do not have periodontal disease to give birth to preterm or low birthweight infants. Between 2000 and 2010, 18.2% of babies born in South Carolina were born premature. South Carolina ranks 47th of the 50 states for low birthweight. The problem is significantly greater in black people and people living in rural South Carolina (March of Dimes, 2010).

Dental disease (cavities) is the most common chronic disease in children in the United States. According to the United States Department of Health and Human Services (USDHHS), dental cavities are five times more common than asthma and hay fever (USDHHS, 2000). Every year across the United States, children miss more than 51 million school hours due to dental problems and visits, and adults lose close to 164 million work hours (CDC, 2011). More than a quarter of all Americans 60 years of age or older have lost all their teeth. Interestingly, edentulism (toothlessness) varies greatly by state. For example, approximately 42% of Americans over age 65 living in West Virginia are toothless, compared with only 13% of those living in California (CDC, 2013). About 1 in 4 nonelderly adults have untreated tooth decay. The rate among low-income adults is twice that for adults with more income (The Kaiser Commission on **Medicaid** and the Uninsured, 2012). An estimated 17 million low-income children go without dental care each year (Pew Centre on States, 2012). Also, more than 64 million Americans have moderate to severe forms of periodontal disease (Eke et al., 2012).

State of Oral Health Care in Rural America

Access to health care has become an extremely important health issue among rural health advocates. Rural populations have fewer dentists, lower dental care utilization, and rates of dental caries and tooth loss than urban populations (Doescher et al., 2009). These **disparities** can be attributed to several factors, including: lack of dentists accepting Medicaid and other subsidized insurance, poverty, geographic location, and absence of coordinated screening and referrals (Fos & Hutchison, 2003). A study published in Access Project (2009) revealed that dental costs were a burden for many families in rural America. Seventy-five percent of households studied

reported having dental out-of-pocket costs, spending an average of $873 annually on dental care and the amount constituted 27% of their overall health out-of-pocket costs. Forty-two percent of the families had dental insurance compared with the 60% of the national population having dental insurance (Pryor, et al., 2009).

Recent studies have highlighted the impact of lack of dental providers in rural America and the overall reliance on Medicaid among people living in rural communities. The Center for Rural Affairs' brief on "Medicaid and Rural America" showed a massive dependence on Medicaid for healthcare access (Bailey, 2012). Sixteen percent of rural residents have Medicaid coverage compared with 13% of urban residents and 35% of rural children are enrolled in Medicaid compared with 28% of urban children. In 2010, 42% or rural children had health insurance coverage through Medicaid and State Child Health Insurance Programs (SCHIP) verses 36% of children nationally (SangNam et al., 2011). Strikingly, rural physicians receive 60% of their revenue from Medicare and Medicaid verses 45% of urban physicians (Bailey, 2012). Thus Rural America not only relies on Medicaid as a major source of healthcare access but also as a major source of revenue for economic stability.

The need for oral health is increasing in rural areas. According to Rural Healthy People, (2010), oral health ranks fifth of 28 priority conditions. The use of nonfluoridated well water is more common in rural areas compared with urban areas, putting the former at greater risk of dental caries (Crosby, 2012). Tobacco use is very common among rural residences in Southeastern America, which predisposes them to oral and pharyngeal cancer, periodontal disease, and caries (US Department of Health and Human Services, 2000).

Disparities exist in oral health needs and outcomes across the various U.S. states. States like Wisconsin, North Dakota, Minnesota, and Massachusetts have high numbers of dental visits, dental Medicaid coverage (**Figure 11-2**),

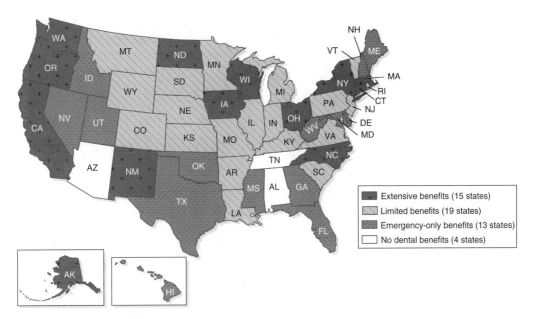

Figure 11-2 2016 Medicaid Coverage of Adult Dental Benefits by State.

Reproduced from Kaiser Family Foundation, Access to Dental Care in Medicaid: Spotlight on Nonelderly Adults, https://www.kff.org/medicaid/issue-brief/access-to-dental-care-in-medicaid-spotlight-on-nonelderly -adults/

and low prevalence of tooth decay while Arkansas, Mississippi, Alabama, and South Carolina have poor oral health outcomes (American Dental Association, 2013).

In America's Health Rankings Senior Report, the United Health Foundation found that 60.6% of rural residents over 65 years old had visited the dentist the previous year compared with 69.5% of the same age group living in urban areas (United Health Foundation, 2018). In 2008, there were 22 generalists (general practice, pediatric, or public health) dentists per 100,000 population in rural areas compared with 30 per 100,000 population in urban areas throughout the United States (Doescher, Keppel, Skillman, Rosenblatt, 2009). Although there are differences in rural oral health delivery across regions, in its report in 2018, the National Advisory Committee on Rural Health and Human Services (NACRHHS) stated that the commonest barriers to oral health in rural America are as follows: geographic location, lack of adequate transportation, higher rate of poverty compared with urban areas, large elderly population, acute provider shortages, state-by-state variability in scope of practice, difficulty finding providers willing to treat Medicaid patients, lack of fluoridated water, and poor oral health education.

Causes of Dental and Oral Diseases and Approaches to Mitigate Poor Oral Health

The oral cavity collects all sorts of bacteria, viruses, and fungi. Although some of them make up the normal flora of the mouth and are generally harmless, they can cause serious health concerns under certain conditions. A diet high in sugar allows acid-producing bacteria to flourish, causing dental cavities.

Bacteria near the gumline thrive in a sticky matrix called *plaque*, which can inflame the gums if it is not removed and subsequently cause inflammation of the gums, called gingivitis. Gingivitis can lead to a more advanced condition of the gum called *periodontitis*. There are many factors that contribute to gingivitis and periodontitis, including:

- Smoking
- Poor brushing habits
- Frequent snacking on sugary foods and drinks
- Diabetes
- The use of medications that reduce the amount of saliva in the mouth
- Family history, or genetics
- Certain infections, such as HIV or AIDS
- Hormonal changes in women
- Acid reflux, or heartburn
- Frequent vomiting due to the acid

Since the Surgeon General's report on oral health in 2000, oral health has been an issue of national concern. In spite of that, oral health has been given a lower priority in healthcare and policy initiatives compared with other issues (USDHHS, 2018). One major limitation to proper oral health care in the United States is that it has been separated from general health care and oral health professionals are trained in separate locations and reimbursed by independent insurance (USHHS, 2018). Although there are some "challenges" not changes. The increase in the use of silver diamine fluoride, which is a less-invasive procedure, has helped reduce the incidence of dental caries (Dye, 2015). In 2011, the Institute of Medicine reported some important steps to combat poor oral health outcomes in rural populations in *Advancing Oral Health in Rural America*. These interventions included the use of dental sealants, fluoride in community water, and community-based programs, usually through educational systems.

The discovery of the link between appropriate levels of fluoride in drinking water and reduced dental caries has led to the promotion of other fluoride vehicles, including salt, milk, toothpastes, gels, and tablets. The CDC's Division of Oral Health reports that community water **fluoridation** is one of the most effective methods to distribute fluoridated water to the population. Drinking fluoridated water reduces dental caries by 25% in both children and adults (Dye, 2015). The use of fluorine in community water systems has a return on investment (ROI) ranging from $28.70 to $35.90 in small and large communities respectively, based on the 2015 report by the US Department of Health and Human Services Federal Panel on Community Water Fluoridation (2015).

Dental **sealants** are thin layers of plastic resin used to fill-up fissures and pits in the teeth to prevent food particles and bacteria from creating a conducive environment for formation of dental caries. (Crosby, 2012). A literature review on the use of resin-based sealants found that they were effective two years after their application; a similar study found effectiveness four years after application (Ahovuo-Saloranta, Forss, Walsh, Nordblad, & Mäkelä, 2017).

In 2018, the U.S Health Resources and Services Administration reported that there are 5,589 areas designated as Dental Health Professional Shortage Areas (DHPSA) in rural and partially rural areas, which accounts for 65% of all designations (Table 11-1). Even with the parts of rural areas not designated as DHPSA, dentists are not obligated to serve Medicaid and CHIP-eligible patients, which further heightens the extent of rural-urban disparity in relation to dental care (Jack, Karina, Joan & Mark, 2017). To address this shortage, **dental therapists** (expanded-function dental hygienists) have been approved to practice in some states; however, the scope of practice varies from state to state, as shown in **Figure 11-3** (Oral Health Workforce Research Center, 2016). However, some concerns have been raised regarding the approval of dental therapists in the performance of certain procedures. These concerns are related to patients' safety and quality of oral care (Adams, 2004).

From Figure 11-3, it can be seen that only Colorado and Oregon allow dental hygienists

Variation in Dental Hygiene Scope of Practice by State

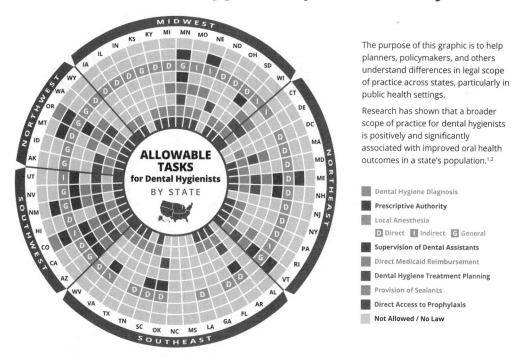

The purpose of this graphic is to help planners, policymakers, and others understand differences in legal scope of practice across states, particularly in public health settings.

Research has shown that a broader scope of practice for dental hygienists is positively and significantly associated with improved oral health outcomes in a state's population.[1,2]

Legend:
- Dental Hygiene Diagnosis
- **Prescriptive Authority**
- Local Anesthesia
  - **D** Direct **I** Indirect **G** General
- **Supervision of Dental Assistants**
- Direct Medicaid Reimbursement
- **Dental Hygiene Treatment Planning**
- Provision of Sealants
- **Direct Access to Prophylaxis**
- Not Allowed / No Law

Dental Hygiene Diagnosis
The identification of oral conditions for which treatment falls within the dental hygiene scope of practice, as part of a dental hygiene treatment plan.

Prescriptive Authority
The ability to prescribe, administer, and dispense fluoride, topical medications, and chlorhexidine.

Local Anesthesia
The administration of local anesthesia.

LEVEL OF SUPERVISION

D **Direct:** The dentist is required to be physically present during the administration of local anesthesia by the dental hygienist.

I **Indirect:** The dentist is required to be on the premises during the administration of local anesthesia by the dental hygienist.

G **General:** The dentist is required to authorize the administration of local anesthesia by the dental hygienist but is not required to be on the premises during the procedure.

Supervision of Dental Assistants
The ability to supervise dental assistants when performing tasks within the dental hygiene scope of practice.

Direct Medicaid Reimbursement
The direct Medicaid reimbursement of dental hygiene services to the dental hygienist.

Dental Hygiene Treatment Planning
The ability of a dental hygienist to assess oral conditions and formulate treatment plans for services within the dental hygiene scope of practice.

Provision of Sealants Without Prior Examination
The ability of a dental hygienist working in a public health setting to provide sealants without prior examination by a dentist.

Direct Access to Prophylaxis from a Dental Hygienist
The ability of a dental hygienist working in a public health setting to provide prophylaxis without prior examination by a dentist.

Not Allowed / No Law

Sources: 1. Langelier M, Baker B, Continelli T. *Development of a New Dental Hygiene Professional Practice Index by State, 2016.* Rensselaer, NY: Oral Health Workforce Research Center, Center for Health Workforce Studies, School of Public Health, SUNY Albany; November 2016. 2. Langelier M, Continelli T, Moore J, Baker B, Surdu S. Expanded Scopes of Practice for Dental Hygienists Associated With Improved Oral Health Outcomes for Adults. *Health Affairs.* 2016;35(12):2207-2215.

http://www.oralhealthworkforce.org/wp-content/uploads/2017/03/OHWRC_Dental_Hygiene_Scope_of_Practice_2016.pdf

This work was supported by the Health Resources and Services Administration (HRSA) of the U.S. Department of Health and Human Services (HHS), under the Health Workforce Research Center Cooperative Agreement Program (U81HP27843). The content and conclusions presented herein are those of the authors and should not be construed as the official position or policy of, nor should any endorsements be inferred by HRSA, HHS or the U.S. Government.

This graphic describes the highest level of practice available to a dental hygienist in a state, including dental hygiene therapy. The graphic is for informational purposes only and scope of practice is subject to change. Contact the applicable dental board or your attorney for specific legal advice.

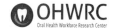
OHWRC
Oral Health Workforce Research Center

Last Updated January 2019.

Figure 11-3 Allowable Tasks for Dental Hygienists by State.

to diagnose oral conditions for which treatment falls within the dental hygiene scope of practice. Six states allow dental hygienists to prescribe, administer, and dispense fluoride topical medications. Fifteen states provide them with the ability to supervise dental assistants when performing dental procedures.

Case Study: Oral Health in South Carolina

Prevalence of Disease and Unmet Needs

Oral health plays an integral role in the overall health of individuals. Tooth decay, which is largely preventable, disproportionately affects minorities, poor and rural children, and is a significant issue in South Carolina (Martin et al., 2010). According to the South Carolina Department of Health and Environmental Control (DHEC), 2008, approximately 405 South Carolina children experience tooth decay before Kindergarten, with half of them being untreated.

Caries and untreated decay are monitored by South Carolina, consistent with the National Oral Health Surveillance System (NOHSS), allowing for comparison with other states and with the nation, as shown in **Figure 11-4**. The figure illustrates that South Carolina falls behind the national average in terms of the prevalence of caries and untreated tooth decay but has still not met the Healthy People 2010 target. Dental caries are not uniformly distributed in South Carolina. Some groups are more likely to experience the disease but less likely to receive treatment. More than half (53.8%) of Black people in South Carolina experience tooth decay compared with 42.4% of White people who experience tooth decay (Healthy People, 2010). Thirty-nine percent of Black people who experience tooth decay go without treatment. Twenty-eight percent of males who experience dental caries in South Carolina are untreated compared with 24% of females who go without treatment (Healthy People, 2010). Only 47.5% of dentists in South Carolina participate in Medicaid or CHIP for child dental services.

Oral Health in Rural South Carolina

According to the United States Census Bureau, in 2010, almost 33.7% of South Carolina's population lives in rural areas. Of the 46 counties in South Carolina, only 15 meet the definition of urban (DHEC, 2010). In 2010, the poverty level of people in rural South Carolina was 18.8%

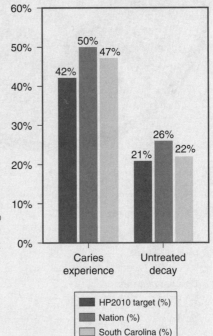

Figure 11-4 Prevalence of Caries and Untreated Tooth Decay in Children.

and the poverty level of children was 27.5% (USDA, 2010). To further complicate the poverty rates in rural South Carolina, there are other barriers, including fewer dentists per population, fewer dentists who participate in Medicaid, and longer travel times and distances to reach healthcare providers compared with urban areas (Martin et al., 2010). Eighty percent of HPSA in South Carolina are found in rural areas (Boynes & Martin, 2016). According to the South Carolina Rural Health Research Centre report in March of 2013, Black children are more likely to have less dental sealants compared with Whites and Hispanics, both in rural and urban South Carolina.

Preventive dental service utilization increased from 71.8% of all children in 2003 to 77.2% from 2011–2012 for all children living in rural South Carolina (Martin, Probst & Jones, 2017). Among

White children, both reported condition of tooth decay and rates for receiving preventive dental visits remained lower among rural than among urban children in the same time period. For children in all other race/ethnic groups, the gap between rural and urban children was smaller (Rural Health Research Centre, 2017). The proportion of children with delayed dental care due to cost was relatively small (less than 3%). The proportion of parents reporting that their child had excellent or very good teeth increased slightly over the period, from 68.6% in 2003 to 70.9% in 2007 and 71.6% from 2011–2012. Urban children tended to have lower incidences of tooth decay, as assessed by their parents (Martin, Probst & Jones, 2017).

Programs and Services to Improve Oral Health in South Carolina

Oral Health Care Needs Assessment

Every five years, DHEC conducts a statewide dental screening to obtain a picture of the dental health of Kindergarten and 3rd grade children in South Carolina. A total of 76 schools in 37 school districts across 29 counties in the state participated in the survey from 2012 to 2013. A variety of dental professionals and school nurses conducted screenings of 6,515 students (SC DHEC, Division of Oral Health Database, 2013). This screening increased knowledge about preventive practices, access to dental care, and helped raise awareness about the connection between a healthy mouth and a healthy body.

SC DHEC School Dental Program

The South Carolina SDPP is composed of four dental programs that enter a yearly Memorandum of Agreement with DHEC to deliver preventive services such as providing sealants in public settings. Programs such as Beaufort-Jasper-Hampton Comprehensive Health Services, Little River Medical Center, Health Promotion Specialists and Classy Smiles, reached 21,888 children in the 2011–2012. During the same year, 9,596 children received one or more sealants on their permanent molars, 20,374 children received fluoride varnish and 20,489 children received prophylactic treatment.

Early Childhood and Oral Health

South Carolina, through a consistent and comprehensive approach, has built support for oral health standards of care. Specific resources have been tapped and targeted assistance has taken place to support these initiatives. Oral Health 101 trainings for health providers; Oral Health Care for Pregnant Women Guidelines; Oral Health for the Young Child; *Oral Health Teacher Activities for the Early Childhood Classroom* booklet (an oral health show that travels across the state to schools and Head start Centers) are some of the resources that have been developed and utilized. These programs are collaborative approaches aimed at improving oral health status of South Carolina's young children.

Tobacco Control

Nearly 14% of South Carolina residents smoke every day, and an additional 7% smoke on at least some days (BRFSS, 2010); this makes tobacco a health issue for all South Carolinians. A quit line has recently been established by the DHEC. The program includes an oral health component where the healthcare provider discusses the impact of tobacco on teeth, gums, breath, and risk of oral cancer with the client.

Conclusion

Since the Surgeon General's report on oral health in 2000, there have been several efforts to improve oral health in the United States. Nevertheless, oral health has persisted as one of the greatest unmet needs in rural America. While some progress has been made in this area, challenges remain. There are still large parts of the US population, especially within rural areas that are considered as HPSA with low and/or no access to dental care.

Although several research findings have linked oral health to general health, oral health has not been a priority in policies and health literacy initiatives compared with other health issues. Dental insurance is lacking in several rural communities across the United States.

To improve dental health, school and community awareness should be created. Increasing oral health literacy in homes, schools, and communities would create awareness of tooth decay and other oral health problems. Community-based fluoridation and school-based sealants have been very effective in improving oral health outcomes in rural communities.

Chapter Summary

Rural populations, which consist of a large percentage of the country's overall population, are expected to increase due to the migration of retired baby boomers. This movement will require much attention to oral health in rural populations as life expectancy increases and elderly people retain their teeth.

Oral health has overall health implications on general health. It affects people before and after birth and can lead to reduced productivity and huge economic loss if it is neglected. However, disparities exist among various states in relation to access to dental care and oral health outcomes.

Rural communities have high oral health conditions and poor oral health outcomes compared with urban areas. These oral health challenges are due to geographic location, lack of adequate transportation, higher rate of poverty compared with urban areas, large elderly population, acute provider shortages, state-by-state variability in scope of practice, difficulty finding providers willing to treat Medicaid patients, lack of fluoridated water, and poor oral health education.

To help mitigate this health issue, some efforts have been put in place by the various states and the federal government. Many communities have received community-based water fluoridation to help improve the fluoride content of water to protect against dental caries.

Resin-based dental sealants have been used at community and school settings to help reduce the incidence of dental caries. Dental therapists/hygienists have been approved to practice in various states. This has helped improve the dental workforce.

Discussion Questions

1. Using knowledge from this chapter, do you think dental health should still be separated from general health or should they be together? Discuss the advantages and disadvantages of both scenarios to convince even the most indifferent policymaker.

2. How can the lessons from South Carolina be generalized to other rural areas? What key factors can be broadened?

Student Activities and Worksheets are available inside the Navigate eBook, included with the printed text. Simply redeem the access code found at the front of the book at www.jblearning.com.

References

Adams, T. L. (2004). Attitudes to independent dental hygiene practice: Dentists and dental hygienists in Ontario. *Journal of the Canadian Dental Association, 70*(8), 535–538.

Ahovuo-Saloranta, A., Forss, H., Walsh, T., Nordblad, A., Mäkelä, M., & Worthington, H. V. (2017). Pit and fissure sealants for preventing dental decay in permanent teeth. *Cochrane Database of Systematic Reviews.*

Retrieved from https://doi.org/10.1002/14651858.CD001830.pub5

Centers for Disease Control and Prevention (CDC). (2013). *Oral health for older Americans. Facts about older adult health.* Retrieved from https://www.cdc.gov/oralhealth/basics/adult-oral-health/adult_older.htm

Cromartie, J., & Nelson, P. (2009). Baby boom migration and its impact on rural America. Economic Research Report No. 79. Washington: Economic Research Service, US Department of Agriculture. Retrieved from https://www.ers.usda.gov/webdocs/publications/46218/9346_err79_1_.pdf?v=41056

Doescher, M., Keppel, G., Skillman, S., & Rosenblatt, R. (2009). Policy brief: The crisis in rural dentistry Seattle: *WWAMI Rural Health Research Center*, University of Washington.

Dye, B. A., Thornton-Evans, G., Li, X., & Iafolla, T. J. (2015). Dental caries and tooth loss in adults in the United States, 2011–2012. CDC *National Center for Health Statistics Data Brief.* Retrieved from https://www.cdc.gov/nchs/data/databriefs/db197.html

Economic Research Service. (2009). Rural population and migration. Washington: US Department of Agriculture; Retrieved from http: //www.ers.usda.gov/Briefing/Population/

Eke, P. I., Dye, B. A., Wei, L., Slade, G. D., Thornton-Evans, G. O., Borgnakke, W. S., . . . Genco, R. J. (2015). Update on prevalence of periodontitis in adults in the United States: NHANES 2009 to 2012. *Journal of Periodontology, 86*(5), 611–622.

Fos, P., & Hutchison, L. (2003). The state of rural oral health: A literature review. *Rural Healthy People 2010: A Companion Document to Healthy People 2010.* Volume 2. College Station: The Texas A & M University System Health Science Center, School of Rural Public Health, Southwest Rural Health Research Center: 131–144.

Health Policy Institute. ADA American Dental Association. (2016). Dentist participation in Medicaid or CHIP. Retrieved from https://www.ada.org/~/media/ADA/Science%20and%20Research/HPI/Files/HPIGraphic_0318_1.pdf?la=en

Hoadley, J., Wagnerman, K., Alker, J., & Holmes, M. (2017). Rural Health Report: Medicaid is a lifeline for small towns and rural communities. *Georgetown University Health Policy Institute. Center for Children and Families.* Retrieved from https://ccf.georgetown.edu/2017/06/06/rural-health-report/

Institute of Medicine of the National Academies. (2011). Advancing oral health in America: Committee on an oral health initiative board on health care services. *The National Academies Press.* Retrieved from https://www.hrsa.gov/sites/default/files/publichealth/clinical/oralhealth/advancingoralhealth.pdf

Kamer, A. R., Craig, R. G., Dasanayake, A. P., Brys, M., Glodzik-Sobanska, L., & de Leon, M. J. (2008). Inflammation and Alzheimer's disease: Possible role of periodontal diseases. *Alzheimer's & Dementia, 4*(4), 242–250.

Krause, D., Mosca, N., & Livingston, M. (2002). Maximizing the dental workforce: Implications for a rural state. (Short Report). *Journal of Dental Hygiene, 77*(4), 253–261.

Langelier, M., Baker, B., Continelli, T., & Moore, J., (2016). A dental hygiene professional practice index by state, 2014. *Oral Health Workforce Research Center.* Retrieved from https://www.chwsny.org/wp-content/uploads/2016/03/DH_Professional_Practice_Index_By_State_2014.pdf

National Rural Health Association. (n.d.). Compendium of rural oral health best practices. *National Rural Oral Health Initiative.* Retrieved from https://www.ruralhealthweb.org/NRHA/media/Emerge_NRHA/Programs/NRHA-Rural-Oral-Health-Compendium.pdf

Pryor, C., Prottas, J., Lottero, B., Rukavina, M., & Knudsin, A. (2009). Issue Brief No. 4: The costs of dental care and the impact of dental insurance coverage (2007 health insurance survey of farm and ranch operators). *The Access Project, 4*, 1–15. Retrieved from https://www.rwjf.org/en/library/research/2009/04/the-costs-of-dental-care-and-the-impact-of-dental-insurance-cove.html

Skillman, S. M., Doescher, M. P., Mouradian, W. E., & Brunson, D. K., (2010). The challenge to delivering oral health services in rural America. *Journal of Public Health Dentistry, 70*(1), S49–S57.

South Carolina, Department of Health and Environmental Control (2010), South Carolina Take Action. The burden of oral disease. Available at https://scdhec.gov/sites/default/files/docs/Health/docs/The%20Burden%20of%20Oral%20Disease%20in%20South%20Carolina.pdf

United Health Foundation. (2018). America's health rankings senior report. Retrieved from https://assets.americashealthrankings.org/app/uploads/ahrsenior18-finalv1.pdf

U.S. Department of Health and Human Services. (2016). Oral Health in America: A Report of the Surgeon General—Executive Summary. Rockville, MD: National Institute of Dental and Craniofacial Research.

U.S. Department of Health and Human Services. U.S. Public Health Service. (2000). Office of the Surgeon General. Oral health in America: A report of the Surgeon General. Rockville, MD: National Institute of Health, National Institute of Dental and Craniofacial Research; p. 33–59.

CHAPTER 12

Cancers in Rural Areas in the United States

Anuli Njoku, DrPH, MPH
Fathima Wakeel, PhD, MPH

LEARNING OBJECTIVES

At the end of this chapter, readers will be able to:

1. Specify cancers that are more prevalent in rural areas.
2. Explore incidence, prevalence, risk, and determinants of cancers in rural areas.
3. Articulate barriers to and best practices for cancer prevention, detection, and control in rural areas.
4. Define primary, secondary, and tertiary levels of care.
5. Learn about racial/ethnic cancer disparities within rural and minority populations.
6. Identify prevalent types of pediatric cancers in rural areas.

KEY TERMS

Cancer
Cancer cluster
Health disparities
Primary prevention
Screening
Secondary prevention
Tertiary prevention

CHAPTER OVERVIEW

Cancer is defined as a collection of related diseases caused by the body's uncontrolled division of cells [National Cancer Institute (NCI), 2015]. Cancer is the second-leading cause of death in the United States, exceeded only by heart disease (Heron, 2016). While cancer death rates have been decreasing nationwide, there is a slower reduction in cancer death rates in the rural United States, driven partly by high death rates from colorectal, prostate, lung, and cervical cancers (Centers for Disease Control and Prevention (CDC), 2018a). Rural communities have higher incidence and death rates for cancers due to a higher prevalence of behavioral risk factors such as poor diet, physical inactivity, alcohol consumption, cigarette smoking, less-frequent adoption of sun safety measures such as sunscreen, and lower human papillomavirus (HPV) vaccination rates, when compared with urban residents (Bodekær et al., 2015; Eberhardt & Pamuk, 2005;

Hartley, 2004; Matthews et al., 2017; CDC, 2018b). Therefore, rural communities have higher morbidity and mortality rates for cancers linked to smoking (e.g., lung and pharyngeal cancers) and higher occurrence of cancers that can be prevented and detected by screening (e.g., colorectal and cervical cancers) (NCI, n.d.-a). While rural areas have lower overall incidence of cancer compared with urban areas, they have higher cancer death rates, with the rural-urban differences in cancer death rates increasing over time (CDC, 2017).

Some of the higher cancer-related incidence and mortality rates can be linked to barriers in accessing healthcare services in rural areas. Cancer disparities are often related to financial barriers (e.g., insufficient or no health insurance coverage), limited public or private transportation, and lack of preventive and screening services (NCI, n.d.-a). Other access to care barriers include terrain, travel time, shortage of healthcare providers, lack of medical specialists, reliance on primary care, and burnout among rural providers due to longer hours, more patient visits, lower net annual incomes, stress, and professional and cultural isolation (Crosby et al., 2012). For example, care for rural cancer patients may be hampered by the limited availability of oncologists, mental health providers, and palliative care specialists (Charlton et al., 2015). This can be caused by transportation barriers, financial issues, and poorer geographic access to services in rural areas. Such access to care barriers can result in unaddressed psychosocial and cancer information needs (Charlton et al., 2015).

The compromised access to care often leads to higher rates of chronic diseases for rural residents. Socioeconomic determinants of rural health differences include lower educational attainment; reliance on low-wage, skilled, or unskilled jobs; higher poverty rates; and prevalence of hazardous jobs (e.g., farming, mining), when compared with urban areas (Crosby et al., 2012; NCI, n.d.-a). Moreover, U.S. rural residents tend to be older, sicker, and more likely to be underinsured or uninsured than their urban counterparts (Meit et al., 2014; Moy et al., 2017). On average, rural populations have more elderly populations and under- or unemployed residents (Crosby et al., 2012). Such factors invariably contribute to higher cancer incidence and death rates (NCI, n.d.-a).

Diversity and Health Disparities in Rural United States

A discussion of cancer in rural areas would be remiss without a mention of health disparities. **Health disparities** are defined as differences in health status among population subgroups that are closely associated with social or economic disadvantage and related to such factors as race or ethnicity, socioeconomic status, gender, religion, and geography [(U.S. Department of Health and Human Services (USDHHS, 2008)]. As discussed, geographically, rural American communities have higher rates of morbidity and mortality and poorer health outcomes compared with urban areas. These rural health disparities are deeply rooted in social, economic, geographic, racial, ethnic, and health workforce factors (Warshaw, 2017).

Moreover, rural American communities are becoming increasingly diverse (Sharp & Lee, 2017). Overall, Hispanics/Latinos are the fastest growing segment of the U.S. rural population (Cromartie, 2018). According to the most recent U.S. census, Hispanics/Latinos comprise 9% (over 6 million) of the rural population, African Americans make up 8% (over 5 million), Native Americans represent 2% (over 1 million), and Asians and Pacific Islanders account for less than 1% (over 700,000) of the rural population (Cromartie, 2018; Housing Assistance Council, 2012). Areas like central Appalachia have seen the Hispanic community grow considerably in the past 15 years, along with a recent arrival of a smaller Haitian community (Warsaw, 2017).

Rural racial and ethnic minority groups face substantial educational, occupational, and income disparities; have less healthcare access and use; are more likely to rate their health as fair or poor (except for Asians or Native Hawaiians/Pacific Islanders), and report less physical activity than their White counterparts (James et al., 2017). A larger percentage of racial/ethnic minority groups live in impoverished rural areas compared with Whites, with rural African Americans and Native Americans/Alaska Natives having the highest rates of poverty (U.S. Department of Agriculture, n.d.). A large percentage of African Americans live in impoverished areas of the Deep South, a cultural and geographic subregion in the Southern United States historically dependent on the use of slaves in agriculture (Warshaw, 2017).

Increasing diversity in rural areas has implications for cancer incidence and prevalence. For instance, at least 74% of all farmworkers identify as Latino/Hispanic (Farm Labor, n.d.). Migrant and seasonal farmworkers may receive sporadic health care and report overexposure to ultraviolet (UV) radiation (Warsaw, 2017). In another example, rural African Americans in the Deep South have lower rates of out migration and are more likely to be in communities that experience rural hospital closures. Furthermore, African Americans have higher rates of cancer morbidity and mortality and comorbid conditions than other rural residents (Warshaw, 2017).

There are also racial and ethnic health disparities in healthcare access and use, health-seeking behaviors, and chronic health conditions among rural adults, which can contribute to higher cancer incidence and death rates. For example, data from the 2012–2015 Behavioral Risk Factor Surveillance System revealed that in rural communities:

- All racial/ethnic minority populations were less likely than non-Hispanic Whites to report having a personal healthcare provider
- Fewer age-eligible Hispanic women (60.1%) reported having had a mammogram in the past 2 years compared with non-Hispanic Whites (73.4%)
- Fewer non-Hispanic Blacks were current with colorectal cancer screenings compared with non-Hispanic Whites

- More non-Hispanic Blacks and American Indian/Alaska Natives (AI/ANs) (40.3% of both groups) than non-Hispanic Whites (36%) reported having multiple chronic health conditions
- Obesity and/or severe obesity was more prevalent among non-Hispanic Blacks and AI/ANs when compared with non-Hispanic Whites (James et al., 2017).

An understanding of these racial and ethnic disparities in health behaviors and outcomes will help inform effective development and evaluation of effective cancer control programs.

Leading Cancers in Rural Areas in the United States

Colorectal Cancer

Colorectal cancer, the unchecked division and survival of abnormal cells in the colon and rectum, is the third-leading cause of cancer death among men and women in the United States and second-leading cause of cancer death when both sexes are combined (American Cancer Society (ACS), 2019a). There were an estimated 101,420 new cases of colon cancer and 44,180 new cases of rectal cancer in the United States in 2019, along with approximately 51,020 colorectal cancer-related deaths in 2019 (ACS, 2019a). Rural areas have generally experienced higher incidence rates for colorectal cancer and late-stage colorectal cancer as well as higher deaths rates related to colorectal cancer compared with urban areas (Henley et al., 2017).

Colorectal cancer risk factors include those related to heredity and family history, personal medical history (e.g., chronic inflammatory bowel disease, diabetes), and behavioral risk (e.g., physical inactivity, diet, overweight and obesity, smoking, alcohol, and medications) (ACS, 2017). Rural communities have a higher prevalence of these behavioral risk factors, contributing to higher cancer incidence and death rates (NCI, n.d.-a).

Colorectal cancer prevention and control can occur at the primary, secondary, and tertiary levels of prevention. **Primary prevention** aims to prevent illness or disease from occurring, **secondary prevention** identifies or detects diseases at their earliest stage, and **tertiary prevention** aims to slow the progression of disease (Snelling, 2014). Primary prevention for colorectal cancer includes increased physical activity, increased fruit and vegetable intake, reduced meat consumption, decreased alcohol intake, and not smoking (ACS, 2017). For persons at average and high risk of colorectal cancer, there are several recommended **screening** or early detection options to examine for and remove polyps (i.e., growths) in the colon (ACS, 2017). The U.S. Preventive Services Task Force (2015) recommends screening for colorectal cancer using fecal occult blood testing, sigmoidoscopy, or colonoscopy for adults, beginning at age 50 years and continuing until age 75 years. Such colorectal cancer screening tests are examples of secondary prevention. Furthermore, colorectal cancer treatment includes imaging, surgical techniques, and chemotherapy (ACS, 2017). The aforementioned are examples of tertiary prevention.

There are several determinants of increased colorectal cancer risk among rural residents. Rural adolescents and adults are more likely to smoke than their urban counterparts (Ziller et al., 2019). Moreover, higher smoking prevalence in rural areas has been linked to increased colorectal cancer mortality rates (Pleis, Ward, & Lucas, 2010; Singh, Miller, & Hankey, 2002). Self-reported obesity has been higher in rural areas compared with large metro areas nationwide (Meit et al., 2014). Leisure time inactivity has been highest in nonmetro counties for residents of all regions, except for the Northeast and women in the Western United States region (Meit et al., 2014). Additionally, cancer screening is

an important part of cancer prevention and control, as it can help detect polyps before they turn into cancer, thus reducing cancer deaths (ACS, 2017). One study using the Centers for Disease Control and Prevention's (CDC's) Behavioral Risk Factor Surveillance System showed that remote rural residents had the lowest screening rates overall (Cole, Jackson, & Doescher, M. (2012a). Data from the National Health Interview Survey revealed that colorectal cancer screening rates were lower in nonmetropolitan counties compared with metropolitan counties (United States Department of Health and Human Services (USDHHS), 2015). Furthermore, higher colorectal cancer death rates in rural areas might indicate lack of access to cancer screening services, follow-up to abnormal tests, quality of care for cancer patients, and cancer survival care (Garcia et al., 2017).

Regarding racial/ethnic disparities in colorectal cancer screening among age-eligible individuals, fewer non-Hispanic Blacks (53.6%), Hispanics (43.4%), and AI/ANs (53.4%) than non-Hispanic Whites (61.7%) reported being up to date with colorectal cancer screenings, according to a CDC report (James et al., 2017). In another study by Cole and colleagues (2012b), rural non-Hispanic Whites (44.3%), rural African American/Blacks (44.8%), rural Hispanic/Latinos (40.8%), rural American Indian/Alaska Natives (46.8%), and rural Asians (39.6%) had lower timely colorectal screening compared with urban non-Hispanic Whites (49.5%; P < .05% for all comparisons). Furthermore, rural Asians were least likely to report use of endoscopy screenings (21.2%) among all groups (Cole, Jackson, & Doescher 2012b). Overall, such rural-urban differences in colorectal cancer incidence and death rates necessitate implementation of evidence-based cancer prevention and control interventions at the individual and population levels to reduce cancer risk factors and increase cancer screening rates (Frieden et al., 2008).

Prostate Cancer

Prostate cancer, a condition in which cells in the prostate gland start to grow uncontrollably, is the most common cancer among American men (after skin cancer) (ACS, 2019b). There were approximately 174,650 new cases of prostate cancer and about 31,620 deaths from prostate cancer in the United States in 2019 (ACS, 2019b). Rural areas tend to have lower incidence rates of prostate cancer but higher deaths rates from prostate cancer (CDC, 2017; Obertova, Brown, Holmes, & Lawrenson, 2012).

Age is the most common risk factor for prostate cancer, and family history also presents an increased risk (CDC, n.d.). Furthermore, African American men are more likely to get prostate cancer than other men and are twice as likely to die from prostate cancer when compared with White men (CDC, n.d.). Other prostate cancer risk factors that have been researched but not clearly established include diet, obesity, smoking, chemical exposures, and sexually transmitted infections (ACS, 2019b).

While prostate cancer cannot be prevented due to risk factors such as age and family history, prostate cancer risk can be lowered by such primary prevention measures as being physically active, maintaining a healthy weight, and having an adequate daily consumption of fruits and vegetables (ACS, 2019b). Screening tests that can detect prostate cancer early include a prostate-specific antigen (PSA) blood test and a digital rectal exam (DRE) (ACS, 2019b). The U.S. Preventive Services Task Force (2018a) recommends that "For men aged 55 to 69 years, the decision to undergo periodic prostate-specific antigen (PSA)–based screening for prostate cancer should be an individual one" that involves informed and shared decision making with their healthcare provider. As an example of tertiary prevention, there are several types of standard treatments for prostate cancer, including watchful waiting or active surveillance, surgery, radiation therapy and radiopharmaceutical therapy, hormone therapy, chemotherapy, biologic therapy, and bisphosphonate therapy. Additionally, new types of treatments are being tested in clinical trials (Prostate Cancer Treatment (PDQ®)–Patient Version, n.d.).

There are various behavioral, socioeconomic, and access to care factors that contribute to prostate cancer incidence and mortality in rural areas. As previously discussed, rural areas report a higher prevalence of behavioral risk factors that can contribute to prostate cancer incidence such as poor diet, physical inactivity, and cigarette smoking (Hartley, 2004; Matthews et al., 2017). Furthermore, studies have shown a relationship between socioeconomic status and prostate cancer mortality (Chu, Miller, & Springfield, 2007; Steenland, Henley, & Thun, 2002). One study showed that men in more deprived groups and rural areas had significantly higher rates of prostate cancer mortality compared with their affluent and urbanized counterparts, with rural African Americans having 22% higher mortality rates compared with their urban counterparts (Singh, Williams, Siahpush, & Mulhollen, 2011). Therefore, behavioral determinants of prostate cancer in rural areas may be determined by socioeconomic factors (Singh, Miller, Hankey, & Edwards, 2003; Kogevinas, Pearce, Susser, & Boffetta, 1997). Access to health services may be a determinant of prostate cancer in rural areas. In one systematic review of the literature, findings suggested that rural men are less likely to be screened for and subsequently less likely to be diagnosed with prostate cancer (Obertova, Brown, Holmes, & Lawrenson, 2012).

Regarding racial and ethnic disparities in prostate cancer mortality, African American men have the highest incidence rate of prostate cancer per 100,000 persons compared with men of other races/ethnicities (176.7 for African American men, 101.9 for White men, 93.4 for Hispanic men, 55.6 for Asian and Pacific Islander men, and 55.4 for American

Indian/Alaska Native men) (NCI, 2016a). African American men also have an increased lifetime risk of prostate cancer death compared with men of other races/ethnicities (4.2% for African American men, 2.9% for Hispanic men, 2.3% for white men, and 2.1% for Asian and Pacific Islander men) (NCI, 2016a).

Demographically, African Americans have the highest rural poverty rates and the highest rates of cancer incidence and deaths, compared with other rural cancer residents (U.S. Department of Agriculture, n.d.; Warshaw, 2017). Health beliefs may influence health-seeking behaviors among rural African American men. One study found that disparity in health status, lack of understanding, tradition, mistrust of the healthcare system, fear, and threat to manhood were common themes about prostate cancer and screening found among rural African American men (Oliver, 2007). Other studies exploring barriers to prostate cancer among rural African American men have identified such factors as distrust of the medical system, poverty, lack of knowledge, inadequate time, fear of test results, and likeliness to seek advice from informal sources, such as family members (Agho, & Lewis, 2001; Diala et al., 2001; Farkas, Marcella, & Rhoads, 2000; Jones, Steeves, & Williams, 2009). A trusting patient-healthcare provider relationship and family involvement in decision making has influenced the decision to obtain prostate cancer screenings among rural African American men (Jones, Steeves, & Williams, 2009). Insight into these factors can help inform effective development of programs to reduce prostate cancer screening disparities.

Lung Cancer

Lung cancer is the second-most common cancer and the most common cause of cancer death in the United States (ACS, 2019c). There are 228,150 estimated new cases of lung cancer in 2019, which accounts for 12.9% of all new cases of cancer and 23.5% of all cancer

deaths (NCI, 2016b). Rural areas have a higher incidence of lung cancer as well as higher rates of deaths attributable to lung cancer, when compared with urban areas (CDC, 2017).

There are several individual and systems-level determinants of lung cancer in rural areas. At the individual level, substantial research has shown that cigarette smoking is a contributory cause for lung cancer in that it is associated with 80–90% of lung cancer deaths; other types of tobacco use, such as cigars and pipes, have also been linked to an increased risk of lung cancer (CDC, 2018c). Although the use of e-cigarettes has been linked to respiratory dysfunction, its link with lung cancer has not been substantiated in epidemiological research; therefore, further research is needed to investigate this potential association (Drummond & Upson, 2014).

Importantly, tobacco use is disproportionately higher in rural communities (28.5%), followed by urban areas (25.1%), small metropolitan areas (22.0%), and large metropolitan areas (18.3%) (Substance Abuse and Mental Health Services Administration, 2017). According to a seminal report from the American Lung Association (ALA) (2015), this significantly higher prevalence is attributable to a variety of individual, interpersonal, community, and systems-level determinants. At the individual level, rural Americans are more likely to use multiple forms of tobacco, including smokeless tobacco. At the interpersonal level, individuals living in rural areas are, therefore, more likely to be exposed to secondhand smoke. At the community level, using tobacco is a social norm in many rural communities and is reinforced by less restrictive tobacco-free policies in public spaces, including restaurants, bars, and workplaces (Huang, et al., 2015). Smokeless tobacco has also been promoted as an alternative in smoke-free locations (Break Free Alliance, 2012) and has been considered a "rite of passage" for males in many rural areas (Nemeth, et al., 2012). At the broader systems level, tobacco companies have targeted rural Americans with images of "rugged individualism, as personified by the Marlboro man (ALA, 2015). Furthermore, as is the case for access to health care in general in rural areas, rural residents have less access to smoking cessation programs and, therefore, fewer resources to help them quit using tobacco.

In addition to cigarette smoking, rural residents have significantly less access to lung cancer screenings, which is a type of secondary prevention compared with their urban counterparts. The United States Preventive Services Task Force (2013) recommends that individuals who have a history of heavy smoking (i.e., smoking a pack of cigarettes each day for 30 years), smoke now or have quit in the past 15 years, and are 50–80 years old get screened for lung cancer. Lung cancer screening entails low-dose computed tomography (also referred to a low-dose CT scan or LDCT), in which an x-ray machine uses low doses of radiation to create images of the lungs (United States Preventive Services Task Force, 2013). Rural individuals are more likely to experience inadequate access to prevention and treatment services due to barriers such as higher rates of poverty, lower health literacy, shortage of healthcare providers, transportation, and distance. Along these lines, population-based research has indicated that only 47.5% of individuals living in rural areas have access to a LDCT screening center within 30 miles, compared with 93.7% of individuals living in urban areas. Similarly, rural residents (22.2%) are also significantly less likely than their urban counterparts (83.2%) to be located within a 30- minute drive of a LDCT screening center. (Eberth, et al., 2018). Additionally, complete surgical resection is the recommended treatment for individuals with stage 1 non-small cell lung cancer (NSCLC) (Manser, et al., 2005; McKenna, et al., 2006; Scott, et al., 2010). Compared with urban individuals, rural individuals who are diagnosed with stage 1 NSCLC had significantly less treatment (i.e., 69% had surgery versus 75% of urban individuals) and significantly lower median survival (i.e., 40 months versus 52 months)

(Atkins, et al., 2017). Based on these individual and system-level determinants of lung cancer, it has been recommended that rural healthcare providers be trained in promoting LDCT screening for their eligible patients and that an integrated strategy incorporating both smoking cessation and screening be used to reduce lung cancer incidence and lung cancer-related deaths in rural settings (Jenkins, et al., 2018; Smieliauskas, et al., 2014; Cardarelli, et al., 2017).

There are also significant racial and ethnic disparities related to lung cancer in the United States and specifically in rural areas. Overall, in the United States, African Americans experience the highest incidence of lung cancer, followed by Whites, American Indians/Alaska Natives, and Asian/Pacific Islanders (CDC, 2010). These disparities in lung cancer incidence are similar and do not appear to broaden within rural settings (Zahnd, et al., 2018). However, rural African Americans and non-Whites in general have been found to be significantly less likely to receive treatment for lung cancer compared with rural Whites (Atkins, et al., 2017). Additionally, in terms of lung cancer prevention, some research suggests that African American long-term smokers have reported significantly lower intention to screen as well as lower actual screening rates than their White counterparts (Carter-Harris, et al., 2018). Further research is needed to examine racial and ethnic disparities in lung cancer screening rates in rural areas.

Cervical Cancer

Cervical cancer used to be one of the most prevalent causes of cancer death among women in the United States (ACS, 2019d). However, with the significant increase in rates of screening through the Pap test, the incidence of cervical cancer was reduced by half between 1975 and 2015 (ACS, 2019e). Additionally, the Human Papillomavirus (HPV) vaccine, which is a type of secondary prevention, has been shown to substantially reduce the risk of cervical cancer among young women in the United States (McClung, et al., 2019). In 2019, it was estimated that there were 13,170 new cases of invasive cervical cancer and that 4,250 women would die from cervical cancer (ACS, 2019e). Data have shown that the incidence and death rates related to cervical cancer are higher in rural counties as well as large central metropolitan counties; furthermore, these rates have undergone a slower decline in rural areas compared with urban areas in the last two decades (CDCa, 2018).

Similar to other types of cancer, there are various individual and systems-level determinants of cervical cancer in rural areas. At the individual level, cigarette smoking is a salient risk factor for cervical cancer; additionally, the risk for cervical cancer is further elevated through daily cigarette smoking and longer duration of smoking (US Department of Health and Human Services, 2001; Roura, et al., 2014; Plummer, et al., 2003). The most important risk factor for cervical cancer, however, is the Human Papillomavirus (HPV), which has been shown to contribute to approximately 90% of cervical cancers (Saraiya, et al., 2015). Furthermore, research has indicated that that there is an interaction effect of cigarette smoking and having HPV, in that HPV-positive women who smoke are twice as likely to get cervical cancer compared with HPV-positive women who have never smoked (Roura, et al., 2014; Plummer, et al., 2003). As discussed earlier, tobacco use is disproportionately higher in rural communities (Substance Abuse and Mental Health Services Administration, 2017).

At the systems level, there are two secondary prevention measures that have been shown to prevent cervical cancer—screening and the HPV vaccine. In terms of screening, the Papanicolao (Pap) test entails examining cells in the cervix for abnormal changes that may signify cervical cancer; in addition, the HPV test directly assesses cervical cells for HPV, which is the most common sexually transmitted infection in the United States (United States

Department of Health and Human Services, 2019). The United States Preventive Services Task Force (2018b) recommends that women between the ages of 21 and 29 years obtain a Pap test every three years and that women aged 30–65 obtain a Pap test every three years, the HPV test every five years, or a Pap test and HPV test together (also known as co-testing) every five years. Due to barriers such as transportation, shortage of healthcare providers, insurance issues, and distance, individuals living in rural areas are less likely to utilize cancer screening services (Casey, et al., 2001; Coughlin, et al., 2002; Doescher and Jackson, 2009). For example, a population-based study by Orwat, et al., (2017) compared cancer screening rates among privately insured urban and rural residents within the same Hospital Referral Region (HRR) and found that cervical cancer screening rates for women visiting rural physicians were lower than their urban counterparts in 55% of HRRs, higher in only 4% of HRRs, and the same in 42% of HRRs.

Along with screening for cervical cancer through the Pap and HPV tests, the HPV vaccine has increasingly become a component of routine clinical care as it can prevent nine strains of HPV and, therefore, 90% of cervical cancers (ACS, 2019f). Based on recommendations by the Advisory Committee on Immunization Practices (ACIP), the routine HPV vaccination series should begin at ages 11–12 for both boys and girls, although it can be initiated as early as age 9; catch-up vaccination is also recommended for all individuals until age 26 years. (Meites, et al., 2019). Despite the importance of the HPV vaccine, the percentage of rural adolescents who received the first dose of HPV vaccine in 2017 was 11 percentage points lower than among their urban counterparts (CDC, 2018b). Along with the previously discussed barriers to seeking and using preventative care in rural areas, including inadequate access to healthcare services, financial constraints, lack of transportation, and distance; there are various additional barriers to obtaining the HPV vaccine that are particularly salient in rural areas such as concerns about vaccine safety and negative effects, lack of awareness about the need for the vaccine, perceived confidentiality issues, and stigma related to the perception that receiving HPV vaccine may encourage sexual activity among adolescents (Gerend, et al., 2013a; Gerend, et al., 2013b; Reiter, et al., 2013; Edwards and Rousseau-Pierre, 2010; Farrell and Romes, 2007; Hershey and Velez, 2009; Vetter and Geller, 2007; Fisher and Brundage, 2009; Lehmann and Benson, 2009). Finally, among other initiatives, two key recommendations that have been shown to increase cervical cancer screening and HPV vaccination rates are cervical cancer education in the community with culturally appropriate health education materials and via multiple means (e.g. phone, videos, text message, etc.) as well as provider-based outreach interventions, such as invitation letters, mailed and phone call reminders, and appointment letters (Musa, et al., 2017).

Within rural areas, there are also significant racial and ethnic disparities in the incidence of and deaths due to cervical cancer. A study by Singh (2012) found that African American women were twice as likely to die from cervical cancer than White women in both urban and rural areas and that cervical cancer mortality decreased less rapidly between 1969 and 2007 among rural African American women than among their urban counterparts. Furthermore, the five-year survival rate for rural African American women with cervical cancer was only 50.8% compared with 60.2% among urban African American women and 71.0% among urban White women (Singh, 2012). Hispanic women in the United States also have significantly high incidence rates of cervical cancer, with a rate twice as high as that of White women; they also have higher cervical cancer mortality rates (3.0/100,000 versus 2.1/100,000) compared with White women (American Cancer Society, 2012). Along these lines, research has suggested that rural Hispanic women are less likely than their urban counterparts to have received a Pap smear in the past three years (Nuno, et al., 2012). Data from population-based registries also indicate that African American and Hispanic rural women have higher incidences of cervical cancer due to unknown causes compared with their urban counterparts (Yu, et al., 2019). Unstaged cancer has been linked to lower survival rates than early stage cancer; hence, further research is needed to explore the mechanisms behind the elevated risk of unstaged cervical incidence among rural African American and Hispanic women (Worthington, et al., 2008; Merrill, et al., 1999; Yu, et al., 2019).

Pediatric Cancers

It is estimated that among the population aged 20 years and younger, 15,000 individuals are diagnosed with cancer annually in the United States (US Cancer Statistics Working Group, 2017). The most common types of pediatric cancers include leukemia, brain and spinal cord tumors, neuroblastoma, Wilms tumor (i.e., cancer of the kidneys), lymphoma, rhabdomyosarcoma, retinoblastoma, and bone cancer (ACS, 2019g). Leukemia (i.e., cancers of the bone marrow and blood), are the most prevalent types of pediatric cancer, constituting almost 30% of all childhood cancers (ACS, 2019g). The second most common type of pediatric cancer is brain and spinal cord tumors, which account for 26% of childhood cancers (ACS, 2019g). Data from the CDC indicates that between 2003 and 2014, there were 171,432 new cases of pediatric cancer, of which the highest incidence rates were found among males (i.e., 181.5 cases per million versus 165.5 cases per million among females); the youngest (ages 0–4 years) and oldest (ages 15–19 years) ends of the pediatric age range (i.e., 228.9 and 213.3 cases, respectively, versus 122.6 cases among children aged 5–9 and 133.0 cases among children aged 10–14); Whites (184.4 compared with 133.3 cases among Blacks); and residents of large metropolitan areas (177.1 compared with 167.2 cases among rural areas) (Siegel, et al., 2018).

Furthermore, research has found that rates of pediatric cancer death do not differ significantly by urban/rural residence, likely due to the high rates of public health insurance among rural children through the Children's Health Insurance Program (CHIP) as well as the widespread national network of pediatric cancer physicians through the Children's Oncology Group, which is supported by the National Cancer Institute (Delavar, et al., 2019). CHIP was enacted in 1997 to provide healthcare coverage for children up to age 19 years from families who could not afford private insurance but whose income levels also exceeded Medicaid eligibility requirements (Centers for Medicare and Medicaid Services, 2019). In 2018, approximately 9.6 million children were enrolled in CHIP; importantly, in 2014, it was estimated that 47% of rural children would be unable to access health care without CHIP or Medicaid (Centers for Medicare and Medicaid Services, 2019; O'Hare, 2014). Additionally, the Children's Oncology Group works with over 200 children's hospitals in 47 states and the District of Columbia, and 90% of pediatric cancer patients in the United States are receiving care from a cancer center affiliated with the Children's Oncology Group, thus helping to elucidate similar cancer survival rates among rural and urban children and adolescents (Delavar, et al.; 2019; Children's Oncology Group, 2019).

Strategies for Cancer Prevention and Control

So far, we have recognized that cancer disparities are present in rural and minority populations. We have also learned about barriers to cancer screenings and prevention among rural residents. These rural-urban differences in cancer incidence and mortality rates encourage implementation of evidence-based cancer prevention and control interventions at the individual and population levels to reduce cancer risk factors and increase cancer screening rates (Frieden et al., 2008).

The CDC (2017) recommends various strategies to reduce disparities in new cancer cases and deaths. These strategies include:

1. **Encourage healthy behaviors that reduce cancer risk**. In rural areas, where there is higher prevalence of cigarette smoking, initiatives are encouraged to stop tobacco initiation, promote tobacco cessation, and eliminate exposure to secondhand smoke. Individuals are advised to limit excessive exposure to ultraviolet rays from the sun and tanning beds and the sun (e.g., sunscreen for outdoor workers such as farmers, migrant workers, and ranchers). Also, healthy eating and physical activity are recommended to prevent and reduce obesity, which is linked to several cancers. For example, farmers' markets can be provided to facilitate an increase of fruit, vegetable, and fiber intake among rural residents.

2. **Increase vaccinations and cancer screenings that prevent cancer or detect it early**. As rural areas have lower vaccination rates, it is recommended that clients receive vaccination against cancer-related diseases such as hepatitis B virus and HPV. Age-appropriate cancer screening tests such as a colonoscopy and Pap tests are also recommended.

3. **Participate in state-level comprehensive control programs**. Comprehensive cancer control programs encourage healthy lifestyles, educate people about cancer symptoms, endorse recommended cancer screenings, improve access to quality cancer care, and support cancer survivors' quality of life.

Another resource in cancer prevention and control is the CDC's National Program of Cancer Registries (NPCR) (CDC, 2019). Cancer registries are important because they collect and share detailed information about cancer patients and the treatments they receive to provide a data-driven foundation for cancer control endeavors in the United States (CDC, 2019). Cancer registries aim to increase screening and awareness in underserved areas such as rural areas, where residents tend to be less likely to be screened for and subsequently less likely to be diagnosed with cancer, more likely to be diagnosed at a later stage, and have higher cancer death rates compared with urban areas (Obertova, Brown, Holmes, & Lawrenson, 2012; (CDC, 2017). Cancer registries also share information about cancer determinants, trends, and treatment with state comprehensive cancer coalitions to determine strategies and solutions (CDC, 2019). An example of a CDC cancer registry in action is the rurally located North Dakota Statewide Cancer Registry (NDSCR) (CDC, 2019; NDSCR, 2014). The NDSCR collects and securely stores information about new cancer cases, cancer treatment, and cancer deaths to analyze cancer trends, support research, improve survival, inform program development and implementation, guide policy efforts, and respond to cancer concerns (NDSCR, 2014). Furthermore, in 2014, a concerned citizen raised concerns to the NDCSR about a high number of people getting cancer in the town. Scientists used their background and knowledge to investigate factors associated with this possible **cancer cluster**, defined as a greater than expected number of cancer cases that occurs within a group of people or in a geographic area (CDC, 2019). The cancer registry helped to ease the county's concerns and ultimately, no link was found between this rural community and the cancer (CDC, 2019).

Another respected source for cancer prevention and control in the United States is the National Cancer Institute's Surveillance, Epidemiology, and End Results (SEER) (NCI, n.d.-b). The SEER program collects information from population-based cancer registries, provides cancer statistics in an attempt to reduce the cancer burden among the U.S. population, and is supported by the Surveillance Research Program (SRP) in the NCI's Division of Cancer Control and Population Sciences (NCI, n.d.-b). Cancer registries regularly collect data on patient demographics, primary tumor site, stage of diagnosis, initial course of treatment, and survival (NCI, 2018). SEER data have been used in numerous peer-reviewed studies and by a vast number of researchers, public health officials, clinicians, cancer registrars, policymakers, community groups, and the general public (Kuo, & Mobley, 2016; NCI, n.d.-b). In terms of delineating rural cancer disparities, SEER data are very versatile and can be used to assess cancer prevention and screening programs, detail disparities by race/ethnicity, geography, gender and other factors, establish the effectiveness of public health interventions, and help translate research into practice and health policy (NCI, 2018). Overall, as a research resource, SEER exists as a foundation for population-based studies that focus on emerging issues in the field of cancer and cancer-related care (Kuo, & Mobley, 2016). SEER also plays a vital role in increasing the scope of scientific research to include various factors such as access to and quality of health care, geographic determinants, and health disparities (NCI, 2018).

Another strategy to address barriers to cancer care in rural areas is to strengthen the rural health workforce. Evidence indicates that there are rural healthcare labor shortages across all providers, including physicians, registered nurses, and mental health professionals (Burrows, Suh, & Hamann, 2008). Critical rural workforce policy issues include rural economic income disparities, recruitment and retention challenges, and underutilized rural workforce development and training; this prompts recommendations for increased health professional training to encourage students to pursue healthcare careers within underserved communities (Rural Health Information Hub, n.d.-a). Bolstering the healthcare workforce is critical to providing access to quality health care in rural areas (Rural Health Information Hub, n.d.-a).

Federal and state resources to help address rural healthcare workforce shortages include funding to support healthcare education and loan repayment and forgiveness programs and policies to allow new or alternate providers to practice in rural areas (Rural Health Information Hub, n.d.-b). There should also be continued funding for workforce pipeline programs that aim to increase the number of health professionals practicing in rural areas (Rural Health Information Hub, n.d.-c).

Mobile clinics and telehealth have also been largely used to address the barriers such as lack of transportation, inadequate healthcare workforce, and lengthy distance required to travel to access health care, which rural residents experience when seeking cancer screening and treatment. Mobile clinics, which are typically housed in vans or recreational vehicles and contain healthcare workers and screening equipment, are often used to offer breast and cervical cancer screening services (Greenwald, et al., 2017). A National Cancer Institute (NCI) study found that mobile clinics were efficient by providing residents with low-cost services, being accessible during nontraditional (e.g., evening) hours, and reaching a greater number of self-referred clients (Brown & Fintor., 1995). Another study found that mobile clinics were an effective way to reach women over age 60 years who may experience difficulty with long travel (Vellozzi, et al., 1996). Furthermore, in terms of cancer treatment, telehealth has played an important role in providing specialist care services to rural residents through audiovisual conference services and has even been found to provide a similarly good, or even better, experience as an office visit (Hede, 2010). Additionally, telehealth has been optimized to provide support services, from psychiatric, nutritional, and palliative care to cancer patients and has been found to result in better pain and depression

symptom scores than usual care as well as higher satisfaction among patients, nurses, and social workers (Doolittle, 1997; Doolittle, et al., 1998; Kroenke, et al., 2010; Satcher, et al., 2014).

It is also important to note the opportunities of living in rural communities that can help promote cancer prevention control. Assets of living in rural communities include aesthetic beauty and physical environments (e.g., water, land formations) that may be conducive to outdoor recreational activities, a strong sense of community, extended families, rich cultural traditions, shared experiences, and tight-knit communities (Crosby, 2012). Rural communities can also display a sense of self-reliance and independence, which can be an asset; self-reliance can serve as a potential barrier to public health efforts if it leads to avoidance of assistance from people outside of the community (Crosby, 2012). Overall, these different resources can be maximized to aid in cancer prevention and control and alleviate rural cancer disparities.

Conclusion

Rural areas experience disparities in sickness, deaths, and screening rates for colorectal, prostate, lung, and cervical cancers compared with urban areas. There are also racial and ethnic disparities for several of these cancers within rural populations. Rural U.S. communities have higher rates of morbidity and mortality and poorer health outcomes and experience greater rates of risky health behaviors compared with urban residents. Overall, there are various behavioral, socioeconomic, demographic, and access to care factors that determine rural cancer disparities. Strategies for cancer prevention and control in rural areas include reducing underlying barriers to care, supporting healthy lifestyles, promoting cancer education, building community partnerships and capacity, and maximizing community resources.

Chapter Summary

- Higher rates of cancer in rural communities are due to a prevalence of cancer-related behavioral risk factors such as cigarette smoking, inadequate diet, physical inactivity, lower vaccination rates, sun exposure, and alcohol intake.
- Rural populations are associated with lower rates of cancer screening, which may lead to later-stage diagnoses, poorer clinical outcomes, and more aggressive treatment.

- There are racial and ethnic cancer disparities in rural areas due to a variety of social, economic, cultural, and historic factors.
- Barriers to cancer screening in rural communities include limited access to health services, lack of transportation, and insufficient or no health insurance coverage.
- Reducing barriers to care, emphasizing community resources, developing collaborations, and increasing community capacity can help promote cancer control and reduce cancer disparities.

Discussion Questions

1. Based on the cancers described in this chapter, describe at least five factors that might contribute to cancer disparities between rural and urban residents. What features of rural environments may serve as protective factors against cancer disparities?
2. Focusing on the cancers described in this chapter, what are the different methods to prevent, reduce the risk of, and/or detect each cancer in rural environments?
3. Discuss some of the salient racial and ethnic disparities in the incidence, mortality, and morbidity rates related to the four cancers described in this chapter.

Student Activities and Worksheets are available for use inside the Navigate eBook, included with the printed text. Simply redeem the access code found at the front of the book at www.jblearning.com.

References

Agho, A. O., & Lewis, M. A. (2001). Correlates of actual and perceived knowledge of prostate cancer among African Americans. *Cancer Nursing, 24*(3), 165–171.

American Cancer Society. (2012). Cancer Facts & Figures for Hispanics/Latinos 2012–2014. https://www.cancer.org/research/cancer-facts-statistics/hispanics-latinos-facts-figures.html

American Cancer Society. (2017). *Colorectal cancer facts & figures 2017–2019.* Retrieved from https://www.cancer.org/content/dam/cancer-org/research/cancer-facts-and-statistics/colorectal-cancer-facts-and-figures/colorectal-cancer-facts-and-figures-2017-2019.pdf

American Cancer Society. (2019a). *Key statistics for colorectal cancer.* Retrieved from https://www.cancer.org/cancer/colon-rectal-cancer/about/key-statistics.html

American Cancer Society. (2019b). *Prostate cancer.* Retrieved from https://www.cancer.org/cancer/prostate-cancer.html

American Cancer Society. (2019c). *Key statistics for lung cancer.* Retrieved from https://www.cancer.org/cancer/non-small-cell-lung-cancer/about/key-statistics.html

American Cancer Society. (2019d). *Key statistics for cervical cancer.* Retrieved from https://www.cancer.org/cancer/cervical-cancer/about/key-statistics.html

American Cancer Society. (2019e). Facts & Figures 2019: US cancer death rate has dropped 27% in 25 years. Atlanta: American Cancer Society.

American Cancer Society. (2019f). HPV Vaccines: What is HPV? Retrieved from https://www.cancer.org/cancer/cancer-causes/infectious-agents/hpv/hpv-vaccines.html

American Cancer Society. (2019g). Types of cancer that develop in children. Retrieved from https://www.cancer.org/cancer/cancer-in-children/types-of-childhood-cancers.html

American Lung Association. (2015). *Cutting Tobacco's Rural Roots: Tobacco Use in Rural Communities.* Chicago: American Lung Association.

Atkins, G. T., Kim, T., & Munson, J. (2017). Residence in rural areas of the United States and lung cancer mortality. Disease incidence, treatment disparities, and stage-specific survival. *Annals of the American Thoracic Society, 14*(3), 403–411.

Bodekær, M., Petersen, B., Philipsen, P. A., Heydenreich, J., Thieden, E., & Wulf, H. C. (2015). Sun exposure patterns of urban, suburban, and rural children: A dosimetry and diary study of 150 children. *Photochemical & Photobiological Sciences, 14*(7), 1282–1289.

Break Free Alliance. (2012). *Addressing Dual Tobacco Use in West Virginia: Report and Recommendations of the Expert Panel.* Health Education Council.

Brown, M. L., & Fintor, L. (1995). U.S. screening mammography services with mobile units: Results from the national survey of mammography facilities. *Radiology, 195,* 529–532.

Burrows, E., Suh, R., & Hamann, D. (2008). Health care workforce distribution and shortage issues in rural America. *National Rural Health Association.* Accessed on July 23, 2020, at https://pdfs.semanticscholar.org/d460/bacf7871b67e044620d170c39b495be179ac.pdf?_ga=2.8565181.947934611.1595553974-807923930.1595553974

Cardarelli, R., Reese, D., Roper, K. L., Cardarelli, K., Feltner, F. J., Studts, J. L., . . . Shaffer, D. (2017). Terminate lung cancer (TLC) study—A mixed-methods population approach to increase lung cancer screening awareness and low-dose computed tomography in Eastern Kentucky. *Cancer Epidemiology, 46,* 1–8. doi 10.1016/j.canep.2016.11.003

Carter-Harris, L., Slaven, J. E., Jr, Monahan, P. O., Shedd-Steele, R., Hanna, N., & Rawl, S. M. (2018). Understanding lung cancer screening behavior: Racial, gender, and geographic differences among Indiana long-term smokers. *Preventive Medicine Reports, 10,* 49–54. doi:10.1016/j.pmedr.2018.01.018

Casey, M. M., Thiede Call, K., & Klingner, J. M. (2001). Are rural residents less likely to obtain recommended preventive healthcare services? *American Journal of Preventive Medicine, 21*(3), 182–188.

Centers for Disease Control and Prevention (CDC). (2017). *New CDC report shows deaths from cancer higher in rural America.* Retrieved from https://www.cdc.gov/media/releases/2017/p0706-rural-cancer-deaths.html

Centers for Disease Control and Prevention. (2018a). *Cancer in rural America.* Retrieved from https://www.cdc.gov/ruralhealth/cancer.html

Centers for Disease Control and Prevention (CDC). (2018b). *Vaccination in rural communities.* Retrieved from https://www.cdc.gov/ruralhealth/vaccines/index.html

Centers for Disease Control and Prevention (CDC). (2018c). *What are the risk factors for lung cancer?* Retrieved from https://www.cdc.gov/cancer/lung/basic_info/risk_factors.htm

Centers for Disease Control and Prevention (CDC). (2019). *National Program of Cancer Registries (NPCR).* Retrieved from https://www.cdc.gov/cancer/npcr/index.htm

Centers for Disease Control and Prevention (CDC). (n.d.). *Who is at risk for prostate cancer?* Retrieved from https://www.cdc.gov/cancer/prostate/basic_info/risk_factors.htm

Charlton, M., Schlichting, J., Chioreso, C., Ward, M., & Vikas, P. (2015). Challenges of rural cancer care in the United States. *Oncology, 29*(9), 633–40. Retrieved from https://pubmed.ncbi.nlm.nih.gov/26384798/

Children's Oncology Group. (2019). About us. Retrieved from https://www.childrensoncologygroup.org/index.php/aboutus

Chu, K. C., Miller, B. A., & Springfield, S. A. (2007). Measures of racial/ethnic health disparities in cancer mortality rates and the influence of socioeconomic status. *Journal of the National Medical Association, 99*(10), 1092–1124.

Cole, A. M., Jackson, J. E., & Doescher, M. (2012a). Urban–rural disparities in colorectal cancer screening: cross-sectional analysis of 1998–2005 data from the Centers for Disease Control's Behavioral Risk Factor Surveillance Study. *Cancer Medicine, 1*(3), 350–356.

Cole, A. M., Jackson, J. E., & Doescher, M. (2012b). Colorectal cancer screening disparities for rural minorities in the United States. *Journal of Primary Care & Community Health, 4*(2), 106–111. doi:10.1177/2150131912463244

Cromartie, J. (2018). *Rural America at a Glance, 2018 Edition* Washington, D.C: United States Department of Agriculture. Retrieved from https://www.ers.usda.gov/publications/pub-details/?pubid=90555

Crosby, R. A., Wendel, M. L., Vanderpool, R. C., & Casey, B. R. (2012). *Rural Populations and Health: Determinants, Disparities, and Solutions.* San Francisco, CA: Jossey-Bass.

Delavar, A., Feng, Q., & Johnson, K. J. (2019). Rural/urban residence and childhood and adolescent cancer survival in the United States. *Cancer, 125*(2), 261–268. https://doi.org/10.1002/cncr.31704

Diala, C. C., Muntaner, C., Walrath, C., Nickerson, K., LaVeist, T., & Leaf, P. (2001). Racial/ethnic differences in attitudes toward seeking professional mental health services. *American Journal of Public Health, 91*(5), 805–807.

Doescher, M. P., & Jackson, J. E. (2009). Trends in cervical and breast cancer screening practices among women in rural and urban areas of the United States. *Journal of Public Health Management Practice, 15*(3), 200–209.

Doolittle, G. (1997). A POTS-based tele-hospice project in Missouri. *Telemedicine Today, 5*, 18–19.

Doolittle, G. C., Yaezel, A., Otto, F., & Clemens, C. (1998). Hospice care using home-based telemedicine systems. *Journal of Telemedicine and Telecare, 4*(Suppl 1), 58–59.

Drummond, M. B. & Upson, D. (2014). Electronic cigarettes: Potential harms and benefits. *Annals of American Thoracic Society, 11*(2), 236–242.

Eberhardt, M., & Pamuk, E. (2004). The importance of place of residence: Examining health in rural and nonrural areas. *American Journal of Public Health, 94*(10), 1682–1686.

Eberth, J. M., Bozorgi, P., Lebrón, L. M., Bills, S. E., Hazlett, L. J., Carlos, R. C., & King, J. C. (2018). Geographic availability of low-dose computed tomography for lung cancer screening in the United States, 2017. *Preventing Chronic Disease, 15*, E119.

Edwards, S. M. & Rousseau-Pierre, T. (2010). Immunizations in adolescents: An update. *Adolescent Medicine: State of the Art Reviews, 21*(2), 173–186.

Fairley, T. L., Tai, E., Townsend, J. S., Stewart, S. L., Steele, C. B., Davis, S. P., & Underwood, J. M. (2010). Racial/ethnic disparities and geographic differences in lung cancer incidence - 38 States and the District of Columbia, 1998-2006. *MMWR Morbidity and Mortality Weekly Report, 59*(44), 1433–1438.

Farkas, A., Marcella, S., & Rhoads, G. G. (1999). Ethnic and racial differences in prostate cancer incidence and mortality. *Ethnicity & Disease, 10*(1), 69–75.

Farm Labor. (n.d.). https://www.ers.usda.gov/topics/farm-economy/farm-labor/. Retrieved May 3, 2020.

Farrell, R. M. & Rome, E. S. (2007). Adolescents' access and consent to the human papillomavirus vaccine. *Pediatrics, 120*(2), 434–437.

Fisher, J. W. & Brundage, S. I. (2009). The challenge of eliminating cervical cancer in the United States: A story of politics, prudishness, and prevention. *Women & Health, 49*(2–3), 246–261.

Frieden, T. R., Myers, J. E., Krauskopf, M. S., & Farley, T. A. (2008). A public health approach to winning the war against cancer. *The Oncologist, 13*(12), 1306–1313.

Garcia, M. C., Faul, M., Massetti, G., Thomas, C. C., Hong, Y., Bauer, U. E., & Iademarco, M. F. (2017). Reducing potentially excess deaths from the five leading causes of death in the rural United States. *MMWR Surveillance Summaries, 66*(2), 1–7.

Gerend, M. A., Shepherd, M. A., and Shepherd, J. E. (2013a). The multidimensional nature of perceived barriers: Global versus practical barriers to HPV vaccination. *Health Psychology, 32*(4), 361–369.

Gerend, M. A., Shepherd, M. A., & Lustria, M. L. (2013b). Increasing human papillomavirus vaccine acceptability by tailoring messages to young adult women's perceived barriers. *Sexually Transmitted Diseases, 40*(5), 401–405.

Greenwald, Z. R., El-Zein, M., Bouten, S., Ensha, H., Vazquez, F. L., & Franco, E. L. (2017). Mobile screening units for the early detection of cancer: A systematic review. *Cancer Epidemiology, Biomarkers & Prevention, 26*(12), 1679–1694.

Hartley, D. (2004). Rural health disparities, population health, and rural culture. *American Journal of Public Health, 94*(10), 1675–1678.

Hede, K. (2010). Teleoncology gaining acceptance with physicians, patients. *Journal of the National Cancer Institute, 102*(20), 1531–1533.

Henley, S. J., Anderson, R. N., Thomas, C. C., Massetti, G. M., Peaker, B., & Richardson, L. C. (2017). Invasive cancer incidence, 2004–2013, and deaths, 2006–2015, in nonmetropolitan and metropolitan counties—United States. *MMWR Surveillance Summaries, 66*(14), 1.

Heron, M. (2018). Deaths: Leading causes for 2016. *National Vital Statistics Reports, 67*(6). Retrieved from https://www.cdc.gov/nchs/data/nvsr/nvsr67/nvsr67_06.pdf

Hershey, J. H. & Velez, L. F. (2009). Public health issues related to HPV vaccination. *J Public Health Management & Practice, 15*(5), 384–392.

Housing Assistance Council. (2012). Race & ethnicity in rural America. *Rural Research Brief, April*, 1283–1288. Retrieved from http://www.ruralhome.org/storage/research_notes/rrn-race-and-ethnicity-web.pdf

Huang, J., King, B. A., Babb, S. D., Xu, X., Hallett, C., & Hopkins, M. (2015). Sociodemographic disparities in local smoke-free law coverage in 10 States. *American Journal of Public Health, 105*(9), 1806–1813.

James, C. V., Moonesinghe, R., Wilson-Frederick, S. M., Hall, J. E., Penman-Aguilar, A., & Bouye, K. (2017). Racial/ethnic health disparities among rural adults—United States, 2012–2015. *MMWR Surveillance Summaries, 66*(23), 1–9.

Jenkins, W. D., Matthews, A. K., Bailey, A., Zahnd, W. E., Watson, K. S., Mueller-Luckey, G., & Patera, J. (2018). Rural areas are disproportionately impacted by smoking and lung cancer. *Preventive Medicine Reports, 10*, 200–203. doi:10.1016/j.pmedr.2018.03.011

Jones, R. A., Steeves, R., & Williams, I. (2009). How African American men decide whether or not to get prostate cancer screening. *Cancer Nursing, 32*(2), 166–172. doi:10.1097/NCC.0b013e3181982c6e

Kogevinas, M., Pearce, N., Susser, M., & Boffetta, P. (eds.) (1997). Social inequalities and cancer. *IARC Scientific Publications, 138*, 1–15.

Kroenke, K., Theobald, D., Wu, J., Norton, K., Morrison, G., Carpenter, J., & Tu, W. (2010). Effect of telecare management on pain and depression in patients with cancer: A randomized trial. *JAMA, 304*, 163–171.

Kuo, T. M., & Mobley, L. R. (2016). How generalizable are the SEER registries to the cancer populations of the USA? *Cancer Causes & Control, 27*(9), 1117–1126. doi:10.1007/s10552-016-0790-x

Lehmann, C. & Benson, P. A. (2009). Vaccine adherence in adolescents. *Clinical Pediatrics, 48*(8), 801–811.

Manser, R., Wright, G., Hart, D., Byrnes, G., Campbell, D., Wainer, Z., & Tort, S. (2005). Surgery for local and locally advanced non-small cell lung cancer. *Cochrane Systematic Reviews. 19CD004699.*

Matthews, K. A., Croft, J. B., Liu, Y., Lu, H., Kanny, D., Wheaton, A. G., . . . Giles, W. H. (2017). Health-related behaviors by urban-rural county classification— United States, 2013. *Morbidity and Mortality Weekly Report Surveillance Summaries, 66*(5), 1–8. doi: http://dx.doi.org/10.15585/mmwr.ss6605a1

McClung, N. M., Gargano, J. W., Bennett, N. M., Niccolai, L. M., Abdullah, N., Griffin, M.R., . . . the HPV-IMPACT Working Group. (2019). Trends in human papillomavirus vaccine types 16 and 18 in cervical precancers, 2008–2014. *Cancer Epidemiology, Biomarkers & Prevention, 28*(3), 602–609.

McKenna, R. J. Jr., Houck, W., & Fuller, C. B. (2006). Video-assisted thoracic surgery lobectomy: Experience with 1,100 cases. *Annals of Thoracic Surgery, 81*(2), 421–426.

Medicaid.gov. (2019). Children's Health Insurance Program (CHIP). Retrieved from https://www.medicaid.gov/chip/index.html

Meit, M., Knudson, A., Gilbert, T., Yu, A. T-C., Tanenbaum, E., Ormson, E., . . . NORC Walsh Center for Rural Health Analysis. (2014). The 2014 Update of the rural-urban chartbook. Retrieved from https://ruralhealth.und.edu/projects/health-reform-policy-research-center/pdf/2014-rural-urban-chartbook-update.pdf

Meites, E., Szilagyi, P. G., Chesson, H. W., Unger, E. R., Romero, J. R., & Markowitz, L. E. (2019). Human papillomavirus vaccination for adults: Updated recommendations of the Advisory Committee on Immunization Practices. *Morbidity and Mortality Weekly Report, 68*, 698–702. Retrieved from https://www.cdc.gov/mmwr/volumes/68/wr/mm6832a3.htm

Moy, E., Garcia, M. C., Bastian, B., Rossen, L. M., Ingram, D. D., Faul, M., . . . Iademarco, M. F. (2017). Leading causes of death in nonmetropolitan and metropolitan areas—United States, 1999–2014. *Morbidity and Mortality Weekly Report—Surveillance Summaries, 66*(1), 1–8.

Musa, J., Achenbach, C. J., O'Dwyer, L. C., Evans, C. T., McHugh, M., Hou, L., . . . Jordan, N. (2017). Effect of cervical cancer education and provider recommendation for screening on screening rates: A systematic review and meta-analysis. *PloS One, 12*(9), e0190661.

National Cancer Institute. (2015). *What is cancer?* Retrieved from https://www.cancer.gov/about-cancer/understanding/what-is-cancer

National Cancer Institute. (2016a). *Cancer stat facts: Prostate Cancer.* Retrieved from https://seer.cancer.gov/statfacts/html/prost.html

National Cancer Institute. (2016b). *Cancer stat facts: Lung and bronchus cancer.* Retrieved from http://seer.cancer.gov/statfacts/html/lungb.html

National Cancer Institute. (2018). *Surveillance, Epidemiology, and End Results (SEER).* Retrieved from https://seer.cancer.gov/about/factsheets/SEER_Overview.pdf

National Cancer Institute. (n.d.-a). *Rural cancer control.* Retrieved from https://cancercontrol.cancer.gov/research-emphasis/rural.html

National Cancer Institute. (n.d.-b). *Surveillance, Epidemiology, and End Results Program.* Retrieved from https://seer.cancer.gov/

Natoinal Cancer Institute. Prostate Cancer Treatment (PDQ®)–Patient Version. (n.d.). Retrieved May 3, 2020, from https://www.cancer.gov/types/prostate/patient/prostate-treatment-pdq#_142

Nemeth, J. M., Liu, S. T., Klein, E. G., Ferketich, A. K., Kwan, M. P., & Wewers, M. E. (2012). Factors influencing smokeless tobacco use in rural Ohio Appalachia. *Journal of Community Health, 37*(6), 1208–1217.

North Dakota Statewide Cancer Registry. (2014). *Welcome to our site.* Retrieved from https://ndcancer.org/

Nuño, T., Gerald, J. K., Harris, R., Martinez, M. E., Estrada, A., & García, F. (2012). Comparison of breast and cervical cancer screening utilization among rural and urban Hispanic and American Indian women in the Southwestern United States. *Cancer Causes & Control, 23*(8), 1333–1341.

Obertova, Z., Brown, C., Holmes, M., & Lawrenson, R. (2012). Prostate cancer incidence and mortality in rural men--a systematic review of the literature. *Rural & Remote Health, 12*(2).

Oliver, J. S. (2007). Attitudes and beliefs about prostate cancer and screening among rural African American men. *Journal of Cultural Diversity, 14*(2), 74–80.

Orwat, J., Caputo, N., Key, W., & De Sa, J. (2017). Comparing rural and urban cervical and breast cancer screening rates in a privately insured population. *Social Work in Public Health, 32*(5), 311–323.

O'Hare, W. P. (2014). Rural children increasingly rely on Medicaid and Child Health Insurance Programs for Health Insurance. Washington, DC: First Focus. Retrieved from https://firstfocus.org/wp-content/uploads/2014/09/Ohare_Draft6.pdf

Pleis, J. R., Ward, B. W., & Lucas, J. W. (2010). Summary health statistics for US adults: National Health Interview Survey, 2009. *Vital and Health Statistics. Series 10, Data from the National Health Survey, 10*(249), 1–207.

Plummer, M., Herrero, R., Franceschi, S., Meijer, C. J., Snijders, P., Bosch, F. X., . . . Muñoz, N. (2003). Smoking and cervical cancer: Pooled analysis of the IARC multi-centric case—control study. *Cancer Causes & Control, 14*, 805–814.

Reiter, P. L., Katz, M. L., & Paskett, E. D. (2013). Correlates of HPV vaccination among adolescent females from Appalachia and reasons why their parents do not intend to vaccinate. *Vaccine, 31*(31), 3121–3125.

Roura, E., Castellsagué, X., Pawlita, M., Travier, N., Waterboer, T., Margall, N., . . . Riboli, E. (2014). Smoking as a major risk factor for cervical cancer and pre-cancer: Results from the EPIC cohort. *Int J Cancer, 135*(2), 453–466.

Rural Health Information Hub. (n.d.-a). Rural Healthcare Workforce. Retrieved May 4, 2020, from https://www.ruralhealthinfo.org/topics/health-care-workforce#workforce

Rural Health Information Hub. (n.d.-b). Scholarships, Loans, and Loan Repayment for Rural Health Professions. Retrieved May 4, 2020, from https://www.ruralhealthinfo.org/topics/scholarships-loans-loan-repayment

Rural Health Information Hub. (n.d.-c). Rural Project Examples: Health workforce pipeline. Retrieved May 4, 2020, from https://www.ruralhealthinfo.org/project-examples/topics/health-workforce-pipeline

Saraiya, M., Unger, E. R., Thompson, T. D., Lynch, C. F., Hernandez, B. Y., Lyu, C. W., . . . HPV Typing of Cancers Workgroup. (2015). HPV Typing of Cancers Workgroup. U.S. assessment of HPV types in cancers: Implications for current and 9-valent HPV vaccines. *Journal of the National Cancer Institute, 107*(6).

Satcher, R. L., Bogler, O., Hyle, L., Lee, A., Simmons, A., Williams, R., . . . Brewster, A. M. (2014). Telemedicine and telesurgery in cancer care: Inaugural conference at MD Anderson Cancer Center. *Journal of Surgical Oncology, 110*(4), 353–359.

Scott, W. J., Allen, M. S., Darling, G., Meyers, B., Decker, M. S., Putnam, J. B., . . . Malthaner, R. A. (2010). Video-assisted thoracic surgery versus open lobectomy for lung cancer: A secondary analysis of data from the American College of Surgeons Oncology Group Z0030 randomized clinical trial. *The Journal of Thoracic and Cardiovascular Surgery, 139*(4), 976–983.

Siegel D. A., Li J., Henley, S. J., Wilson, R. J., Buchanan Lunsford, N., Tai, E., . . . Van Dyne, E. A. (2018). Geographic variation in pediatric cancer incidence—United States, 2003–2014. *MMWR Morbidity and Mortality Weekly Report, 67*(25), 707–713. DOI: http://dx.doi.org/10.15585/mmwr.mm6725a2external icon

Singh, G. K. (2012). Rural-urban trends and patterns in cervical cancer mortality, incidence, stage, and survival in the United States, 19502008. *Journal of Community Health, 37*, 217–223.

Singh, G. K., Miller, B. A., & Hankey, B. F. (2002). Changing area socioeconomic patterns in US cancer mortality, 1950–1998: Part II—lung and colorectal cancers. *Journal of the National Cancer Institute, 94*(12), 916–925.

Singh, G. K., Miller, B. A., Hankey, B. F., & Edwards, B. K. (2003). Area socioeconomic variations in US cancer incidence, mortality, stage, treatment, and survival, 1975–1999. *NCI Cancer Surveillance Monograph Series, 4.*

Singh, G. K., Siahpush, M., & Williams, S. D. (2012). Changing urbanization patterns in US lung cancer mortality, 1950–2007. *Journal of Community Health, 37*, 412–420.

Singh, G. K., Williams, S. D., Siahpush, M., & Mulhollen, A. (2011). Socioeconomic, rural-urban, and racial inequalities in US cancer mortality: Part I—All cancers and lung cancer and Part II—colorectal, prostate, breast, and cervical cancers. *Journal of Cancer Epidemiology.*

Smieliauskas, F., MacMahon, H., Salgia, R., & Shih, Y. C. (2014). Geographic variation in radiologist capacity and widespread implementation of lung cancer CT screening. *Journal of Medical Screening, 21*(4), 207–215. doi 10.1177/0969141314548055

Snelling, A. (2014). *Health Promotion.* San Francisco: John Wiley & Sons, Inc.

Steenland, K., Henley, J., & Thun, M. (2002). All-cause and cause-specific death rates by educational status for two million people in two American Cancer Society cohorts, 1959–1996. *American Journal of Epidemiology, 156*(1), 11–21.

Substance Abuse and Mental Health Services Administration. (2017). *Results from the 2016* Rockville, MD: Substance Abuse and Mental Health Services Administration, Center for Behavioral Health Statistics and Quality.

U.S. Cancer Statistics Working Group. (2017). United States cancer statistics: 1999–2014 incidence and mortality web-based report. Atlanta, GA: US Department of Health and Human Services, CDC; National Cancer Institute. Retrieved from https://www.cdc.gov/uscs

U.S. Department of Health and Human Services, Centers for Disease Control and Prevention & National Center for Chronic Disease Prevention and Health Promotion. (2001). *Women and smoking: A report of the Surgeon General.* Rockville, MD: U.S. Dept. of Health and Human Services, Public Health Service, Office of the Surgeon General.

U.S. Department of Health and Human Services. (2008). The Secretary's Advisory Committee on National Health Promotion and Disease Prevention Objectives for 2020. Phase I report: Recommendations for the framework and format of Healthy People 2020 [Internet]. Section IV: Advisory Committee findings

and recommendations. Retrieved from http://www
.healthypeople.gov/sites/default/files/PhaseI_0.pdf

U.S. Department of Health and Human Services. (2015).
Agency for Healthcare Research and Quality. 2014
National Healthcare Quality & Disparities Report
Chartbook on Rural Health Care. AHRQ Pub. No.
15–0007–9-EF. Rockville, MD. Retrieved from https://
www.ahrq.gov/sites/default/files/wysiwyg/research
/findings/nhqrdr/chartbooks/qdr-ruralhealth
chartbook-update.pdf

U.S. Preventive Services Task Force. (2013). *Lung cancer:
Screening.* Retrieved from https://www.uspreventive
servicestaskforce.org/Page/Document/Update
SummaryFinal/lung-cancer-screening

U.S. Preventive Services Task Force. (2016). *Final recommendation statement. Colorectal cancer: Screening.* Retrieved from https://pubmed.ncbi.nlm.nih
.gov/27304597/

U.S. Preventive Services Task Force. (2018a). *Prostate
cancer: Screening.* Retrieved from https://pubmed.ncbi
.nlm.nih.gov/29801017/

U.S. Preventive Services Task Force. (2018b). *Cervical cancer: Screening.* Retrieved from https://www
.uspreventiveservicestaskforce.org/Page/Document
/UpdateSummaryFinal/cervical-cancer-screening

United States Department of Agriculture. (n.d.). *Rural
poverty & well-being.* Retrieved from https://www
.ers.usda.gov/topics/rural-economy-population
/rural-poverty-well-being/

United States Department of Health and Human Services.
(2019). Pap and HPV tests. Retrieved from https://
www.womenshealth.gov/a-z-topics/pap-hpv-tests

Vellozzi, C. J., Romans, M., & Rothenberg, R. B. (1996).
Delivering breast and cervical cancer screening services to underserved women: Part I. Literature review
and telephone survey. *Women's Health Issues, 6*(2),
65–73.

Vetter, K. M. and Geller, S. E. (2007). Moving forward:
Human papillomavirus vaccination and the prevention of cervical cancer. *Journal of Women's Health,
16*(9), 1258–1268.

Warsaw, R. (2017, October 31). *Health disparities
affect millions in rural U.S. communities.* Retrieved
from https://www.aamc.org/news-insights/health
-disparities-affect-millions-rural-us-communities

Yu, L., Sabatino, S. A., & White, M. C. (2019). Rural–
urban and racial/ethnic disparities in invasive cervical
cancer incidence in the United States, 2010–2014.
Preventing Chronic Disease, 16, E70.

Zahnd, W., James, A. S., Jenkins, W. D., Izadi, S. R.,
Fogleman, A., Steward, D., . . . Brard, L. (2018). Rural-
urban differences in cancer incidence and trends in
the United States. *Cancer Epidemiology, Biomarkers &
Prevention: A Publication of the American Association
for Cancer Research, Cosponsored by the American
Society of Preventive Oncology, 27*(11), 1265–1274.

Ziller, E. C., Lenardson, J. D., Paluso, N. C., Talbot, J. A.,
& Daley, A. (2019). Rural–urban differences in the
decline of adolescent cigarette smoking. *American
Journal of Public Health, 109*(5), 771–773.

CHAPTER 13

Environmental Health in Rural Regions of the United States

Salma Haidar, PhD, MPH
Rebecca Uzarski, PhD
Ruben Juarez, MPH

LEARNING OBJECTIVES

At the end of this chapter, readers will be able to:

1. Compare and contrast three common types of private wells.
2. Describe factors influencing well-water quality.
3. Identify common contaminants in well water and related risks.
4. Describe the term "criteria pollutants."
5. Identify and describe measures of air quality in rural areas.
6. Identify the health effects of the major air pollutants in rural areas.
7. Identify the environmental effects of the major air pollutants in rural areas.
8. Introduce the unique concerns of hazardous waste in rural regions.
9. Identify electronic waste and the major health concerns they pose.
10. Describe agribusiness and its influence on rural health.
11. Identify emerging and endemic zoonotic diseases in rural regions.
12. Describe causative agent and disease burden and impacts of zoonotic diseases on humans and animals.
13. Describe environmental impacts of zoonotic diseases.

KEY TERMS

Agribusiness
Air Pollution
Aquifer
Endemic
Environment
Hazardous Waste
Sewer system
Water Contaminants
Well Water
Zoonotic Diseases

CHAPTER OVERVIEW

This chapter will investigate environmental causes associated with water quality, air quality, waste generation and disposal, agricultural practices, and zoonosis that disproportionally affect residents in rural America.

Introduction

According to the Centers for Disease Control and Prevention (CDC), approximately 46 million Americans (15% of the U.S. population) currently live in rural areas. Rural residents are at higher risk of death than the rest of the U.S. population due to demographic, environmental, economic, and social factors (U.S. Environmental Protection Agency [EPA], 2019). The five leading causes of deaths in rural America in 2014 were heart disease, cancer, unintentional injuries, chronic respiratory disease, and stroke (EPA, 2019). It appears that environmental factors play an important role in affecting the health of the rural residents. Exposure to environmental determinants of disease in rural settings differ significantly from urban areas. Some rural areas have characteristics that put residents at higher risk of death, such as long travel distances to specialty and emergency care or exposures to specific environmental hazards. In addition, "Rural Americans tend to have higher rates of cigarette smoking, high blood pressure, and obesity. Rural residents report less leisure-time physical activity and lower seatbelt use than their urban counterparts. They also have higher rates of poverty, less access to health care, and are less likely to have health insurance. All of these factors can lead to poor health outcomes" (EPA, 2017b).

Water Quality

The United States Environmental Protection Agency (EPA) is responsible for protecting public health through regulation of drinking **water contaminants**. However, the Safe Drinking Water Act (SDWA) protects public water systems serving a minimum of 25 persons or 15 service connections. Approximately 15 million rural households (43 million people) use small private wells serving one or a few homes. Therefore, private water supplies in rural communities are largely untested and unprotected by the EPA under federal safety regulations. Recent estimates by the United States Geological Survey (USGS) indicate that over 20% of these private systems have one or more contaminants at levels of a potential health concern (USGS, 2009).

Determinants of Water Quality in Rural Communities

Drinking water quality depends on the water source, nature of the soil surrounding the **aquifer**, construction and depth of the **well**, a properly maintained **sewer system**, and well placement or location.

Water Source

Large-scale public water systems typically utilize surface water from reservoirs, lakes, or rivers for drinking water. Surface water quality can be affected by area land use. Surface runoff from surrounding industry and agriculture contributes to the poor water quality of surface water and requires extensive treatment prior to consumption. Wells drilled into aquifers provide ground water for small-scale and private drinking water systems in rural communities. Ground water is considered higher quality but can be affected by surface runoff, agricultural practices, and leachate from **waste** disposal sites (CDC and USHUD, 2006).

Soil Composition

Soil composition surrounding ground water aquifers plays a critical role in water sanitation. Surface water containing suspended microorganisms, chemicals, or naturally occurring elements will seep through overlying soils to reach the ground water. Composition and thickness of the overlying materials will determine the extent of removal of microorganisms and **pollutants**. Clay, sand, and gravel provide the most efficient filter of ground water compared with limestone, rock, and lava formations. Limited filtration from coarse soil or insufficient soil depth will increase the likelihood of contamination (EPA, 2019d).

Well Construction and Depth

Private drinking water well construction and depth are determinants of water quality. Dug wells, common before 1950, were constructed by digging with a shovel or backhoe to a depth of 10 to 30 feet. The wells were lined with brick or tile but lacked an impermeable casing. Shallow with a large circumference, dug wells are often contaminated with surface water. Driven wells are constructed by driving a pipe into the ground to a depth of 30 to 50 feet. Shallow with an impenetrable casing, driven wells are often contaminated easily due to the proximity to the surface. Modern wells are drilled to depths ranging from 100 to 1,000 feet. Increased depth and continual casing of drilled wells provides the lowest risk of contamination (USGS, 2016). The type of well (dug, driven, or drilled)

present in rural communities, as shown in **Figure 13-1**, is a result of the age of the infrastructure and the depth of the water table or aquifer.

Sewer Systems

While urban localities generally create a centralized public **sewer system** that removes sewage and wastewater from homes to treatment plants. In rural communities, adequate wastewater removal requires a decentralized sewer system. A decentralized sewer system has four major features: 1) a pipe system leading wastewater out of homes; 2) a septic tank that separates solid and liquid waste; 3) a drain field, or an area below the surface where water can flow down through; and 4) soil that will filter out microbial contaminants before the water reaches ground water (EPA, n.d.i.). Within the septic tank, waste can be divided into three categories: scum (oily wastes), effluent (the liquid waste), and sludge (solid waste) (EPA, n.d.i). Although this is the classic decentralized sewer system layout, other systems are commercially available for residents (**Figure 13-2**) with geological features

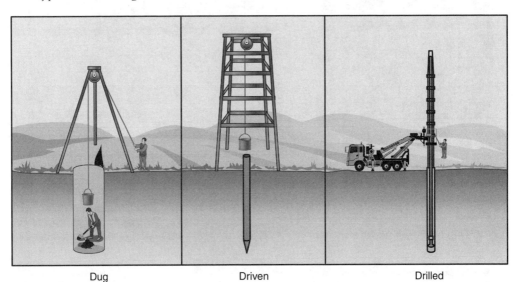

| Dug | Driven | Drilled |

Figure 13-1 Dug, Driven, and Drilled Wells.

Waller, R. M. (2016). Ground water and the rural homeowner. Retrieved from https://pubs.usgs.gov/gip/gw_ruralhomeowner/gw_ruralhomeowner_new.html.

that do not make this traditional system possible or feasible. A properly maintained system prevents ground water contamination; however, a majority of septic systems are at least three decades old, increasing the likelihood of system failure and drinking water contamination (EPA, 2005).

Well Placement

Finally, the safety of a private well depends on the location of the well with respect to possible pollution sources. The EPA recommends a minimum distance of 50 feet between a private well and septic tank, septic leach field, or livestock yard. Private wells should be placed at least 100 feet from liquid manure storage, fertilizer storage and handling, or petroleum storage sites. Manure stacks should be separated from private wells by at least 250 feet (CDC, 2009; EPA, 2019d). These distances are recommendations and may vary with individual sites. Ultimately, a safe distance should be the maximum space with consideration given to geology, topography, economics, and land ownership.

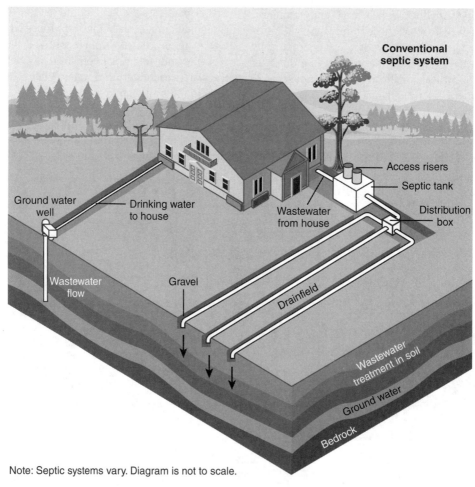

Note: Septic systems vary. Diagram is not to scale.

Figure 13-2 Conventional Septic System.

Environmental Protection Agency. (n.d.g). Septic systems: Types of septic systems. Retrieved from https://www.epa.gov/septic/types-septic-systems.

Common Contaminants in Private Wells

Ground water wells can be polluted by human or animal fecal contaminants, naturally occurring substances, and chemicals associated with current or historic land use. Waterborne disease and outbreak data (Benedict, et al., 2017) indicate that fecal contaminants (bacterial, viral, and parasitic) were the leading cause of outbreaks in private wells (**Table 13-1**).

Fecal contaminants can enter private wells through failing septic systems, sewage overflows, storm water contamination, agricultural runoff, or after flood events (CDC, 2009). Shallow wells are vulnerable to flooding, especially dug or driven wells. The most common fecal contaminants found in private wells are briefly described below:

> *Hepatitis A (HAV)* is a human viral disease that infects the liver. Symptoms of infection include fatigue, nausea, and jaundice.

Table 13-1 **Most Common Causes of Outbreaks in Private Wells (CDC, 2015a)**

Top 6 Causes—Outbreaks in Individual (Private) Water Systems—Wells
Top Causes of Outbreaks in Wells
1. Hepatitis A
2. *Giardia*
3. *Campylobacter, E.Coli* (tie)
4. *Shigella*
5. *Cryptosporidium Salmonella* (tie)
6. Arsenic Gasoline, Nitrate, Phenol, Selenium (tie)

Centers for Disease Control and Prevention. (2015a). Overview of water-related diseases and contaminants in private wells. Retrieved from: https://www.cdc.gov/healthywater/drinking/private/wells/diseases.html.

Giardia is a human and animal parasite. Giardia is surrounded by a protective outer shell that increases survival in the environment and resists chlorination. A symptom of infection includes diarrhea.

Campylobacter is a bacterium carried in the intestines of cows, chickens, and other animals. Symptoms include bloody diarrhea, fever, and abdominal cramps. Campylobacter is the most common bacterial cause of human diarrheal illness in the United States.

Escherichia coli (E. coli) is a bacterium common in the environment and the intestines of people and animals. Most strains of *E. coli* are harmless; however, some cause diarrheal illness.

Shigella is a bacterium present in the human intestine. Symptoms of infection include diarrhea, fever, and stomach cramps.

Cryptosporidium is a parasite present in the intestines of infected humans and animals. Cryptosporidium has a protective outer shell that promotes survival in the environment and resists chlorination. Symptoms of infection include watery diarrhea, fever, and stomach cramps. Cryptosporidium is the leading cause of waterborne disease in humans in the United States.

Salmonella is a bacterium present in the intestines of humans and animals. Symptoms of infection include diarrhea, fever, and stomach cramps.

The remaining top causes of waterborne disease outbreaks in private wells result from a combination of naturally occurring and anthropogenic sources (CDC, 2015a). In some cases, these contaminants result from historical land use, improper waste disposal, or unsuitable well construction. The composition and health effects of the most common pollutants are described below:

Arsenic in private wells may result from natural deposits, agricultural fertilizers, or industrial waste. Consumption of arsenic in drinking water may cause stomach irritation, nausea, vomiting, and fatigue. With continued exposure, tingling in the hands and feet and patches of darkened skin may develop. With chronic exposure, the risk of skin cancer increases.

Gasoline is automotive fuel derived from petroleum that contains approximately 150 different chemicals in small amounts. Many of these chemicals are hydrocarbons and volatile organic compounds. Because chemicals that penetrate ground water will vary, health effects are largely unclassifiable.

Nitrate occurs naturally in the environment and is a component of inorganic fertilizers. Consumption of high levels of nitrate in drinking water can interfere with the ability of blood to carry oxygen to the tissues. Exposure may cause a decrease in blood pressure, increase in heart rate, and headaches. Infants who consume formula prepared with nitrate-contaminated water are a particularly sensitive population.

Phenol is produced naturally and in the manufacture of plastics. Additional uses include consumer products (i.e., mouthwash) and household cleaning products. Phenol has been found in surface water, soil, and sediment. Phenol in the soil is likely to migrate into ground water. Consumption of phenol may cause gastrointestinal damage. Laboratory animals exposed to phenol orally displayed muscle tremors and difficulty walking.

Selenium is naturally occurring in the soil, used as a nutritional supplement in livestock, and has a variety of uses in industry. While low levels of selenium are required for maintaining health, high levels have been associated with nausea, vomiting, and diarrhea. Chronic exposure to selenium causes hair loss and numbness in the hands and feet.

In addition to being safe to drink, water should be appealing. Secondary contaminants are responsible for aesthetic changes in odor, taste, or color of the water; cosmetic changes able to cause changes in skin or tooth coloration; and technical effects that may have economic consequences related to staining of household fixtures or corrosion of pipes. Secondary contaminants described in **Table 13-2** do not pose a human health risk but cause various water quality issues (EPA, 2017c). The USEPA recommends maximum contaminant levels (MCL) of secondary contaminants but does not enforce compliance.

Tips from the Field: Health Professional Expert Advice

Prevent Well Water Pollution

Well Maintenance

The USEPA (2017d) recommends protecting private drinking water sources from pollution by following proper well maintenance, never disposing chemicals in a dry well, and checking with the local health department to ensure that contaminants are at a safe distance.

Test Private Wells Annually

The USEPA (2017d) recommends testing private wells annually for coliform bacteria, nitrate, total dissolved solids, and pH.

Table 13-2 Secondary Contaminants and Effects (EPA, 2017c)

Contaminant	Secondary MCL	Noticeable Effects above the Secondary MCL
Aluminum	0.05 to 02 mg/L*	colored water
Chloride	250 mg/L	salty taste
Color	15 color units	visible tint
Copper	1.0 mg/L	metallic taste; blue-green staining
Corrosivity	Non-corrosive	metallic taste; corroded pipes/fixtures staining
Fluoride	2.0 mg/L	tooth discoloration
Foaming agents	0.5 mg/L	frothy; cloudy; bitter taste; odor
Iron	0.3 mg/L	rusty color; sediment; metallic taste; reddish or orange staining
Manganese	0.05 mg/L	black to brown color; black staining; bitter metallic taste
Odor	3 TON (threshold odor number)	"rotten-egg"; musty or chemical smell
pH	6.5–8.5	low pH: bitter metallic taste; corrosion high pH: slippery feel; soda taste; deposits
Silver	0.1 mg/L	skin discoloration; graying of the white part of the eye
Sulfate	250 mg/L	salty taste
Total Dissolved Solids (TDS)	500 mg/L	hardness; deposits; colored water; staining; salty taste
Zinc	5 mg/L	metallic taste

*mg/L is milligrams of substance per liter of water.

Environmental Protection Agency. (2017c). Secondary drinking water standards: Guidance for nuisance chemicals. Retrieved from https://www.epa.gov/dwstandardsregulations/secondary-drinking-water-standards-guidance-nuisance-chemicals.

Wells should be tested immediately if there are known ground water problems in the area; changes including area construction or flooding; or any noticeable changes in water quality. **Table 13-3** outlines common reasons to test private wells.

Where to Test Water from Private Wells

Individuals with private wells concerned about contaminants should have their water tested by a state-certified laboratory. Laboratory information is available through the local health department.

Septic System Maintenance

A properly maintained system prevents ground water contamination. The USEPA recommends avoiding disposal of chemicals in a septic system, inspecting the system every three years, and pumping every five years.

Table 13-3 Common Reasons to Test Private Wells

Conditions or Nearby Activities:	Test for:
Recurring gastro-intestinal illness	Coliform bacteria
Household plumbing or service lines that contain lead	pH, lead copper
Radon in indoor air or region is radon rich	Radon
Corrosion of pipes, plumbing	Corrosion, pH, lead
Nearby areas of intensive agriculture	Nitrate, nitrite, pesticides, coliform bacteria
Coal or other mining operations nearby	Metals, pH, corrosion
Gas drilling operations nearby	Chloride, sodium, barium, strontium
Dump, junkyard, landfill, factory, gas station or dry-cleaning operation nearby	Volatile organic compounds, total dissolved solids, pH, sulfate, chloride, metals
Odor of gasoline or fuel oil, and near gas station or buried fuel tanks	Volatile organic compounds
Objectionable taste or smell	Hydrogen sulfide, corrosion, metals
Stained plumbing fixtures, laundry	Iron, copper, manganese
Salty taste and seawater, or a heavily salted roadway nearby	Chloride, total dissolved solids, sodium
Scaly residues, soaps don't leather	Hardness
Rapid wear of water treatment equipment	pH, corrosion
Water softener needed to treat hardness	Manganese, iron
Water appears cloudy, frothy or colored	Color, detergents

United States Environmental Protection Agency. 2017, December 15. Protect Your Home's Water. Retrieved August 1, 2019, from https://www.epa.gov/privatewells/protect-your-homes-water#welltestanchor

Air Quality

Most air contaminants originate from human-made sources such as power plants, factories, and transportation vehicles and are concentrated in urban areas. However, rural areas are subject to local sources of pollution as well as secondary effects from urban areas.

Primary Source: Backyard Burning and Crop Residue Burning

Household Waste Burning.

Backyard Burning

Although less common than in past decades, some rural residents opt to burn their waste on their property as a practical way of reducing its volume, a practice generally called backyard burning (as depicted in **Figure 13-3**). Open-air fire pits, burn boxes, outdoor stoves, and boilers are used to set fire to refuse such as paper products, food waste, plastic material, and yard waste (EPA, 2016a). Colloquially referred to as "burn barrels," the use of metal drums has been a common practice to address waste management in sparsely populated communities in

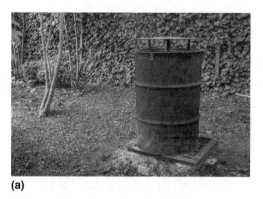
(a)

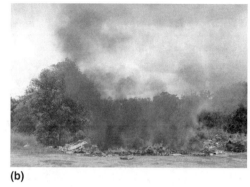
(b)

Figure 13-3 **(a)** Burn Barrell. **(b)** Open Burning.

(a) © Alexander Denisenko/Shutterstock. **(b)** © kittirat roekburi/Shutterstock.

the United States (EPA, 2016a). However, due to the increased presence of highly processed materials and the increased presence of plastics in products and packaging, this practice is highly discouraged. **Exhibit 13-1** demonstrates examples of some challenges faced by the Minnesota Department of Natural Resources regarding backyard burning (Goetzman, 2016).

Studies investigating resulting exposures from burning such materials have shown that it can introduce a wide range of hazards to humans and the surrounding environment. Dioxins are the primary contaminant, but backyard burning also includes polycyclic aromatic hydrocarbons (PAHs), volatile organic compounds (VOCs), hexachlorobenzene, and heavy metals.

Currently, there are no accurate measures indicating the frequency or quantity of household or outdoor wastes burned in rural America (EPA, n.d.b.). As awareness of the health hazards posed by backyard burning has increased, regulations on burning trash have been established. Although most states ban the practice of backyard burning completely as management for municipal solid waste, some states allow it. A survey by Lemieux et al., (2000) in Illinois estimated that up to 50% of rural residents partake in this practice. A Minnesota survey showed similar results, with 45% of rural residents stating they burned

at least some household waste (Minnesota Pollution Control Agency, n.d.).

Dioxins refers to the chemical 2,3,7,8-tetrachlorodibenzo-P-dioxin (TCDD) (National Center for Biotechnology Information, n.d.). Dioxin has also been commonly adopted as a general term encompassing polychlorinated dibenzo-p-dioxin (PCDDs), polychlorinated dibenzofurans (PCDFs or furans), and dioxin-like polychlorinated biphenyls (PCBs) (Zhang, Buekens, & Li, 2017). Backyard burning, along with burnings in farming and forestry, is estimated to be responsible for generating approximately 50% of these chemicals (Zhang, Buekens, & Li, 2017). Compared with controlled waste incinerators, the generation of these chemicals can be several times higher in quantity when backyard burning practices are used (WLSSD, 2015). Dioxins and furans are products of incomplete combustion, which backyard burning conditions provide, as temperature, oxygen, and other factors cannot be controlled to minimize dioxin generation (Zhang, Buekens, Li, & 2017).

Exhibit 13-1 Backyard Burning in Minnesota

Sparking Changes

When [Minnesota Department of Natural Resources] (MDNR) conservation officers and local law enforcement authorities write a ticket for illegal burning, it's typically a misdemeanor, with fines seldom topping $2,000. The [Minnesota Pollution Control Agency] (MPCA) focuses on investigating larger-scale violations and can issue civil penalties starting at $3,500. Spring and fall—when people tend to do cleaning, decluttering, and yard work—are the busiest periods.

DNR conservation officer Paul Kuske takes a keen personal interest in trash burning. "It's a pet peeve of mine. I hate the smell of burning garbage," he says. "And it's incredible how much backyard burning goes on in this state."

For years, Kuske taught a class on illegal burning at the DNR's conservation officer training academy, urging recruits to take burning violations as seriously as those involving fish and game. He puts those lessons to use on his home turf, a central Minnesota county with many farms and rural residences as well as lake homes and cabins. "Morrison County has a real vast history of burning," he says.

On one Fourth of July weekend, Kuske came across a group of partiers ready to toss a match into a huge fire pit containing three mattresses and a living-room chair. He has discovered burn barrels being used right next to propane tanks.

As Kuske drives around peeking into burn barrels, he also knocks on doors and chats with property owners, amiably reminding them that burning garbage isn't OK and discussing other options for disposal. Most are receptive, but a few seem guarded and uneasy. One man, after Kuske prods him for information about his trash burner, answers with a staged Germanic accent, only half-jokingly, "I know noth-ink."

MPCA inspector Jake Brady works in the part of the state where the MPCA investigates more illegal burning than anywhere else: the south. Based in Rochester, Brady covers a 20-county area. Only two counties in his area have enacted a "no-burn" resolution to close a loophole allowing farmers to burn agriculture-related waste. The loophole, say Brady and his colleagues, creates confusion about burning laws and fuels an erroneous perception that farmers and their rural neighbors can burn just about anything. Inspectors once found a charred horse carcass in the rubble of a garbage fire. Brady describes investigating a property that had become a dump-and-burn site for debris from foreclosed homes.

Most of Brady's tips about illegal burning come in by phone. Many tipsters are reporting their neighbors and don't want to be identified. About half of the trash burners Brady investigates have valid burn permits to burn plant material or untreated wood, but they have violated permit terms by tossing garbage into the mix.

Unlike Kuske, Brady doesn't carry a badge or a sidearm, so he sometimes asks local law enforcers for backup when he senses that a confrontation with a burner might turn threatening.

"When you start talking plastics and other kinds of toxic materials, most people understand it. And I'm pretty sure a majority of them know it's bad," says Brady. "Usually, by the end of the conversation, they're saying, 'We apologize, we didn't really understand the effects, we'll stop this now.'"

(Goetzman, 2016)

Goetzman, Keith. (2016). A Burning problem: Torching garbage has serious consequences for the environment— yet it's a Minnesota habit that's been hard to break. Minnesota Department of Natural Resources. Retrieved from https://www.dnr.state.mn.us /mcvmagazine/issues/2016/may-jun/illegal-burning .html.

Health effects of dioxins result from bioaccumulation in fat tissue. TCDD is classified as a carcinogen by the World Health Organization (WHO, 2016). Animal testing and accidental exposures to humans have demonstrated links between dioxins and dioxin-like chemicals with health effects, including cancer, weight loss, heart disease, blood abnormalities, immunosuppression, reproductive health issues, birth defects, liver damage, and lung impairments. Additionally, individuals exposed to PCDD/PCDF-containing smoke have been shown to experience increased levels of headaches, nausea, skin rashes (known as chloracne for high dioxin exposures), and exacerbation of pulmonary conditions such as emphysema and asthma (EPA, 2016a).

Environmental effects of dioxins and furans result from the persistence and bioaccumulation when introduced to soil or bodies of water. When produced through incineration, dioxins and furans can concentrate on surrounding soil or vegetation, increasing in concentration with more exposure. If washed into a nearby river, lake, or pond, the chemicals can be taken up by fish and concentrated further (EPA, 2003).

Polycyclic Aromatic Hydrocarbons (PAHs) are a classification of chemicals generated with the combustion of gasoline, oil, wood, tobacco, and coal (CDC, 2017a). Although it is not certain what health outcomes PAHs produce in outdoor conditions, when commercially produced as naphthalene, PAHs has been known to cause eye, nose, and throat irritation; liver and blood conditions; and cancer (CDC, 2017a).

Volatile Organic Compounds (VOCs) are carbon-based chemicals found in solids and liquids that readily react with the air (EPA, n.d.h.). Health effects of VOCs include headaches and irritation of the eyes, nose, and throat. Additionally, they may cause harm to the liver, kidneys, and the central nervous system (n.d.h.). Certain VOCs are potential or confirmed carcinogens. ***Hexachlorobenzene*** is a chemical once produced and used as a pesticide against fungi (CDC, 2015b). Exposure to high levels of hexachlorobenzene may produce neurological effects, including shaking, muscle weakness, and convulsions (CDC, 2015b). Additionally, skin sores can develop, as well as poor functioning of the liver and thyroid. Fat tissue can store this compound, and long-term exposure can result in the intensification of short-term effects (CDC, 2015b). This substance is thought to be carcinogenic, since experiments on animals have demonstrated a link to liver, kidney, and thyroid cancer.

Heavy Metals such as mercury, lead (see air quality section), chromium, and arsenic (see water quality section) can also be found in backyard burning. General effects of exposure to these metals include headaches, neurological damage, cognitive impairment, and altered function of the kidneys, lungs, reproductive, immune, and cardiovascular systems (EPA, n.d.d.; EPA, n.d.a.).

Crop Residue Burning

Crop residue burning contributes to local air pollution in rural environments. Once crops are harvested, a variety of left-over materials remain such as stalks, shoots, leaves, and seedcases (Soccol et al., 2019). Farmers may choose to burn the crop waste as a practical way of managing the material. Nationwide, more than 1.2 million hectares of farmland are incinerated every year to manage crop residue. For comparison, this is equivalent to more than 40%

of the area consumed by naturally occurring wildfires annually (McCarty, Korontzi, Justice, & Loboda, 2009). When harvested products undergo partial processing for market or utility reasons, processing waste may also be fated for incineration. (Estrellan & Iino, 2010).

The five states that incinerate the most agricultural residues are Florida, Arkansas, Idaho, California, and Texas, which averaged between 79,000 hectares to over 319,000 hectares burned every year between 2003 and 2007 (McCarty, 2009). In terms of emissions, crop residue incineration is a source of atmospheric methane (CH_4), nitrous oxide (N_2O), carbon monoxide (CO), and nitrites (NO_x) (EPA, 2019c). The health and environmental significance of these air contaminants is discussed below under Criteria Pollutants. More effective farm production, as well as expanded crop residue practice, has resulted in higher emission levels, as reflected in the 82% increase in methane and 72% increase in nitrous oxide observed from 1990 to 2017. The crops that produce the highest levels of emissions from residue incineration include sugarcane, wheat, rice, and blue grass (McCarty, 2011).

Secondary Source: Criteria Air Pollutants

Criteria Air Pollutants

Since the Clean Air Act was established in 1970, the EPA defined National Ambient Air Quality (NAAQS) standards for six common pollutants known as the "criteria pollutants" associated with a variety of human health and environmental effects. These pollutants include particulate matter, ozone, sulfur dioxide, nitrogen dioxide, carbon monoxide, and lead (EPA, 2017b). There were major revisions made to the Clean Air Act in 1977 and 1990. These revisions aimed to improve the effectiveness of recognizing additional pollutants such as acid rain and greenhouse gases (EPA, 2017b).

In 2002, Congress provided funding to the CDC to establish the National Environmental Public Health Tracking Program. From 2008–2012, the CDC used three measures of air quality to assess the air quality in the nation. These measures were: 1) the number of days with levels of particulate matter ($PM_{2.5}$) greater than allowed by the U.S. Environmental Protection Agency National Ambient Air Quality Standards (NAAQS) in the average for a 24-hour period; 2) the annual mean of average ambient concentrations of $PM_{2.5}$ measured in micrograms per cubic meter; and finally 3) the number of days with the 8-hour maximum average ozone, which exceed NAAQS levels. The findings of this study are shown by urban-rural classification. The results showed that the air quality measures improved as the area became more rural (CDC, 2018). However, the secondary effects of criteria pollutants from urban air drift to rural environments is described below:

Particulate Matter (PM) is also called *particle pollution*. According to the EPA, this includes a mixture of solid and liquid particles found in the air. These particles that can be very small and cannot be seen by the naked eye "fine particles or $PM_{2.5}$," or large "coarse particle or PM_{10}" such as dust, smoke, soot, or dirt. The major components of PM include sulfate and nitrate compounds, carbon, and crustal materials such as soil and ash. In 2003, a report by EPA showed that $PM_{2.5}$ was higher in rural areas in the eastern part of the United States. This high concentration was attributed to emission sources such as power plants, natural sources, and urban pollution, which was transported hundreds of miles (EPA, 2004). In general, both PM_{10} and $PM_{2.5}$ have been improving nationwide and their levels have been decreasing everywhere. However, sulfates that account for 25–55% of $PM_{2.5}$ and produced mostly by power plants has been found to be similar in urban and rural areas (EPA, 2004).

Health effects of PM are greater with small particle size ($PM_{2.5}$ or less) since they can be inhaled more deeply in the lungs than coarse particles. Short-term effects (exposure for hours or days) can cause decreased lung functions, cardiac arrhythmias, and heart attack. Long-term effects (exposure for many years) can cause decreased lung function, chronic bronchitis, and premature death. The effects are worse on sensitive and high-risk populations, including people with heart and lung diseases, the elderly, and children (EPA, 2003).

Environmental Effects of PM are the contribution to haze and reduced visibility in the United States (EPA, 2018b). PM can also affect vegetation and causes soiling and erosion damage to structures, including culturally important objects such as monuments and statues (EPA, 2003).

Sulfur dioxide (SO_2), in addition to other sulfur oxide gases, is most concerning for air quality due to chemical reactions resulting in the formation of PM (Department of the Environment and Heritage, 2005; EPA, 2019d). Most SO gases (99%) are formed because of human activities such as the burning of fossil fuels and industrial activities; although there are some natural sources such as volcanic activities that contribute to the formation of these gases (EPA, 2019d). Natural sources of sulfur oxides cannot be underestimated. According to data from the United Nations Environmental Program in 1983, 80–288 million tons of sulfur oxide per year worldwide came from natural sources, compared with only 69 million tons related to human sources (Marja, 2011). Lefohn and Shadwick (1991) report that the concentration of SO_2 had declined in rural areas in the United States. More recent studies have estimated the approximate generation of SO_2 from crop residue burning in rural areas to be more than 4 gigagrams (Gg) annually (McCarty, 2011).

Health effects associated with exposure to SO_2 include difficulty breathing. Since SO_2 contributes to the formation of $PM_{2.5}$, health effects of high levels of SO_2 mimic PM exposure described above (EPA, 2019d).

Environmental Effects of high concentrations of SO_2 cause the formation of other sulfur oxides (SO_x). Together, SO_2 and SO_x contribute to PM pollution and to the formation of acid rain that is very harmful to the ecosystem and buildings and structures. In addition, SO_x decreases the growth of trees and plants and destroys foliage (EPA, 2019d).

Ozone "is a gas composed of three atoms of oxygen (O_3)" (EPA, 2018a). Stratospheric ozone, which is found in the upper atmosphere, is a very beneficial factor for health as it provides protection from ultraviolet rays. However, ground ozone is considered a harmful air pollutant and the major component of "smog" (EPA, 2018a). Ground ozone is usually created as a chemical reaction between oxides of nitrogen (NO_x) and volatile organic compounds

(VOC), combined with heat and sun in urban areas. Still, ozone can be transported for a long distance by winds and as a result, can affect rural areas (EPA, 2018a).

Health effects resulting from inhalation of ozone include, chest pain, coughing, throat irritation, airway inflammation, and reduced lung function. It can also exacerbate symptoms of bronchitis, emphysema, and asthma and increase the need for medical care. Other high-risk populations include, children, elderly, outdoor workers, and people with reduced intake to vitamins C and E. (EPA, 2018a)

Environmental Effects of ozone include harming vegetation such as forests and parks by reducing photosynthesis, slowing the growth of plants, and increasing the risk of the plants to get diseases and damage from insects (EPA, 2018a).

Nitrogen dioxide (NO_2) is a gas that is produced by burning fossil fuel used in cars, trucks, buses, power plants, and off-road equipment (EPA, 2016d). Human activity, including burning crop residue material is a contributor of nitrogen oxide (NO_2). An average of 10.6 Gg of NO_2 per year were generated from 2003 to 2007 (McCarty, 2011) via crop burning. Additionally, NO_2 can be produced from natural sources such as volcanoes, oceans, biological decay, and lightning strikes. Natural sources account for 20–90 million tons per year worldwide compared with 24 million tons produced from human sources (Marja, 2011).

Health effects of NO_2 depend on the duration of exposure. Short-term exposure can cause coughing, wheezing, difficulty breathing, and increased visits to emergency departments. This is especially a problem for those with asthma. Long-term exposure can cause asthma and lung infections specifically in high-risk populations such as children and the elderly (EPA, 2016d).

Environmental Effects of NO_2, along with other gases such as nitrous acid and nitric acid (also known as nitrogen oxides (NOx), can cause haze and acid rain. These would affect many rural areas, including coastal waters, national parks, and the ecosystems such as the lakes and forests (EPA, 2016d).

Carbon monoxide (CO) is a colorless and odorless gas produced by combustion. The main source of CO in outdoor air is vehicles such as cars, trucks, and other machineries that burn fossil fuels. For that reason, most of CO in outdoor air is found in urban areas in the United States (EPA, 2016b). However, burning agricultural residue from crops, including wheat, rice, and sugar cane resulted in an average CO generation of 232 Gg per year (Estrellan & Iino, 2010; McCarty, 2011).

Health effects of CO include dizziness, confusion, unconsciousness, and death. These effects occur only at high levels of exposure typically in indoor environments. Nevertheless, people with heart or lung conditions are more vulnerable to elevated CO levels in the environment and can suffer from chest pain (EPA, 2016b).

Environmental effects of CO are minimal.

Lead is a heavy metal that contributes to air pollution. According to the EPA, "major sources of lead in the air are ore and metals processing and piston-engine aircraft operating on leaded aviation fuel. Other sources are waste incinerators, utilities, and lead-acid battery manufacturers. The highest air concentrations of lead are usually found near lead smelters" (EPA, 2016c). Many regulatory efforts were established by the EPA to reduce exposure to lead. These regulations included the removal of lead from gasoline. As a result, the levels of lead in the air have declined 98% between 1980 and 2014 (EPA, 2016c). A potential lead source in rural regions includes the informal incineration of household waste, especially if they include electronic waste (discussed below) (Gullett et al., 2007).

Health effects of lead result from the impairment of multiple physiological systems, including nervous, kidney, immune, reproductive, developmental, and cardiovascular systems (EPA, 2016c). Lead is especially harmful to children and can contribute to behavioral and learning issues and lowered IQ.

Environmental Effects of lead result from deposition in soil, dust, and water. Lead can cause decreased growth in plants and animals and

neurological effects in vertebrates (EPA, 2016c). The deposits of lead in soil will not decompose so it will stay in the environment for years (EPA, 2016c).

Refer to **Exhibit 13-2** to learn about the effect of secondary sources of air pollution on the U.S. National Parks.

Tips from the Field: Health Professional Expert Advice

Backyard Burning: Best Practices

Understand State and Local Regulations and Recommendations

Backyard burning rules and regulations vary from state to state, with many entirely prohibiting the practice of backyard burning for household waste disposal. In states with no such ban, community-level ordinances may step in to restrict the activity or may only permit the burning of household waste under specific conditions and authorization. Most states will allow the burning of specific materials and vegetative debris, such as paper products, cardboard, foliage, shrubbery, grass, and branches. It is important to become

---

Exhibit 13-2 National Park Service

According to the National Park Service: "Over the last 30 years air quality has improved significantly in national parks and across the U.S. This is great news because parks need clean air. It is essential for the health of our visitors and employees, clean clear views of park scenery, and a healthy natural environment. But, we also know that almost all national parks are still affected by air pollution" (National Park Service, 2019). The National Park Service monitors the air quality in real time and on an annual basis to check for conditions and trends over time. Some of the conditions concerning visibility, secondary air pollutants (ozone, nitrogen, and sulfur) are shown below (National Park Service, 2019).

(continues)

Exhibit 13-2 National Park Service   (*continued*)

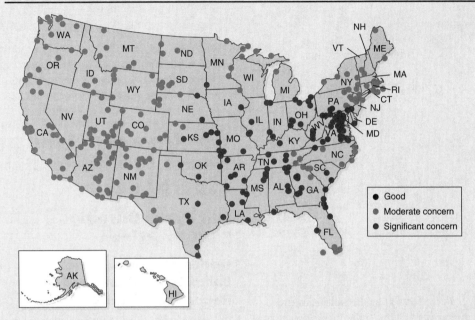

Visibility Conditions

National Park Service. (n.d.). NPS air conditions and trends. Retrieved from https://www.nps.gov/gis/storymaps/mapseries/v2/index.html?appid=73d71b11d2c044b9ab50cd2972de077e.

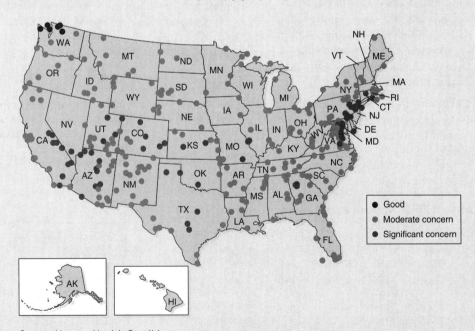

Ozone: Human Health Conditions

National Park Service. (n.d.). NPS air conditions and trends. Retrieved from https://www.nps.gov/gis/storymaps/mapseries/v2/index.html?appid=73d71b11d2c044b9ab50cd2972de077e.

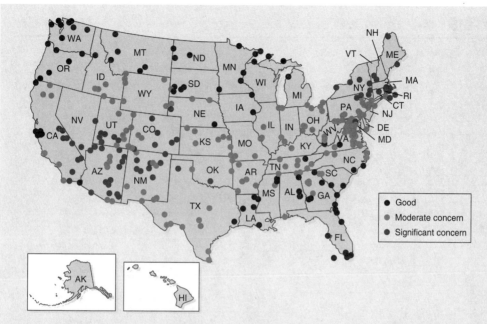

Ozone: Vegetation Health Conditions

National Park Service. (n.d.). NPS air conditions and trends. Retrieved from https://www.nps.gov/gis/storymaps/mapseries/v2/index.html?appid=73d71b11d2c044b9ab50cd2972de077e.

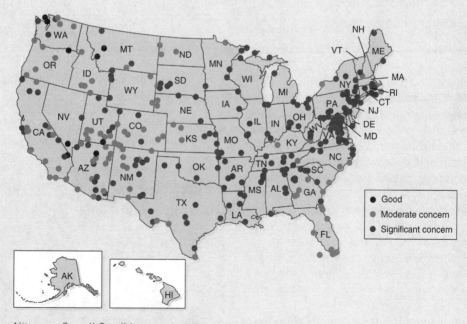

Nitrogen: Overall Conditions

National Park Service. (n.d.). NPS air conditions and trends. Retrieved from https://www.nps.gov/gis/storymaps/mapseries/v2/index.html?appid=73d71b11d2c044b9ab50cd2972de077e.

(continues)

Exhibit 13-2 National Park Service (continued)

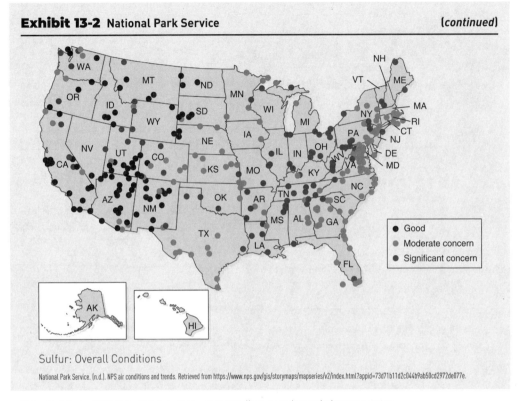

Sulfur: Overall Conditions

National Park Service. (n.d.). NPS air conditions and trends. Retrieved from https://www.nps.gov/gis/storymaps/mapseries/v2/index.html?appid=73d71b11d2c044b9ab50cd2972de077e.

National Park Service. (2019). Air Quality in Parks. Retrieved from https://www.nps.gov/subjects/air/airqualityparks.htm.

familiar with state and local regulations that may provide specific guidelines for items that can and cannot be incinerated. **Figure 13-4** shows unsafe practices for backyard burning.

Although it would be best for people to refrain from burning wastes, there may be strategies that can help to reduce the risk of wildfires, injury, and minimize exposure to harmful chemicals when burning nonhousehold wastes. Although not optimal, following certain specifications in constructing a burn barrel can reduce potential harms. Some states such as Alaska, mandate specific burn barrel design and practices, as described below (Alaska Department of Natural Resources, n.d.):

Recommended Burn Barrel Design (see **Figure 13-5**):

- A 55-gallon metal barrel.
- Vents equally spaced on the lower half of the barrel.

- The top of the barrel and the vents should be covered by 5/8-inch metal mesh.
- Located at least 50 feet from a utility tunnel and 30 feet from a building.

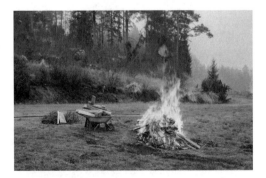

Figure 13-4 "A person cleaning out a shed burned a pile of wood scraps and decided to throw on a mattress."

© BM-W/Shutterstock.

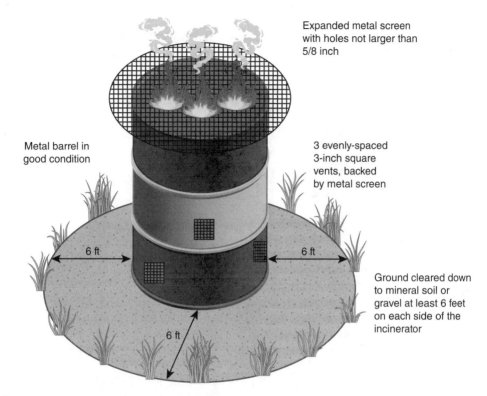

Figure 13-5 Recommended Burn Barrel Design.

Alaska Department of Natural Resources. (n.d.). Burn barrel specifications, debris pile requirements, and lawn burning. Retrieved from https://dnr.alaska.gov/burn /specifications.

- Remove all materials and vegetation at least 6 feet all around the barrel.

Best Practices:

- Items only allowed to be burned: paper, cardboard with no wax, untreated wood, and vegetative wastes.
- Items NOT to burn: household waste, plastics, rubber, Styrofoam, and items containing asbestos.
- Close monitoring and ensuring high strength in flames so that as much combustion takes place.
- Not burning when wind speeds are higher than 10 mph.
- Be aware of additional or temporary restrictions or prohibitions at the local level.

Exhibit 13-3 is an example of community education effort to teach residents about possible backyard burning hazards.

Solid Waste Management in Rural Communities

In 2017, the United States, comprising a little more than four percent of the globe's population (7.53 billion), is one of the top producers of waste. The United States generated the highest levels of waste in 2017, reaching more than 267.8 million tons of municipal solid waste (MSW) (EPA, 2019e). On a daily basis, an American resident generates almost 4.5 lbs. of MSW. Not surprisingly, cities and other highly populated areas produce the majority of waste, since they hold the vast majority of the country's population. Nevertheless, waste management in rural America, where 15% of the population resides, has unique characteristics and needs in order to achieve and maintain adequate environmental health.

Exhibit 13-3 Community Education on Backyard Burning Solid Waste Management in Rural Communities

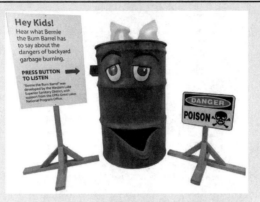

"Bernie the Burn Barrel" and related materials developed by the Western Lake Superior Sanitary District with support from the EPA's Great Lakes National Program Office.

A pioneer in understanding the dangers that garbage present and its common use by rural residents, the Western Lake Superior Sanitary District sought out to create an educational campaign that would discourage the practice in 2001. "Bernie the Burn Barrel" became the face of an educational campaign, finding himself in newspaper and television advertisements, posters, informational material, and a traveling prop for local events (see image below) (WLSSD, 2015). Since then, this effort to educate the public about the harm of burn barrels has spread to other states across the nation.

The Minnesota Pollution Control Agency developed a "Don't Burn Your Garbage" toolkit to discourage rural residents from setting fire to their household waste. It is publicly available (Minnesota Pollution Control Agency, n.d.). The toolkit consists of a number of educational materials that span a number of media. This includes informational material with details about the potential harms of burning garbage, a slide presentation, templates for local ordinances banning trash burning, and research materials (Minnesota Pollution Control Agency, n.d.). Radio announcements, an animated short video, and the "Bernie the Burn Barrel" event prop (picture below) are also available.

Data from Western Lake Superior Sanitary District. (2005). Clearing the air: Tools for reducing residential garbage burning. Retrieved from: https://wlssd .com/wp-content/uploads/2015/08/Clearing-the-Air-download-vs.pdf.

The establishment of the Environmental Protection Agency in 1970 provided the foundation for waste management regulation that largely enforces waste management systems across the United States (EPA, 2018c). Failing to closely monitor waste can present numerous issues for human health, and rural America presents particular waste management challenges. In addition to burning waste (discussed above), common concerns for this segment of the country include disposal of hazardous waste and electronic waste (e-waste).

Hazardous Waste

Hazardous wastes are solid wastes that are reactive, combustible, toxic, or corrosive in nature (EPA, 2019a). Federal law dictates that all individuals and organizations that generate waste are required to assess whether the waste is hazardous or not. Under the Resource Conservation and Recovery Act (RCRA), the material must first meet the definition of a solid waste, as well as three other conditions (**Figure 13-6**) (EPA, 2019a). First, the

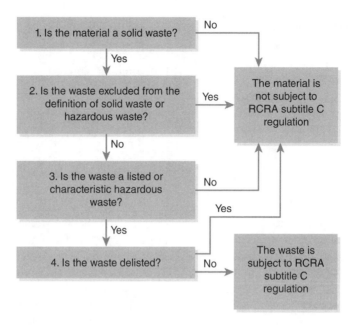

Figure 13-6 The Hazardous Waste Identification Process.

United States Environmental Protection Agency. (2019a). Defining hazardous waste: Listed, characteristic and mixed radiological wastes. Retrieved from https://www.epa.gov/hw/defining-hazardous-waste-listed-characteristic-and-mixed-radiological-wastes

term solid waste does not reflect the physical characteristics of a hazard, because wastes in liquid and sludge form may still be considered a solid waste. Second, certain wastes are not included in the definition of solid waste, which may not be a reflection on their level of harm but may be due to the logistical impracticality of monitoring their disposal. Third, the waste must either be listed as a hazardous waste or possess the qualities of one. If a waste is included as a delisted waste, they are not hazardous, and their disposal is under the jurisdiction of other regulation(s) (EPA, 2019a). Additionally, the EPA has amassed four lists that name specific wastes that are considered hazardous; they are referred to as the F, K, P, and U lists.

In rural areas, hazardous wastes are present in many forms in homes and as part of farming, including as paint, solvents, oils, cleaning products, preservatives, adhesives, and pesticides (Harris, Hoffman, &

Mazac, n.d.). Careful management, storage, and disposal of these items are important to avoid direct exposure, as well as to prevent contamination of water sources, soil, and the surrounding environment.

Tips from the Field: Health Professional Expert Advice

Hazardous Waste Management

Know Your State and Local Hazardous Waste Regulations and Resources

Learn about local hazardous material recycling, rules, accepted items, and suggestion on how to handle specific wastes. Reach out to inquire about further questions or concerns (Harris, Hoffman, & Mazac, n.d.).

Use Necessary Amounts of Hazardous Products

Minimize hazards by reducing the production of hazardous waste and practice proper recycling when they are generated (Harris, Hoffman, & Mazac, n.d.).

Safe Use

- Work with hazardous materials in areas and on surfaces that minimize chances of chemicals spilling on the ground, to the soil, and ultimately ground water.
- Keep a spill kit conveniently available and understand how to properly use all items in it.

Safe Storage

- Store hazardous materials and chemicals 150 feet from water sources, at the same level or downhill (Harris, Hoffman, & Mazac, n.d.).
- Keep containers to refill with leftover amounts of the product or in case of leaking. This may include antifreeze, oil, solvents, paint, etc.
- Adequately separate and prevent exposure of different types of chemical products and wastes to avoid chemical reactions.

Safe Disposal

Rinse pesticide containers three times and follow administration instructions to apply the solution to fields at the indicated rate.

e-Waste

The United States generates the second-highest quantity of electronic waste after China (Balde et al., 2017). Electronic waste (e-waste) is the stream of waste composed of electronic equipment and devices, as well as their parts, when deemed no longer usable. Categories of e-waste include (Balde et al., 2017):

1. "Temperature exchange equipment" (refrigerators, air conditioners, etc.)
2. Screens (TVs, laptops, tablets, etc.)
3. Lamps and bulbs
4. Large appliances (washers, driers, stoves, office printers, etc.)
5. "Small equipment" (microwaves, ovens, cameras, toys, personal medical machines, etc.)
6. "Small IT and telecommunication equipment" (home computers, small calculators, cell phones, etc.).

The lifecycle of e-waste products, as well as the proper recycling methods, varies, even among items in the same category (Balde et al., 2017). Once these electronics are discarded; however, proper recycling can salvage reusable components. Various components, such as plastics, steel, aluminum, copper, gold, and silver are difficult to extract from the earth, to produce, or simply exist in a limited quantity. In 2016, the world created approximately 45 MT (million tons) of electronic waste, only one-fifth of which was adequately recycled (Balde, et al., 2017).

E-waste has the greatest potential to harm rural communities when improperly disposed of in landfills, dumps, or as material in backyard burning. Since electronic products vary widely in their internal components, even within categories, their hazard potential also varies significantly. A wide variety of chemical hazards is present in e-waste, including persistent organic pollutants; dioxins and dioxin-like chemicals; and heavy metals such as lead, chromium, mercury, cadmium, nickel, lithium, and more (Grant et al., 2013). Studies that recreate the burning of electric circuits and wires find that burn barrel practices release high concentrations of polychlorinated dibenzodioxins and dibenzofurans (PCDD/PCDFs), as well as particulates of bromine, tin, copper, and more than 200 times the permitted concentration of lead produced in regulated incinerators (Gullett et al., 2007).

The production of e-waste is projected to increase, which presents an opportunity for decision makers to help improve the way these wastes are generated and recycled. A major factor in this generation is the use of information and communication technology (ICT) items (cell phones, tables, etc.) at increasing rates (Balde et al., 2017). Not surprisingly, very limited data on e-waste disposal exists in rural communities. Urban and suburban localities generally have some formal e-waste collection services established. However, systems in rural America largely rely on volunteer-based programs, which can vary widely between rural communities.

Federal legislation does not require tracking or providing disposal guidelines for e-waste (Schumacher & Agbemabiese, 2019). Approximately one-half of the states in the United States have legislation addressing e-waste, but not all types of waste from electronics are managed (EPA, n.d.f.). Nevertheless, certain products, due to the hazardous potential of internal components, fall under the jurisdiction of environmental regulations at the federal level. The lead content in cathode ray tubes (CRT) in older versions of television and computer monitors, for example, may be high enough for these devices to be considered hazardous waste under the Resource Conservation and Recovery Act (RCRA) (EPA, n.d.f.).

Individual state regulations may provide procedures for disposal. Michigan, for instance, has an "Electronic Waste Takeback Program" that requires manufacturers to track and have a recycling program for computers, electronic tablets, printers, and monitors (MDEGE, n.d.). Other categories of e-waste may still be destined for the landfill. **Exhibit 13-4** also provides a short description of an e-waste program in Alaska known as the "Backhaul Alaska" project which specifically addresses the need to safely discard e-waste in rural regions.

Commercial Agribusiness

Once virtually self-sufficient and self-reliant, farms have become integrated in several other systems, markets, and industries. Noticing the increased interconnectedness between the agricultural sector and other industries in the development of the modern economy, Davis & Goldberg (1957) proposed the term "Agribusiness" to frame this vast network of increasingly interrelated and interdependent fields. As such, **agribusiness** is related

Exhibit 13-4 Backhaul Alaska: Hazardous Waste Management in Alaskan Rural Communities

For those in remote regions, proper storage and collection pose the largest risk to environmental health, and various programs have attempted to address these needs. Sparsely populated areas, which are also geographically difficult to reach, do not lend themselves to efficient hazardous waste collection. However, waste management programs have been proposed as potentially effective and financially feasible. One such program is the EPA-funded "Backhaul Alaska" project, which began its trial stage in 2018 and will operate for 10 years (Backhaul Alaska, n.d.). Collaborating with over two dozen towns across Alaska, this program seeks to coordinate the removal of electronic waste, fluorescent light bulbs, and lead acid batteries from these sites (Backhaul Alaska, n.d.). The project also encourages waste prevention by providing waste management information to rural waste generators.

Modified from Backhaul Alaska. (n.d.). Overview. Retrieved from http://www.backhaulalaska.org/

to a wide number and variety of fields, including farming practices, research, economics, manufacturing, policy, and more. As a generalization, Commercial Agribusiness examines how goods move from production, processing, distribution, and the market, as well as the factors that help or hinder these processes.

Analyses have demonstrated an increase in agricultural product demand. Between 2005 and 2050, the predicted world population increase will be accompanied with a 100% increase in demand for calories from foods derived from crops (Tilman, Balzer, Hill, & Befort, 2011). The 2017 Census of Agriculture (USDA, 2019) reported the number of U.S. farms at approximately 2 million and noted an increase in large and small farms, while mid-sized farms decreased in number. Large farms (generating $5 million sales) were less than 1% of all farms but comprised more than one-third of all sales.

Small farms (sales less than $50,000) made up 76% of all farms, yet their combined sales added up to 3% of overall sales. Collectively, the United States devotes 40% of its land to agriculture. Farm distribution is depicted in **Figure 13-7**. States with the highest sales in agriculture products were California, Iowa, and Texas. The top ranked commodities include cattle and calves, corn, poultry and eggs, soybeans, and milk. The prevalence of farms in rural communities creates unique environmental exposures.

Exposures in Farming Communities

In addition to unique occupational hazards in rural communities (discussed in Chapter 14), residents may also experience a variety of health concerns due to the impact of agribusiness on water quality, air quality, agricultural waste generation, and zoonotic disease risk.

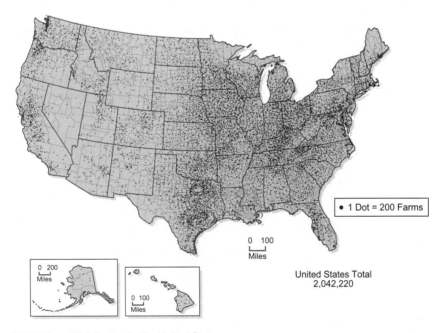

Figure 13-7 Farm Distribution in the United States.

United States Department of Agriculture. (2019). 2017 Census of Agriculture: United States Summary and State Data. Retrieved from https://www.nass.usda.gov/Publications/AgCensus/2017/Full_Report/Volume_1,_Chapter_1_US/usv1.pdf

Water Quality

Of the 1.1 billion pounds of pesticides used annually, 90% are associated with agricultural application. Furthermore, herbicides account for 60% of pesticide usage. The herbicide glyphosate is the #1 ranked pesticide in the agricultural market sector. Glyphosate use has increased in recent history (Benbrook, 2016). Estimated glyphosate application in 2016 is depicted in **Figure 13-8**. When mixed with other inactive ingredients, it makes up the well-known and commercially available glyphosate-based products RangerPro and RoundUp. In the environment, soil bacteria break down the herbicide, but this degradation process does not occur in water, which increases the likelihood of water contamination from runoff.

Health Effects of glyphosate have become a concern in recent years. Although considered harmless for many years, potential health effects, including carcinogenic potential have

become more pronounced. The EPA has stated that "there are no risks to public health when glyphosate is used in accordance with its current label and that glyphosate is not a carcinogen" (EPA, 2019b). Although previously in accordance with the EPA's decision, the European Food Safety Authority (EFSA) in 2019 cited epidemiologic evidence suggesting neurological effects on children and proclaimed that there was no acceptable minimum level of exposure for the chemical (EFSA, 2019). Additionally, the World Health Organization's International Agency for Research on Cancer (IARC) classified glyphosate a Group 2A compound, indicating that it is "probably carcinogenic to humans" (IARC, 2015). These differing conclusions among the IARC and the EPA regarding the health effects of glyphosate have been noted and are likely due to the evidence considered by each analysis (Benbrook, 2019). The EPA's analysis centered on the effects of glyphosate

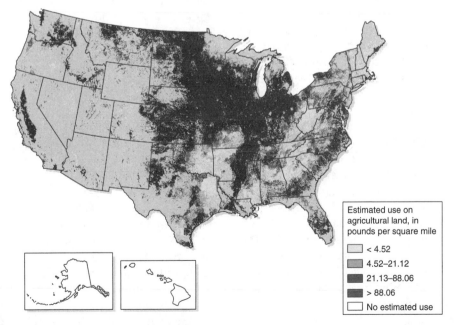

Figure 13-8 Estimated Agricultural Use for Glyphosate, 2016.

United States Geological Survey. (2018). Estimated Annual Agricultural Pesticide Use. Retrieved from https://water.usgs.gov/nawqa/pnsp/usage/maps/show_map.php?year=2016&map=GLYPHOSATE&hilo=L

agricultural product consumers, not on the occupational handling of pesticides on farms or evidence pertaining to residential drift exposure. This appraisal only made a conclusion on pure glyphosate and placed considerable importance on industry-collected data. Alternatively, the IARC placed more weight on both high exposure circumstances (occupational) and examined glyphosate-based pesticides containing additional inactive ingredients.

Air Quality

Generally, rural communities experience better air quality compared with urban communities. Overall, cities are host to higher rates of respiratory issues, especially asthma and allergies. Studies conducted in Europe show a lower burden of respiratory conditions in rural areas compared with more urbanized localities (Ege et al., 2011; Genuneit, 2012; Horak et al., 2014; Parsons, Beach, & Senthilselvan, 2017). In fact, a number of these studies are regularly cited as supporting the Hygiene Hypothesis, which states that childhood exposure to a diversity of microscopic agents (bacteria, viruses, fungi) imparts an immunological defense against allergies. Thus, a growing body of evidence suggests there is a protective effect to living by farms as it pertains to allergies and asthma.

Despite these proposed respiratory benefits related to rural residence, farming practices in the United States may have an opposite effect, posing a risk to respiratory health. Compared with European animal farms, American farms have larger and more densely packed animal operations. Accompanying this intensification in farming productivity is the increased generation of animal wastes and particulate matter that affect nearby rural inhabitants. Moreover, these exposures can further intensify symptomology for individuals with existing respiratory conditions.

Concentrated animal feeding operations (CAFOs) are large animal farms that house livestock to produce meat, milk, eggs, and more, pose a concern to residential air quality. The USDA estimates that around 450,000 CAFOs are established across the country (USDA, n.d.). CAFOs are categorized by the number and size of the livestock kept, or the use of pits or bodies of water for waste disposal (Hribar, 2010). From these animal farms, winds can carry "dusts, bacteria, mold, hydrogen sulfide, ammonia, methane, pharmaceutical residues, and animal dander" (Mirabelli et al., 2006). Some of these airborne particles are viable organisms (fungi, bacteria, and viruses), or their fragments and byproducts (dander, dust, mycotoxins, endotoxins, ammonia, etc.), and referred to as bioaerosols (Dungan, 2010). Farms with high density of livestock can produce high quantities of bioaerosols, which can be carried by wind to residents in the surrounding area (Dungan, 2010).

Health Effects near CAFOs in the United States include higher levels of asthma than expected among children for rural regions. Pavilonis, Sanderson, and Merchant (2013) found asthma among children and prescribed medication for asthma and asthma symptoms were more likely among children exposed to CAFOs. Iowa children living in swine farms that use antibiotics have been found to have high asthma or asthma-like symptoms (Merchant et al., 2005). Another study in Iowa found similar prevalence of asthma symptoms in rural counties as cities in the region (Chrischilles et al., 2004). In addition to residences, Sigurdarson and Kline (2006) found that children attending schools 0.5 miles or closer to an CAFO had more than five times the odds of having diagnosed asthma compared with students in schools more than 10 miles away from an CAFO (Sigurdarson & Kline, 2006).

Children are more highly impacted by exposure due to body size and underdeveloped immune systems. Certain social determinants also influence exposure to CAFOs. Researchers Mirabelli et al., (2006) analyzed 339 North Carolina public schools, and found lower social economic status were more likely in close proximity to swine CAFOs, and to a lesser extent, schools with more children of color (Mirabelli et al., 2006).

Studies involving respiratory issues of American adults residing near CAFOs demonstrate similar negative health effects. Exploring the relationship between animal farm proximity and asthma-related conditions, Rasmussen, et al., (2017) found a 29% increased chance of hospitalization and 11% increased chance of corticosteroid medication prescription for residents within 3 miles of an industrial animal farm. In Wisconsin, when comparing adults living 5 miles from a CAFO, those within 1.5 miles had more than two times the odds of asthma, nasal and lung allergies, and uncontrolled asthma, as well as an increased use of medication for asthma and a noted decrease in lung function (Schultz, Peppard, Gangnon, & Malecki, 2019).

Agricultural Waste

In term of quantities, more agricultural waste is created in the United States than municipal solid waste (Pichtel, 2005). The major components of this waste include crop residue/particulates (see air quality), manure from livestock, and pesticide use and storage (see water quality and air quality).

There are largely two ways of characterizing farm animal waste: dry and liquid form. This is in reference to the moisture content in the manure that provides the waste's characteristics and has important implications relating to hazardous gasses when managing its storage. Certain gasses such as ammonia (NH_3), carbon dioxide (CO_2), hydrogen sulfide (H_2S), methane (CH_4), and nitrous oxide (N_2O) are associated with manure storage

units and can be harmful to humans in sufficient concentrations (Pichtel, 2005; EPA, 2019c). Improper storage and failure to heed precautions have resulted in negative acute health effects, specially affecting children and older individuals.

For liquid manure storage, there is generally a higher potential for harm. Precautions must be taken when liquid manure undergoes agitation, a process in which water is introduced to contained waste in order to create a slurry waste substance that is more easily pumped out of its container. This is occasionally done for the pits directly under livestock habitat areas, for example. The agitation in waste material during this process may expose people to toxic levels of ammonia, hydrogen sulfide, methane, and carbon dioxide. Methane production is at a higher concern when manure is in a position to promote anaerobic processes, such as when held in lagoons, ponds, tanks, or pits. Due to the increased number of CAFOs, as well as other regulations overlooking the administration of manure nutrients on farmland, the storage of manure in liquid form is being used increasingly (EPA, 2019c).

Manure can also accumulate in areas that will minimize the chance of runoff or not be too close to bodies of water. The two major options here are called stockpiling and dry stacking, where methane is not generated in high levels due to more exposure to oxygen during the decomposition. Although less likely to be harmful, nitrous oxide can leach to underground water reservoirs and flow into bodies of water as runoff.

Zoonotic Diseases in Rural Settings

Due to higher frequent exposure to animals, residents in rural communities are at higher risk of **zoonotic** diseases, or conditions contracted from animals (LeJeune & Kersting, 2010).

The One Health Zoonotic Disease Prioritization (OHZDP) Workshop was held in December of 2017 and was organized by the U.S. Centers for Disease Control and Prevention (CDC), the U.S. Department of Agriculture (USDA), and the U.S. Department of the Interior (DOI). This workshop identified eight zoonotic diseases from a list of emerging and **endemic** zoonoses using reportable disease lists, reports, and data on zoonotic diseases of concern (CDC Workshop, 2017). The list included zoonotic influenza viruses, salmonellosis, West Nile virus, plague, emerging coronaviruses, rabies virus, brucellosis, and Lyme disease (**Table 13-4**). Refer to **Exhibit 13-5** for more details.

Table 13-4 Top 8 Zoonotic Diseases in the United States (CDC Workshop, 2017)

1. Zoonotic influenza (zoonotic influenza A viruses)

2. Salmonellosis (*Salmonella* species)

3. West Nile virus (Flaviviridae, *Flavivirus*)

4. Plague (*Yersinia pestis*)

5. Emerging coronaviruses (Coronaviridae; i.e., severe acute respiratory syndrome [SARS-CoV] and Middle East respiratory syndrome [MERS-CoV])

6. Rabies (Rhabdoviridae, *Lyssavirus*)

7. Brucellosis (*Brucella* species)

8. Lyme disease (*Borrelia burgdorferi*)

Centers for Disease Control and Prevention (CDC). One Health Zoonotic Disease Prioritization. (2017). Prioritizing zoonotic diseases for multisectoral, One Health collaboration in the United States: Workshop summary. Retrieved from https://www.cdc.gov/onehealth /pdfs/us-ohzdp-report-508.pdf.

Exhibit 13-5 Profiles of the Top 8 Zoonotic Diseases in the U.S. Information

Profiles of the Top 8 Zoonotic Diseases in the U.S. Information taken from the workshop summary report of Prioritizing Zoonotic Diseases for Multisectoral, One Health Collaboration in the United State, 2017. For more information and to review the full report, please visit https://www.cdc.gov /onehealth/pdfs/us-ohzdp-report-508.pdf

1. Zoonotic Influenza

Causative Agent
- Influenza A viruses normally maintained in domestic and wild animals but that can be transmitted between animal species, including humans. Disease Burden and Impacts

Human Disease Burden
- Some animal influenza viruses are zoonotic and occasionally infect humans, although sustained human-to-human transmission requires host adaptation. This includes certain avian H5, H7,

and H9 viruses and swine influenza viruses that may infect humans (referred to as "variant" viruses when infecting humans and designated with letter "v" including H3N2v, H1N1v, and H1N2v.

- In the United States, no human infections with any avian influenza A H5 or H9 viruses have been identified to date. One human infection with avian-origin influenza A (H7N2) virus was reported in 2016, in a person with prolonged unprotected exposure to the respiratory secretions of infected cats at an animal shelter experiencing an outbreak of H7N2 virus in cats. This virus was ultimately characterized to be of avian-origin.
- Influenza viruses that circulate in swine such as H3N2 may cause sporadic human disease, with limited human-to-human transmission. From 2005 to 2017, 468 human infections of variant viruses (mainly H3N2v) were recorded in the United States.
- In the United States, the largest zoonotic disease outbreak of recent years was the 2009 H1N1 pandemic, which led to an estimated 60.8 million human cases and over 12,000 human deaths in the United States.

Environmental Impacts

- USDA and the DOI's U.S. Geological Survey (USGS) actively coordinate with other federal, state, and tribal wildlife, agricultural, and human health agencies to understand avian influenza introductions from foreign sources. They also look at introduction into poultry production operations and distribution across the landscape among host species, including dynamics within and among biotic and abiotic reservoirs. This aids natural resource managers, agricultural officials, and the poultry industry in understanding this disease.
- A 2015 USGS ground water study identified three wells and one lagoon that were positive for the matrix gene indicative of influenza A virus, with one well positive for H5 virus, suggesting that it is possible for avian influenza viruses to be transported to ground water.
- Outbreaks of HPAI can affect wild bird populations, which could have a negative impact on recreational activities related to wildlife resources, such as tourism and hunting.

2. Salmonellosis

Causative Agent

- *Salmonella* species (bacteria)

Human Disease Burden

- Salmonellosis is one of the most important foodborne diseases in the United States. It sickens an estimated 1.2 million people annually, approximately 400 cases per 100,000 persons per year, most of which are not laboratory-confirmed. It also leads to approximately 23,000 hospitalizations and 450 deaths.
- In 2017, FoodNet data indicated that *Salmonella* was responsible for an estimated 17 laboratory-confirmed illnesses per 100,000 persons in the United States.
- In 2017, 48 U.S. multistate *Salmonella* outbreaks were linked to contact with backyard poultry, resulting in 1,120 laboratory-confirmed illnesses, 249 hospitalizations, and 1 death. That same year, contact with pet turtles resulted in 76 laboratory-confirmed illnesses and 30 hospitalizations.
- Multi-drug resistant (MDR) strains of *Salmonella* have been detected in food, environmental sampling, and human case outbreaks. These are associated with more severe illness and more adverse outcomes.

Environmental Impacts

- *Salmonella* has been found in high levels in surface water used for irrigation, which may be connected to produce-related outbreaks.

(continues)

Exhibit 13-5 *(continued)*

---

3. West Nile Virus (WNV)

Causative Agent

- Flaviviridae, *Flavivirus*

Human Disease Burden

- Between 2014 and 2016, incidence has remained around 0.40/100,000 population. Case fatality rate is approximately 6%. In 2017 alone, there were 1,937 cases, 1,293 neuroinvasive cases, and 115 deaths reported to CDC. The disease is most common in mid-to-late summer. Neuroinvasive disease can cause long-term disability. Human incidence can vary considerably among years or regions of the United States due to climate and weather conditions that support enzootic transmission (the virus amplifies among birds and mosquitoes). There is evidence that as many as 70 unreported cases of WNV occur for every reported case. Immunity among avian amplifiers also regulates transmission levels.

Environmental Impacts

- The original WNV outbreak led to a marked decrease in the crow population in the United States, which as of 2007, was still recovering. There continues to be concern regarding the impact of WNV on the persistence and recovery of grouse and wild turkey populations. Other bird species, such as black-billed magpie and black-capped chickadee, appear to have been less severely affected or to have returned to normal more rapidly. Without the use of an experimental DNA vaccine among the endangered California Condor population, it is likely that this species would have become extinct due to WNV infections.

4. Plague

Causative Agent

- *Yersinia pestis* (bacteria)

Human Disease Burden

- From 1965 to 2012, a median of 8 cases of plague were reported in the United States annually. During this time period, the human case fatality rate was approximately 13%. Although the endemic burden is small, pneumonic plague has epidemic potential. Yersinia pestis is a potential bioterrorist agent and is classified as a tier 1 biological agent on the HHS Select Agents and Toxins list.

Environmental Impacts

- Plague can cause up to 90% mortality in prairie dog colonies, leading to local extinction. Black-footed ferrets are also susceptible to the disease, and direct mortality as well as loss of the prairie dog food supply are major obstacles to population recovery. Many other sensitive species, such as badger, swift fox, mountain plover, burrowing owl, and others, are associated with the habitat or prey base that prairie dogs provide, and thus are also affected by plague on the landscape.

5. Emerging Coronaviruses

Causative Agent

- Coronaviridae- Examples include severe acute respiratory syndrome-associated coronavirus (SARS-CoV) and Middle East respiratory syndrome coronavirus (MERS-CoV).

Human Disease Burden

- There have been two travel-acquired cases of MERS-CoV in the U.S. in 2014, neither of which was fatal. During the 2002-2003 SARS outbreak, there were 27 probable cases in the United States, none of which were fatal.

Environmental Impacts
- There is no evidence that either MERS-CoV or SARS-CoV has the potential to cause a significant environmental impact. Contact with wildlife may have been associated with the 2003 SARS outbreak in China.

6. Rabies Virus

Causative Agent
- Rhabdoviridae, *Lyssavirus*

Human Disease Burden
- It is estimated that U.S. citizens experience a potential rabies exposure at a rate of 140 exposures per 100,000 persons each year (40,000 – 50,000 exposures annum). Post-exposure prophylaxis costs an average of $4,500 U.S. dollars (USD) per person, for an estimated national PEP expenditure of at least $225 million. Compulsory rabies vaccination of domestic pets is a critical component for preventing human deaths and is estimated to cost pet owners more than $30 million per year.
- Overall, rabies control costs in the United States exceed $510 million annually.
- Despite relatively frequent human rabies exposures in the United States, human deaths are relatively uncommon due to accessible post-exposure treatment. There have been an average of 2.8 cases per year from 2003–2015.
- Globally, rabies causes approximately 60,000 deaths annually, more than any other zoonotic pathogen.

Environmental Impacts
- The USDA APHIS Wildlife Services conducts a wildlife rabies control program targeting raccoons in the Eastern United States and foxes along the U.S. Mexico border. This program distributes more than 10 million oral rabies vaccine (ORV) baits to prevent expansion of the endemic zone. An economic evaluation of rabies prevention data indicates that for every dollar spent on a coyote ORV program in Texas, between $4 and $13 USD are saved.
- The domestic dog-coyote variant of rabies was successfully eliminated from the United States in 2008 as a result of an ORV baiting program in Texas, proving that ORV of wildlife can successfully eliminate terrestrial rabies.
- Rabies is considered a threat to endangered populations of carnivores in Africa.

7. Brucellosis

Causative Agent
- *Brucella* species (bacteria)

Human Disease Burden
- Incidence in the United States is 0.4 cases per million. There are approximately 100 cases per year reported in the United States, with the highest numbers reported by California, Texas, Arizona, and Florida. Brucellosis is rarely fatal if treated; in untreated cases, case fatality rate ranges from <2 to 5%. Death is usually caused by endocarditis or meningitis. Most cases recover in 2-4 weeks, although a minority of patients become chronically ill, and relapse can occur even in successfully treated cases. Most human cases are acquired overseas or due to consumption of infected milk products.

Environmental Impacts
- Brucellosis affects populations of bison and elk. Yellowstone bison birth rates are significantly lower for seropositive Yellowstone bison. The population impacts on elk are less well studied, but brucellosis is known to cause abortion.

(continues)

Exhibit 13-5   *(continued)*

---

8. Lyme disease

Causative Agent
- *Borrelia burgdorferi* (bacteria)

Human Disease Burden
- *Borrelia burgdorferi*, an obligatory zoonosis, is the most common vector-borne pathogen in the United States. During 2004-2016, more than 400,000 cases were reported to CDC, but these might represent as little as 10% of true incidence. The range of the principal vector, the tick Ixodes scapularis, has been expanding and the number of cases rising, representing a substantial burden on state and local health department resources in high incidence states. Lyme disease is rarely fatal, but the economic cost of testing, treatment, and lost productivity is a major national burden. Even with treatment, a small percentage of cases experience posttreatment Lyme disease syndrome and experience symptoms such as fatigue and muscle aches that can last for more than 6 months.

Environmental Impacts
- It is not well understood what the impacts of Lyme disease and efforts to manage ticks are on ecology and wildlife health. Deer population control measures have been instituted in many locations in the northeastern United States due to rampant Lyme disease, but more research is needed to understand the relationship between deer populations and human Lyme disease cases.
- The desirability of housing near natural areas and the increasing attraction of outdoor recreation might be increasing human exposure to infected tick bite.
- Environmental changes may lead to increased range of the tick vector. Forest fragmentation is associated with increased infection prevalence in ticks.

Discussion Questions

1. Explain actions for preventing well water contamination.
2. Describe conditions that require a well water test.
3. Research a recent example of drinking water contamination in a rural community.
4. What are the most important air pollutants seen in rural United States?
5. Describe the human and environmental impacts of three of the air pollutants in rural areas in the United States.
6. List the five zoonotic diseases seen in the United States and describe their human and environmental impact.
7. How do agricultural practices affect the health of surrounding communities in terms of air quality?
8. Look up the "Don't Burn Your Garbage" toolkit on the Minnesota Pollution Control Agency website. How would you incorporate this into a local event in your community?
9. Visit your state and local community environmental websites. What regulations and restrictions do they have on backyard burning?
10. What are the four main characteristics of a hazardous waste?

Additional Readings

- Friis, R. H. (2018). Essentials of Environmental Health (Essential Public Health) (3rd Ed.), Sudbury, MA: Jones and Bartlett.
- Zimeri, A. (2017). Introduction to Environmental Health: A Global Perspective (2nd Ed.), San Diego, CA: Cognella Academic Publishing.
- Levy, B. Wegman, D. Baron, S. and R. Sokas. (2017). Occupational and Environmental Health (7th Ed.), New York, NY: Oxford University Press.

Student activities and worksheets are available for use inside the Navigate eBook, included with the printed text. Simply redeem the access code found at the front of the book at www.jblearning.com.

References

Agency for Toxic Substances & Disease Registry. (2015b). Public health statement for hexachlorobenzene. Retrieved from https://www.atsdr.cdc.gov/phs/phs.asp?id=625&tid=115

Airborne Toxic Control Measure to Reduce Emissions of Toxic Air Contaminants from Outdoor Residential Waste Burning. (2004). Section 93113, title 17. Retrieved from https://ww2.arb.ca.gov/resources/documents/outdoor-residential-waste-burning-0

Alaska Department of Natural Resources. (n.d.). Burn barrel specifications, debris pile requirements, and lawn burning. Retrieved from https://dnr.alaska.gov/burn/specifications

Australian Government Department of Agriculture, Water and the Environment. (2005). Sulfur dioxide (SO_2). Retrieved from https://www.environment.gov.au/protection/publications/factsheet-sulfur-dioxide-so2

Backhaul Alaska. (n.d.). Overview. Retrieved from http://www.backhaulalaska.org/

Baldé, C. P., Forti, V., Gray, V., Kuehr, R., & Stegmann, P. (2017). The global e-waste monitor 2017: Quantities, flows and resources. United Nations University, International Telecommunication Union, and International Solid Waste Association. Retrieved from https://collections.unu.edu/view/UNU:6341

Benbrook, C. M. (2016). Trends in glyphosate herbicide use in the United States and globally. *Environmental Sciences Europe, 28*(3).

Benbrook, C. M. (2019). How did the US EPA and IARC reach diametrically opposed conclusions on the genotoxicity of glyphosate-based herbicides? *Environmental Sciences Europe, 31*(2).

Benedict, K. M., Reses H., Vigar, M., Roth, D. M., Roberts, V. A., Mattioli M., . . . Hill, V. R. 2017. Surveillance for waterborne disease outbreaks associated with drinking water — United States, 2013–2014. *MMWR Morbidity and Mortality Weekly Report, 66*(44), 1216–1221.

Centers for Disease Control and Prevention (CDC). (2009). Well siting & potential contaminants. Retrieved from https://www.cdc.gov/healthywater/drinking/private/wells/location.html

Centers for Disease Control and Prevention (CDC). (2015a). Overview of water-related diseases and contaminants in private wells. Retrieved from https://www.cdc.gov/healthywater/drinking/private/wells/diseases.html

Centers for Disease Control and Prevention (CDC). (2017a). Polycyclic aromatic hydrocarbons (PAHs) factsheet. Retrieved from https://www.cdc.gov/biomonitoring/PAHs_FactSheet.html

Centers for Disease Control and Prevention (CDC). (2017b). Rural Americans at higher risk of death from five leading causes: Demographic, environmental, economic, social factors might be key to difference. Retrieved from https://www.cdc.gov/media/releases/2017/p0112-rural-death-risk.html

Centers for Disease Control and Prevention (CDC). (2018). National environmental public health tracking: history. Retrieved from https://www.cdc.gov/nceh/tracking/background.htm

Centers for Disease Control and Prevention (CDC). (2019). Rural health: Leading causes of death in rural America. Retrieved from https://www.cdc.gov/ruralhealth/cause-of-death.html

Centers for Disease Control and Prevention (CDC). One Health Zoonotic Disease Prioritization. (2017). Prioritizing zoonotic diseases for multisectoral, One Health collaboration in the United States: Workshop summary. Retrieved from https://www.cdc.gov/onehealth/pdfs/us-ohzdp-report-508.pdf

Centers for Disease Control and Prevention (CDC) and U.S. Department of Housing and Urban Development. (2006). Healthy housing reference manual. Retrieved from https://www.cdc.gov/nceh/publications/books/housing/housing_ref_manual_2012.pdf

Chrischilles, E., Ahrens, R., Kuehl, A., Kelly, K., Thorne, P., Burmeister, L., & Merchant, J. (2004). Asthma prevalence and morbidity among rural Iowa schoolchildren. *Journal of Allergy and Clinical Immunology, 113*(1), 66–71.

Davis, J. G. & Whiting, D. (2013). Choosing a soil amendment. Retrieved from https://extension.colostate.edu/topic-areas/yard-garden/choosing-a-soil-amendment/

Davis, J. H., & Goldberg, R. A. (1957). Concept of agribusiness.

Dungan, R. S. (2010). Board-invited review: Fate and transport of bioaerosols associated with livestock operations and manures. *Journal of Animal Science, 88*(11), 3693–3706.

Ege, M. J., Mayer, M., Normand, A. C., Genuneit, J., Cookson, W. O., Braun-Fahrländer, C., . . . von Mutius, E. (2011). Exposure to environmental microorganisms and childhood asthma. *New England Journal of Medicine, 364*(8), 701–709.

Estrellan, C. R., & Iino, F. (2010). Toxic emissions from open burning. *Chemosphere, 80*(3), 193–207.

European Food Safety Authority (EFSA). (2015). Glyphosate: EFSA updates toxicological profile. Retrieved from https://www.efsa.europa.eu/en/press/news/151112

Genuneit, J. (2012). Exposure to farming environments in childhood and asthma and wheeze in rural populations: A systematic review with meta-analysis. *Pediatric Allergy and Immunology, 23*(6), 509–518.

Goetzman, Keith. (2016). A Burning problem: Torching garbage has serious consequences for the environment—yet it's a Minnesota habit that's been hard to break. Minnesota Department of Natural Resources. Retrieved from https://www.dnr.state.mn.us/mcvmagazine/issues/2016/may-jun/illegal-burning.html

Grant, K., Goldizen, F. C., Sly, P. D., Brune, M. N., Neira, M., van den Berg, M., & Norman, R. E. (2013). Health consequences of exposure to e-waste: A systematic review. *The Lancet Global Health, 1*(6), e350–e361.

Gullett, B. K., Linak, W. P., Touati, A., Wasson, S. J., Gatica, S., & King, C. J. (2007). Characterization of air emissions and residual ash from open burning of electronic wastes during simulated rudimentary recycling operations. *Journal of Material Cycles and Waste Management, 9*(1), 69–79.

Harris, B. L., Hoffman, D. W., & Mazac, F. J. (n.d.). Reducing contamination by improving hazardous waste management. Retrieved from https://blackland.tamu.edu/decision-aids/texasyst/reducing-contamination-by-improving-hazardous-waste-management/

Horak, E., Morass, B., Ulmer, H., Genuneit, J., Braun-Fahrländer, C., von Mutius, E., & GABRIEL Study Group. (2014). Prevalence of wheezing and atopic diseases in Austrian schoolchildren in conjunction with urban, rural or farm residence. *Wiener Klinische Wochenschrift, 126*(17–18), 532–536.

Hribar, C. (2010). Understanding concentrated animal feeding operations and their impact on communities. Retrieved from https://stacks.cdc.gov/view/cdc/59792

International Agency for Research on Cancer. (2015). IARC Monographs Volume 112: Evaluation of five organophosphate insecticides and herbicides. World Health Organization, Lyon.

Jochum, K. (2006). State fair's eco experience shows the way to conserve. *MPRNews,* Retrieved from org/story/2006/08/23/greenexpo

Lefohn, A. S., & Shadwick, D. S. (1991). Ozone, sulfur dioxide, and nitrogen dioxide trends at rural sites located in the United States. *Atmospheric Environment. Part A. General Topics, 25*(2), 491–501.

LeJeune, J., & Kersting, A. (2010). Zoonoses: An occupational hazard for livestock workers and a public health concern for rural communities. *Journal of Agricultural Safety and Health, 16*(3), 161–179.

Lemieux, P. M., Lutes, C. C., Abbott, J. A., & Aldous, K. M. (2000). Emissions of polychlorinated dibenzo-p-dioxins and polychlorinated dibenzofurans from the open burning of household waste in barrels. *Environmental Science & Technology, 34*(3), 377–384.

Majra, J. P. (2011). Air quality in rural areas. In *Chemistry, Emission Control, Radioactive Pollution and Indoor Air Quality.* IntechOpen.

Maryland Department of the Environment (2019). Regulation of open burning of solid waste: What you need to know. Retrieved from https://mde.maryland.gov/programs/LAND/SolidWaste/Documents/Open_Burning_Facts.pdf

McCarty, J. L. (2011). Remote sensing-based estimates of annual and seasonal emissions from crop residue burning in the contiguous United States. *Journal of the Air & Waste Management Association, 61*(1), 22–34.

McCarty, J. L., Korontzi, S., Justice, C. O., & Loboda, T. (2009). The spatial and temporal distribution of crop residue burning in the contiguous United States. *Science of the Total Environment, 407*(21), 5701–5712.

Merchant, J. A., Naleway, A. L., Svendsen, E. R., Kelly, K. M., Burmeister, L. F, Stromquist, A. M., . . . & Chrischilles, E. A. (2005). Asthma and farm exposures in a cohort of rural Iowa children. *Environmental health perspectives, 113*(3), 350–356.

Michigan Department of Environment, Great Lakes, and Energy. (2019). Open burning regulations in Michigan. Retrieved from https://www.michigan.gov/documents/deq/deq-aqd-open-burning-brochure_273553_7.pdf

Minnesota Pollution Control Agency. (n.d.). Don't burn your garbage toolkit. Retrieved from https://www

.pca.state.mn.us/waste/dont-burn-your-garbage-toolkit

Mirabelli, M. C., Wing, S., Marshall, S. W., & Wilcosky, T. C. (2006). Race, poverty, and potential exposure of middle-school students to air emissions from confined swine feeding operations. *Environmental Health Perspectives, 114*(4), 591–596.

National Center for Biotechnology Information. Compound summary: 2,3,7,8-Tetrachlorodibenzo-p-dioxin (n.d.). Retrieved from https://pubchem.ncbi.nlm.nih.gov/compound/2_3_7_8-Tetrachlorodibenzo-P-dioxin

National Park Service. (2019). Air quality in parks. Retrieved from https://www.nps.gov/subjects/air/airqualityparks.htm

National Park Service. (n.d.). NPS air conditions and trends. Retrieved from https://www.nps.gov/gis/storymaps/mapseries/v2/index.html?appid=73d71b11d2c044b9ab50cd2972de077e

Parsons, M. A., Beach, J., & Senthilselvan, A. (2017). Association of living in a farming environment with asthma incidence in Canadian children. *Journal of Asthma, 54*(3), 239–249.

Pavilonis, B. T., Sanderson, W. T., & Merchant, J. A. (2013). Relative exposure to swine animal feeding operations and childhood asthma prevalence in an agricultural cohort. *Environmental Research, 122*, 74–80.

Pichtel, J. Waste management practices: Municipal, Hazardous, and Industrial. (2005). Taylor and Francis Group LLC. ISBN, *10*, 0-8493.

Rasmussen, S., Casey, J. A., Bandeen-Roche, K., & Schwartz, B. S. (2017). Proximity to industrial food animal production and asthma exacerbations in Pennsylvania, 2005–2012. *International Journal of Environmental Research and Public Health, 14*(4), 362.

Schultz, A. A., Peppard, P., Gangnon, R. E., & Malecki, K. M. (2019). Residential proximity to concentrated animal feeding operations and allergic and respiratory disease. *Environment International, 130*, 104911.

Schumacher, K. A., & Agbemabiese, L. (2019). Towards comprehensive e-waste legislation in the United States: Design considerations based on quantitative and qualitative assessments. *Resources, Conservation and Recycling, 149*, 605–621.

Sigurdarson, S. T., & Kline, J. N. (2006). School proximity to concentrated animal feeding operations and prevalence of asthma in students. *Chest, 129*(6), 1486–1491.

Soccol, C. R., Faraco, V., Karp, S. G., Vandenberghe, L. P., Thomaz-Soccol, V., Woiciechowski, A. L., & Pandey, A. (2019). Lignocellulosic bioethanol: Current status and future perspectives. In *Biofuels: Alternative Feedstocks and Conversion Processes for the Production of Liquid and Gaseous Biofuels* (pp. 331–354).

Tilman, D., Balzer, C., Hill, J., & Befort, B. L. (2011). Global food demand and the sustainable intensification of agriculture. *Proceedings of the National Academy of Sciences of the United States of America, 108*(50), 20260–20264.

United States Department of Agriculture. (2019). 2017 Census of Agriculture: United States Summary and State Data. Retrieved from https://www.nass.usda.gov/Publications/AgCensus/2017/Full_Report/Volume_1,_Chapter_1_US/usv1.pdf

United States Department of Agriculture. Natural Resources Conservation Service. (n.d.) Animal Feeding Operations (AFO) and concentrated animal feeding operations (CAFO). Retrieved from https://www.nrcs.usda.gov/wps/portal/nrcs/main/national/plantsanimals/livestock/afo/

United States Environmental Protection Agency. (2003). The hidden hazards of backyard burning. Retrieved from https://www.epa.gov/dioxin/dioxins-produced-backyard-burning

United States Environmental Protection Agency. (2004). The particle pollution report: Current understanding of air quality and emissions through 2003. Retrieved from https://www.epa.gov/sites/production/files/2017-11/documents/pp_report_2003.pdf

United States Environmental Protection Agency. (2005). Handbook for managing onsite and clustered (decentralized) wastewater treatment systems. An introduction to management tools and information for implementing EPA's management guidelines. Retrieved from https://nepis.epa.gov/Exe/ZyPURL.cgi?Dockey=20017K2G.txt

United States Environmental Protection Agency. (2016a). Backyard burning. Retrieved from https://archive.epa.gov/epawaste/nonhaz/municipal/web/html/index-3.html

United States Environmental Protection Agency. (2016b). Carbon monoxide (CO) pollution in outdoor air: Basic information about carbon monoxide (CO) outdoor air pollution. Retrieved from https://www.epa.gov/co-pollution/basic-information-about-carbon-monoxide-co-outdoor-air-pollution#What%20is%20CO

United States Environmental Protection Agency. (2016c). Lead: Lead in outdoor air. Retrieved from https://www.epa.gov/lead/lead-outdoor-air

United States Environmental Protection Agency. (2016d). Nitrogen dioxide (NO_2) pollution: Basic information about NO_2. Retrieved from https://www.epa.gov/no2-pollution/basic-information-about-no2#What%20is%20NO2

United States Environmental Protection Agency. (2017b). Clean air act overview: Clean air act requirements and history. Retrieved from https://www.epa.gov/clean-air-act-overview/clean-air-act-requirements-and-history

United States Environmental Protection Agency. (2017c). Secondary drinking water standards: Guidance for nuisance chemicals. Retrieved from https://www.epa.gov/dwstandardsregulations/secondary-drinking-water-standards-guidance-nuisance-chemicals

United States Environmental Protection Agency. (2017d). Protect your home's water. Retrieved from https://www.epa.gov/privatewells/protect-your-homes-water#welltestanchor

United States Environmental Protection Agency. (2018a). Ground-level ozone pollution: Ground-level ozone basics. Retrieved from https://www.epa.gov/ground-level-ozone-pollution/ground-level-ozone-basics#wwh

United States Environmental Protection Agency. (2018b). Particulate matter (PM) pollution: Particulate matter (PM) basics. Retrieved from https://www.epa.gov/pm-pollution/particulate-matter-pm-basics

United States Environmental Protection Agency. (2018c). About EPA: Our mission and what we do. Retrieved from https://www.epa.gov/aboutepa/our-mission-and-what-we-do

United States Environmental Protection Agency. (2019a). Defining hazardous waste: Listed, characteristic and mixed radiological wastes. Retrieved from https://www.epa.gov/hw/defining-hazardous-waste-listed-characteristic-and-mixed-radiological-wastes

United States Environmental Protection Agency. (2019b) Glyphosate. Retrieved from https://www.epa.gov/ingredients-used-pesticide-products/glyphosate

United States Environmental Protection Agency. (2019c). Inventory of U.S. Greenhouse Gas Emission and Sinks: 1990-2017. Retrieved from https://www.epa.gov/sites/production/files/2019-04/documents/us-ghg-inventory-2019-main-text.pdf

United States Environmental Protection Agency. (2019d). Publications that support private water well safety. Retrieved from https://www.epa.gov/privatewells/publications-support-private-water-well-safety

United States Environmental Protection Agency. (2019d). Sulfur dioxide (SO_2) pollution: Sulfur dioxide basics. Retrieved from https://www.epa.gov/so2-pollution/sulfur-dioxide-basics#what%20is%20so2

United States Environmental Protection Agency. (2019e). National Overview: Facts and Figures on Materials, Wastes and Recycling. Retrieved from https://www.epa.gov/facts-and-figures-about-materials-waste-and-recycling/national-overview-facts-and-figures-materials

United States Environmental Protection Agency. (n.d.a). Basic Information about lead air pollution. Retrieved from https://www.epa.gov/lead-air-pollution/basic-information-about-lead-air-pollution#how

United States Environmental Protection Agency. (n.d.b). Guide to the facts and figures report about materials, waste and recycling. Retrieved from https://www.epa.gov/facts-and-figures-about-materials-waste-and-recycling/guide-facts-and-figures-report-about-materials

United States Environmental Protection Agency. (n.d.c). Health and environmental effects of particulate matter (PM). Retrieved from https://www.epa.gov/pm-pollution/health-and-environmental-effects-particulate-matter-pm

United States Environmental Protection Agency. (n.d.d). Health Effects of exposures to mercury. Retrieved from https://www.epa.gov/mercury/health-effects-exposures-mercury

United States Environmental Protection Agency. (n.d.e). Ozone trends. Retrieved from https://www.epa.gov/air-trends/ozone-trends. https://www.epa.gov/air-trends/ozone-trends

United States Environmental Protection Agency. (n.d.f.). Regulations, initiatives and research on electronics stewardship. Retrieved from https://www.epa.gov/smm-electronics/regulations-initiatives-and-research-electronics-stewardship

United States Environmental Protection Agency. (n.d.g.). Septic systems: Types of septic systems. Retrieved from https://www.epa.gov/septic/types-septic-systems

United States Environmental Protection Agency. (n.d.h.). Volatile organic compounds' impact on indoor air quality. Retrieved from https://www.epa.gov/indoor-air-quality-iaq/volatile-organic-compounds-impact-indoor-air-quality#Health_Effects

United States Environmental Protection Agency. (n.d.i.). A homeowner's guide to septic systems. Retrieved from https://www3.epa.gov/npdes/pubs/homeowner_guide_long.pdf

United States Geological Survey. (2009). Contaminants in 20 percent of U.S. private wells. Retrieved from https://www.usgs.gov/media/audio/contaminants-20-percent-us-private-wellschemicals

United States Geological Survey. (2017). Census of Agriculture: 2017 census Ag atlas maps - farms. Retrieved from https://www.nass.usda.gov/Publications/AgCensus/2017/Online_Resources/Ag_Atlas_Maps/17-M207.php

United States Geological Survey. (2018). Estimated annual agricultural pesticide use: Pesticide use maps. Retrieved from https://water.usgs.gov/nawqa/pnsp/usage/maps/show_map.php?year=2016&map=GLYPHOSATE&hilo=L

Waller, R. M. (2016). Ground water and the rural homeowner. Retrieved from https://pubs.usgs.gov/gip/gw_ruralhomeowner/gw_ruralhomeowner_new.html

Western Lake Superior Sanitary District. (2005). Clearing the air: Tools for reducing residential garbage burning. Retrieved from https://wlssd.com/wp-content/uploads/2015/08/Clearing-the-Air-download-vs.pdf

West Virginia Department of Environmental Protection. (n.d.). Open burning: Know the law about open burning. Retrieved from https://dep.wv.gov/daq/CandE/OpenBurningBrochure/Pages/default.aspx

White, S. S., & Birnbaum, L. S. (2009). An overview of the effects of dioxins and dioxin-like compounds on vertebrates, as documented in human and ecological epidemiology. *Journal of Environmental Science and Health*, Part C. *Environmental Carcinogenesis & Ecotoxicology Reviews, 27*(4), 197–211. doi:10.1080/10590500903310047

World Health Organization. (2016). Dioxins and their effects on human health. Retrieved from https://www.who.int/news-room/fact-sheets/detail/dioxins-and-their-effects-on-human-health.mpca

World Health Organization. (2018). Household air pollution and health. Retrieved from https://www.who.int/news-room/fact-sheets/detail/household-air-pollution-and-health

Zhang, M., Buekens, A., & Li, X. (2017). Open burning as a source of dioxins. *Critical Reviews in Environmental Science and Technology, 47*(8), 543–620.

CHAPTER 14

Occupational Health and Safety Considerations in Rural Agricultural Operations

Tunde M. Akinmoladun, PhD, DAAS, FRSPH

LEARNING OBJECTIVES

At the end of this chapter, the student or reader will be able to:

1. Learn a brief history of the Occupational Safety and Health Administration (OSHA) and its evolution.
2. Understand the types of farming-related hazards, accidents, and injuries.
3. Learn some farm safety lessons from abroad.
4. Understand OSHA farm work regulations.
5. Identify solutions to prevent or curtail farming-related accidents, injuries, and death.

KEY TERMS

Farm hazards
Heat stress
National Institute for Occupational Safety and Health (NIOSH)
Occupational Safety and Health Act (OSHACT)
Occupational Safety and Health Administration (OSHA)
Pesticide exposure

CHAPTER OVERVIEW

The chapter addresses a brief history of Occupational Safety and Health Administration (OSHA), its functions, the law that created it, and different types of hazards associated with agricultural operations. Statistics on farming hazards, injuries, and deaths, types of agricultural work and workers, and regions mostly affected in the United Sates are illustrated in Figures 14-1 to 14-3. Typical farm equipment and vehicles used are listed, including their safety and management concerns. Farming continues to be one of the most hazardous occupations in the United States, inspite of laws promulgated by congress, and regulations developed and enforced by OSHA. OSHA's oversight does not extend to small family farms with less than 10 employees who are usually made up of mostly family members. Such farms are only visited when safety concerns are reported by employees or when there are reported accidents, and/ or fatalities.

The rest of the chapter focuses on heat stress, and different routes of environmental and occupational exposure to pesticides. Additionally, case studies are presented as an exercise for written and oral discussion to end the chapter. In conclusion, primary prevention is the best and most effective solution to agricultural operations, and related human and ecological consequences as exemplified in the Hierarchy of Controls in Figure 14-6.

Introduction

The **Occupational Safety and Health Act (OSHAct)** of 1970 facilitated public and workplace awareness of the real and potential hazards of different workplaces. The OSHAct was signed into law by President Richard M. Nixon in 1970 and enforced through regulations developed by the **Occupational Safety and Health Administration, (OSHA)** a division of the Department of Labor, since 1971. The Act empowered OSHA to develop standards for different industries and to have them published as part of Volume 29 of the Code of Federal Regulations (29 CFR). For General Industry, it is 29 CFR 1910; for Construction, 29 CFR 1926; Maritime, 29 CFR 1915, 1917, and 1918; and Agro work, 29 CFR 1928 (OSHA, n.d.). OSHA regulates most private workplaces with at least 10 employees directly or indirectly through approved states' plans. State approved plans could be as stringent as federal OSHA or better but must not contradict federal OSHA. Also, federal, local, and state agencies and educational institutions must comply with workplace regulations as promulgated under the OSHAct.

U.S. Workplace Safety Statistics

The Bureau of Labor Statistics (BLS) reported approximately 4,690 workplace deaths in 2010 and 4,836 in 2015, a slight death increase attributed to increased population. The estimated cost of workplace injuries and death to date is about $275 billion annually, and many are preventable and controllable with appropriate safety measures. Healthy people 2020 has targeted reducing work-related deaths and injuries in all industries for full-time workers from 4.0 per 100,000 in 2007 to about 3.6 by 2020; and for agricultural and forestry-related deaths, a targeted reduction from 27.0 per 100,000 in 2007 to 24.3 per 100,000 by 2020 for full-time workers (OSHA, n.d.).

Agriculture, Agro Business, and Employees

Farming is one of the most hazardous occupations in the United States and the world. Farmers and family members often experience a higher rate of work-related injuries and deaths than their counterparts in other industries. According to the **National Institute for Occupational Safety and Health (NIOSH)** (2019), approximately 2,050,000 people were engaged in full-time agricultural work in 2017. NIOSH statistics in 2017 put farm workers' deaths at 416, representing approximately 20.4 deaths per 100, 000 (NIOSH, 2019).

Table 14-1 illustrates an estimated number of adults, 20 years and older, who worked on U.S. farms in 2001, 2004, 2009, 2012, and 2014, according to Occupational Injury Surveillance of Production Agricultural Survey (OISPA). In **Table 14-2** according to OISPA survey for the same period as above shows adults 20 years and older who worked on U.S. farms by region. **Table 14-3** by OISPA in the same survey period illustrates adults 20 years and older who worked on U.S. farms by type of adult worker and type of farm (NIOSH, 2018).

Table 14-1 National Estimates of Adults (20 Years and Older) Who Work on U.S. Farms by Type of Adult Worker

Table AD-1. National Estimates of Adults (20 Years and Older) Who Work on U.S. Farms by Type of Adult Worker

Type of Adult Worker	2001	2004	2009	2012	2014
Household	4,440,318	3,535,666	3,526,321	3,651,077	3,345,829
Hired	2,991,806	1,759,246	1,158,502	1,170,301	1,304,643
Visitor	6,714,769	9,446,234	7,825,982	18,966,134	17,617,405
Total (1)	14,146,893	14,741,146	12,510,805	23,787,512	22,267,877

1 Estimates may not sum to total due to rounding

Occupational Injury Surveillance of Production Agricultural Survey, 2001, 2004, 2009, 2012 and 2014.

Table 14-2 National Estimates of Adults (20 Years and Older) Who Work on U.S. Farms by Type of Adult Worker and Region

Table AD-2. National Estimates of Adults (20 Years and Older) Who Work on U.S. Farms by Type of Adult Worker and Region

Region	Type of Adult Worker	2001	2004	2009	2012	2014
Northeast	All working adults	926,955	1,053,530	872,316	1,520,455	1,551,198
	Household	290,969	240,202	250,964	254,231	244,686
	Hired	150,596	104,501	60,675	89,969	90,636
	Visitor	485,389	708,826	560,678	1,176,255	1,215,876
Midwest	All working adults	5,063,872	4,781,879	4,878,584	9,003,457	8,732,421
	Household	1,658,956	1,334,159	1,277,756	1,334,852	1,180,134
	Hired	925,758	455,687	394,519	321,375	352,993
	Visitor	2,479,157	2,992,033	3,206,308	7,347,229	7,199,294
South	All working adults	5,670,004	6,214,480	4,799,546	9,301,240	8,303,144
	Household	1,872,372	1,455,557	1,449,812	1,472,086	1,351,303
	Hired	1,102,830	567,377	439,195	438,016	418,657
	Visitor	2,694,801	4,191,547	2,910,540	7,391,138	6,533,184

(continues)

Table 14-2 National Estimates of Adults (20 Years and Older) Who Work on U.S. Farms by Type of Adult Worker and Region *(continued)*

Table AD-2. National Estimates of Adults (20 Years and Older) Who Work on U.S. Farms by Type of Adult Worker and Region

Region	Type of Adult Worker	2001	2004	2009	2012	2014
West	**All working adults**	**2,486,064**	**2,691,257**	**1,960,358**	**3,962,359**	**3,681,114**
	Household	618,021	505,747	547,789	589,907	569,706
	Hired	812,621	631,682	264,113	320,941	442,358
	Visitor	1,055,422	1,553,828	1,148,456	3,051,512	2,669,050
Total (1)	**All working adults**	**14,146,893**	**14,741,146**	**12,510,805**	**23,787,512**	**22,267,877**
	Household	4,440,318	3,535,666	3,526,321	3,651,076	3,345,829
	Hired	2,991,806	1,759,246	1,158,502	1,170,301	1,304,643
	Visitor	6,714,769	9,446,234	7,825,982	18,966,134	17,617,405

1 Estimates may not sum to total due to rounding

Occupational Injury Surveillance of Production Agriculture Survey, 2001, 2004, 2009, 2012 and 2014.

Table 14-3 National Estimates of Adults (20 Years and Older) Who Work on U.S. Farms by Type of Adult Worker and Type of Farm

Table AD-3. National Estimates of Adults (20 Years and Older) Who Work on U.S. Farms by Type of Adult Worker and Type of Farm

Type of Farm	Type of Adult Worker	2001	2004	2009	2012	2014
Crop	**All working adults**	**6,071,414**	**7,761,528**	**6,397,035**	**12,059,934**	**11,136,836**
	Household	1,805,658	1,674,727	1,659,983	1,720,782	1,602,684
	Hired	1,677,073	1,235,513	695,332	750,617	822,499
	Visitor	2,588,683	4,851,287	4,041,720	9,588,535	8,711,654
Livestock	**All working adults**	**7,305,588**	**6,979,618**	**6,113,770**	**11,727,578**	**11,131,041**
	Household	2,476,525	1,860,938	1,866,339	1,930,294	1,743,145
	Hired	992,395	523,733	463,169	419,684	482,145
	Visitor	3,836,668	4,594,946	3,784,262	9,377,600	8,905,751
Unknown	**All working adults**	**769,891**	**0**	**0**	**0**	**0**
	Household	158,135	0	0	0	0

	Hired	322,338	0	0	0	0
	Visitor	289,418	0	0	0	0
Total (1)	**All working adults**	**14,146,893**	**14,741,146**	**12,510,805**	**23,787,512**	**22,267,877**
	Household	4,440,318	3,535,666	3,526,321	3,651,076	3,345,829
	Hired	2,991,806	1,759,246	1,158,502	1,170,301	1,304,643
	Visitor	6,714,769	9,446,234	7,825,982	18,966,134	17,617,405

1 Estimates may not sum to total due to rounding

Occupational Injury Surveillance of Production Agriculture Survey, 2001, 2004, 2009, 2012 and 2014.

Most Prevalent Agricultural Accidents, Injuries, and Causes

Agriculture remains one of the most hazardous industries in the United States according to BLS in 2010 (OSHA, n.d.). In 1998, the National Coalition for Agricultural Safety and Health (NCASH) reported that the tractor was the predominant machine of traumatic death and disabling injury, due mostly to tractors overturning or rolling over. In 1998, NCASH also reported that other injuries were due to inadequate farm building design, livestock handling, farm motor vehicle accidents, electrocution, falls, and mechanical suffocations (NCASH, 1998). **Table 14-4** illustrates the largest identifiable sources of all injuries, where tractors, trucks, and harvesting machines accounted for about half of all fatalities combined. **Table 14-5** shows that overturning vehicles, being run over by vehicles, and body part being caught by running equipment accounted for almost 40% of all agricultural deaths between 1992 and 1998. In 2001, the region of the United States with the highest proportion of injuries was the Midwest, accounting for 45% of all injuries; the West at 25%; South at 22%; and Northeast at 8%. It is reasonable to conclude that the

Table 14-4 Production Agriculture Deaths by Source of Injury, 1992–1998, the Census of Fatal Occupational Injuries (CFOI)

Source of injury	Deaths	%
Tractors	1,510	37
Trucks	390	9.6
Harvesting machines	180	4.4
Mowing machines	150	3.7
Animals	144	3.5
Other Agricultural machines	129	3.2
Ground	121	3.0
Bullets	115	2.8
Loaders	75	1.8
Trees, logs	74	1.8
Other sources	1,194	29.3

Reproduced from Hard, D., Myers, J., & Gerberich, S. G. (2001). Traumatic injuries in agriculture. Agricultural Safety and Health Network (Ash-net). Retrieved from https://nasdonline.org/1828/d001773/traumatic-injuries-in-agriculture.html

more a region is engaged in agriculture, the greater the risk of accident, injury, and death (Hard, Myers, & Gerberich, 2001).

Table 14-5 Production Agriculture Deaths by Type of Injury Event, 1992–1998, the Census of Fatal Occupational Injuries (CFOI)

Table 5. Production Agriculture Deaths by Type of Injury Event, 1992–1998, The Census of Fatal Occupational Injuries (CFOI)		
Type of Injury Event	Deaths	%
Overturning vehicle/machine	1,051	25.8
Fall from & run over by Vehicle/Machine	298	7.3
Caught in running equipment	277	6.8
Struck by falling object	234	5.7
Run over (pedestrian)	211	5.2
Fall to lower level	173	4.2
Struck by rolling objects	136	3.3
Assault by animal	129	3.2
Suicide	88	2.2
Caught in a collapsing material	80	2.0
All other events	1,405	3.4

NASD Traumatic Injuries in Agriculture (1992–1998) as cited in Hard et al., 2001.

Tractor Rollovers, and Why?

The following diagrams illustrate what typical tractors look like, and what happens when they roll over. When a tractor rolls over, it means it has lost its center of gravity. The center of gravity is defined as an equal weight of distribution. That is, the weight of a tractor is distributed equally in front and back. **Figure 14-1** is a diagram depicting a tractor's center of gravity. **Figure 14-2** and **Figure 14-3** are diagrams with a tractor's center of gravity and a shifted center of gravity, respectively. **Figure 14-4** are actual tractors' photos of side and rear rollovers. When there is a shifted or lost center of gravity, there is a rollover, and rollovers account for most of the injuries and deaths on American farms (Smith, 2005). In 2010, the NIOSH concluded that approximately 4.8 million tractors on U.S. farms were not equipped with a rollover protection structure (ROPS), that the average age of tractors on U.S. farms was about 26 years, and that most of the tractors had no protective device or structure. New or modern tractors are designed to prevent rollovers by a wide base of stability and lower center of gravity (Murphy et al., 2010). On October of 1976, OSHA passed a regulation ensuring that all tractors built after October of 1976 must have ROPS, and that all farm employers must ensure that farm employees use seatbelts on ROPS tractors (OSHA, 2005).

Although the issues with farm equipment and machines get the most attention in agro safety because they are responsible for most accidents and fatalities, some attention must be focused on farm pesticide application and routes of exposure and **heat stress** as well.

Pesticide Exposure and Consequences

Pesticides such as atrazine, glyphosate, chlorpyrifos, etc., are commonly used in the United States and around the world and are toxic to farm workers, their families, nearby residents, and the environment. In 2017, farms in the United States spent more than $17.5 billion on pesticides. That was an average of about $37 for every acre of land treated, translating to an increase of about $27 per acre from the 1997 figure (National Agricultural Statistics Service, 2019a).

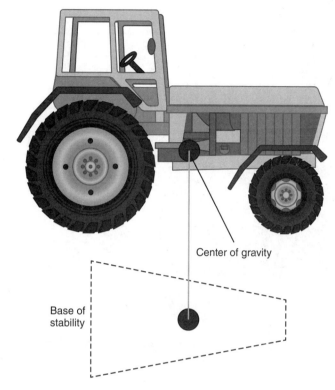

Center of gravity

Base of
stability

Figure 14-1 A Tractor's Base of Stability.

Smith, D.W. (2005). Safe tractor operation: Rollover protection. Texas A&M Agrilife Extension. Retrieved from https://agrilifeextension.tamu.edu/library/disasters-safety/safe-tractor-operation-rollover-prevention/

In spite of prolific application of pesticides, many farm workers lack training in the use of personal protective equipment (PPE), and in the safe storage and handling of pesticides and other farm chemicals, according to the United States Environmental Protection Agency (EPA), and the United States Department of Agriculture (USDA) (EPA, 2015). Also, instructions on safe use of pesticides are sometime ignored by farm workers due to a language barrier, especially if the instruction is written in a language foreign to the farm workers. It is also not unusual to find some pesticide containers with missing labels according to the EPA and USDA (EPA, 2015; Nadakavukaren, 2011).

Based on OSHA regulations, it is incumbent on employers to train employees on the safety of the chemical(s) they handle and must make sure that instruction labels are readable and affixed to the chemical container(s). They must also have the material safety data sheets (MSDS) available onsite. Not complying with all of the above enhances the risk of workers being exposed, which may result in health consequences.

Farm size often dictates how pesticides are applied to crops and land, whether by hand spraying from a pesticide containing tank or by spraying using tractors with attached tanks, or by aerial dusting. **Figure 14-5** below illustrates crop dusting in action on a big farm.

Regardless of how pesticides are used, there are three major categories of exposures:

1. Primary Occupational Exposure—includes inhalation followed by skin absorption when crops such as fruits and vegetables are picked or harvested by bare hands. Accidental ingestion can

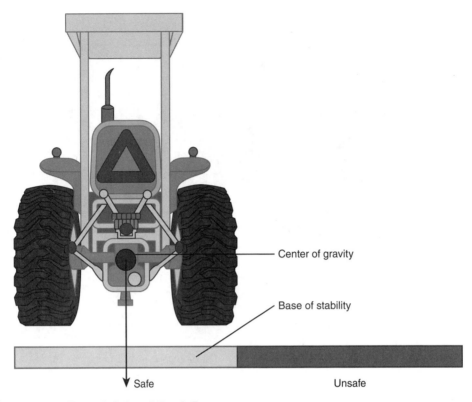

Figure 14-2 A Tractor's Safe and Unsafe Zones.

Smith, D.W. (2005). Safe tractor operation: Rollover protection. Texas A&M Agrilife Extension. Retrieved from https://agrilifeextension.tamu.edu/library/disasters-safety/safe-tractor-operation-rollover-prevention/

occur when chemically soaked hands are used to eat and smoke.

2. Secondary Exposure—Occurs when farm workers take work apparel and shoes home, thus exposing family members who may be children, the elderly, pregnant women, and the infirmed. This exposure impacts the most vulnerable population.

3. Tertiary Exposure—a consequence of aerial crop spraying or dusting, which spreads pesticide to nearby homes and surroundings, including pollution of ground and surface water. After all, air and water have no boundaries.

Heavy reliance on pesticides is not the optimal solution for dealing with agricultural pests. There are alternatives known as integrated pest management (IPM) that can be used in combination with a small amount of pesticides. As a result of heavy reliance on pesticides today, thousands of workers suffer from symptoms of acute pesticide poisoning such as persistent cough, wheezing, asthma, and dermatitis, etc. Chronic **pesticide exposure** has been associated with devastating health issues such as skin and lung cancer, depression, diabetes, anencephaly, anophthalmia, Parkinson's disease, and dementia, etc. (Kim, Kabir, & Jahan, 2017).

Heat Exposure and Consequences

Over the past 30 years, exposure to extreme heat has been documented as a contributing factor to weather-related deaths in the United States (National Weather Service, 2019).

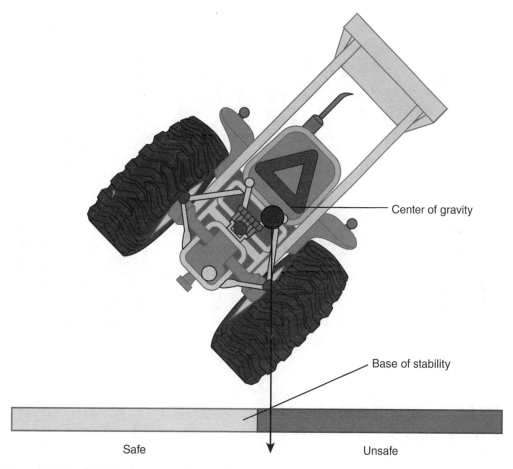

Figure 14-3 A Tractor's Shifted Center of Gravity.

Smith, D.W. (2005). Safe tractor operation: Rollover protection. Texas A&M Agrilife Extension. Retrieved from https://agrilifeextension.tamu.edu/library/disasters-safety/safe-tractor-operation-rollover-prevention/

Between 1992 and 2017, heat was estimated to be responsible for an average of 2,700 serious injuries, and 30 deaths per year among all U.S. workers (Tanglis & Devine, 2018). Farm workers die of heat-related causes at roughly 20 times the rate of workers in all other civilian occupations (CDC, 2008). Many states do not have worker heat protection regulations, except for California and Washington State (National Agricultural Statistics Service, 2019b). This is an astonishing fact, demanding national attention to save the lives of farm workers, especially during the summer season.

Controlling and Preventing Accident, Injury, and Death on the Farm

Environmental and occupational health measures, if practiced on farms, will definitely make a big dent in reducing and preventing farm casualties. However, preventive and control measures must include elimination, substitution, engineering, and administrative controls, as **Figure 14-6** depicts (NIOSH, 2015).

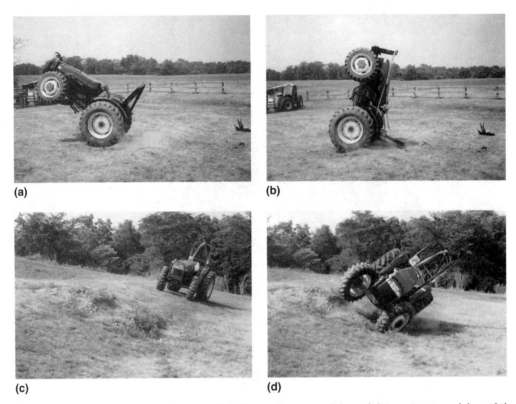

Figure 14-4 Actual Pictures of Rear and Side Tractor Overturns. **(a)** and **(b)** Rear Overturn. **(c)** and **(d)** Side Overturn.

Courtesy of Pennsylvania State University © 2020.

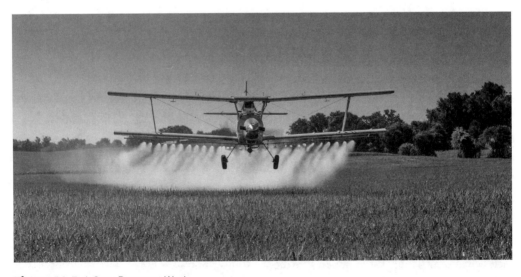

Figure 14-5 A Crop Duster at Work.

© Grindstone Media Group/Shutterstock

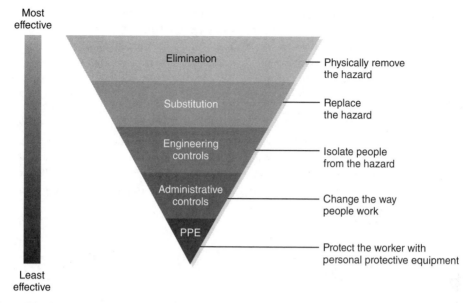

Figure 14-6 Hierarchy of Controls.

National Institute for Occupational safety and Health (NIOSH). (2015). Hierarchy of controls. Centers of Disease Control and Prevention. Retrieved from https://www.cdc.gov/niosh/topics/hierarchy/default.html

1. Elimination—simply phasing out structures and/or equipment that pose as hazards.
2. Substitution—use of safe alternatives like replacing hazardous chemicals or pesticides with safe or safer ones with fewer health and ecological consequences. Elimination and substitution are considered most effective in curtailing hazards but are difficult to implement in an existing operation. Both are more cost-effective in the design/implementation stage of an operation since they will not incur change in equipment.
3. Engineering controls—good for controlling workers' exposure in an existing workplace. That is, in the postdesign and during the operation stage to remove or prevent hazards to employees. For example, retrofitting an old tractor to prevent rollover.
4. Administrative controls—are more adaptable to corporate farms with many employees and in nonagricultural work. They may include job rotation, frequent

work breaks, safety meetings, and workplace exercise and wellness initiatives. etc.
5. Personal Protective Equipment (PPE)—includes use of gloves, eye goggles, aprons, coveralls, ear muffs, respirators, dust masks, safety shoes, helmets, etc., to prevent and/or control hazardous exposures.

Chapter Summary and Conclusion

Fatal and nonfatal accidents, injuries, and deaths associated with agricultural production are major public health problems necessitating a multifaceted approach. The approaches must include safety education/training and dissemination of information during employment orientation and throughout employment. Additionally, employees must be trained on the appropriate use of farm equipment and machines and personal protective equipment (PPE). Additionally, there must be improved rule making and enforcement at state and federal levels to monitor child labor, especially on family-owned farms. Promotion of workplace hygiene and sanitation to prevent primary, secondary, and tertiary exposure to farm chemicals, etc., are also very important to safeguard the health and safety of employees and their families.

In the final analysis, control and prevention of **farm hazards** must be everyone's business. Farm work and hazards should not be out of sight and out of mind, since rural community economic development and sustainability depends on the safety and productivity of farm workers.

It is a fact that a healthy worker is a productive worker. The consequences of inadequate protection of life, health, and safety on the farm are lost productivity and revenue, and, in turn, legal and medical liabilities, etc. Primary prevention, which is the goal of public health, is always better and cheaper than cure or treatment. In other words, "pay me now, or pay me more later." This maxim still holds true today, and will tomorrow and forever.

Discussion Questions

Case Studies

1. A farmer was preparing a pesticide to spray on his orchard. He was following the manufacturer's instructions closely because he knew that the substance was highly toxic. He always used gloves when handling chemicals to protect his hands and he preferred single-use gloves that he could throw away after each use. He had a box of medical gloves purchased from the supermarket and they were of excellent quality. However, a couple of hours after using them he came down with a severe rash on his hands: redness, pain, heat, and swelling.

   a. What should the farmer have done? He should have carried out a simple risk assessment to determine: What could go wrong? • Skin irritation; • ingestion; • inhalation of mists; • exposure to toxicity. What is the likelihood of this happening? High, taking into account: • unsuitability of gloves and personal protective equipment in general. What are the possible consequences (severity)? • Irritation, inflammation, illness, anaphylactic shock, and death. What control measures should the farmer have taken to reduce the risk? He should have: • Read and followed the safety information on the container and consulted the safety data sheet; • Selected the appropriate gloves, taking into account their specifications such as permeation rate, breakthrough time, and degradation; • Selected and used all relevant PPE (face protection, gloves, shoes, and overalls).

2. A 58-year-old female farmer was manually picking tobacco from a small plot she owned after her paid worker became sick. She had been collecting corn manually well before she had hired the worker. As time passed, it became warmer and very sunny. She was not accustomed to the task and was getting tired. She lost consciousness. Her husband found her lying there five hours later. What should the farmer have done? The farmer should have carried out a simple risk assessment of the site to determine:

   a. What could go wrong? • Dehydration, heat/sunstroke from warm weather; • Stings and bites from reptiles, insects, and rodents; • Unable to communicate with other people in case of an accident. What is the likelihood of any of these happening? High, taking into account: • The lady farmer's age; • Lone working; • Exposure to extremely warm weather; • The omission of safe practices. What are the possible consequences (severity)? • Injury, loss of consciousness, death. What measures should she have taken to reduce the risks?

She should have: • Not been working alone; • Selected cooler hours of the day and avoided working close to midday; • Ensured that she drank plenty of liquids to prevent dehydration; • Had a means of communicating and advised someone about the expected time she would return; • Waited for the worker to recover.

3. A farmer who decided that his cotton picker was not worth repairing dumped it near his field. The site soon became the playground for schoolboys from the neighboring village. After prolonged corrosion and wear, the cab of the cotton picker collapsed when six boys were playing inside. They all suffered scratches and bruises and one was hospitalized with a tetanus infection because a rusty piece of metal had pierced his leg.

   a. What should the farmer have done? The farmer should have carried out a simple risk assessment to determine: What could go wrong? • Injuries to children using it as a play area; • The public injured by contact with equipment; • Pest nesting. What is the likelihood of this happening? High, taking into account: • Uncontrolled access to the site; • Individual's and especially children's curiosity; • Gradual corrosion of equipment; • Pest infestation in abandoned machinery structures. What are the possible consequences (severity)? • Injury, tetanus infection (potentially fatal). What control measures should he have taken if he had assessed the situation in advance? He could have: • Prevented access to the site; • Disposed of the machinery; • Asked a professional to decommission/recycle the equipment; • Sold the equipment as scrap metal. When disposing of equipment, you are still responsible for it.

4. A.J. had worked for a potato farmer for many years. Her job was to harvest potatoes, put them in boxes, and place the boxes on trucks. She had been doing this job for 15 years. She is now suffering from spine disorders and is claiming compensation from her former employer for her current health problem.

   a. What should the farmer have done? The farmer should have carried out a simple risk assessment of the potato harvesting activities to determine: What could go wrong? • Chronic spine, muscle, and back problems. What is the likelihood of this happening? High, taking into account: • Lifting and carrying of weights; • Repetitive bending; • Poor posture; • Long working hours. What are the possible consequences (severity)? • Chronic spine, muscle, and back problems. If the farmer had assessed the situation beforehand, what control measures should he have taken? He should have: • Automated the process as much as possible; • Arranged for ergonomic containers if these had to be lifted by workers; • Ensured that lifting and twisting actions were eliminated from the system of work; • Assessed the ability and suitability of each employee; • Arranged for adequate breaks and time for rest; • Provided training for his workers on the correct lifting techniques to be used in the task; • Ensured that the weights lifted and hours worked by individuals did not exceed their ability; • Provided health surveillance—the workers' health should have been monitored periodically.

5. A six-year-old grandson was visiting his grandparents during the summer holidays. He always loved going to the field with his granddad who would leave him to wander around the farm, sit on the tractor, gather potatoes, or play with his grandma's chickens and rabbits. Out of sight of his grandparents as he was playing by the pond, he slipped, fell in the pond, and drowned. The pond was not fenced.

   a. What should the farmer have done? The farmer should have carried out a simple risk assessment of his site to determine: What could go wrong? • Drowning in the pond; • Entanglement in moving parts of machinery; • Accident involving tractor or other vehicles or equipment; • Consumption of inedible/harmful substances; • Falls from height while climbing. What is the likelihood of any of these happening? High, taking into account: • The child's curiosity; • His unfamiliarity with the site; • Lack of supervision. What are the possible consequences (severity)? • Injury, death. What control measures should the farmer have taken to reduce the risks? He should have: • Fenced the pond and other hazardous areas; • Spoken to the child about farm hazards and set out some simple rules; • Not left the child unattended on the farm.

6. A worker at a pig farm was assigned to clean the feedstuff silos so that they could be refilled the next day. He was supposed to undertake the job with a coworker. Due to a sudden illness of the coworker, he decided to proceed alone. While descending inside the silo, he fell and hit his head against the side of the silo. He was found dead seven hours later.

   a. What should the farmer have done? He should have carried out a simple risk assessment to determine: What could go wrong? • Worker being injured while working in the silo; • Worker becoming trapped in the silo with no assistance available; • Falls from height. What is the likelihood of any of these happening? High, taking into account: • The worker was working alone. What are the possible consequences (severity)? • Injury, coma, death. What control measures should the farmer have taken if he had assessed the situation beforehand? He should have: • Replaced the sick coworker; • Provided the workers with a safety method statement; • Supervised the work at frequent intervals.

European Commission. (2012). Protecting health and safety of workers in agriculture, livestock farming, horticulture, and forestry.

Student Activities and Worksheets are available for use inside the Navigate eBook, included with the printed text. Simply redeem the access code found at the front of the book at www.jblearning.com.

Additional Reading

- Ackerman, F., Whited, M., & Knight, P. (2014). Would banning atrazine benefit farmers? *International Journal of Occupational and Environmental Health, 20*(1), 61–70.
- Alonso, L. L., Demetrio, P. M., Etchegoyen, M. A., & Marino, D. J. (2018). Glyphosate and atrazine in rainfall and soils in agro productive areas of the pampas region in Argentina. *Science of the Total Environment, 645,* 89–96.
- Annett, R., Habibi, H. R., & Hontela, A. (2014). Impact of glyphosate and glyphosate-based herbicides on the freshwater environment. *Journal of Applied Toxicology, 34*(5), 458–479.
- Barberis, C. L., Carranza, C. S., Magnoli, K., Benito, N., & Magnoli, C. E. (2019). Development and removal ability of non-toxigenic *Aspergillus* section *Flavi* in presence of atrazine, chlorpyrifos and endosulfan. *Revista Argentina de Microbiologia, 51*(1), 3–11.
- Boily, M., Sarrasin, B., DeBlois, C., Aras, P., & Chagnon, M. (2013). Acetylcholinesterase in honey bees (Apis *mellifera)* exposed to neonicotinoids, atrazine and glyphosate: Laboratory and field experiments. *Environmental Science and Pollution Research, 20*(8), 5603–5614.
- Bronars, Stephen. (2015). *A vanishing breed: How the decline in US farm laborers over the last decade has hurt the U.S. economy and slowed production on American farms.* Partnership for a New American Economy. Retrieved from http://research.newamericaneconomy.org/wp-content/uploads/2015/08/PNAE_FarmLabor_August-3-3.pdf
- California Department of Pesticide Regulation (CDPR). (2019). *California pesticide illness query (CalPIQ).* Retrieved from https://apps.cdpr.ca.gov/calpiq
- Calvert, G. M., Beckman, J., Prado, J. B., Bojes, H., & Schwartz, A. (2009). *Occupational heat illness in Washington State: Technical report 59-2–2010.* Olympia, Washington. Department of Labor and Industries.
- Calvert, G. M., Karnik, J., Mehler, L., Beckman, J., Morrissey, B., Sievert, J., . . . Moraga–McHaley, S. (2008). Acute

pesticide poisoning among agricultural workers in the United States, 1998–2005. *American Journal of Industrial Medicine, 51*(12), 883–898. https:// doi.org/10.1002/ajim.20623

- Choudhary, E., & Vaidyanathan, A. (2014). Heat stress illness hospitalizations— environmental public health tracking program, 20 states, 2001–2010. *Morbidity and Mortality Weekly Report, 63*(13), 1–10. Retrieved from https://www.cdc.gov/mmwr /preview/mmwrhtml/ss6313a1.htm

- Clemens, M. A. (2013). *International Harvest: A Case Study of How Foreign Workers Help American Farms Grow Crops and the Economy: A Report by the Partnership for a New American Economy and the Center for Global Development*. The Partnership for a New American Economy. Retrieved from https://www.cgdev.org/sites/default /files/international-harvest.pdf

- García, J., Ventura, M. I., Requena, M., Hernández, A. F., Parrón, T., & Alarcón. (2017). Association of reproductive disorders and male congenital anomalies with environmental exposure to endocrine active pesticides. *Reproductive Toxicology, 71*, 95–100. https://doi.org/10.1016/j .reprotox.2017.04.011

- Gliessman, S., & Tittonell, P. (2015). Agroecology for food security and nutrition. *Agroecology and Sustainable Food Systems, 39*(2), 131–33. https://doi.org/10.10 80/21683565.2014.972001

- Gordon, C. J., & Leon, L. R. (2005). Thermal stress and the physiological response to environmental toxicants. *Reviews on Environmental Health, 20*(4), 235–64. https://doi.org/10.1515/REVEH .2005.20.4.235

- Guild, A., & Figueroa, I. (2018). The neighbors who feed us: Farmworkers and government policy—challenges and solutions. *Harvard Law & Policy Review, 13*, 157.

- Guirguis, K., Gershunov, A., Tardy, A., & Basu, R. (2014). The impact of recent heat waves on human health in California. *Journal of Applied Meteorology and Climatology, 53*(1), 3–19. https://doi .org/10.1175/JAMC-D-13-0130.1

- Hernandez, T., & Gabbard, S. (2018). *Findings from the National Agricultural Workers Survey (NAWS) 2015–2016: A demographic and employment profile of United States farmworkers. Research Report No. 13*. Rockville, MD: JBS International for the U.S. Department of Labor, Employment and Training Administration, Office of Policy Development and Research. https://www.doleta.gov/naws/research /docs/NAWS_Research_Report_13.pdf

- Houbraken, M., van den Berg, F., Butler Ellis, C. M., Dekeyser, D., Nuyttens, D., De Schampheleire, M., & Spanoghe, P. (2016). Volatilisation of pesticides under field conditions: Inverse modelling and pesticide fate models. *Pest Management Science, 72*(7), 1309–1321. https://doi .org/10.1002/ ps.4149

- Hyland, C., & Laribi, O. (2017). Review of take-home pesticide exposure pathway in children living in agricultural areas. *Environmental Research, 156*, 559–570. https:// doi. org/10.1016/j.envres.2017.04.017

- Jackson, L. L., & Rosenberg, H. R. (2010). Preventing heat-related illness among agricultural workers. *Journal of Agromedicine, 15*(3), 200–215. https://doi .org/10.1080/105992 4X.2010.487021

- Johnson, R. J., Wesseling, C., & Newman L. S. (2019). Chronic kidney disease of unknown cause in agricultural communities. *The New England Journal of Medicine, 380*(19), 1843–1852. https://doi .org/10.1056/NEJMra1813869

- Karl, T. R., & Knight, R. W. (1997). The 1995 Chicago heat wave: How likely is a recurrence? *Bulletin of the American Meteorological Society, 78*(6), 1107–1120. https://doi.org/10.1175/1520-0477

- Kim, K. H., Kabir, E., & Jahan, S. A. (2017). Exposure to pesticides and the associated human health effects. *Science of the Total Environment, 575*, 525–535. https://

doi.org/10.1016/j.scitotenv.2016.09.009

- Lacey, T. A., Toossi, M., Dubina, K. S., & Gensler, A. B. (2017). Projections overview and highlights, 2016–26. *Monthly Labor Review.* https://doi.org/10.21916/mlr.2017.29

- Lam, M., Krenz, J., Palmández, P., Negrete, M., Perla, M., Murphy-Robinson, H., & Spector, J. T. (2013). Identification of barriers to the prevention and treatment of heat-related illness in Latino farmworkers using activity-oriented, participatory rural appraisal focus group methods. *BMC Public Health, 13*(1), 1004. https://doi.org/10.1186/1471-2458-13-1004

- Lambar, E. F., & Thomas, G. (2019). The health and well-being of North Carolina's farmworkers: The importance of inclusion, accessible services and personal connection. *North Carolina Medical Journal, 80*(2), 107–112. https://doi.org/10.18043/ncm.80.2.107

- Lane, D., Murdock, E., Genskow, K., Betz, C. R., & Chatrchyan, A. (2019). Climate change and dairy in New York and Wisconsin: Risk perceptions, vulnerability, and adaptation among farmers and advisors. *Sustainability, 11*(13), 3599. https://doi.org/10.3390/su11133599

- Leigh, J. P., Du, J., & McCurdy, S. A. (2014). An estimate of the U.S. government's undercount of nonfatal occupational injuries and illnesses in agriculture. *Annals of Epidemiology, 24*(4), 254–259. https://doi.org/10.1016/j.annepidem.2014.01.006

- Leigh, J. P., McCurdy, S. A., & Schenker, M. B. (2001). Costs of occupational injuries in agriculture. *Public Health Reports, 116*(3), 235–248. https://doi.org/10.1093/phr/116.3.235

- Linder, M. (1987). Farm workers and the fair labor standards act: Racial discrimination in the new deal. *Texas Law Review, 65,* 1335–1339

- Mackay, D., Giesy, J. P., & Solomon, K. R. (2014). Fate in the environment and long-range atmospheric transport of the organophosphorus insecticide, chlorpyrifos and its oxon. *Ecological Risk Assessment for Chlorpyrifos in Terrestrial and Aquatic Systems in the United States,* 35–76. https://doi.org/10.1007/978-3-319-03865-0_3

- Martin, P., Hooker, B., Akhtar, M., & Stockton, M. (2016). How many workers are employed in California agriculture? *California Agriculture, 71*(1), 30–34. https://doi.org/10.3733/ca.2016a0011

References

Bourguet, D., & Guillemaud, T. (2016). The hidden and external costs of pesticide use. *Sustainable Agriculture Reviews, 19,* 35–120. https://doi.org/10.1007/978-3-319-26777-7_2

Centers for Disease Control and Prevention (CDC). (2008). Heat-related deaths among crop workers—United States, 1992–2006. *MMWR Morbidity and Mortality Weekly Report, 57*(24), 649–653.

Chemical Hazards Emergency Medical Management (CHEMM). (2020). *Personal protective equipment (PPE).* U.S. Department of Health and Human Services. Retrieved from https://chemm.nlm.nih.gov/ppe.htm

Environmental Protection Agency (EPA). (2015). Pesticides: Agricultural worker protection standard revisions. *Federal Register, 80*(221), 67496–67574.

European Commission. (2012). *Protecting health and safety of workers in agriculture, livestock farming, horticulture and forestry.* Retrieved from https://osha.europa.eu/en/publications/protecting-health-and-safety-workers-agriculture-livestock-farming-horticulture-and

Frazier, L. M. (2007). Reproductive disorders associated with pesticide exposure. *Journal of Agromedicine, 12*(1), 27–37. https://doi.org/10.1300/J096v12n01_04

Hard, D. L., Myers, J., & Gerberich, S. G. (2001). *Traumatic injuries in agriculture.* Agricultural Safety and Health Network (Ash-net). Retrieved from https://nasdonline.org/1828/d001773/traumatic-injuries-in-agriculture.html

Kim, K. H., Kabir, E., & Jahan, S. A. (2017). Exposure to pesticides and the associated human effects. *Science of the Total Environment, 575*, 525–535. https://doi .org/10.1016/Jscitotenv.2016.09.009

Murphy, D. J., Myers, J., McKenzie, E. A. Jr., Cavaletto, R., May, J., & Sorensen, J. (2010). Tractors and rollover protection in the United States. *The National Institute for Occupational Safety and Health (NIOSH), 15*(3), 249–263.

Nadakavukaren, A., & Caravanos, J. (2011). *Our Global Environment: A Health Perspective* (7th ed.). Long Grove, IL: Waveland Press, Inc.

National Agricultural Statistics Service (NASS). (2019a). *Percentage of chemicals used on American farms*. Retrieved from https://quickstats.nass.usda.gov

National Agricultural Statistics Service (NASS). (2019b). *Quick Stats*. Retrieved from https://quickstats.nass. usda.gov

National Coalition for Agricultural Safety and Health (NCASH). (1998). *National ag safety database*. Retrieved from https://nasdonline.org/about.php

National Institute for Occupational Safety and Health (NIOSH). (2015). *Hierarchy of controls*. Centers of Disease Control and Prevention (CDC). Retrieved from https://www.cdc.gov/niosh/topics/hierarchy /default.html

National Institute for Occupational Safety and Health (NIOSH). (2018). *Occupational injury surveillance of production agriculture (OISPA) survey*. Centers for Disease Control and Prevention. Retrieved from https:// www.cdc.gov/niosh/topics/aginjury/oispa/default .html

National Institute for Occupational Safety and Health (NIOSH). (2019). *Agricultural safety*. Retrieved from https://www.cdc.gov/niosh/topics/aginjury/

National Weather Service (NWS). (2019). *79-year list of severe weather fatalities*. Retrieved from https://www .weather.gov/media/hazstat/79years.pdf

Northeast Center for Occupational Safety and Health. (2020). *Tractor stability*. Retrieved from http://www .necenter.org/agriculture/past-research/?id=32

Occupational Safety and Health Administration (OSHA). (2005). *Roll-over protective structures (ROPS) for tractors used in agricultural operations*. United States Department of Labor. Retrieved from https://www .osha.gov/laws-regs/regulations/standardnumber /1928/1928.51

Smith, D. W. (2005). *Safe tractor operation: Rollover protection*. Texas A&M Agrilife Extension. Retrieved from https://agrilifeextension.tamu.edu/library /disasters-safety/safe-tractor-operation-rollover -prevention/

Tanglis, M., & Devine, S. (2018). *Extreme heat and unprotected workers: Public citizen petitioned OSHA to protect millions of workers who labor in dangerous temperatures*. Retrieved from https://www.citizen.org/wp-content /uploads/migration/extreme_heat_and_unprotected _workers.pdf

United States Department of Labor. Occupational Safety and Health Administration (OSHA). (n.d.). *Employer responsibilities*. Retrieved from https://www.osha.gov /as/opa/worker/employer-responsibility.html

CHAPTER 15

Mental Health in Rural America

Mark J. Minelli, PhD, MA, MPA
Fathima Wakeel, PhD, MPH

LEARNING OBJECTIVES

At the end of this chapter, readers will be able to:

1. Describe the adverse health effects of tobacco use.
2. Discuss the key determinants of greater tobacco use in rural areas.
3. Discuss the maternal and child implications of tobacco use in rural areas.
4. Describe the adverse health effects of tobacco use.
5. Describe one way to provide screening for alcohol abuse in rural areas.
6. Discuss the potential public health and medical implications of the legalization of marijuana in some states.
7. Identify the three historical trends of opioid use in the United States.
8. Discuss key determinants of higher opioid overdose death rates in rural areas.
9. Identify various treatment options for behavioral health and substance abuse disorders.

KEY TERMS

Delta-9-tetrahydrocannabinol (THC)
Heroin
Medication-Assisted Treatment (MAT)
Naloxone
Opioid Use Disorder (OUD)

CHAPTER OVERVIEW

Behavioral health and substance use disorders seem to be branches from the same tree. As there are books on either topic to attempt to cover all conditions in one chapter is not the purpose of this book. Here, the authors have focused the reading on some of the major issues facing public health in America in both rural and urban settings.

Tobacco

Tobacco use is the leading preventable cause of morbidity and mortality in the United States, resulting in approximately 480,000 deaths per year (U.S. Health and Human Services [USDHHS], 2014). Tobacco use is causally linked to a wide range of chronic diseases, including cancers (specifically lung, liver, and colorectal cancers), cardiovascular disease, respiratory illnesses, adverse reproductive outcomes, diabetes, and impaired immune function (USDHHS, 2014). According to the USDHHS Food and Drug Administration (2018), tobacco products comprise cigarettes, cigars, dissolvables, nicotine gels, hookah tobacco, pipe tobacco, roll-your-own tobacco, smoke tobacco (including dip, snuff, snus, and chewing tobacco), vapes, e-cigarettes, hookah pens, and other Electronic Nicotine Delivery Systems (ENDS).

Importantly, tobacco use is disproportionately higher in rural communities (28.5%), followed by urban areas (25.1%), small metropolitan areas (22.0%), and large metropolitan areas (18.3%) (Substance Abuse and Mental Health Services Administration, 2017). According to a seminal report from the American Lung Association [ALA] (2015), this significantly higher prevalence is attributable to a variety of individual, interpersonal, community, and systems-level determinants. At the individual level, rural Americans are more likely to use multiple forms of tobacco, including smokeless tobacco; men from rural areas are two times more likely as their counterparts in metropolitan areas to use smokeless tobacco. At the interpersonal level, individuals living in rural areas are, therefore, more likely to be exposed to secondhand smoke. At the community level, using tobacco is a social norm in many rural communities and is reinforced by less restrictive tobacco-free policies in public spaces, including restaurants, bars, and workplaces (Huang, et al., 2015). Smokeless tobacco has also been promoted as an alternative in smoke-free locations (Break Free Alliance, 2012) and has been considered a "rite of passage" for males in many rural areas (Nemeth, et al., 2012). At the broader systems level, tobacco companies have targeted rural Americans with images of "rugged individualism, as personified by the Marlboro man (ALA, 2015). Furthermore, as is the case for access to health care in general in rural areas, rural residents have less access to smoking cessation programs and, therefore, fewer resources to help them quit using tobacco. Additionally, low socioeconomic status has been strongly linked to risky health behaviors such as tobacco use, and rural Americans are more likely to live below the poverty line and have higher unemployment rates than their urban counterparts.

Tobacco use is also a critical maternal and child health issue in rural areas. Women in rural communities are more than twice as likely (27.4%) as urban women (11.2%) to smoke during pregnancy (ALA, 2015). Prenatal smoking has been strongly linked to a multitude of adverse pregnancy and birth outcomes, including low birthweight, preterm birth, sudden infant death syndrome, and placental abruption (Ananth, et al., 1996; Floyd, et al., 1991; Anderson, et al., 1992; Ness, et al., 1999, and long-term child outcomes, such as impaired physical, cognitive, and behavioral development and childhood obesity (Levin & Slotkin, 1998; Naeye & Peters, 1984; Rantakallio & Koiranen, 1987; Roy, Seidler & Slotkin, 2002; Wakschlag & Keenan, 2001; Wakschlag, et al., 1997; Oken, et al., 2008). Furthermore, across the United States, tobacco use, specifically e-cigarette use, has dramatically risen among middle- and high-school students (USDHHS Centers for Disease Control and Prevention, 2019). In rural communities, the normalization of tobacco use has resulted in tobacco users serving as role models for many youth (ALA, 2015). Hence, rural youths have been found to be three times more likely than their urban and suburban counterparts to smoke (Lutfiyya, et al., 2008), with 37.4% of adolescents in rural settings being daily smokers (ALA, 2015). Along with the actual use of tobacco, exposure to secondhand smoke among youth is disproportionately higher among rural youth (with a prevalence range of 33.1%–35.0%) compared with urban youth (24.4%) (USDHHS, 2011).

Alcohol Abuse Screening and Treatment

The distance that clients need to go to reach professional substance use disorder programs in rural areas can be a concern for both the client and the healthcare providers. One way to access validated screening instruments is by using the internet. Available tools are the CAGE (often used by healthcare professionals as it is a quick screening survey), the Michigan Alcoholism Screening Test (MAST), and the Alcohol Use Disorders Identification Test (AUDIT). If these tools indicate a concern for alcohol abuse, reaching out to a substance use disorder program or local Alcoholics Anonymous group could be beneficial.

Gfroerer, et al., (2007) found that rural substance users reported more alcohol use than their urban counterparts. This also goes with the data of admission rates for alcohol use as the primary drug of choice is higher in rural than urban drug abuse clients. There may be a number of variables of why alcohol abuse rates seem to be more prevalent in a rural than urban setting. With this information available to human service delivery programs, alcohol treatment, intervention, and prevention programs should plan accordingly.

Rural substance users have reported more alcohol use than their urban counterparts (Gfroerer, et al., 2007). This also goes with the data of admission rates for alcohol use as the primary drug of choice is higher in rural than urban drug abuse clients. There may be a number of variables to explain why alcohol

abuse rates seem to be more prevalent in a rural than urban setting. With this information available to human service delivery programs, alcohol treatment, intervention, and prevention programs should plan accordingly.

The National Institute on Alcohol Abuse and Alcoholism has a factsheet on "Alcohol Facts and Statistics," which covers the epidemiology of alcohol use in the United States. It can be found on their website: https://www.niaaa.nih.gov.

Marijuana

The landscape is changing in rural and urban America concerning marijuana as more states continue to legalize medical and recreational use of this drug. Public opinion appears to be changing as additional states come on board with these sweeping changes while federal law still classifies marijuana as an illegal substance. While decreased criminal charges should result from these changes, there are significant public health concerns due to the potential abuse of the drug. Although there will be increased economic incentives for states through tax revenue, the social problems created by additional public usage may counter balance spending for police, emergency room visits, and substance-abuse treatment programs.

There are two main types of marijuana: *Cannabis indica* and *Cannabis sativa* (Small & Cronquist, 1976). *Cannabis sativa* is known more for a high, or psychoactive effects, while *Cannabis indica* has been used for pain reduction and as a sedative (Hillig, Mahlberg, Paul, 2004).

Public safety is one issue as there appears to be a relationship between impaired driving and levels of the active ingredient **delta-9-tetrahydro-cannabinol (THC)** (Lenne et al., 2010, Hartman & Huestis, 2013, Hartman, et al., 2015). We are also seeing increased potency levels of THC in marijuana over the years (Mehmedic et al., 2010).

Educationally, reduced rates of graduating have been noted in users versus nonusers

(Macleod et al., 2004). This appears to be related to the amotivational syndrome (a lack of desire to complete tasks) as a result of drug abuse, which could be tied to increased unemployment, lowered income levels, increased welfare dependence, increased criminal behavior, and lowered life satisfaction (Fergusson & Boden, 2008; Brook et al., 2013).

Medically, the relationship with chronic bronchitis and the regular or chronic use of marijuana has been documented and the drug is often used in a similar manner as smoking cigarettes (Tashkin, 2013; Owen, Sutter, Albertson, 2014). Addiction to the drug is another concern for medical and other human service workers, which can negatively impact the lives of those affected (Hasin et al., 2015).

Determinants of Opioid Abuse

Opioid abuse is a rapidly growing epidemic in the United States. Opioids comprise prescription pain medications (e.g., oxycodone, hydrocodone, codeine, morphine, etc.) and illegal drugs such as **heroin** and synthetically created fentanyl (Centers for Disease Control and Prevention (CDC), 2018). As opioid use results in a euphoric sensation along with pain relief, opioids can often be misused, thus leading to **Opioid Use Disorder (OUD)**, which is defined as a "problematic pattern of opioid use that causes significant impairment or distress" (CDC, 2018). In 2017 itself, drug overdoses claimed the lives of over 70,000 people, thereby becoming a leading cause of injury-related death in the United States (CDC, 2018). Prescription or illegal opioids were implicated in approximately 68% of these deaths (CDC, 2018). Furthermore, there was a sixfold increase in the number of opioid-related overdose deaths between 1999 and 2017. The country has experienced three significant surges in opioid use within the past three decades: 1) Increase in opioids prescriptions in the 1990s, resulting in increased

overdose deaths; 2) Increase in heroin-related overdose deaths beginning in 2010; and 3) Increase in overdose deaths related to synthetic opioids, such as illicitly manufactured fentanyl (IMF) (Kolodny et al., 2015; Scholl et al., 2019).

Although residents of rural communities engage in less opioid use than their urban counterparts, they currently experience higher rates of opioid overdose deaths; they have also experienced a significantly higher rise (325%) in these deaths between 1999 and 2015 compared with urban residents (198%) (Mack et al., 2017). This disparity may be due to several factors. First, data indicate that individuals who live in the most rural areas are 87% more likely to receive an opioid prescription versus individuals who live in large central metropolitan areas (Garcia et al., 2019). This trend has been attributed to several potential risk factors related to rural settings, including increased prescription opioid use and misuse at earlier ages; a higher population of older individuals, who are more likely to experience chronic pain and be prescribed opioids; and differences in state prescription drug monitoring programs as well as the adherence of healthcare providers to prescribing guidelines (Keyes et al., 2014; Monnat and Rigg, 2016; Click et al., 2018; Rutkow, et al., 2015). Second, rural residents are more likely to face various obstacles in accessing treatment, specifically medication-assisted treatment (MAT), for OUD, including a shortage of opioid treatment programs (i.e., affecting almost 89% of large rural counties), fewer services offered in these programs, and greater distances to travel for obtaining treatment (Pullen & Oser, 2014; Johnson et al., 2018; Dick et al., 2015). Along these lines, in the case of a drug overdose, **naloxone**, an opioid antagonist medication, may not be readily accessible in many rural settings, and emergency medical services may not be allowed to administer it in some states or may not have the required training to do so (Faul et al., 2015). Third, from an upstream perspective, greater economic stress related to high rates of poverty and unemployment as well as the significant shortage of necessary mental health resources in rural communities probably contribute to self-medication through misuse of prescription opioids and use of illicit opioids such as heroin and fentanyl (Keyes et al., 2014; Dasgupta et al., 2018).

Abuse of Heroin Progression

Through a qualitative research design, Dygert and Minelli (1993) interviewed over 200 prisoners through small group educational sessions to illicit their views on the signs and symptoms of heroin abuse progression. Although this study was done in the 1990s, recovering heroin addicts today believe that this still follows their progress from use to abuse of heroin (following educational sessions presenting this model). The model was broken down into three phases of use/abuse with the following signs and symptoms.

In the early addiction phase, users are introduced to other users and curiosity about using heroin. When it came to experimentation with the drug provided by peers, users felt they were still in control. With the euphoric feelings provided by heroin, users felt the need to increase their usage. This increased use of heroin lead to involvement within the drug subculture and buying and selling. As dependence started to develop, users started to accept intravenous use of heroin as a way of life.

During the middle addiction phase, increased tolerance and daily use lead to physical dependency. Family problems often developed due to dysfunctional relationships and disruption of family life. Job problems may also surface with increased absenteeism, poor job performance, and potential loss of jobs. The criminal justice system may also become involved due to criminal activities to fund their drug habit. Finally, overall social life

structure would become chaotic for the users and they would lose self-respect and develop feelings of guilt.

The late phase of addiction brings additional criminal activities to support ongoing drug usage. Long-term use of heroin would show deterioration of health and hygiene and disregard for living a healthy lifestyle. Regardless of the overall consequences, drug use would continue. The three final choices in this struggle of addiction are to seek help and become drug-free, incarceration, or death.

Treatment and Prevention of Opioid Abuse and Opioid-related Deaths

Medication-assisted Treatment (MAT) has been regarded as the most effective way to treat Opioid Use Disorder (OUD). MAT combines behavioral therapy and counseling with medications, including methadone, buprenorphine, or naltrexone (CDC, 2017). Opioid Treatment Programs (OTPs), which must be accredited by the Substance Abuse and Mental Health Services Administration (SAMHSA), have been available in 48 states from 2015 and are able to administer MAT to individuals experiencing OUD (SAMHSA, 2019). The CDC also recommends providing targeted MAT to individuals in criminal justice settings and emergency departments (CDC, 2018). Overall, treatment and recovery for OUD may take months or even years, depending on the individual's health and level of addiction, stressors, and resources (e.g., financial, social, etc.) (SAMHSA, 2019).

Although treatment and recovery are critically important components of the reduction of OUD, public health efforts have increasingly focused on front-end preventative efforts to reduce opioid abuse and overdose deaths in the population. Naloxone, which is an opioid agonist medication, can be administered to individuals experiencing an opioid overdose to reverse its potentially fatal effects (CDC, 2018). As part of its seminal 2018 report titled, "Evidence-based Strategies for Preventing Opioid Overdose: What's Working in the United States," the CDC recommends developing targeted naloxone distribution programs, in which first responders, healthcare providers, and laypeople (e.g., restaurant or bar staff) are trained in naloxone administration to quickly address an opioid overdose, especially in areas (e.g., rural settings) where emergency assistance may not be readily accessible (CDC, 2018). The CDC also suggests that access to naloxone and referrals for MAT be integrated into syringe exchange programs, through which drug users can exchange contaminated needles for clean needles in order to prevent the spread of infections (CDC, 2018). Furthermore, expanded access to mental health services through their integration with primary care (thus also reducing stigma) and through telehealth have become increasingly important, particularly in rural settings (Rural Health Information Hub, 2019). Finally, some preemptive strategies that have been recommended to prevent opioid misuse and abuse include increased provider and patient education about the impact of opioid misuse and proper disposal techniques for unused opioids, use of Prescription Drug Monitoring Programs (PDMP) to curb inappropriate prescriptions of opioids as well as doctor or pharmacy shopping (i.e., when drug users move from provider to provider to solicit unnecessary prescriptions or from pharmacy to pharmacy to fill such prescriptions), and the establishment of community disposal sites for unused opioids (Mattson et al., 2018; Hahn, 2011). **Table 15-1** reviews many treatment modalities for behavioral health and substance use disorders.

Table 15-1 **Treatment Modalities for Behavioral Health and Substance Use Disorders**

1. Self-help groups—based on the model of Alcoholics Anonymous (AA) founded in the 1930s by Bill W. and Dr. Bob. Most self-help groups utilize a similar format and can cover a wide variety of topics from substance use disorders to behavioral health issues. Website for further information can be found at www.aa.org/

2. Outpatient counseling/psychotherapy—can offer individual, group, and family counseling services based in a variety of community settings (community mental health services, hospitals, agencies, etc.).

3. Residential programs/inpatient hospitalization—patients live at these programs for a period of time and the programs are staffed by a variety of specialists and generalists (at hospitals or other free-standing facilities).

4. Medical detoxification—a process and setting in which patients are medically supervised through withdrawal from alcohol or other drugs.

5. Day treatment programs—not considered an inpatient facility. Patients may spend the day with trained behavioral health staff for supportive care services.

6. Pharmacological interventions—medications that treat specific behavioral health and substance use disorders often combined with psychotherapy (referred to as MAT). For example, MAT for opioid use disorder combines behavioral therapy and counseling with the use of medications, including methadone, buprenorphine, or naltrexone.

7. Complementary and alternative services (CAM)—A wide variety of alternative therapies, herbs, over-the-counter medications, etc.

8. Relapse prevention programs—may offer therapies or drug free activities to assist patients as they cope with the stress of daily life and support to remain alcohol- and drug-free.

9. Telecommunication technology—uses telehealth, telemedicine, or telepsychiatry to provide health care and health information to large and underserved areas.

From: Mental Health America (n.d.). *Mental health treatments*. Retrieved from www.mentalhealthamerica.net/types-mental-health-treatments.; Minelli, M. (2013). Drugs of abuse: A quick information guide. Champaign, IL: Stipes Publishing Co.;
Benavides-Vaello, S., Strode, A., & Sheeran, B.C. (2013). Using technology in the delivery of mental health and substance abuse treatment in rural communities: A review. *Journal of Behavioral Health Services & Research*, 40, 111–120.

Chapter Summary

Behavioral health and substance use disorders are very common issues and concerns in rural communities. Lack of adequate service delivery resources and expertise to help people with recovery from addictions and behavioral health problems is a common theme in rural America. With some severity of problems even higher in rural areas, this only adds to the hardship.

Even with the country facing the COVID-19 pandemic, substance use disorder overdoses, depression, and suicides are still active and ongoing issues. This chapter sheds light on some of our ongoing struggles facing our nation in rural regions of the United States.

Discussion Questions

1. Discuss the current problems related to e-cigarette use and teenagers.
2. Make a list of famous people who have overdosed. Then, create a list of people you may know who have overdosed. Discuss the relationships and stories of the people on your lists.
3. Discuss the reasons why it may be difficult to find behavioral health services in rural countries.
4. In small groups, research the behavioral health services within a rural county. Present your findings to the classroom for further discussion.

Student Activities and Worksheets are available for use inside the Navigate eBook included with the printed text. Simply redeem the access code found at the front of the book at www.jblearning.com.

References

American Lung Association. (2015). Cutting tobacco's rural roots: Tobacco use in rural communities. Retrieved from https://www.cdc.gov/tobacco/disparities/geographic/index.htm

Ananth, C. V., Savitz, D. A., & Luther, E. R. (1996). Maternal cigarette smoking as a risk factor for placental abruption, placenta previa, and uterine bleeding in pregnancy. *American Journal of Epidemiology*, 144(9), 881–889. doi:10.1093/oxfordjournals.aje.a009022

Anderson, H., Bland, J., & Peacock, J. (1992). The effect of smoking on fetal growth. In D. Poswillo & E. Alberman (Eds.), *Effects of Smoking on the Fetus,* *Neonate, and Child* (8th ed., 89-105). New York, NY: Oxford University Press Inc.

Break Free Alliance. (2012). *Addressing dual tobacco use in West Virginia: Report and recommendations of the expert panel*. Executive summary. Retrieved from https://dhhr.wv.gov/wvdtp/Resources/reports/Documents/WV-Dual-TobUse-ExpertPanel%20ExecSum-04-12.pdf

Brook, J. S., Lee, J. Y., Finch, S. J., Seltzer, N., & Brook, D. W. (2013). Adult work commitment, financial stability, and social environment as related to trajectories of marijuana use beginning in adolescence. *Substance*

Abuse, 34(3), 298–305. doi:10.1080/08897077.2013.775092

Center for Behavioral Health Statistics and Quality. (2012). A comparison of rural and urban substance abuse treatment admissions. *The Treatment Episode Data Set (TEDS) Report*. Retrieved from https://www.samhsa.gov/sites/default/files/teds-short-report043-urban-rural-admissions-2012.pdf.

Centers for Disease Control and Prevention (CDC). (2017). *Treat opioid use disorder*. U.S. Department of Health and Human Services, CDC National Center for Injury Prevention and Control. Retrieved from https://www.cdc.gov/drugoverdose/prevention/treatment.html

Centers for Disease Control and Prevention (CDC). (2018). *Evidence-based strategies for preventing opioid overdose: What's working in the United States*. National Center for Injury Prevention and Control, Centers for Disease Control and Prevention, U.S. Department of Health and Human Services. Retrieved from http://www.cdc.gov/drugoverdose/pdf/pubs/2018-evidence-based-strategies.pdf

Centers for Disease Control and Prevention (CDC). (2018). *Opioid overdose*. Retrieved from https://www.cdc.gov/drugoverdose/epidemic/index.html

Click, I. A., Basden, J. A., Bohannon, J. M., Anderson, H., & Tudiver, F. (2018). Opioid prescribing in rural family practices: A qualitative study. *Substance Use and Misuse, 53*(4), 533–540. doi:10.1080/10826084.2017.1342659

Dasgupta, N., Beletsky, L., & Ciccarone, D. (2018). Opioid crisis: No easy fix to its social and economic determinants. *American Journal of Public Health, 108*(2), 182–186. doi:10.2105/AJPH.2017.304187

Dick, A. W., Pacula, R. L., Gordon, A. J., Sorbero, M., Burns, R. M., Leslie, D., & Stein, B. D. (2015). Growth in buprenorphine waivers for physicians increased potential access to opioid agonist treatment 2002–11. *Health Affairs, 34*(6), 1028–1034. doi:10.1377/hlthaff.2014.1205

Dygert, S., & Minelli, M. (1993). Heroin abuse progression chart. *Addiction & Recovery, 13*(2), 27–31.

Ewing, J. A. (2020). *CAGE questions for alcohol use*. MD+ Calc. Retrieved from https://www.mdcalc.com/cage-questions-alcohol-use

Faul, M., Dailey, M. W., Sugerman, D. E., Sasser, S. M., Levy, B., & Paulozzi, L. J. (2015). Disparity in naloxone administration by emergency medical service providers and the burden of drug overdose in US rural communities. *American Journal of Public Health, 105*(S3), e26–e32. doi:10.2105/AJPH.2014.302520

Fergusson, D. M., & Boden, J. M. (2008) Cannabis use and later life outcomes. *Addiction, 103*(6), 969–976. doi:10.1111/j.1360-0443.2008.02221.x

Floyd, R. L., Zahniser, S. C., Gunter, E. P., & Kendrick, J. S. (1991). Smoking during pregnancy:

Prevalence, effects, and intervention strategies. *Birth: Issues in Perinatal Care, 18*(1), 47–53.

García, M. C., Heilig, C. M., Lee, S. H., Faul, M., Guy, G., Iadermarco, M. F., . . . Gray, J. (2019). Opioid prescribing rates in nonmetropolitan and metropolitan counties among primary care providers using an electronic health record system—United States, 2014–2017. *MMWR Morbidity and Mortality Weekly Report, 68*(2), 25–30.

Gfroerer, J. C., Larson, S. L., & Colliver, J. D. (2007). Drug use patterns and trends in rural communities. *The Journal of Rural Health, 23*(Suppl 1), 10–15.

Hahn, K. L. (2011). Strategies to prevent opioid misuse, abuse, and diversion that may also reduce the associated costs. *American Health & Drug Benefits, 4*(2), 107–114.

Hartman, R. L., & Huestis M. A. (2013). Cannabis effects on driving skills. *Clinical Chemistry, 59*(3), 478–492. doi:10.1373/clinchem.2012.194381

Hartman, R. L., Brown, T. L., Milavetz, G., Spurgin, A., Pierce, R. S., Gorelick, D. A., . . . Huestis, M. A. (2015). Cannabis effects on driving lateral control with and without alcohol. *Drug and Alcohol Dependence, 154*, 25–37. doi:10.1016/j.drugalcdep.2015.06.015

Hasin, D. S., Saha, T. D., Kerridge, B. T., Goldstein, R. B., Chou, S. P., Zhang, H., . . . Grant, B. (2015). Prevalence of marijuana use disorders in the United States between 2001-2002 and 2012-2013. *JAMA Psychiatry, 72*(12), 1235–1242. doi:10.1001/jamapsychiatry.2015.1858

Hillig, K. W., & Mahlberg, P. G. (2004). A chemotaxonomic analysis of cannabinoid variation in *cannabis* (cannabaceae). *American Journal of Botany, 91*(6), 966–975. doi:10.3732/ajb.91.6.966

Huang, J., King, B. A., Babb, S. D., Xu, X., Hallett, C., & Hopkins, M. (2015). Sociodemographic disparities in local smoke-free law coverage in 10 states. *American Journal of Public Health, 105*(9), 1806–1813.

Johnson, Q., Mund, B., & Joudrey, P. J. (2018). Improving rural access to opioid treatment programs. *The Journal of Law, Medicine & Ethics, 46*(2), 437–439. doi:10.1177/1073110518782951

Keyes, K. M., Cerdá, M., Brady, J. E., Havens, J. R., & Galea, S. (2014). Understanding the rural-urban differences in nonmedical prescription opioid use and abuse in the United States. *American Journal of Public Health, 104*(2), e52–e59.

Kolodny, A., Courtwright, D. T., Hwang, C. S., Kreiner, P., Eadie, J. L., Clark, T. W., & Alexander, G. C. (2015). The prescription opioid and heroin crisis: A public health approach to an epidemic of addiction. *Annual Review of Public Health, 36*, 559–574.

Lenné, M. G., Dietze, P. M., Triggs, T. J., Walmsley, S., Murphy, B., & Redman, J. R. (2010). The effects of cannabis and alcohol on simulated arterial driving: Influences of driving experience and task demand.

Accident; Analysis & Prevention, 42(3), 859–866. doi:10.1016/j.aap.2009.04.021

Mack, K. A., Jones, C., & Ballesteros, M. (2017). Illicit drug use and drug overdose in metropolitan and non-metropolitan areas - United States. *MMWR Morbidity and Mortality Weekly Report, 66*, 1–12.

Macleod, J., Oakes, R., Copello, A., Crome, I., Egger, M., Hickman, M., . . . Davey Smith, G. (2004). Psychological and social sequelae of cannabis and other illicit drug use by young people: A systematic review of longitudinal, general population studies. *The Lancet, 363*(9421), 1579–1588. doi:10.1016/S0140-6736(04)16200-4

Mattson, C. L., O'Donnell, J., Kariisa, M., Seth, P., Scholl, L., & Gladden, R. (2018). Opportunities to prevent overdose deaths involving prescription and illicit opioids, 11 states, July 2016–June 2017. *MMWR Morbidity and Mortality Weekly Report, 67*(34), 945–951. http://dx.doi.org/10.15585/mmwr.mm6734a2external icon

Mehmedic, Z., Chandra, S., Slade, D., Denham, H., Foster, S., Patel, A. S., . . . ElSohly, M. A. (2010). Potency trends of Δ9-THC and other cannabinoids in confiscated cannabis preparations from 1993 to 2008. *Journal of Forensic Sciences, 55*(5), 1209–1217. doi:10.1111/j.1556-4029.2010.01441.x

Monnat, S. M. & Rigg, K. K. (2016). Examining rural/urban differences in prescription opioid misuse among US adolescents. *The Journal of Rural Health, 32*(2), 204–218.

Nemeth, J. M., Liu, S. T., Klein, E. G., Ferketich, A. K., Kwan, M. P., & Wewers, M. E. (2012). Factors influencing smokeless tobacco use in rural Ohio Appalachia. *Journal of Community Health, 37*(6), 1208–1217. doi:10.1007/s10900-012-9556-x

Pullen, E. & Oser, C. (2014). Barriers to substance abuse treatment in rural and urban communities: Counselor perspectives. *Substance Use & Misuse, 49*(7), 891–901. doi:10.3109/10826084.2014.891615

Rural Health Information Hub. (2019). *Integration of mental health services in primary care settings.* Retrieved from https://www.ruralhealthinfo.org/toolkits/substance-abuse/2/care-delivery/mental-health-integration

Rutkow, L., Chang, H. Y., Daubresse, M., Webster, D. W., Stuart, E. A., & Alexander, G. C. (2015). Effect of Florida's prescription drug monitoring program and pill mill laws on opioid prescribing and use. *JAMA Internal Medicine, 175*(10), 1642–1649. doi:10.1001/jamainternmed.2015.3931

Scholl, L., Seth, P., Kariisa, M., Wilson, N., & Baldwin, G. (2019). Drug and opioid-involved overdose deaths—United States, 2013–2017. *MMWR Morbidity and Mortality Weekly Report, 67*(51–52), 1419–1427.

Small, E., & Cronquist, A. (1976). A practical and natural taxonomy for cannabis. *Taxon, 25*(4), 405–435. doi:10.2307/1220524

Substance Abuse and Mental Health Services Administration. (2011). *Treatment episode data set (TEDS): 1999-2009. National admissions to substance abuse treatment services* (DASIS Series S-56, HHS Publication No. SMA 11-4646). Substance Abuse and Mental Health Services Administration. Retrieved from https://www.dasis.samhsa.gov/dasis2/teds_pubs/2009_teds_rpt_natl.pdf

Substance Abuse and Mental Health Services Administration. (2017). *Results from the 2016 National Survey on Drug Use and Health: Detailed tables.* Rockville, MD: Substance Abuse and Mental health Services Administration, Center for Behavioral Health Statistics and Quality.

Substance Abuse and Mental Health Services Administration. (2020). *Medication and counseling treatment.* Retrieved from https://www.samhsa.gov/medication-assisted-treatment/treatment

Substance Abuse and Mental Health Services Administration. (2020). *Recovery and recovery support.* Retrieved from https://www.samhsa.gov/find-help/recovery

Tashkin, D. P. (2013). Effects of marijuana smoking on the lung. *Annals of the American Thoracic Society, 10*(3), 239–247. doi:10.1513/AnnalsATS.201212-127FR

U.S. Department of Health and Human Services. (2014). *The health consequences of smoking—50 years of progress: A report of the surgeon general.* Atlanta, GA: Centers for Disease Control and Prevention.

U.S. Department of Health and Human Services. Burden of cigarette use in the U.S.: Current cigarette smoking among U.S. adults aged 18 years and older. U.S. Department of Health and Human Services, Centers for Disease Control and Prevention, National Center for Chronic Disease Prevention and Health Promotion, Office on Smoking and Health, 2014 [Accessed February 12, 2019].

U.S. Food and Drug Administration. (2020). *Products, ingredients & components.* Retrieved from https://www.fda.gov/tobacco-products/products-guidance-regulations/products-ingredients-components

PART 4

Health Disparities Among Special Populations

CHAPTER 16

Rural Public Health for Migrant Workers

Siew Li Ng, PhD, MA
Chun-Fang Frank Kuo, PhD, MS
Xiao Shiang Lee, MA
Wei Wen Megan Chow, BA

LEARNING OBJECTIVES

At the end of this chapter, readers will be able to:

1. Describe the immigration path and distribution patterns of migrant workers across the United States.
2. Identify the physical and mental health concerns of migrant workers as well as the key challenges they face when living in rural areas.
3. Explain the reasons behind the under-utilization of healthcare services among migrant workers.
4. Distinguish the similarities and differences in experiences faced by different subgroups and age groups within the migrant worker community.
5. Evaluate current efforts and suggestions provided to improve quality of life and increase accessibility of care for migrant workers.

KEY TERMS

Barriers to access health services
Mental health
Migrant workers
Physical health

CHAPTER OVERVIEW

This chapter begins with a brief introduction of the definitions of migrant workers as well as their country of origin and typical settlement patterns within the United States. Focusing on migrant workers in the rural areas, the subsequent sections of the chapter cover a wide range of physical and **mental health** practices that migrant workers have and concerns that they face. Finally, the chapter highlights the barriers that contribute to the health concerns they faced before concluding with suggestions to tackle the barriers identified.

Introduction

According to the United Nations Convention on the Rights of Migrants, the term "migrant worker" refers to someone who is currently involved or will be involved in work, who will be compensated, in a foreign State where this person is not a citizen; this is similar to what was defined by the International Labour Organization (Usher, 2004). Migrant workers are also sometimes referred to as foreign workers, expatriates or guest workers.

As of 2018, there are approximately 28.2 million foreign-born individuals working in the United States, which is about 17.4% of the total workforce, as estimated by the Bureau of Labor Statistics (2019, May 16). This number includes refugees, temporary residents, and undocumented immigrants. Approximately 47.7% of this population are individuals identified as Hispanic/Latinx (a more gender-neutral term for Latino and Latina), one-quarter (25.1%) is identified as Asians, 16.6% as White, and 9.5% as Black. For those aged 25 years and above, approximately 21.2% had not completed high school. The statistics also suggest that migrant workers were less likely than nonmigrant workers to have some college degree.

Although the report did not include information to distinguish between those in urban and rural areas, it did provide information on types of employment. Compared with non-migrant workers, **migrant workers** were more likely to be in the service industry; natural resources; construction and maintenance industry; and production, transportation, and material-moving industry (Bureau of Labor Statistics, 2019, May 16). They were also less likely to be in managerial, sales, and professional positions. On average, they also make less money than native-born residents. In addition, they are likely to be more vulnerable to discrimination in pay, especially for undocumented workers as they are at risk of being reported to the immigration authorities.

Statistics for Migrant Workers in Rural Areas

The migrant worker population in the United States is diverse as the migrant workers originate from various locations around the world. Studies suggest that the majority of them are predominantly from Mexico (e.g., Farmer & Slesinger, 1992; Frank, Liebman, Ryder, Weir, & Arcury, 2013; Hansen & Donohoe, 2003). Other notable places of origin include the Central American and Hispanic nations, and the Caribbean region—such as Barbados, Cuba, Haiti, and Jamaica. Additionally, Asians, Blacks, and rural Whites from Florida and other southeastern states make up the rest of the demographic composition.

Exhibit 16-1 Hispanic versus Latinx

Generally, Hispanic refers to individuals from Spanish-speaking countries, including those from Latin America or Spain, whereas Latinx refers to individuals who are born in or with ancestors from Latin America. (Encyclopaedia Britannica, n.d.) These categories indicate a person's place of origin or ancestry and not his or her race. A Hispanic or Latinx person can be of any race. (Encyclopaedia Britannica, n.d.) However, these two terms are often used interchangeably. In many surveys conducted, the categories for Hispanic and Latinx are sometimes combined, which makes it difficult to differentiate these individuals (Lopez, Krogstad, & Passel, 2020). Furthermore, some individuals (e.g., White Hispanic) may be forced to choose either "White" or "Hispanic" in some surveys. There is still an ongoing dispute over the usage of these terms due to its imperfect categorization. The terms used in this chapter are based on actual terms used in the sources of the information cited. For example, the term "Hispanic" may be used to represent both Hispanic and Latinx if the researchers or writers did not differentiate them.

In 2003, a survey on foreign-born individuals in the country from the U.S. Department of Commerce indicated that 53% of foreign-born residents were from Latin America, followed by Asia (25%), Europe (14%), and others (8%; Larsen, 2007). More recent data show ethnic composition specific to hired farmworkers across the United States. The U.S. Department of Labor's 2015–2016 National Agricultural Workers Survey collected data from 5,342 farmworkers, which estimated that 76% of farmworkers and their families were foreign-born, and were from Mexico (69%), Central America (6%), and others, including South America, the Caribbean, Asia, and the Pacific Islands (1%; Hernandez & Gabbard, 2018). The report also indicated that approximately 83% of these farmworkers were Hispanic.

Physical Health

Diet

Migrant workers in the United States commonly do not have proper nutritional intake. This may be due to a lack of resources such as cooking facilities, financial means, and time (Farmer & Slesinger, 1992). A lack thereof then poses a challenge for one's own meal preparation. Subsequently, migrant workers may sometimes prefer convenience food over healthy nutritious meals. This leads to an overconsumption of such food, which may not necessarily be beneficial for their health over time as convenience food, or processed food, have little to no nutritional value, and also contain high levels of sugar and sodium (Poti, Mendez, Ng, & Popkin, 2015). Some qualitative accounts from Hispanic migrant workers in Pennsylvania mentioned that they consumed more fast food and junk food, as well as bought more canned food since their arrival in the United States (Cason, Nieto-Montenegro, & Chavez-Martinez, 2006). They cited a lack of time as one of the reasons for these food choices because they were busy working long hours; hence, they relied partly on convenience when deciding what they eat. Moreover, some of the migrant workers also stated that they consume fewer fresh fruits and vegetables because they felt the prices were generally more expensive than those in their home countries (Cason et al., 2006).

Substance Use

In addition to having insufficient nutrients, migrant workers appeared to have a tendency to indulge in smoking and drinking behaviors. When it comes to drinking, their alcohol consumption is typically in high frequency and quantity, with some to the extent of having at least five drinks in one sitting (Alderete, Vega,

---

Exhibit 16-2 Migration Paths of Farmworkers

Historically, there are three major migration paths that migrant workers follow from south to north: Western Stream, Midwest Stream, and Eastern Stream (Farmer & Slesinger, 1992). First, the Western Stream—heading toward the west coast—begins from Mexico, southern Texas, Arizona, and California to Oregon and Washington. Second, starting from Mexico and southern Texas, the Midwest Stream passes through Arizona, Colorado, Kansas, and Missouri to get to Minnesota, Wisconsin, and Michigan. Finally, the Eastern Stream begins from southern Florida along the east coast to New York. It was common for migrant workers, especially those in the agriculture industry, to move seasonally between places as they follow the harvest season (Farmer & Slesinger, 1992). Many Mexicans and Hispanics were centered in Western and Midwest streams. As for the Eastern stream, most workers there were rural Blacks, Hispanics, nonHispanic Whites from southeastern states, Filipinos, Haitians, and Jamaicans. Since the 1980s, more Southeast Asians are settling around the Eastern and Western streams (Farmer & Slesinger, 1992).

Kolody, & Aguilar-Gaxiola, 2000). Between 2008 and 2010, Sánchez (2015) studied 278 Latinx migrant workers, particularly in south Florida, and found that 64.4% ($N = 179$) of them had consumed alcohol within 30 days prior to their initial assessment interview. Among them, nearly half (49.7%; $N = 89$) reported having five or more drinks per occasion, with beer as the standard choice of alcoholic beverage. When analyzing the frequency of heavy drinking of those 89 participants, slightly more than one-third (34.8%) reported drinking on a weekly basis or even more often than that. Interestingly, in spite of the high frequency and quantity being reported, only a small percentage (13.4%) of those who consumed alcohol ($N = 179$) is indicative of potential alcohol abuse and dependence.

Compared with their drinking behaviors, there is a lower likelihood of smoking prevalence among migrant workers. In general, the smoking prevalence statistics were comparably lower for immigrants (13.4%) than for native-born residents (22.6%; Baluja, Park, & Myers, 2003). Based on the farmworker sample in south Georgia ($N = 405$), the majority (71.4%) had never engaged in smoking while the remaining percentage consists of current and former smokers (Fleischer et al., 2013). Nevertheless, smoking remains a high-risk behavior and a risk factor for tobacco use and eventual health problems.

Sleep

Another common health pattern is poor sleep quality. Poor levels of sleep quality have been documented through several studies among migrant farmworkers in various parts of the country, ranging from 17% in North Carolina (Sandberg et al., 2016) to 20% in Texas (Shipp et al., 2009). Other findings also include reports of having less than eight hours of sleep per night (Shipp et al., 2009) and elevated daytime sleepiness (Sandberg et al., 2012). This becomes a concern given that migrant workers typically have long working hours and strenuous working conditions, which puts them at an increased risk for occupational injuries. Poor sleep quality was also correlated to poor health indicators as well as high levels of musculoskeletal pain, depressive symptoms, and anxiety (Sandberg et al., 2014).

Physical Activity and Body Weight

Furthermore, research has shown that immigrants and refugees in the United States tend to have a lack of physical activity compared with the nonimmigrant population (Wieland et al., 2015). One possible explanation is attributed to the shifting trend in sedentary lifestyles (e.g., watching television, playing video games, etc.) because people are becoming increasingly more dependent on technological devices. It was also stated that more time was spent outdoors when in their home country compared with when they were in the United States, which could have allowed opportunities to be physically active (Wieland et al., 2015). In addition, time constraints due to work demands also reduce the likelihood of these individuals exercising. After spending long hours at work, not only is the available time for physical activity reduced but the energy level is also reduced. They would likely experience fatigue, after which they would feel too tired and disheartened to get involved with more physical activities like exercise and sports. Although the study by Wieland et al., (2015) was based on a small urban area in Minnesota, it is expected that similar effects can also be observed in rural migrant communities elsewhere considering that the nature of their work can be more physically intense.

A combination of poor diet and sleep, alcohol consumption, and a lack of exercise may have resulted in deteriorating health conditions among migrant workers. For instance, Mexican farmworkers showed health declines within the first few years after their arrival in the United States (Villarejo, 2003). Some even reported gaining weight since starting work in the United States mainly due to dramatic changes in their diet and lifestyle (Cason et al., 2006). In fact, higher obesity rates are typically observed among those of Hispanic descent (Velasco-Mondragon, Jimenez, Palladino-Davis, Davis, & Escamilla-Cejudo, 2016). This can be seen across all age groups as Hispanic children, youth, and adults were more likely to be obese than their non-Hispanic White counterparts. In terms of gender differences, females were more prone to be obese than males. However, between foreign-born Hispanics and native-born Hispanics, the obesity rates were significantly different at 36.3% and 47.1%, respectively (Dominguez et al., 2015) and higher degrees of acculturation correlated with greater body weight across all migrant groups (Barcenas et al., 2007).

To understand what underlies the obesity epidemic among the Hispanic population in the United States, several contributing factors will be discussed as follows (e.g., Pan, Sherry, Njai, & Blanck, 2012; Rosado, Johnson, McGinnity, & Cuevas, 2013; Velasco-Mondragon, Jimenez, Palladino-Davis, Davis, & Escamilla-Cejudo, 2016). First, there is a significant relationship between food insecurity and obesity. Food insecurity, which is the state of having limited access to sufficient and nutritious food, is usually associated with low-income households. People experiencing food insecurity may have difficulties in maintaining a nutritionally rich diet, so they may find themselves consuming high-calorie, low-nutrient, low-cost foods. This can then lead to excessive caloric intake, contributing to the development of obesity. In general, foreign-born residents are more likely to encounter healthcare inequalities and are less likely to receive preventative counseling.

Parents decidedly play a role in shaping their children's eating behaviors. Hispanic mothers have a tendency to feed their children indulgently as there is a cultural connotation that thinness is unhealthy, hence cultivating a preference for children to be heavier (Lindsay, Sussner, Greaney, & Peterson, 2011; Power,

O'Connor, Fisher, & Hughes, 2015). As a result, these mothers may fail to recognize their children as overweight or subsequently obese. Additionally, the promotion of high-calorie, low-nutrient foods and beverages are especially being marketed and targeted toward children, which increases the likelihood of childhood obesity. Finally, a study by Rosado, Johnson, McGinnity, and Cuevas (2013) indicated that a parent's body mass index (BMI) is predictive of a child's BMI. Based on a sample of Latinx migrant farmworkers in rural southwest Florida ($N = 472$), approximately 83% of parents were either overweight or obese whereas the percentage of their children who fell within these two categories was nearly half (47%).

Morbidity & Mortality

The leading causes of death for migrant workers are cancer, heart disease, and unintentional injuries (Velasco-Mondragon et al., 2016). Farmworkers have a high mortality rate from injuries. As they only seek healthcare services when they are suffering from extreme pain or chronic illness, it could have been too late as the prognosis of their condition would have worsened (Villarejo, 2003).

Chronic Illness

For migrant workers in the United States, one of the most prevalent chronic illnesses is diabetes. In comparison, Hispanics (12.8%) have a higher incidence of diabetes than non-Hispanic Whites (7.6%; Centers for Disease Control and Prevention; CDC, 2014). The percentage breakdown of diabetes diagnoses within the Hispanic subgroups in 2012 is as follows: 14.8% for Puerto Ricans, 13.9% for Mexicans, 9.3% for Cubans, and 8.5% for Central and South Americans (CDC, 2014).

Other chronic illnesses include cardiovascular diseases, hypertension (high blood pressure), and cancer (Velasco-Mondragon et al., 2016). In relation to incidence of cancer among Hispanic men, the most common cancers are prostate (22%), colorectal (11%), and lung (9%). As for Hispanic women, the most common cancer types are breast (29%), thyroid (9%), colorectal (8%), and uterine (8%).

Obesity is another chronic health concern, which is particularly prevalent among the Hispanic migrant communities. Substance abuse, especially alcohol and tobacco, are also commonly identified in the migrant populations (Farmer & Slesinger, 1992; Frank et al., 2013; Villarejo, 2003). Excessive alcohol consumption is associated with gastrointestinal bleeding and acute withdrawal symptoms (Watson, Mattera, Morales, Kunitz, & Lynch; 1985) as well as fatty liver disease (Velasco-Mondragon et al., 2016).

Prevalence of chronic illnesses also varies according to locations in the United States (Villarejo, 2003). For instance, in California, obesity and high serum cholesterol were reported with high rates of prevalence among the farmworkers. Meanwhile, it was respiratory diseases for the farmworkers in Indiana whereby increased chronic respiratory symptoms such as coughing, wheezing, and sputum production were indicated. Villarejo and his colleagues' (2010) study indicated that although there was an increase in prevalence of chronic disease among immigrant farmworkers in California, there was a lack of healthcare access, which could be attributed to a lack of knowledge on workplace protection.

All in all, the leading cause of death for Hispanics in the United States is cancer, followed by cardiovascular diseases (Velasco-Mondragon et al., 2016). When it comes to cancer deaths, the main cause for men is lung (17%), seconded by liver (12%), followed lastly by colorectal (11%). On the other hand, breast (16%), lung (13%), and colorectal (9%) are the main causes of cancer deaths among women. Despite that, Hispanics generally have a 30% lower mortality rate due to cancer and 25% lower due to cardiovascular disease than non-Hispanic Whites. Factors that

can influence these differences in mortality rates include age, first-generation migrant status, healthy immigrant effects (e.g., Hispanic Mortality Paradox—a phenomenon in which Hispanic immigrants have relatively better health outcomes than non-Hispanic immigrants), origin country, late-stage detection and diagnosis, and access to preventive and diagnostic health care (Velasco-Mondragon et al., 2016).

Environment

Migrant workers are, more often than not, exposed to hazardous working environments due to the high-risk nature of jobs they hold. Some examples of tasks are operating machinery, handling agricultural pesticides, and working with livestock. Among all private industry sectors in 2018, agriculture, forestry, and fishing industries had the highest injury and illness rate at 5.3 per 100 workers (Bureau of Labor Statistics, 2019, November 7). Due to the fact that they had to work with below-par safety measures and that they may be unskilled at times, it would explain why they have a higher risk of mortality from occupational injuries such as respiratory and skin complications in addition to eye and musculoskeletal conditions (Carballo & Nerukar, 2001; Velasco-Mondragon et al., 2016; Villarejo, 2003).

Exposure to chemicals and dangerous machinery could lead to traumatic injuries like chemical burns and bone fractures (Frank et al., 2013). Particularly in the agriculture industry, workers have a higher risk of exposure to harmful levels of agricultural pesticides, in which prolonged exposure can lead to symptoms like headache, fatigue, and nausea. Those with extended contact with tobacco leaves may exhibit green tobacco sickness, which is a kind of nicotine poisoning. Besides that, workers are more prone to dehydration, heat stress, and heat stroke if they are constantly working under extreme heat. Other hazards also include road safety, poor weather conditions, and sleep deprivation.

Why do such injuries happen? A common obstacle for migrant workers is the command of language. When language is a barrier for them, difficulties in understanding the safety instructions and potential risks may arise (Anthony, Martin, Avery, & Williams, 2010; Carballo & Nerukar, 2001).

Infectious Disease

Sexually transmitted diseases (STD), urinary tract infections (UTI), and tuberculosis (TB) are prevalent infectious diseases in the migrant population (Frank et al., 2013; Hansen & Donohoe, 2003; Villarejo, 2003). Albarrán and Nyamathi (2011) suggest that Mexican migrant workers' increased risk in HIV infection are likely due to unprotected sex, multiple sexual partners, limited access to healthcare services, lay injection practices, as well as sex between men.

One's living conditions can also compromise his or her health. Migrant workers often live in overcrowded and unsanitary housing, making them more vulnerable to infectious diseases (Hansen & Donohoe, 2003). Moreover, with the limited access to clean water and septic systems, urinary tract infection becomes another concern for the migrant populations (Hansen & Donohoe, 2003).

Lack Preventive Care

Most migrant workers fall under the low-income class. As a result, they are unable to afford the premiums for health insurance and choose to seek medical services only when their symptoms become severe (Farmer & Slesinger, 1992; Villarejo, 2003). Without the insurance to pay for medical services, this means that they are also unlikely to receive vaccination, rendering them vulnerable to various health risks. Children of migrant parents typically receive some form of vaccination, however, at a delayed point in time (Farmer & Slesinger, 1992; Villarejo, 2003).

Self-Treatment

Generally, migrant workers are likely to perform self-treatment where they would attempt to medicate themselves without professional medical supervision (Anthony et al., 2010). This could be due to challenges faced by migrant workers when they try to seek medical attention. Examples of these challenges include sick leave being prohibited by their employer, no transportation means, an inability to stop work, and a lack of money for medical care (Cooper, Burau, Frankowski, Shipp, Del Junco, & Whitworth, 2006). Common self-treatment of migrant workers are home remedies and over-the-counter treatments for injuries and using folk or herbal remedies for illnesses. At times, migrant workers may not even seek treatment but only rest (Anthony et al., 2010). When migrant workers do seek professional help, they often do not discuss their use of home remedies and alternative care to their healthcare providers (Poss, Pierce, & Prieto, 2005). This can be dangerous and a concern as this information is important to healthcare providers for an accurate diagnosis and subsequent treatment.

Oral Health

Oral health care is one of the areas often neglected among migrant workers for several reasons. Dental care can be costly and visiting the dentist can be challenging due to limited clinic hours and a lack of transportation. Additionally, migrant workers' dissatisfaction with past experiences and long waiting times can be off-putting for them to seek dental care. Other obstacles include language barriers, workers' immigration status, and limited insurance coverage. Finally, a lack of awareness and discrimination can further discourage migrant workers from visiting dental health clinics (Hansen & Donohoe, 2003; Frank et al., 2013). As a result, a majority of migrant workers' dental problems are left untreated, where they often have missing or

---

Exhibit 16-3 Maternal Care Among Migrant Workers

Maternal care among migrant workers are generally underdeveloped. Expecting mothers in the migrant community who work at jobs that require high physical demands can be at risk of overexertion, dehydration, and even exposure to harmful chemicals in their (Frank et al., 2013). As a result, these expecting mothers may be at an increased risk for spontaneous abortion, premature delivery, and abnormal pre- or postnatal development. In addition to these, poor diet, a lack of prenatal care support, as well as low socioeconomic status (Frank et al., 2013) often increase risk for both mother and child.

For migrant workers, poorer sexual education, a lack of understanding and access to contraceptives sometimes increase cases of unwanted pregnancies where they may later seek an abortion. In Spain, requests for abortion are two times higher among migrant workers than Spanish women (Carballo & Nerukar, 2001). This lack of sexual education and access to health care can be attributed to challenges presented in terms of differences in language medium, environmental circumstances, accessibility of knowledge, and social status (Carballo & Nerukar, 2001; Villarejo, 2003).

Although the Patient Protection and Affordable Care Act and enhanced Medicaid for perinatal care are in place to improve access to health care for those living in the United States, yet barriers still exist between migrant workers and obtaining care. Some reasons cited for the lack of access include not being "poor enough" to meet the requirement to qualify for Medicaid without any structured perinatal care and being unable to afford the coverage offered by the ACA (Valesco-Mondragon et al., 2016). Furthermore, those who were born outside of the United States may not be eligible for Medicaid coverage. Many migrant workers without insurance would only seek help when complications arise or when they are in labor. Lesser attention is also paid to children's health among migrant workers, and this is associated with poverty as well as a lack of health insurance and a regular physician (Smith, Kreutzer, Goldman, Casey-Paal, & Kizer, 1996).

---

broken teeth or periodontal disease (Villarejo, 2003). Similarly, for children of migrant workers, a large number of their dental cases are also left untreated (Nurko, Aponte-Merced, Bradley, & Fox, 1998).

Mental Health

Stress, Anxiety, and Depression

Stress is one of the strongest and most consistent predictors of poor mental health. Many migrant workers constantly operate at high stress levels daily (Frank et al., 2013), facing many stressors as they work in a foreign country. A study conducted in Northern California found that approximately 57.8% ($N = 102$) of day laborers experienced elevated stress levels (Duke, Bourdeau, & Hovey, 2010). As

migrant workers typically engage in hard physical work that not only pays minimally but also lacks job security, they often need to worry about meeting basic needs for themselves and their families in their home countries. Moreover, when migrant workers come to the United States, they need to abide by the immigration policies and procedures, which can be a very stressful process. The mental health of Latinx in the United States has been found to be closely related to the immigration policy restrictions (Hatzenbuehler, Prins, Flake, Philbin, Frazer, Hagen, & Hirsch, 2017). In addition to the physical concerns stated above, other stressors that migrant workers face include separation from friends and family, rejection from local communities, social exclusion, stigma, discrimination, and fear of deportation.

High stress levels, especially chronic stress, may contribute to manifestation of a

---

Exhibit 16-4 Acculturative Stress

Acculturation is a process of change that happens when two or more cultures come into contact, where balancing and adjustment of cultures occurs when one acquires new practices or values and adapts to a new environment Berry (2004). This is a common process that takes place for immigrants who move to a new country where cultural values and practices are often different from their own. As one moves to a new place and tries to assimilate into another culture, the person often faces multiple stressors as they go through the acculturation process. For example, he or she may be forced to separate from family members, have to face the possibility of deportation, and experience rejection from the dominant culture due to his or her immigrant or ethnic minority status. As a result, the person may experience elevated levels of stress during this process. Acculturative stress, a term coined by Berry (1970), refers to the psychological impact and stress as a result of acculturation. Acculturative stress has been found to be associated with various mental health concerns experienced by immigrants, which will be described in the sub-sections under mental health.

---

variety of problems such as physical illnesses, increased anger, anxiety, depression, low self-esteem, alienation, suicidality, psychosomatic complaints, substance abuse, and a lack of self-confidence (Carballo & Nerukar, 2001; Gonzales, Suárez-Orozco, & Dedios-Sanguineti, 2013; Hansen & Donohoe, 2003). According to a study done with farmworkers in the Midwest region, approximately 37.8% of their participants scored at or above the cutoff score that indicates a risk of depression against an expected percentage of 18% estimated from the general population (Hovey & Magaña, 2000). As for anxiety, it was 28.9% (farmworkers) against 16% (estimated number from the general population). Similar results were found in a study done in Nebraska where 45.8% of 200 migrant farmworkers were identified to be depressed and more than 30% of them experienced high levels of stress (Ramos, Su, Lander, & Rivera, 2015).

Elevation in stress, anxiety, or depression levels is not uncommon among migrant workers. Some studies suggest that certain occupations may present more physical and mental health risks for migrant workers. Results from Arcury and colleagues (2018) suggested that farmworkers may experience greater anxiety and stress compared with non-farmworkers in a sample consists of Latinx workings in North Carolina. Furthermore, employed farmworkers and non-farmworkers experienced

greater anxiety and stress than those who were unemployed (Arcury, Sandberg, Talton, Laurienti, Daniel, & Quandt, 2018). Agriculture, being a hazardous industry due to repeated exposure to dangerous chemicals, machinery, extreme weather, and livestock, is likely one of the main contributing factors to the significant mental health concerns observed among this specific migrant worker population. Rural Latinx farmworkers utilize community health clinics and private practices for their health concerns. Farmworkers tend to seek health care when they experience elevated depressive symptoms (Georges, Alterman, Gabbard, Grzywacz, Shen, Nakamoto, Carroll, & Muntaner, 2013).

Stigma and Discrimination

Stigma

Individuals who do not conform to the normative or dominant culture are likely stigmatized. Stigma is a phenomenon where a person's attribute, visible or not, is severely discredited by others in the society (Goffman, 1963). In the case of migrant workers, many aspects of their lives may be perceived as nonconforming; for example, their appearance, language used, traditional cultural values, and dietary practices, among others. When such attributes are made known in migrant workers and perceived by others in the dominant cultural group, migrant workers may be rejected or discriminated due to their immigrant status as long as they are stigmatized. Stigmatization has been found to be related to many physical and mental health issues within the minority community such as anxiety, depression, and chronic physical illnesses.

In addition to stigmatization against migrant workers due to their statuses, migrant workers themselves may have their own stigmas that affects their mental well-being. Despite the increasing effort for mental health awareness, mental disorders are still highly stigmatized by the general public and more so by migrant workers' community. They are often unwilling to attribute symptoms to a mental disorder. Mental health services are rarely available in rural areas, and if they are, migrant workers face additional challenges on seeking help due to cultural and language barriers (Kirmayer et al., 2011).

Stigmatization against mental disorders reduces the likelihood of mental health conditions receiving a proper diagnosis, which further limits treatment options. A review by Kirmayer and colleagues (2011) found that migrant workers are also sometimes reluctant to share or disclose personal and emotional problems to others outside of their family as they are concerned about feelings of shame, being labeled as mentally unstable, or bringing scrutiny to their family. In cases in which they perceive their problems to be psychological in nature, they are probably unwilling to seek medical treatment. Furthermore, migrant women sometimes fear that seeking treatment will cause them to lose authority over their children and this further discourages them from seeking help from mental health providers.

Discrimination

Discrimination refers to the unfair or prejudicial treatment of individuals based on their characteristics such as race, gender, or socioeconomic status (American Psychological Association, 2020). Many migrant workers face discrimination where they are unfairly treated than nonimmigrants. Often exploited due to their immigrant status, employers at work may take advantage of migrant workers due to actual or perceived lack of legal protection for these individuals (Moyce & Schenker, 2018). Discrimination against migrant workers could be in the form of failure to implement appropriate safety measures; physical, verbal, or sexual abuse; working longer hours; delayed payment; or withholding of food (Kirmayer et al., 2011; Moyce & Schenker, 2018; Snipes, Cooper, & Shipp, 2018). These actions often bring about a negative impact on migrant workers' lives. Snipes, Cooper, and Shipp (2018) conducted ethnographic fieldwork in which Latinx farmworkers were interviewed about their experience with injury and discrimination in which many were left untreated and pressured to continue working despite being injured. One farmworker said, "The only thing I wish I could change is that they treat us like people and not like animals," which effectively captures how they perceived being treated by their employers.

At the state or national levels, policies are often created to improve the physical and mental well-being of ethnic minorities. However, some policies can indirectly lead to more harm in the migrant worker population if they inadvertently perpetuate social exclusion, which leads to discrimination. For example, Hardy and colleagues (2012) found that Latinx were less likely to apply for services that they are qualified for and experienced more fear and decreased mobility following the passage of Arizona Senate Bill 1070. Instead of making residents feel safer, there was a general increase in fear of deportation, being separated from their children, and losing jobs, among others. Such fears indirectly affected their **physical health** because they had limited opportunities to exercise and access healthier food options (Hardy, Getrich, Quezada, Guay, Michalowski, & Henley,

Isolation

Exhibit 16-5 Additional Information on Arizona Senate Bill 1070

U.S. Federal law requires any foreign individuals to possess necessary documentation at all times whereas Arizona Senate Bill 1070 (S.B. 1070) requires that law enforcement officers attempt to determine an individual's status and suggests that they can detain or arrest those under reasonable suspicion that they may be illegal immigrants. This act also imposes penalties on anyone suspected of sheltering, employing, or transporting undocumented immigrants.

Migrant workers also face social and physical isolation as they are separated from their friends and family back home if they work at a job that often requires long hours. This lack of social support and living near poverty on top of needing to constantly relocate and fearing unemployment are additional obstacles that migrant workers face. Being away from familiar people and environment are also challenges as they have to learn to adapt to new routines and value systems. Feelings of isolation are often associated with poorer mental and physical health such as higher prevalence of stress, substance abuse, and sexually transmitted diseases (Carballo & Nerukar, 2001; Frank et al., 2013; Hansen & Donohoe, 2003).

2012). Undocumented immigrants are often deterred from seeking help. The restrictions that are experienced in people's lives impact their mental health. Hatzenbuehler and colleagues (2017) found that more exclusionary immigration policies leads to poorer mental health, especially among Latinx.

Violence

Domestic or family violence within the migrant worker population, as a health problem, has been receiving more attention over the

Exhibit 16-6 Mental Health of Children and Youth of Migrant Workers

Children of migrant workers often experience stressors that unfavorably affect their physical and mental health. Some of them may be separated from their family before they are reunited with their parents in a foreign environment. Their parents' undocumented status, constant fear of separation and deportation, and acculturative stress may negatively affect their mental well-being.

In the process of relocation and acculturation, they experience various stressors and disruptions to their emotional and educational development, which contribute to social withdrawal, depression, anxiety, and somatic symptoms (Kirmayer et al., 2011; Sirin, Ryce, Gupta & Rogers-Sirin, 2013). This increases their risk of developing psychopathological disorders, including posttraumatic stress disorder, depression, anxiety, and conduct disorder (Kirmayer et al., 2011). In addition, they may experience an identity crisis, racism and discrimination, language and educational barriers, social isolation, as well as financial difficulties that contribute to their self-blame and internalized shame (Gonzales, Suarez-Orozco, & Dedios-Sanguineti, 2013). Those who are unaccompanied and have an unstable living environment are at high risk for mental health concerns.

However, some children of migrant workers do exceptionally well compared with their native-born peers, surpassing them in terms of aspiration and academic achievement (Kirmayer et al., 2011). Despite having experienced war or political tension at their home country, they have relatively good mental and physical health. For others, programs such as the Deferred Action for Childhood Arrivals (DACA) program (Siemons, Raymond-Flesh, Auerswald, & Brindis, 2017) helps undocumented immigrant youth to reduce stress and improve mental health. It also helps to increase access to resources, support, mental health services, and health insurance. Adolescents have also reported feeling a greater sense of autonomy and sense of belonging after having gone through this program (Siemons et al., 2017).

years. Although this phenomenon is difficult to be recognized by healthcare workers due to language and cultural differences within these families, female leaders, sometimes the spouses of abusive men, have since brought the issue to light to be addressed (Villarejo, 2003). Women and children are among the most susceptible to domestic abuse and mistreatment at home. Domestic violence is a serious health problem as it not only affects the present but also the well-being and growth of children who grow up in such a household. Past research has indicated that exposure to violence is connected with poorer mental health, emotional issues such as low self-esteem, feelings of hopelessness, distrust of others, and behavioral problems such as absenteeism and even carrying weapons (Fantuzzo & Mohr, 1999; Villarejo, 2003).

Overall, many migrant workers suffer from poor mental health due to stressors such as unstable employment, low income, rejection and discrimination from the dominant cultural group, and a political climate of anti-immigration. These psychosocial and individual factors impact occupational health in multicultural workforces (Capasso, Zurlo, & Smith, 2018). There are needs for mental health services especially for farmworkers in rural areas and a comprehensive approach to treat and prevent mental health issues (Grzywacz, 2009). Mental health outreach may be useful to improve farmworkers quality of life and reduce healthcare utilization (Georges, Alterman, Gabbard, Grzywacz, Shen, Nakamoto, Carroll, & Muntaner, 2013).

Barriers to Health Care for Migrant Workers

Language Barrier

Language barrier is one of the main factors that impedes migrant workers from receiving appropriate physical and mental healthcare services in the United States. The English language is not a native language to most migrant workers, who come from different parts of the world. Only about 1 in 10 migrant workers claim that they can speak or read English fluently (Villarejo, 2003). In fact, many of them are functionally illiterate in both English and their native language, particularly among farmworkers (Arcury & Quandt, 2007). Although many agencies try to accommodate by including Spanish translations for application forms or instructions needed, it is still difficult for migrant workers to use healthcare services when they are not literate in Spanish, even if it is their native language. Furthermore, due to the lack of language skills, migrant workers may find it challenging to apply for and purchase insurance, especially when they have to complete application forms (Farmer & Slesinger, 1992).

Generally, there is a lack of trained healthcare providers who are bilingual, especially in rural areas. As there are limited linguistically-appropriate services, many medical staff are not able to communicate directly with their patients. Migrants workers may request nonmedical staff members or friends to translate; however, they may sometimes be embarrassed about their physical or mental health condition. If these translators are not properly trained, there is also a risk of mistranslation, where the meanings of words or instructions may be misconstrued. Mistranslations or incomplete information will likely affect the quality of the diagnosis and subsequently treatment will be affected (Cristancho, Garces, Peters, & Mueller, 2008; Derose, Escarce, & Lurie, 2007). As a result, a lower quality of care may be provided and these experiences may influence healthcare-seeking behaviors, where migrant workers may avoid seeking treatment or will not adhere to a treatment regimen (Documét & Sharma, 2004), especially if they feel embarrassed or do not fully understand the medical instructions given. Thus, the language barrier could present multiple challenges to migrant workers from receiving appropriate healthcare services.

Cultural Differences in Understanding Health

Cultural differences in terms of understanding and approaching health care also pose as a barrier to migrant workers from receiving healthcare services in the United States. Such variation in cultural values and practices often result in a wide variety of differences in terms of health-seeking behaviors e.g., traditional healing methods, vaccination, foreign healthcare system, and treatment follow-up practices.

Vaccination and Traditional Healing Methods

Generally, migrant workers are less likely or show delay in acquiring vaccination(s). Depending on their country of origin, they appear to hold beliefs that are different from western medical models, especially in terms of treatment regimen. Some tend to follow their traditional healing methods instead of going to healthcare providers for treatment. For example, Hispanics believe receiving injections is not only beneficial to health but also superior to orally administered treatment (McVea, 1997); hence, many would choose to receive injections of vitamins or antibiotics from a lay person over a conventional treatment modality offered in the United States and do not adhere to the treatment regimen prescribed by medical professionals (Villarejo, 2003).

Migrant workers may also be more comfortable in using traditional methods to alleviate medical concerns over western medicine (Arcury & Quandt, 2007). There are many Hispanic and Latinx who believe in folk or traditional healing. Unfortunately, the use of traditional medicine may hamper the use of conventional medical treatment if taken together. However, the use of these traditional methods are not usually made known to physicians who attend to the patients. These medical professionals are also unlikely to be knowledgeable about the differences in understanding health when treating the foreign workers (Villarejo, 2003).

Foreign Healthcare System and Follow-up Treatment

Migrant workers, especially those who have recently arrived and are less socially integrated those who have may lack trust and knowledge of the U.S. healthcare system (Kemppainen, Kemppainen, Skogberg, Kuusio & Koponen, 2017). As a result, they may be more comfortable in returning to their own country to seek treatment where there are no language and cultural barriers between doctors and patients, and the doctors are more aware of their cultural concerns (Kemppainen et al., 2017; Villarejo, 2003). Often, treatment received in their home country is also more cost-effective. However, migrant workers are often not able to travel home frequently, which results in a delay in treatment, and thus increases the likelihood of a poorer prognosis. This also reduces the likelihood that they are able to attend any follow-up treatment in their home country after the initial visit.

Access to Services

Accessibility of healthcare services poses another challenge for migrant workers. Multiple factors contribute to the **barriers to access health services** for these individuals, e.g., a lack of resources, transportation issues, poverty, health insurance availability, health assistance programs, and discrimination. As a result, many are not able to receive appropriate health care which subsequently lowers their quality of life.

Lack of Resources

There have been many changes in the rural healthcare system over the years with the introduction of new technologies and dissemination methods. Despite these efforts and improvements, available resources in rural areas remain relatively inadequate to cater to the needs of their residents (Ricketts, 2000). For example, there are fewer options for hospitals and clinics, limited clinic hours, insufficient medical facilities, a shortage of professional staff or specialists, insufficient mental health services, and a lack of advocacy- and community-based organizations (Derose et al., 2007; Frank et al., 2013). The demand for specialty care is rarely met in rural communities where most farmworkers work and live (Ricketts, 2000). Hospital and medical facilities in rural areas also usually lack effective medical interpretation services. As a majority of migrant workers speak Spanish and little English, the lack of appropriate translation services lowers the quality of care offered, which contributes to a general sense of dissatisfaction of the patients (Cristancho et al., 2008).

Transportation Issues

Migrant workers often do not have a car and they need to rely on public transportation to access health clinics that are often located far from where the workers live (Frank et al., 2013). Public transportation, however, may not be available to those who live in rural or new areas (Cristancho, Garces, Peters & Mueller, 2008; Farmer & Slesinger, 1992). In cases in which they do exist, migrant workers may lack sufficient funds to commute to the health clinics. Individuals who own a car have concerns over high gasoline prices, especially when they have to travel out of town for specialist's care (Cristancho et al., 2008). Moreover, migrant workers are sometimes subjected to constant relocation, which complicates the ability to monitor their progress, and inaccessibility of health care further inhibits preventative care or regular check-ups (Arcury & Quandt, 2007).

Poverty

The high cost of healthcare services in the United States often deters migrant workers from seeking treatment as many migrant workers are living near or below the poverty level, which makes it difficult for them to pay for such services (Cristancho et al., 2008; Hansen & Donohoe, 2003). Although some of them are able to pay for the consultation's fee for the doctor's visit, some participants at a focus-group discussion expressed that they may not be able to afford the medications prescribed for their condition (Cristancho et al., 2008). In addition, these researchers also found that many female migrant workers are unable to afford regular screening programs for women due to the costs.

Migrant workers, especially those recently arrived, may not understand the healthcare system in the United States, which contributes to their reluctance in accessing the available services. For example, they may not understand the different services available and may visit the emergency department at hospitals for mild health-related issues when other, more affordable options are available. They may also not be aware of where they can go to ask for help in navigating through the healthcare system in the United States (Cristancho et al., 2008).

Health Insurance

Insurance coverage is important in the United States due to relatively high costs of healthcare services. However, migrant workers generally have lower rates of having health insurance (Carrasquillo, Carrasquillo, & Shea, 2000; Derose et al., 2007; Villarejo, 2003). Migrant workers who have a low income, recently arrived, and limited English capacity are more likely to be uninsured (Cristancho et al., 2008). The lack of health insurance is a huge challenge as it makes it difficult for them to afford health care in general. Utilization of healthcare services is typically low among immigrants; dental and vision care are even lower.

Having illegal statuses or a lack of documentation makes it difficult for migrant workers to get health insurance (Arcury &

Quandt, 2007; Carrasquillo et al., 2000). Immigrants have few public benefits; however, benefits such as Medicaid, State Children's Health Insurance Program (SCHIP), and Medicare are not available for those without legal documentation (Frank et al., 2013). Some individuals who fled their own country—e.g., undocumented immigrants from Guatemala and El Salvador—for political reasons but were not granted refugee status are then not entitled to these benefits (Carrasquillo et al., 2000). Due to the fear of deportation, losing their job or putting future security at risk, undocumented migrant workers avoid healthcare services for fear of being reported to the authorities (Arcury & Quandt, 2007; Carrasquillo et al., 2000; Derose et al., 2007).

When immigrants want to apply for insurance, they may lack the knowledge to navigate through the healthcare system, which prevents them from being insured (Cristancho et al., 2008). The differences that exist among different insurance plans, policies, and eligibility criteria could create more difficulty for migrant workers. For example, Medicaid eligibility varies according to states, and this creates confusion and ambiguity for them to fully be aware of what is available to them. Immigrants who are not citizens of the United States were less likely to receive government insurance than native-born or naturalized immigrants (Carrasquillo et al., 2000). Language barriers and unclear instructions also make it difficult for them to comprehend the insurance plans. Some are also deterred from getting health insurance due to the high costs associated with it and limited coverage of the plans (Cristancho et al., 2008).

When the application is finally submitted, there are factors that impact the likelihood of approval of migrant workers' insurance applications such as income level, time residing in the United States, and residency status (Carrasquillo et al., 2000; Cristancho et al., 2008). For example, legal immigrants are not eligible for publicly funded services such as Medicaid for the first five years of residence (Derose, Escarce & Lurie, 2007). For those who are in the process of applying for a legal status, without proper documentation, they do not have access to employer-provided health insurance (Frank et al., 2013).

Few migrant workers are insured through their employment (Cristancho et al., 2008). Some employers are less likely to apply for health insurance for immigrants from Central America, the Caribbean, Vietnam, and Korea compared with those from Europe, India, and the Philippines. Among immigrants, employers are least likely to apply for health insurance for Mexicans (Carrasquillo et al., 2000). Even if insured, farmworkers usually do not get paid time-off to see a doctor (Arcury., & Quandt, 2007). They work long hours, fear losing their pay or job, and do not have sick leave (Arcury & Quandt, 2007; Farmer & Slesinger, 1992). These factors make it less likely for them to use the available services.

A study done by Cristancho and colleagues (2008) found that most pregnant women and children were insured through Medicaid. However, those who have Medicaid perceived that they were treated differently from those who held private insurance. In addition, they also expressed concerns that most healthcare providers in rural areas were not accepting Medicaid patients; as a result, these migrant workers had to travel to other cities to get access to needed services.

Health Assistance Programs

There are a number of public and private health assistance programs delivering healthcare services to migrant workers who struggle to access these services on their own. For example, programs such as Migrant Health Program and Community Health Center (CHC) are designed to provide health services to migratory and seasonal farmworkers and their families as well as to individuals from medically underserved areas, respectively

(Frank et al., 2013). Organizations such as the National Center for Farmworker Health and National Association of Community Health Centers were founded to improve the health of local communities, some focusing on assisting specific populations (e.g., farmworkers, pregnant women and their children). Many of these programs provide services regardless of one's immigration status. However, not all hospitals or clinics accept these health assistance programs, and many of them do not cover all family members. As there are a number of programs available, there could also be confusion with these different programs. Difficulties in accessing services may then create more frustration among migrant workers and their families.

Discrimination

Discrimination is another barrier contributing to migrant workers' health concerns. As mentioned previously, many migrant workers experience prejudicial and unjust treatment. Immigrants are often discriminated against due to their differences in physical appearance, cultural values and practices, language and communication styles, accent, and skin tone (Derose, Escarce & Lurie, 2007). Non-immigrants may perceive these individuals as overburdening the healthcare system and taking away the opportunities for these health services from those they perceive as more deserving. As a result of discrimination, they are often socially isolated and excluded, and they may be treated unequally when they try to access healthcare services (e.g., Carballo & Nerukar, 2001; Cristancho et al., 2008; Kirmayer et al., 2011). With discriminating actions and stereotypical attitudes targeted at immigrants, these individuals are more likely to avoid healthcare systems in the United States, which contributes to an underutilization of health services among the migrant population (Cristancho et al., 2008; Documét & Sharma, 2004; Kemppainen et al., 2017).

Suggestions

Education and Training
Health Concerns

The lack of knowledge on health has contributed to physical and mental health concerns that migrant workers experience. For example, they may not be aware of the consequences of certain dietary patterns, risky behaviors (e.g., sharing needles), chronic illnesses, or prolonged depression, and thus fail to seek early treatment or preventative care. It is, therefore, important to educate them on both physical and mental health concerns typical to this population (Hansen & Donohoe, 2003). Education and campaigns could be done on preventative care; early detection; and treatment at their homes, workplaces, or community centers. At their workplaces, training could be done to reduce injuries for work that involve intensive physical labor.

As mental health conditions are still highly stigmatized in some immigrant populations, it is vital to clarify any misconceptions surrounding this topic. Migrant workers generally experience multiple stressors that contribute to poorer mental well-being. Thus, it is important to promote the importance of mental health and provide psychological resources with different mental health interventions to help them develop productive coping strategies (Kirmayer et al., 2011). The focus could also be on increasing community participation and civic engagement to help create a sense of belongingness and community within this population. This is especially important in rural areas where they tend to be more isolated with less support. These interventions will likely help the migrant workers to reduce anxiety (Gonzales, Orozco & Sanguineti, 2013) and improve general well-being. A qualitative study found that patients in Yuma County, Arizona, preferred that the community health center provides support groups, information on mental health resources, and talks to address stigma concerns (Ingram, Schachter, Guensey de Zapien, Herman, & Carvajal, 2014).

Healthcare System

Migrant workers sometimes find it difficult to navigate through the U.S. healthcare system, which can be very different from those from their home country. As a result, they tended to avoid accessing health services due to the frustrations and confusion of the system available. Illiteracy and the language barrier further complicate this process as they may be deterred by the application forms or medical instructions that are given in a language with which they are not familiar. Therefore, it is recommended to help migrant workers to learn about the U.S. healthcare system, including differences that may exist between the U.S. system and the one from their home country.

Language and Cultural Considerations

Ineffective medical interpretation services and the hospital staffs' lack of cultural understanding of patients' traditional values and practices also deter migrant workers from accessing health services. Poor communication between physicians and their minority patients likely negatively affects the quality of care provided. Therefore, education and training are also needed for healthcare providers, especially those in rural areas where many migrant workers reside. These providers could be educated on the implicit biases and prejudices they may have to reduce the likelihood of discriminatory actions. In addition, they could also be trained in differential cultural understanding of health and communication with patients who may not be proficient in English.

Medical Training

Migrant workers, especially farmworkers, are frequently exposed to a hazardous environment when they have to manage heavy machinery or chemicals and livestock. Constant exposure to such environmental factors increases the likelihood of specific medical illnesses (e.g., animal-acquired infections, musculoskeletal injuries, or respiratory diseases). Through training, migrant health care can be included in the curriculum for medical, nursing, and dental schools. This helps to enhance the recognition, management, and reporting of illnesses common among migrant workers (Hansen & Donohoe, 2003).

Improving Accessibility
Public Health Infrastructure

Hansen and Donohoe (2003) recommended for a stronger public health infrastructure to help improve migrant and seasonal farmworkers' healthcare needs. Suggestions provided include improving the information-tracking system to assist in communication among providers, increasing preventative care services (e.g., accident prevention, family planning, etc.), increasing the number of healthcare providers for underserved populations, as well as training on language and cultural competencies among providers. They also recommended to improve worker protection via legislation to eliminate a hazardous work environment and unsanitary living conditions.

Migrant workers also struggle to obtain health insurance due to high costs and their immigration status. In order to ensure health protection, policymakers could focus on providing more affordable health care to those who may or may not have health insurance. For example, individuals of certain income levels could be subsidized for seeking healthcare services. More community clinics that offer low-cost basic services could be established in rural areas, where patients could be referred to other specialized services if needed. Furthermore, eligibility criteria for health insurance and government funded programs could be reviewed and modified to increase accessibility to these programs that are designed to assist these individuals.

Use of Technology

Geographic distance often presents challenges to migrant workers in rural areas to access services in a regular and timely manner. In addition to increasing the availability of services in rural areas (e.g., establishing community clinics) when possible, alternative methods in providing services could also be considered. For instance, telehealth as well as mobile health clinics could be utilized to deliver healthcare services to locations that are difficult to reach. As there are often high costs related to using mobile units and equipment, community outreach workers or lay health workers could be recruited to provide some basic services to rural communities (Frank et al., 2013; Hansen & Donohoe, 2003).

In terms of telehealth, health-related information could be conveyed using cell phones as the majority of individuals now own one. A study done by Price and colleagues (2013) showed that approximately 81% of migrant farmworkers ($N = 80$) own a cell phone and have the ability to send and receive text messages. These individuals responded positively to using their cell phone to receive health-related messages, which would likely help improve treatment adherence, monitoring of health conditions, as well as changing medications.

Conclusion

Migrant workers experience various chronic stressors throughout their lives, starting from the immigration process to moving to the United States before settling and adapting to a new environment. The stress of acculturation, financial shortage, and hazardous work environment, among other stressors, contribute to an increased risk in developing physical and mental health concerns. In general, their immigration status and the lack of access to health services create many barriers to their well-being. Policies and government-funded programs have been designed to assist and improve their well-being; however, much help is still needed for this underserved population. Their continuous hard work contributes to the U.S. economic growth, yet many still continue to struggle to make ends meet and suffer from a poor quality of life. A comprehensive approach to help them access the healthcare system would be the responsibility of different levels of government, society, and communities. Therefore, a cooperative and integrative approach, comprehensive policies, and effective programs would be in need to help the migrant workers.

Among those different agencies and programs, first of all, it is important to have assessments, surveys, or focus group to know the specific problems and needs of migrant workers and their families. This is important as factors such as occupational types, country of origin, age, sex, and residing states influence their needs and highlight their unique struggles associated with these factors. Results of such an assessment would then guide the development of programs and services needed to serve this population. Secondly, it is imperative to have continuous evaluation of the effectiveness and outcome of the different services, where any changes and improvements done to the program will be evidence-based. Thirdly, the delivery of the program needs to be adequately planned and carried out. Proper trainings for providers are important to ensure linguistic and cultural appropriateness in serving this population. Finally, it will also be beneficial to cooperate with international or global organizations to develop a network and platform for experience sharing and knowledge application to improve the well-being of migrant workers.

More research in this area will be needed to monitor and study the changes of trends and new strategies to support this underserved population. Cooperation from all parties—e.g., policymakers, employers, nonimmigrants, immigrants—is essential to help improve the public health infrastructure and reduce the unnecessary stressors that affect their health. As a society, it is imperative to think about how to provide an inclusive and supportive atmosphere to help this population to adapt and settle in a new country.

Chapter Summary

A migrant worker refers to someone who is currently involved or will be involved in work, who will be compensated, in a foreign state where this person is not a citizen. To date, there are approximately 28.2 million foreign-born individuals working in the United States. The majority of them are from Mexico, with much smaller groups from Central America, South America, the Caribbean, Asia, and the Pacific Islands. Most are Hispanic.

Many migrant workers experience numerous physical health concerns, including an unhealthy diet; chronic illnesses such as diabetes, cancer, hypertension and cardiovascular disease, and substance use. Poor sleep patterns, hazardous work, and unsanitary living conditions also contribute to their poorer physical health. Many of them prefer to treat themselves with over-the-counter medications rather than seeking professional help. They are also less likely to engage in preventative care, which often leads to late detection of diseases and poorer oral health. For women, maternal care is typically underdeveloped.

Acculturative stress refers to the psychological impact and stress as a result of acculturation, and it has been found to be associated with various mental health concerns experienced by immigrants. It is not uncommon for migrant workers to experience discrimination, coupled with being stigmatized due to their minority status; many experience isolation, societal rejection, and a lack of social support. As a result, these contribute to an increased risk of them developing mental health concerns such as stress, anxiety, and depression. Children and youth of migrant workers also experience their fair share of stressors such as being separated from families and have a constant fear of deportation. However, some do exceptionally well, if not better than their native-born peers in terms of aspirations and academic achievement.

Despite these physical and mental health concerns, many migrant workers struggle to access the healthcare system due to various barriers experienced. These barriers include the language barrier, cultural differences in understanding health, limited resources (e.g., financial and transportation issues), difficulty in obtaining health insurance, and discrimination. Some also actively avoid accessing healthcare services due to a fear of deportation, especially when they are without legal documentation.

Based on the barriers identified, some suggestions are offered. It was recommended that education and training programs are provided for both migrant workers and healthcare providers to tackle concerns such as a lack of knowledge on health in general and having linguistically and culturally insensitive healthcare services. Accessibility could be improved by having a stronger public health infrastructure and integrating the use of technology in the delivery of healthcare services.

Finally, more research is needed to be done to better identify the struggles and needs of migrant workers. Evidence-based programs could be developed and evaluated to help address their health concerns and improve their general well-being. As a society, cooperation is needed from all parties, who have the social responsibility to better support and assist this underserved population.

Discussion Questions

Self-Test Questions

1. What is the definition of migrant workers?
2. Describe the migration paths of farm-workers.
3. What are the major physical health concerns of migrant workers?
4. Identify the major mental health concerns highlighted in this chapter.
5. What is acculturative stress and how might it affect migrant workers' mental health?
6. What are the unique challenges that migrant workers in rural areas face compared with their nonrural counterparts?
7. Explain why legal/documented migrant workers may be afraid to access healthcare services.
8. Describe the suggestions and current efforts that are in place to serve the migrant worker population.

Group Discussions

1. If you are a foreigner who would like to work in the United States, what are the pros and cons that you will have to consider when it comes to adapting to a new country? Do take into account immigration policies as well as concerns related to living in a rural area.
2. As healthcare providers may have biases against and negative attitudes toward migrant workers due to their minority status, what are some strategies that could help reduce prejudice and promote awareness among healthcare providers? Discuss.

Student Activities and Worksheets are available inside the Navigate eBook, included with the printed text. Simply redeem the access code found at the front of the book at www.jblearning.com.

References

Albarrán, C. R., & Nyamathi, A. (2011). HIV and Mexican migrant workers in the United States: A review applying the vulnerable population's conceptual model. *Journal of the Association of Nurses in AIDS Care, 22*(3), 173–185. http://dx.doi.org/10.1016/j.jana.2010.08.001

Alderete, E., Vega, W. A., Kolody, B., & Aguilar-Gaxiola, S. (2000). Lifetime prevalence of and risk factors for psychiatric disorders among Mexican migrant farmworkers in California. *American Journal of Public Health, 90*(4), 608–614. http://dx.doi.org/10.2105/ajph.90.4.608

American Psychological Association (2020). *Discrimination: What it is, and how to cope.* Retrieved December 3, 2019, from https://www.apa.org/topics/discrimination.

Anthony, M. J., Martin, E. G., Avery, A. M., & Williams, J. M. (2010). Self-care and health-seeking behavior of migrant farmworkers. *Journal of Immigrant and Minority Health, 12*(5), 634–639. http://dx.doi.org/10.1007/s10903-009-9252-9

Arcury, T. A., Sandberg, J. C., Talton, J. W., Laurienti, P. J., Daniel, S. S., & Quandt, S. A. (2018). Mental health among Latina farmworkers and other employed Latinas in North Carolina. *Journal of Rural Mental Health, 42*(2), 89–101. http://dx.doi.org/10.1037/rmh0000091

Arcury, T. A., & Quandt, S. A. (2007). Delivery of health services to migrant and seasonal farmworkers. *Annual Review of Public Health, 28*, 345–363.

Baluja, K. F., Park, J., & Myers, D. (2003). Inclusion of immigrant status in smoking prevalence statistics. *American Journal of Public Health, 93*(4), 642–646. http://dx.doi.org/10.2105/AJPH.93.4.642

Barcenas, C. H., Wilkinson, A. V., Strom, S. S., Cao, Y., Saunders, K. C., Mahabir, S., . . ., Bondy, M. L. (2007). Birthplace, years of residence in the United States, and obesity among Mexican-American adults. *Obesity, 15*(40), 1043–1052.

Berry, J. W. (1970). Marginality, stress and ethnic identification in an acculturated Aboriginal community. *Journal of Cross-Cultural Psychology, 1*(3), 239–252.

Berry, J.W. (2004). *Acculturation. Encyclopedia of Applied Psychology*, 1, 27-34. https://doi.org/10.1016/B978-0-12-809324-5.05455-9

Bureau of Labor Statistics, U.S. Department of Labor (2019, May 16). Foreign-born workers: Labor force characteristics—2018. *BLS.* Retrieved from https://www.bls.gov/news.release/pdf/forbrn.pdf

Bureau of Labor Statistics, U.S. Department of Labor (2019, November 7). Employer-reported workplace injuries and illnesses - 2018. BLS. Retrieved from http://www.bls.gov/news.release/pdf/osh.pdf

Capasso, R., Zurlo, M. C., & Smith, A. P. (2018). Ethnicity, work-related stress and subjective reports of health by migrant workers: A multi-dimensional model. *Ethnicity & Health, 23*(2), 174–193. http://dx.doi.org/10.1080/13557858.2016.1258041

Carballo, M., & Nerukar, A. (2001). Migration, refugees, and health risks. *Emerging Infectious Diseases, 7*(3 Suppl), 556–560. http://dx.doi.org/10.3201/eid0707.017733

Carrasquillo, O., Carrasquillo, A. I., & Shea, S. (2000). Health insurance coverage of immigrants living in the United States: Differences by citizenship status and country of origin. *American Journal of Public Health, 90*(6), 917–923.

Cason, K., Nieto-Montenegro, S., & Chavez-Martinez, A. (2006). Food choices, food sufficiency practices, and nutrition education needs of Hispanic migrant workers in Pennsylvania. *Topics in Clinical Nutrition, 21*(2), 145–158.

Centers for Disease Control and Prevention. (2014). *National Diabetes Statistics Report: Estimates of diabetes and its burden in the United States, 2014.* Atlanta, GA: Centers for Disease Control and Prevention, US Department of Health and Human Services.

Cooper, S., Burau, K. E., Frankowski, R., Shipp, E. M., Del Junco, D. J., & Whitworth, R. E. (2006). A cohort study of injuries in migrant farm worker families in South Texas. *Annals of Epidemiology, 16*(4), 313–320. http://dx.doi.org/10.1016/j.annepidem.2005.04.004

Cristancho, S., Garcés, D. M., Peters, K. E., & Mueller, B. (2008). Listening to rural Hispanic immigrants in the Midwest: A community-based participatory assessment of major barriers to health care access and use. *Qualitative Health Research, 18*(5), 633–646.

Derose, K. P., Escarce, J. J., & Lurie, N. (2007). Immigrants and health care: Sources of vulnerability. *Health Affairs, 26*(5), 1258–1268. http://dx.doi.org/10.1377/hlthaff.26.5.1258

Documét, P. I., & Sharma, R. K. (2004). Latinos' Health Care Access: Financial and Cultural Barriers. *Journal of Immigrant Health, 6*(1), 5–13. doi:10.1023/b:joih.0000014638.87569.2e

Dominguez, K., Penman-Aguilar, A., Chang, M. H., Moonesinghe, R., Castellanos, T., Rodriguez-Lainz, A., . . ., Schieber, R. (2015). Vital signs: Leading causes of death, prevalence of diseases and risk factors, and use of health services among Hispanics in the United States—2009–2013. *MMWR Morbidity and Mortality Weekly Report, 64*(17), 469–78.

Duke, M. R., Bourdeau, B., & Hovey, J. D. (2010). Day laborers and occupational stress: Testing the Migrant Stress Inventory with a Latino day laborer population. *Cultural Diversity and Ethnic Minority Psychology, 16*(2), 116–122. http://dx.doi.org/10.1037/a0018665

Encyclopaedia Britannica. (n.d.). What's the difference between Hispanic and Latino? In *Encyclopaedia Britannica.* Retrieved December 4, 2019, from https://www.britannica.com/story/whats-the-difference-between-hispanic-and-latino

Fantuzzo, J. W., & Mohr, W. K. (1999). Prevalence and effects of child exposure to domestic violence. *The Future of Children, 9*(3), 21–32.

Fleischer, N. L., Tiesman, H. M., Sumitani, J., Mize, T., Amarnath, K. K., Bayakly, A. R., & Murphy, M. W. (2013). Public health impact of heat-related illness among migrant farmworkers. *American Journal of Preventive Medicine, 44*(3), 199–206.

Frank, A. L., Liebman, A. K., Ryder, B., Weir, M., & Arcury, T. A. (2013). Health care access and health care workforce for immigrant workers in the agriculture, forestry, and fisheries sector in the southeastern US. *American Journal of Industrial Medicine, 56*(8), 960–974. http://dx.doi.org/10.1002/ajim.22183

Georges, A., Alterman, T., Gabbard, S., Grzywacz, J. G., Shen, R., Nakamoto, J., . . . Muntaner, C. (2013). Depression, social factors, and farmworker health care utilization. *The Journal of Rural Health, 29*(s1), s7–s16.

Gonzales, R. G., Suárez-Orozco, C., & Dedios-Sanguineti, M.C. (2013). No place to belong: Contextualizing concepts of mental health among undocumented immigrant youth in the United States. *American Behavioral Scientist, 57*(8), 1174–1199. http://dx.doi.org/10.1177/0002764213487349

Grzywacz J. G. (2009). Mental health among farmworkers in the Eastern United States. In: Quandt S., Arcury T. (Eds.) Latino Farmworkers in the Eastern United States. Springer, New York, NY.

Hansen, E. E., & Donohoe, M. (2003). Health issues of migrant and seasonal farmworkers. *Journal of Health Care for the Poor and Underserved, 14*(2), 153–164.

Hardy, L. J., Getrich, C. M., Quezada, J. C., Guay, A., Michalowski, R. J., & Henley, E. (2012). A call for further research on the impact of state-level immigration policies on public health. *American Journal of Public Health, 102*(7), 1250–1253. http://dx.doi.org/10.2105/AJPH.2011.300541

Hatzenbuehler, M. L., Prins, S. J., Flake, M., Philbin, M., Frazer, M. S., Hagen, D., & Hirsch, J. (2017).

Immigration policies and mental health morbidity among Latinos: A state-level analysis. *Social Science & Medicine, 174*, 169–178. http://dx.doi.org/10.1016/j.socscimed.2016.11.040

Health Outreach Partners. (2013). *Understanding Health Concerns and Barriers to Accessing Care Among Underserved Populations.* Retrieved from https://outreach-partners.org/2013/11/01/understanding-health-concerns-and-barriers-to-accessing-care-among-underserved-populations/

Hernandez, T. & Gabbard, S. (2018). *Findings from the National Agricultural Workers Survey (NAWS) 2015–2016: A Demographic and Employment Profile of United States Farmworkers* (Research Report No. 13). Retrieved from https://www.doleta.gov/naws/research/docs/NAWS_Research_Report_13.pdf

Hovey, J. D. & Magaña, C. (2000). Acculturative stress, anxiety, and depression among Mexican immigrant farmworkers in the Midwest United States. *Journal of Immigrant Health, 2*(3), 119–131. doi: 10.1023/A:1009556802759

Ingram, M., Schachter, K. A., Guernsey de Zapien, J., Herman, P. M., & Carvajal, S. C. (2015). Using participatory methods to enhance patient-centred mental health care in a federally qualified community health center serving a Mexican American farmworker community. *Health Expectations, 18*(6), 3007–3018. http://dx.doi.org/10.1111/hex.12284

Kemppainen, L., Kemppainen, T., Skogberg, N., Kuusio, H., & Koponen, P. (2017). Immigrants' use of health care in their country of origin: The role of social integration, discrimination and the parallel use of health care systems. *Scandinavian Journal of Caring Science, 32*(2), 1–9. doi: 10.1111/scs.12499

Kirmayer, L. J., Narasiah, L., Munoz, M., Rashid, M., Ryder, A. G., Guzder, J., . . . Pottie K. (2011). Common mental health problems in immigrants and refugees: General approach in primary care. *CMAJ, 183*(12), E959–E967. http://dx.doi.org/10.1503/cmaj.090292

Larsen, L. J. (2004). *The foreign-born population in the United States: 2003.* Retrieved from https://www.census.gov/prod/2004pubs/p20-551.pdf

Lindsay, A. C., Sussner, K. M., Greaney, M. L., & Peterson, K. E. (2011). Latina mothers' beliefs and practices related to weight status, feeding, and the development of child overweight. *Public Health Nursing, 28*(2), 107–118. doi: 10.1111/j.1525-1446.2010.00906.x

Lopez, M. H., Krogstad, J. M., & Passel, J. S. (2020). *Who is Hispanic?* Retrieved from https://www.pewresearch.org/

Moyce, S. C. & Schenker, M. (2018). Migrant workers and their occupational health and safety. *Annual Review of Public Health, 39*, 351–365. http://dx.doi.org/10.1146/annurev-publhealth-040617-013714

Nurko, C., Aponte-Merced, L., Bradley, E. L., & Fox, L. (1998). Dental caries prevalence and dental health care of Mexican-American workers' children. *Journal of Dentistry for Children, 65*(1), 65–72.

Pan, L., Sherry, B., Njai, R., & Blanck, H. M. (2012). Food insecurity is associated with obesity among US adults in 12 states. *Journal of the Academy of Nutrition and Dietetics, 112*(9), 1403–1409. http://dx.doi.org/10.1016/j.jand.2012.06.011

Poss, J., Pierce, R., & Prieto, V. (2005). Herbal remedies used by selected migrant farmworkers in El Paso, Texas. *The Journal of Rural Health, 21*(2), 187–191. http://dx.doi.org/10.1111/j.1748-0361.2005.tb00081.x

Poti, J. M., Mendez, M. A., Ng, S. W., & Popkin, B. M. (2015). Is the degree of food processing and convenience linked with the nutritional quality of foods purchased by US households? *The American Journal of Clinical Nutrition, 101*(6), 1251–1262. http://dx.doi.org/10.3945/ajcn.114.100925

Power, T. G., O'Connor, T. M., Fisher, J. O., & Hughes, S. O. (2015). Obesity risk in children: The role of acculturation in the feeding practices and styles of low-income Hispanic Families. *Childhood Obesity, 11*(6), 715–721. http://dx.doi.org/10.1089/chi.2015.0036

Price M, Williamson D, McCandless R, Mueller M, Gregoski M, Brunner-Jackson B, Treiber E, Davidson L, Treiber F. (2013). Hispanic migrant farm workers' attitudes toward mobile phone-based telehealth for management of chronic health conditions. *Journal of Medical Internet Research, 15*(4): e76. http://dx.doi.org/10.2196/jmir.2500

Ramos, A. K., Su, D., Lander, L, & Rivera, R. (2015). Stress factors contributing to depression among Latino migrant farmworkers in Nebraska. *Journal of Immigrant and Minority Health, 17*(6), 1627–1634. http://dx.doi.org/10.1007/s10903-015-0201-5

Ricketts T. C. (2000). The changing nature of rural health care. *Annual Review of Public Health 21*, 639–657.

Rosado, J. I., Johnson, S. B., McGinnity, K. A., & Cuevas, J. P. (2013). Obesity among Latino children within a migrant farmworker community. *American Journal of Preventive Medicine, 44*(3), S274–S281. http://dx.doi.org/10.1016/j.amepre.2012.11.019

Sandberg, J. C., Grzywacz, J. G., Talton, J. W., Quandt, S. A., Chen, H., Chatterjee, A. B., & Arcury, T. A. (2012). A cross-sectional exploration of excessive daytime sleepiness, depression, and musculoskeletal pain among migrant farmworkers. *Journal of Agromedicine, 17*(1), 70–80. http://dx.doi.org/10.1080/1059924X.2012.626750

Sandberg, J. C., Nguyen, H. T., Quandt, S. A., Chen, H., Summers, P., Walker, F. O., & Arcury, T. A. (2016). Sleep quality among Latino farmworkers in North Carolina: Examination of the job control-demand-support model. *Journal of Immigrant and Minority*

Health, 18(3), 532–541. http://dx.doi.org/10.1007/s10903-015-0248-3

Sandberg, J. C., Talton, J. W., Quandt, S. A., Chen, H., Weir, M., Doumani, W. R., . . . Arcury, T. A. (2014). Association between housing quality and individual health characteristics on sleep quality among Latino farmworkers. *Journal of Immigrant and Minority Health, 16*(2), 265–272. doi:10.1007/s10903-012-9746-8

S.B. 1070, 49th Leg., 2d Reg. Sess. (Ariz. Apr. 23, 2010). https://www.azleg.gov/legtext/49leg/2r/bills/sb1070s.pdf

Shipp, E. M., Cooper, S. P., del Junco, D. J., Delclos, G. L., Burau, K. D., Tortolero, S., & Whitworth, R. E. (2009). Chronic back pain and associated work and non-work variables among farmworkers from Starr County, Texas. *Journal of Agromedicine, 14*(1), 22–32. http://dx.doi.org/10.1080/10599240802612539

Siemons, R., Raymond-Flesh, M., Auerswald, C. L., & Brindis, C. D. (2017). Coming of age on the margins: Mental health and wellbeing among Latino immigrant young adults eligible for Deferred Action for Childhood Arrivals (DACA). *Journal of Immigrant and Minority Health, 19*(3), 543–551. http://dx.doi.org/10.1007/s10903-016-0354-x

Sirin, S. R., Ryce, P., Gupta, T., & Rogers-Sirin, L. (2013). The role of acculturative stress on mental health symptoms for immigrant adolescents: A longitudinal investigation. *Developmental Psychology, 49*(4), 736–748. http://dx.doi.org/10.1037/a0028398

Slesinger, D. P. (1992). Health status and needs of migrant farm workers in the United States: A literature review. *The Journal of Rural Health, 8*(3), 227–234. http://dx.doi.org/10.1111/j.1748-0361.1992.tb00356.x

Smith, M. W., Kreutzer, R. A., Goldman, L., Casey-Paal, A., & Kizer, K. W. (1996). How economic demand influences access to medical care for rural Hispanic children. *Medical Care, 34*(11), 1135–1148. http://dx.doi.org/10.1097/00005650-199611000-00007

Snipes, S. A., Cooper, S. P., & Shipp, E. M. (2017). "The only thing I wish I could change is that they treat us like people and not like animals": Injury and discrimination among Latino farmworkers. *Journal of Agromedicine, 22*(1), 36–46. doi: 10.1080/1059924X.2016.1248307.

Sánchez, J. (2015). Alcohol use among Latino migrant workers in South Florida. *Drug and Alcohol Dependence, 151,* 241–249. http://dx.doi.org/10.1016/j.drugalcdep.2015.03.025

Usher, E. (2004). Migration and labour. In Usher, E. (Ed.). *Essentials of migration management: A guide for policy makers and practitioners.* Geneva: United Nations Publications.

Velasco-Mondragon, E., Jimenez, A., Palladino-Davis, A. G., Davis, D., & Escamilla-Cejudo, J. A. (2016). Hispanic health in the USA: A scoping review of the literature. *Public Health Reviews, 37,* 31. http://dx.doi.org/10.1186/s40985-016-0043-2

Villarejo, D. (2003). The health of U.S. hired farm workers. *Annual Review of Public Health, 24,* 175–193. http://dx.doi.org/10.1146/annurev.publhealth.24.100901.140901

Villarejo, D., McCurdy, S. A., Bade, B., Samuels, S., Lighthall, D., & Williams III, D. (2010). The health of California's immigrant hired farm workers. *Special Issue: Migration and Occupational Health, 53*(4), 387–397. http://dx.doi.org/10.1002/ajim.20796

Watson, J., Mattera, G., Morales, R., Kunitz, S. J., & Lynch, R. (1985). Alcohol use among migrant laborers in western New York. *Journal of Studies on Alcohol and Drugs, 46*(5), 403–411.

Wieland, M. L., Tiedje, K., Meiers, S. J., Mohamed, A. A., Formea, C. M., Ridgeway, J. L., . . . Sia, I. G. (2015). Perspectives on physical activity among immigrants and refugees to a small urban community in Minnesota. *Journal of Immigrant and Minority Health, 17*(1), 263–275. http://dx.doi.org/10.1007/s10903-013-9917-2

Worby, P. A., & Organista, K. C. (2007). Alcohol use and problem drinking among male Mexican and Central American immigrant laborers: A review of the literature. *Hispanic Journal of Behavioral Sciences, 29*(4), 413–455.

Additional Reading

- Bekteshi, V. & Kang, S. (2018). Contextualizing acculturative stress among Latino immigrants in the United States: A systematic review. *Ethnicity & Health, 23,* 1–18. http://dx.doi.org/10.1080/13557858.2018.1469733

- Kumar, B. N. & Diaz, E. (Eds.) (2019). *Migrant Health: A primary care perspective.* Boca Raton, FL: CRC Press.

- Schenker M. B. (2010). A global perspective of migration and occupational health. *American Journal of Industrial Medicine, 53(4),* 329–337.

- Sweileh, W. M., Wickramage, K., Pottie, K., Hui, C., Roberts, B., Sawalha, A. F., & Zyoud, S. H. (2018). Bibliometric analysis of global migration health research in peer-reviewed literature (2000–2016). *BMC Public Health, 18,* 777. http://dx.doi.org/10.1186/s12889-018-5689-x

CHAPTER 17

Adolescent Health in Rural Areas

Joseph N. Inungu, MD, DrPH, MPH
Livingstone Aduse-Poku, MPH

LEARNING OBJECTIVES

At the end of this chapter, readers will be able to:

1. Describe how living in rural areas impacts adolescent health.
2. Understand adolescent development and changes that come with it.
3. Explain rural adolescent behaviors influencing health.
4. Appreciate the trends of adolescent health in rural areas.
5. Illustrate ways to improve adolescent health in rural areas.

KEY TERMS

Adolescents
Behaviors
Disparities
Transition

CHAPTER OVERVIEW

There are almost 42 million **adolescents** between the ages of 10 and 19 years in the United States, making up 12.9% of the population (United States Census Bureau, 2017). The percentage of adolescents in the United is expected to decrease to 11.3% as the population ages although the number of adolescents is expected to rise to 44 million by 2050 (United States Census Bureau, 2017).

Adolescence is a period of **transition** from childhood to adulthood. This transition is marked by physical (hormonal changes and development), cognitive (changes in the way the brain functions), emotional (how adolescents process emotions and stress), social (changes in familial, social, and romantic relationships), morals and values (how adolescents regard their place in the world). Adolescents are generally healthier than other age groups but of high public health concern. Adolescents go through several psychosocial challenges that affect their health. Also, many health problems that cause morbidity and mortality in adulthood start during adolescence, making it pertinent to put in place health programs and strategies that influence **behaviors** affecting health.

Place of residence or where adolescents live is an important factor that affects their health. Most adolescents in the United States live in urban areas (U.S Census, 2018). Children living in urban areas have access to playgrounds, community and recreational centers, and parks, although they are more prone to violent crimes compared with children living in rural areas (U.S. Department of Health and Human Services, 2015).

Rural youths face barriers to accessing health due to provider shortage and transportation challenges; however, both rural and urban adolescents are equally likely to have health insurance (Ferdinand et al., 2015). The 1998 Institute of Medicine (IOM) report *America's Children: Health Insurance and Access to Care* found that uninsured children "are more likely to be sick as newborns, less likely to be immunized as preschoolers, less likely to receive medical treatment when they are injured, and less likely to receive treatment for illness such as acute or recurrent ear infections, asthma and tooth decay" (IOM, 1998: 3). Adolescents in rural areas are more likely to be obese, smoke, and commit suicide than youth in urban areas (Fontanella, 2015).

Adolescent Development

Adolescence is a period of rapid change, including a flood of hormonal and rapid psychological development. It is also a period of dependency and preparation for adulthood, which is reinforced by social changes, including economic restructuring and changing cultural norms about parenting (Goldin & Katz, 2008). Most people, especially parents, find it very difficult to understand the nature of adolescents. Adults often do not accept that that adolescence is a period of stress and storm. As a result, it is likely that problems that are inherent to adolescence are dismissed rather than seeing as signs of significant psychological and social problems that can be modified (Ferdinand et al., 2015).

The period of adolescence is marked by biological, psychological, and social development. During adolescence, the endocrine and reproductive systems develop. In adolescent females, puberty changes may begin as early as 8 years old with the first stages of breast development and height spurts, which commonly occur between age 9.5 to 14.5 years, with menarche occurring between ages 10.5 to 15.5 years. In males, the testicles begin to enlarge between 10.5 and 13.5 years of age. Adolescent physical growth and sexual maturation can be influenced by gender, race, body mass, environmental factors, and overall health status (Steinberg, 2014).

Scientists have recently been studying why adolescents become more reckless as they develop critical thinking skills. One explanation is that adolescence is a period of heightened sensitivity, social influences, and greater propensity toward emotional stimulation (Crosnoe & Johnson, 2011). However, neurological research by Dahl and Spear (2004), using Magnetic Resonance Imaging (MRI) suggests that increased risky behavior during adolescence reflects different rates of growth in the brain's socioemotional and cognitive systems. After puberty, dopamine receptors increase rapidly in regions that control sensation-seeking systems, which encourages behaviors that bring sensory rewards such as peer approval. (Steinberg, 2008). Evidence indicates that engaging in some level of dangerous behavior engenders peer esteem and popularity. (Allen et al., 2005; Kreager & Staff, 2009).

Adolescents undergo lots of psychological development. These changes strengthen adolescent's decision-making ability that will help them flourish now and in the future. Psychological development can occur in three forms: growing new brain cells, pruning some of the extra growth, and strengthening connections (Steinberg, 2014). Adolescence marks one of the stages when the brain produces a large number of cells at a faster rate. As the brain cells grow, the brain trims down extra-growth based on the part the adolescent actively uses; adolescents are, therefore, able to easily access information they use most (USDHHS, 2019). The brain fortifies the connection between cells by wrapping a special fatty acid around cells to protect and insulate them, enabling adolescents to recall information faster (USDHHS, 2019). This process enhances learning, abstract thinking, advanced reasoning, and metacognition. Adolescence is, therefore, the ideal time in a person's life to gain and maintain new skills.

Although the stereotype of adolescence emphasizes mood swings and emotional outburst, adolescents have a quest for emotional and social competence (Steinberg, 2014). Emotional competence is the ability to perceive, assess, and manage one's emotions whiles social competence is the capacity to be sensitive and effective in relating to other people (Child Development Institute, 2008). Emotional and social development in adolescents take place in four areas: self-awareness, social awareness, self-management, and peer relationships (Child Development Institute, 2008). Self-awareness centers on adolescents learning to recognize and name their emotions. Without this awareness, adolescents may grow withdrawn, depressed, or pursue such numbing behaviors such as alcoholism and other substance abuse. While it is important that youth recognize their own emotions, they must strive to take in account the feelings of others. This is social awareness. Adolescents are also expected to monitor and regulate their emotions. This self-management involves developing reasoning and abstract thinking skills and considering how these emotions bear on longer- term goals. Social and emotional development also involves establishing and maintaining healthy, rewarding relationships based on cooperation, effective communication, and the ability to resolve conflict (American Psychological Association, 2010). These social skills are fostered by involvement in a peer group. Adolescents generally prefer to spend an increasing amount of time with their friends rather than their family.

Adolescent Behaviors Influencing Health

Rural settings may influence adolescent health risk behaviors. In a study describing the health risk behaviors among adolescents attending rural, suburban, and urban schools in suburban New York, a consistent pattern emerged from the analysis of the data, with rural residents most at risk of tobacco, sexual activity, illegal substances, and carrying weapons (Atav, & Spencer, 2002).

Alcohol use among adolescents in the United States has declined since its peak in 1990. Almost one in five 8th, 10th, and 12th grade students (19%) reported drinking alcohol within a month in 2019 (Johnston et al., 2019). In the same year, 4% of 8th graders, 9% of 10th graders, and 14% of 12th grade students reported binge drinking within a week (Johnston et al., 2019). An analysis using the 2002 through 2004 National Survey of Drug Use found that rural adolescents were more likely to use alcohol and cocaine than their urban peers, with no significant difference found across other drug types (Lambert, Gale, & Hartley, 2008). Related to alcohol use, rural adolescents were more likely to report binge drinking, heavy drinking, and driving under the influence (Johnson, Mink, Harun, Moore, Martin, & Bennett, 2003).

In 2017, male high school students (57%) were more likely to report 60 minutes of physical activity on five or more days in the past weeks than female high school students (37 percent) (Centers for Disease Control and Prevention, 2018). A recent meta-analysis reporting data on adolescents aged 10 to 17 years found that adolescents in nonmetropolitan areas have 28% greater odds of obesity than adolescents in metropolitan areas (Johnson & Johnson, 2016). This difference in obesity may be a result of a disparity in physical activities. Nevertheless, a study (Adolescents Committed to Improvement of Nutrition and Physical Activity) by the Centers for Disease Control and Prevention (CDC), conducted from 2014 through 2017, reported that dietary intake and physical activity level by measures of rurality were small, inconsistent in direction, and unable to explain the **disparities** in obesity observed in urban and rural areas (CDC, 2019).

Most people begin smoking in adolescence (CDC, 2019). In a study by Johnson et al., (2019), approximately 46% of 8th, 10th, and 12th grade students in the United States reported smoking cigarettes within a month; less than 1% of adolescents reported smoking at least a half pack a day. Vaping or e-cigarette use has increased exceedingly among the youth in the past couple of years, prompting the Surgeon General to declare youth e-cigarette use an epidemic (United States Department of Health and Human Services, 2018). In 2018, 19% of 8th, 10th, and 12th grade students reported vaping within a month (Johnson at al. 2019). Substances that can be vaped include nicotine, marijuana, and flavoring; although their long-term consequences are still being studied, long-term vaping is considered harmful to youth (U.S. Department of Health and Human Services, 2016). A study by Michael, Pesko, Adam & Robarts, (2017) found a fourfold increase in e-cigarette use from 2013 to 2014 but a slower rate of increased use in rural areas. Urban youth cigarette smokers are twice as likely as rural cigarette smokers to also use e-cigarettes (Noland et al., 2018). This difference is due to the increased use of e-cigarettes instead of traditional tobacco in urban areas.

Opioids include heroin, fentanyl, oxycodone, hydrocodone, cocaine, and morphine. In 2017, President Trump declared the opioid crisis a public health emergency. Opioid abuse among adolescents is mostly in the form of prescription drug misuse; in 2018, 1% of 12th graders reported misusing prescription opioids within the past month and 3% reported using prescription opioids inappropriately in the past year (Substance Abuse and Mental Health Services Administration, 2018).

There is evidence that abuse of prescription opioids has increased more in rural areas compared with urban areas, although the availability of prescription opioids has increased in all areas (McDonald, Carlson, & Izrael, 2012). Specifically, per-capita sales indicate that states with large rural populations such as West Virginia are among the highest prescribers of opioid analgesics (McDonald, Carlson, & Izrael, 2012).

There has been a recent increase in the incidence of gun violence in the United States. In August 2019, 31 people were killed in a mass shooting in El Paso, Texas, and Dayton, Ohio. Fifteen-to-nineteen-year-old adolescents in urban areas are hospitalized for firearm assaults at a rate eight times higher than 15–19-year-old adolescents in rural areas (Herrin, Gaither, Leventhal, & Dodington, 2018; Nance, Denysenko, & Durbin, 2002). Urban and low-income youth are more likely to witness gun violence than suburban and higher-income youth (Stein, Jaycox, Kataoka, Rhodes, & Vestal, 2013). A study by Siegel et al., (2019), found that universal background checks resulted in a 13% decline in urban firearm homicide rates, while laws that disqualify people in violent misconduct convictions from purchasing firearms came with a 30% decrease in rates of gun violence in rural areas.

Trends of Adolescent Health in Rural Areas

Rising adolescent health issues such as road traffic accidents (RTAs), substance abuse disorders, and mental health problems pose an increased cause for apprehension in countries that have otherwise boosted child health and have reduced maternal mortality (Patton et al., 2009). Also, compounding the problems of adolescent health risks such as tobacco use, obesity, physical inactivity, and substance use are the issues of an aging population and a convergence to a disease burden dominated by noncommunicable diseases in later years (Jamison et al., 2013).

Almost half (45%) of adolescents aged 12–17 years had at least one chronic health condition in 2016–2017, with 25% having two or more conditions in the United States (Child and Adolescent Health Measurement Initiative, 2017). Asthma is the single most common cause of chronic disease in adolescents affecting 23% of children in 2017 (Centers for Disease Control and Prevention, 2018). Recent studies have shown that the prevalence of rural adolescent asthma is similar to suburban and urban prevalence (Valet et al., 2011; Ownby, Tingen, Havstad, Waller, Johnson, Joseph, 2015; Fedele, Barnett, Everhart, Lawless, Forrest, 2016). The pattern of distribution appears to be more closely correlated with socioeconomic factors than geographic location. Factors such as race/ethnicity, socioeconomic status, indoor smoking, and other environmental exposures have shown a more accurate pattern of distribution (Keet et al., 2015). Asthma is an important health problem with management problems requiring locally appropriate interventions for rural children, adolescents, and their families.

Research has revealed that most mental health issues begin during adolescent years (Boyd et al., 2006). During the 2018 Youth Risk Behavior Surveillance by the CDC, it was found that 32% of adolescents feel so sad or hopeless that they stopped doing some usual activities almost every day for two or more weeks in a row during the past year (CDC, 2018). Almost 6 in 10 youths aged 12–17 years who are diagnosed with major depressive episode do not receive treatment (Substance Abuse & Mental Health Services Administration, 2018). There is growing evidence in the literature that indicates that the prevalence of depression is similar in both rural and urban areas (Black, Roberts, & Li-Leng, 2012). Nevertheless, people assume that factors associated with comprised mental health among rural residents include deprivation and lack of access to healthcare services. Untreated depression can lead to serious consequences such as suicide. The good news is that prompt intervention before symptoms get more serious and effective treatments can help.

Attention Deficit Hyperactive Disorder (ADHD) is the most common neurodevelopmental disorder diagnosed in childhood with symptoms, including inattention and hyperactivity leading to functional impairment (Perou et al., 2013). The 2018 Youth Risk Behavior Surveillance (CDC, 2018), revealed that 13% of adolescents between the ages of 12 and 17 years had experienced ADHD at one point in their lives (CDC, 2018). Adolescents living in rural areas are more likely to be diagnosed with ADHD and less likely to receive behavioral therapy compared with children in urban areas (Melissa et al., 2018; Danielson, Bitsko, Ghandour, et al., 2018). Untreated ADHD often interferes with peer relationships.

Another issue worth considering among adolescents is teenage pregnancy. In 2017, a total of 194,377 babies were born to women aged 15–19 years (CDC, 2017). United States teen pregnancy is substantially higher than other industrialized countries, and geographic disparities in teen birth rates exist (Sedgh, Finer, Bankole, Eilers, & Singh, 2015). The teen birth rate is nearly one-third in rural areas than that in urban areas of the United States, and teen pregnancy rates have had a much slower decline in rural counties over the past decade (Sedgh, Finer, Bankole, Eilers, & Singh, 2015). Barriers to contraceptive services have been implicated as the reason for this pattern.

An estimated 20.6% of all 12- to 19-year-olds were obese between 2015 and 2016. Hispanics (25.8%) and non-Hispanic Blacks (22.0%) had higher obesity prevalence than non-Hispanic Whites (14.1%), whereas non-Hispanic Asians (11.0%) had lower obesity prevalence than non-Hispanic Blacks and Hispanics (Hales, 2017). Childhood obesity has been attributed to several factors, including societal changes that have contributed to decreased physical activity levels, increased time spent with sedentary activities, and increased consumption of foods and beverages that are high in calories, sugar, and fat, but low in nutrients (Story et al., 2009).

Improving Adolescent Health in Rural Areas

Adolescents living in rural areas face many obstacles in the way of accessing health. In order to ensure that adolescents have access to high-quality care, a number of approaches have to be taken to improve health services for adolescents, improve workforce distribution for providing adolescent-related services, and enhance support for adolescent health services. These can be accomplished by using strategies such as improving training in adolescent health, increasing the number of racially and ethnically diverse professionals working with adolescents, developing approaches to overcome adolescents' barriers to access, and providing adolescent-focused health services.

The impact of the environment on adolescent health cannot be overemphasized. Environments refer to the formal and informal settings where adolescents spend most of their time, including the family, schools, neighborhoods, religious organizations, and other community settings. An emphasis on comprehensive approaches to ensure environmental changes and a concentration on the more proximal settings of family, school, and neighborhoods where adolescents spend most of their time are highly recommended (American Medical Association, Department of Adolescent Health, 2010) These can be realized by using these strategies: improving the social conditions of families, strengthening the role of community institutions in the lives of adolescents, implementing specific anti-discrimination measures, and reducing exposure to unhealthy conditions, including violence.

Schools play a vital role in the lives of adolescents. To achieve the goal of increased service provision and coordination of care, policies are needed to comprise health and educational objectives and resources required to augment the ability of schools to offer on-site services or access to off-site services. Promoting educational policies that encourage success for all students, linking schools with families, establishing school-based and school-linked health centers is highly recommended.

Rural areas pose several health challenges to adolescent health. To deal with these problems it is required that individuals and communities come up with innovative ideas. Some of the approaches are telehealth and telemedicine. These strategies involve using telecommunications technology to provide health services to patients who live in remote areas. Both telehealth and telemedicine involve the delivery of clinical care, with telehealth having the added advantage of providing health education. Adolescents in rural areas usually avoid care due to embarrassment, confidentiality concerns, and transportation difficulties, making the use of telehealth and telemedicine very necessary (Elliott & Larson, 2004).

In a prospective study conducted in 2016, the researchers evaluated the use of telehealth to teach reproductive health to 55 female students at two high schools in West Virginia, where teen pregnancy rates are high (Yoost et al., 2017). High-definition teleconferencing equipment was used to deliver eight 60-minute sessions over the course of one month. This led to an increase (from 38% to 70%) in HPV vaccination and 91.8% of the participants reported that telehealth was very effective as a teaching tool (Yoost et al., 2017). This model can be adopted to reach adolescents in other rural communities with limited resources and health providers.

Conclusion

The rural adolescent in the 21st century is faced with several challenges that affect health. This is compounded by challenges such as transportation barriers, limited access to health insurance and provider shortages. It is, therefore, imperative that adequate attention be given to rural adolescents in order to meet their physical, cognitive, emotional, and social needs during this important stage of their lives.

Chapter Summary

- The period of adolescence involves lots of changes, including an inundation of hormonal and quick psychological growth. The transition is marked by physical, cognitive, emotional, and social changes.
- Adolescents living in rural areas face challenges such as health provider shortages, transportation challenges, limited access to health insurance, obesity, and are more likely to smoke and commit suicide.
- Rural adolescents are influenced by certain behaviors that affect health. Rural adolescents are more likely to engage in binge drinking, heavy drinking, and driving under influence of alcohol.
- Although disparities in obesity have been seen in rural and urban areas, dietary intake and physical activities have been unable to explain this difference.
- Vaping has recently been on the rise among adolescents in the United States and has been declared an epidemic by the Surgeon General. Opioid abuse among adolescents is mostly in the form of prescription drug use. President Trump declared the opioid crisis a public health emergency in 2017.
- Urban and low-income youth are more likely to witness gun violence compared with suburban and higher-income youth.
- There is a very high rate of asthma, depression, ADHD, teenage pregnancy, and obesity among rural youth.
- Improving adolescent health in rural areas include an emphasis on comprehensive approaches to ensure environmental changes, promoting educational policies that encourage success for all students, and proper use of telehealth and telemedicine.

Discussion Questions

1. Why is the study of adolescent health important in a textbook on Rural Health?
2. Discuss the influence of the rural setting on adolescent health risk behaviors.
3. What are the determinants for contraceptive use among unmarried youth in the higher institution?
4. Discuss and contract the use e-cigarette between urban and rural adolescents.
5. Discuss and contract the prevalence of obesity by ethnicity and place of residence.
6. Discuss the prevalence and risk factors for gun violence among adolescents in the United States.
7. Discuss two evidence-based interventions to improve the health of adolescents in rural areas.
8. How can schools contribute to improving the health of adolescents in rural areas?

> *Student Activities and Worksheets are available inside the Navigate eBook, included with the printed text. Simply redeem the access code found at the front of the book at www.jblearning.com.*

References

Atav, S., & Spencer, G. A. (2002). Health risk behaviors among adolescents attending rural, suburban, and urban schools: A comparative study. *Family and Community Health, 25*(2), 53–65.

Black, G., Roberts, R., & Li-Leng, T. (2012). Depression in rural adolescents: Relationships with gender and availability of mental health services. *Rural and Remote Health, 12,* 2092.

Boyd, C. P., Hayes, L., Nurse, S., Aisbett, D., Francis, K., Newnham, K., & Sewell, J. (2011). Preferences and intention of rural adolescents toward seeking help for mental health problems. *Rural and Remote Health,* 11, 1582.

Centers for Disease Control and Prevention (CDC). (2018). Youth risk behavior surveillance—United States, 2017. *MMWR Morbidity and Mortality Weekly Report,* 67(8), 1–479. Retrieved from https://www.cdc.gov /healthyyouth/data/yrbs/pdf/2017/ss6708.pdf - PDF

Centers for Disease Control and Prevention (CDC). (2019). *Youth and tobacco use.* Retrieved from https:// www.cdc.gov/tobacco/data_statistics/fact_sheets /youth_data/tobacco_use/index.htm

Data Resource Center for Child & Adolescent Health Measurement Initiative. (2017). *2016-17 National Survey of Children's Health* [Data query]. Retrieved from http://www.childhealthdata.org/browse/survey

Elliott, B. A., & Larson, J. T. (2004). Adolescents in midsized and rural communities: Foregone care, perceived barriers, and risk factors. *Journal of Adolescent Health,* 35(4), 303–309.

Fedele, D. A., Barnett, T. E., Everhart, R. S., Lawless, C., & Forrest, J. R. (2016). Comparison of asthma prevalence and morbidity among rural and nonrural youth. *Annals of Allergy, Asthma & Immunology,* 117(2), P193– P194. e1.

Herrin, B. R., Gaither, J. R., Leventhal, J. M., & Dodington J. (2018). Rural versus urban hospitalizations for firearm injuries in children and adolescents. *Pediatrics,* 142(2), e20173318.

Johnson, A. O., Mink, M. D., Harun, N., Moore, C. G., Martin, A. B., & Bennett, K. J. (2008). Violence and drug use in rural teens: National prevalence estimates from the 2003 Youth Risk Behavior Survey. *Journal of School Health,* 78(10), 554–561.

Johnson, J., & Johnson, A. M. (2015). Urban-rural differences in childhood and adolescent obesity in the United States: A systematic review and meta-analysis. *Childhood Obesity,* 11(3), 233–241.

Johnston, L. D., Miech, R. A., O'Malley, P. M., Bachman, J. G., Schulenberg, J. E., & Patrick, M. E. (2019). *Monitoring the Future National Survey Results on Drug Use 1975-2018: Overview, Key Findings on Adolescent Drug Use.* Ann Arbor: Institute for Social Research, University of Michigan. Retrieved from http://www .monitoringthefuture.org//pubs/monographs/mtf -overview2018.pdf - PDF

Keet, C. A., McCormack, M. C., Pollack, C. E., Peng, R., McGowan, E., & Matsui, E. C. (2015). Neighborhood poverty, urban residence, race/ethnicity, and asthma: Rethinking the inner-city asthma epidemic. *Journal of Allergy and Clinical Immunology,* 135(3), 655–662.

Lambert, D., Gale, J. A., & Hartley D. (2008). Substance abuse by youth and young adults in rural America. *The Journal of Rural Health,* 24(3), 221–228.

McDonald, D. C., Carlson, K., & Izrael D. (2012). Geographical variation in opioid prescribing in the U.S. *The Journal of Pain,* 13(10), 988–996.

Danielson, M. L., Bitsko, R. H., Ghandour, R. M., Holbrook, J. R., Kogan, M., D., & Blumberg, S. J. (2018). Prevalence of parent-reported ADHD diagnosis and associated treatment among U.S. children and adolescents, 2016. *Journal of Clinical Child & Adolescent Psychology,* 47(2), 199–212. doi:10.1080/153744 16.2017.1417860

Nance, M. L., Denysenko, L., Durbin D. R. (2002). The rural-urban continuum: Variability in statewide serious firearm injuries in children and adolescents. *Archives of Pediatrics and Adolescent Medicine,* 156(8), 781–785.

Hales, C. M., Carroll, M. D., Fryar, C. D., & Ogden, C. L. Prevalence of obesity among adults and youth: United States, 2015–2016. *NHS Data Brief, 288,* 1290.

National Research Council (US) and Institute of Medicine (US) Committee on Children, Health Insurance, and Access to Care, Edmunds, M., & Coye, M. J. (Eds.). (1998). *America's children: Health insurance and access to care.* National Academies Press (US).

Noland, M., Rayens, M. K., Wiggins, A. T., Huntington-Moskos, L., Rayens, E. A., Howard, T., & Hahn, E. J. (2018). Current use of e-cigarettes and conventional cigarettes among US high school students in urban and rural locations: 2014 National Youth Tobacco Survey. *American Journal of Health Promotion,* 32(5), 1239–1247.

Ownby, D., Tingen, M., Havstad, S., Waller, J. L., Johnson, C. C., & Joseph, C. L. (2015). Comparison of asthma prevalence among African American teenage youth attending public high schools in rural Georgia and urban Detroit. *Journal of Allergy and Clinical Immunology, 136(3),* 595–600. e3.

Perou R., Bitsko, R. H., Blumberg, S.J., Pastor, P., Ghandour, R. M., Gfroerer, J. C., . . . Huang, L. N. (2013). Mental health surveillance among children—United States, 2005–2011. *Morbidity and Mortality Weekly Report MMWR Supplement, 62(2),* 1–35.

Sedgh, G., Finer, B., Bankole, A., Eilers, M. A., & Singh, S. (2015). Adolescent pregnancy, birth, and abortion rates across countries: Levels and recent trends. *Journal of Adolescent Health,* 56(2), 223–230.

Stein, B. D., Jaycox, L. H., Kataoka, S., Rhodes, H. J., Vestal, K. D. (2003). Prevalence of child and adolescent exposure to community violence. *Clinical Child and Family Psychology Review,* 6(4), 247–264.

Story, M., Sallis, J. F., & Orleans, C. T. (2009). Adolescent obesity: Towards evidence-based policy and environmental solutions. *Journal of Adolescent Health,* 45(3), S1–S5.

Substance Abuse and Mental Health Services Administration. (2018). *Key substance use and mental health* indicators in the United States: Results from the 2017 *National Survey on Drug Use and Health* (HHS Publication No. SMA 18-5068, NSDUH Series H-53). Rockville, MD: Center for Behavioral Health Statistics and Quality, Substance Abuse and Mental Health Services Administration. Retrieved from https://www.samhsa.gov/data/

Substance Abuse & Mental Health Services Administration. (2018). *Results from the 2017 National Survey on Drug Use and Health: Detailed tables. Table 9.6B [Data set].* Retrieved from https://www.samhsa.gov/data/sites/default/files/cbhsq-reports/NSDUHDetailedTabs2017/NSDUHDetailedTabs2017.pdf - PDF

United States Department of Health and Human Services. (2016). *E-Cigarette use among youth and young adults: A report of the Surgeon General.* Atlanta, GA: U.S. Department of Health and Human Services, Centers for Disease Control and Prevention, National Center for Chronic Disease Prevention and Health Promotion, Office on Smoking and Health. Retrieved from https://e-cigarettes.surgeongeneral.gov/documents/2016_SGR_Exec_Summ_508.pdf

United States Department of Health and Human Services. (2018). *Surgeon General releases advisory on E-cigarette epidemic among youth.* Washington, DC: U.S. Department of Health and Human Services. Retrieved from https://www.hhs.gov/about/news/2018/12/18/surgeon-general-releases-advisory-e-cigarette-epidemic-among-youth.html

Valet, R. S., Gebretsadik, T., Carroll, K. N., Wu, P., Dupont, W. D., Mitchel, E. F., & Hartert, T. V. (2011). High asthma prevalence and increased morbidity among rural children in a Medicaid cohort. *Annals of Allergy, Asthma & Immunology. 106*(6), 467–473. doi:10.1016/j.anai.2011.02.013

Yoost, J., Whitley Starcher, R., King-Mallory R. A., Hussain, N., Hensley, C. A., & Gress T. W. (2017). The use of telehealth to teach reproductive health to female rural high school students. *Journal of Pediatric and Adolescent Gynecology. 30*(2), 193–198.

CHAPTER 18

Aging Populations in Rural United States

Eileen E. MaloneBeach, PhD

Han-Jung Ko, PhD

Mikiyasu Hakoyama, PhD

LEARNING OBJECTIVES

At the end of this chapter, readers will be able to:

1. Describe demographic trends that are impacting health care for older adults living in rural areas.
2. Identify challenges in obtaining effective and quality health care specific to rural older adults compared with urban/suburban counterparts.
3. Identify assets specific to rural older adults in obtaining health care.
4. Discuss the motivations for and against aging in place for rural older adults.
5. Describe major threats to health and well-being of rural older adults.
6. Describe the use of information technology in delivering health care to older adults living in rural areas.
7. Describe caregiving for rural older adults living with impairments.
8. Evaluate proposed solutions for improving rural health care and brainstorm new ideas.

KEY TERMS

Access to services
Ageism
Aging in place
Developmental changes
Health care
Quality of life
Rural older adults
Usual source of health care

CHAPTER OVERVIEW

This chapter discusses the health and **health care** of American older adults who live in rural places. Today, as always, the world is changing, and rural conditions are included in the changes. Moreover, the rate of change is accelerating, and change necessitates adaptation. Failing to adapt to changes can jeopardize one's health and well-being. Some adaptations are short-lived and potentially expensive and ultimately ineffective. Others may lead to long-term improvements.

Determining which changes to adapt to and how to adjust poses serious challenges for older adults, their families, their communities, their nation's policies, and for the world.

The positive and negative aspects of rurality will be discussed throughout the chapter. We aim to demonstrate the enduring and impending threats to rural health for older adults as well as efforts to address them, perhaps by borrowing ideas from other countries that are confronted with similar concerns. In this chapter, you will be asked to critically analyze the past and to consider and propose solutions for a projected and ever-changing future.

Introduction

As we grow older, numerous **developmental changes** take place physically, cognitively, and socioemotionally. Developmental changes include weakened muscles and bones, changed weight, slowed cognitive functioning, diminished immune response, and limited sensory ability. Developmental changes in late life are normal and expected but they do not mean that every older individual is subject to health crises. Health problems are neither developmental nor inevitable for older adults. By nature, the older we grow, the more likely we are to be at risk for multiple health problems (i.e., comorbidities). However, most older adults remain healthy and able until very late in life.

In late life, changes in health conditions can lead to decline or limitations in older adults' ability to maintain an optimal or acceptable **quality of life**. The changes, combined with life-style choices, genetic predispositions, and limited access to health care, may lead to health problems, such as heart disease, stroke, diabetes, cancer, osteoporosis, and depression. Some of these health problems are more prevalent among the rural elderly than their urban counterparts.

Some researchers argue that limited resources and unavailability of services account for some of the urban/rural health disparities (CMS, 2019; Cohen, Greasey, & Sabik, 2018; Purtle, et al., 2019). The rural elderly, however, are not necessarily disadvantaged in every aspect of life. For example, they are more likely than their urban counterparts to breathe cleaner air (Strosnider, Kennedy, Monti, Yip, 2017), experience less noise and light pollution, to grow their own vegetables, fruits, and meat, and to be surrounded by neighbors who are more likely to know and check up on each other (Buys, et al., 2015). However, environmental factors can be critical determinants of how aging manifests with age (DeGroot, et al., 2018).

In this chapter, we will focus on public health issues associated with older adults by taking into specific consideration how rurality may influence health and quality of life of older adults. We first demonstrate the demographics of rural aging, comparing the resources of individuals and communities between rural and urban areas. We then discuss normal age-related developmental changes before examining the disparities in health and health behaviors due to rurality. Proposals for optimal rural aging will be discussed, including **aging in place**, and improving availability of rural health care and services. Moreover, we advocate for addressing **ageism** to better create an aging-friendly environment for current older adults and future generations to come. Finally, we offer case studies to apply knowledge gained in this chapter and to brainstorm better solutions.

Demographics of Rural Aging

Older adults (age 65+) comprise 15% of the U.S. population; in the 21st century, the elderly portion of the population increased while other age groups receded in relative size (Smith and Trevelyan, 2019). More than 46 million Americans reside in rural areas (CDC, 2017). At any age, rural Americans are at higher risk of dying from heart disease, cancer, unintentional injury, chronic lower respiratory disease, and stroke than their urban counterparts. Rural deaths, nearly 50% higher than the deaths of urban elders, can be attributed, in part, to opioid overdoses and vehicular accidents. Overall, rural Americans tend to be older and sicker than urban dwellers (CDC, 2017). Concurrently, the rural population has decreased in size, as younger people leave farms and small communities to seek employment in cities; the older generation of adults is more likely to remain in place, resulting in rural communities with larger populations of persons over 65 years. The number of those over 85 years is increasing even more rapidly (Hirsch, 2019). As a result, localized population aging has become common.

More older adults in rural areas are below the poverty threshold than their urban counterparts (Peltzer, Phaswana-Mafuy, & Pengpid, 2019). Poverty is a major factor for poorer health outcomes (Dai, et al., 2019). The rates of heart disease, diabetes, vision and hearing impairments, and repeated falls are significantly higher for low-income **rural older adults** than for suburban and urban elders (Yoo, et al., 2016). Moreover, rural ethnic minorities experience more poverty and rates of comorbidity than white rural elders and urban elders (De Trinidad Young, et al., 2018). This is a growing inequity as rural populations have become increasingly more ethnically diverse in recent years (Torres-Gil & Demko, 2019).

Adult Development in Late Life

Hearing

Sensory acuity begins to decline around midlife. Nearly two-thirds of older adults aged 70+ yeares in the United States suffer from hearing loss and men are at a higher risk for hearing impairments than women (Curhan, Willett, Grodstein, Curhan, 2019). Although hearing loss is an expected developmental change associated with aging, its impact on quality of late life is significant.

Hearing is a critical element of balance; hearing loss can lead to falls (Lin & Ferrucci, 2012) and inhibit movement on a daily basis. It affects driving ability, walking, and numerous physical activities (Hickson, Wood, Chaparro, Lacherez, & Marszalek, 2010).

Limited hearing also impairs communications (Bae, et al., 2018). Persons who are hearing impaired may not be able to track conversations, which leads to feeling excluded and fear of looking foolish for saying something that is a non sequitur. In the context of health care, information provided by healthcare professionals may not be understood or heard (Blustein & Weinstein, 2016). The person does not comprehend what is going on around them, receives less cognitive stimulation, and potentially appears to be confused. In some unfortunate instances, persons with hearing impairment have been diagnosed mistakenly as developing dementia, specifically Alzheimer's disease (Chang, Kim, Haeng, Mook-Jung, Oh, 2019; Ford, et al., 2018).

At this time, little research has investigated urban-rural disparities in hearing ability in late life. One can speculate that those in agribusiness, especially men who are exposed to loud machinery for long periods of time across numerous years, as are many factory workers and laborers. These elderly are more likely to suffer hearing loss based on work-related exposure to noise, whereas younger cohorts have learned to limit exposure and to use ear protection.

Vision

Like hearing loss, vision impairment significantly affects quality of life. Visual impairment in older adults is also a major sensory-related public health concern; 17% of adults 65+ years reported "vision trouble" and 6.6% are legally blind (Owsley and McGwin, 2010). Vision impairment is associated with falls and significantly contributes to lost independence (Niigata, et al., 2018).

Visual impairment, particularly in combination with hearing impairment, makes driving increasingly hazardous. For older adults, impaired vision also results in reduced leisure activities, which jeopardizes psychosocial well-being. The loss of driving ability is a major fear associated with vision impairment. Ceasing to drive symbolizes the loss of autonomy, independence, and self-worth (Owsley, et al., 2010). Regular eye examination is crucial to maintaining healthy vision; yet, more than 40% of older adults with moderate to extreme visual impairment see little or no reason for routine eye examination. In rural areas, a lack of eye-care specialists poses added challenges for older adults who do seek check-ups (National Center for Health Statistics, 2012). This suggests that public health professionals emphasize messaging regarding preventive hearing and vision health care. Perhaps messaging that highlights losses, such as driving and reading, would convince rural elders of the importance of routine examinations. Alternately, emphasizing that attention to one's hearing and vision may increase the potential to continue favorite activities well into very old age.

Oral Health

The oral health of rural older adults also suffers; approximately 20% of older adults no longer have their natural teeth (Dye, Thornton-Evans, and Iafolla, 2015) and more than two-thirds have gum disease (Eke, et al., 2015). Preventive dental checkups are imperative to lower the risk for oral disease and tooth loss. Having a usual source of health care is also linked to more attention to general health (Caldwell, Lee, and Cagney, 2017). Hamano, Takeda, Tominaga, Sundquist, and Nabika (2017) found that those who had dental checkups within the previous year were less likely than their counterparts without routine checkups to have major tooth loss and frequent dental visits lower the odds of complete tooth loss. Overall, rural older adults are

at a higher risk of poorer oral health, as they tend to have fewer preventive dental checkups while having more complete tooth loss than their urban counterparts. The contrast in urban/rural oral health among older adults is shown to be explained, in part, by fewer dental visits, lower likelihood of a usual source of health care, fewer numbers of dental care providers, and greater travel times (Eke, et al., 2019; Hamano, et al., 2017).

Most older adults are insured through Medicare; however, Medicare does not cover routine dental or vision care. More than 70% of older adults aged 65+ years have no dental insurance and the older the individuals are, the less likely they are to have dental insurance. More rural residents tended not to have dental insurance coverage than their urban residents, making cost another barrier. In addition to urban/rural disparities in dental care, ethnic differences have been found. Rural African American older adults were less likely to have a usual source of health care and far less likely to have had a recent dental visit than their urban and rural whites and urban African American counterparts (Caldwell, Lee, and Cagney, 2017). Moreover, Hispanics are less likely to have dental insurance than their white, African American, or Asian Americans elderly counterparts (Kramarov, 2019). Loss of insurance and reduced income due to retirement may account for reduced dental visits, which subsequently influences older residents' oral health.

Furthermore, lack of preventive dental care is linked to numerous other health issues.

Urban/Rural Health Disparities in Late Life

Of all age groups, older adults have the poorest health. Moreover, rural older adults have higher rates of chronic disease and depression than urban elders (Purtle, et al., 2019). In addition, they report worse physical health than their counterparts residing in urban areas and are likely to suffer more comorbidity, including obesity and physical inactivity, diabetes, falls, Alzheimer's disease and dementia illnesses, and depression (de Melo, et al., 2019).

Overweight/Obesity and Physical Inactivity

Rural older adults are more physically inactive and overweight or obese than their urban or suburban counterparts (Prakash, Bihari and Kumar, 2016). More than two thirds of older adults in the U.S. are overweight and obesity rates are higher in rural areas than in urban areas (CDC, 2018; Cohen, Cook, Kelley, Foutz, & Sando, 2016). Obesity negatively impacts both physical and mental health in older adults and can be a precursor to diabetes, hypertension, cancers, depression, and sleep disorders (Cohen, Greaney, & Sabik, 2018). Obesity is also a risk factor for frailty and institutionalization and is linked to increased healthcare costs (Biener, Cawley, & Meyerhoefer, 2018; Tremmel, Gerdtham, Nilsson, & Saha, 2017).

A study of obesity and geographic effects found that urban-rural obesity prevalence varied across regions, rurality, and states. In several states, obesity prevalence was linearly oriented toward rurality: the more rural the area, the higher the prevalence of obesity. However, for the U.S. overall, obesity showed a curvilinear relationship to population density: the relationship was weakest for the most rural and the most urban elders. Those in intermediate settings had the highest obesity rates (Cohen et al., 2018).

However, a recent meta-analysis by de Groot, et al. (2019) found that triglycerides and total cholesterol levels favored rural elders; they emphasized the role of the built environment in interpreting the differences. Built environments impact life-style choices, activity levels, and diets, to the benefit of rural elders (Jeffery, Muhajarine, & Hackett, 2018). Nevertheless, the damage of obesity to physical health is more significant among rural

elderly than their urban counterparts (Batsis, Whiteman, Lohman, Scherer & Bartels, 2017), indicating that from a public health perspective, locality needs to be taken into consideration. Overall, it is imperative for weight-related issues to be a major rural public health concern.

Diabetes

Diabetes is the seventh leading cause of death in the United States. Its prevalence rate among rural older adults is 26.8% (N=14.3 million), which is 17 times greater than in older adults in urban areas (Callaghan, Towne, Bolin, & Ferdinand, 2017). Older diabetics tend to have lower health status than age-matched peers and suffer more hypertension, cerebrovascular disease dementia and other chronic conditions (Sinclair, Conroy, and Bayer, 2008). Rural diabetes sufferers (76.3%) are less likely to have their blood sugar under control than their urban counterparts (84.5%).

Furthermore, rural people with diabetes are slightly less likely to have had a blood sugar or blood pressure test within the past year.

Diabetes is mentioned frequently in this chapter, first, because it is related to so many other health conditions and is a common comorbidity in older adults. Second, it is prevalent, particularly in rural areas. As such, the cause of death may be attributed to any one of the comorbidities, potentially leading to underreporting diabetes.

Falls

Falls are the leading cause of fatal and nonfatal injuries among older adults (persons aged ≥65 years). From 2007 to 2016, a 31% in the rate of falls was reported; 30,000 deaths occurred because of falls (Burns and Kakara, 2018). Annual percentage change in deaths from falls appear similar between urban (2.2 to 3.4%) and rural adults (2.8 to 3.3%); however, the prevalence rates tend to be higher in rural areas. In light of the deaths attributed to falls, nonfatal falls may seem trivial. However, they result in dependence, immobilization, and decreased function. Hip fractures had a 22% mortality rate at one-year post fall and cervical fractures had a 24.5% mortality rate also at one year.

While falls themselves are dangerous, falls induce fear of future falling. The related anxiety may lead to avoidance behaviors, including physical activities and even the autonomous performance of basic activities of daily living (ADL) and instrumental activities of daily living (IADL). Anxiety related to fear of falling, when persistent, may lead to depression (Painter, et al., 2012). Preventive measures, for example, fall prevention screening (Cho et al., 2018), fall risk reduction programs (Jones et al., 2015), and balance-oriented exercise programs such as yoga and Tai Chi (Hamrick, Mross, Christopher, & Smith, 2017), are effective approaches to decreasing falls. However, options to participate in these programs are more limited in rural areas (Weber, White, & Mclivried, 2008): travel times are longer, costs pose barriers to participation, and the small numbers of attendees make programs expensive to run (Smith & Morton, 2009).

Furthermore, obesity and a lack of physical activity heighten older adults' risk of unintentional injuries specifically caused by falls (Mitchell, Lord, Harvey, & Close, 2014, Tremmel et al., 2017). More than 25% of older adults in the United States fall each year, a quarter of whom sustain injuries. Moreover, the prevalence of falls leading to injuries has increased (Bergen, Stevens, & Burns, 2016; Burns and Kakara, 2018). Among older adults, for both men and women, those 75+ years are at a higher risk of fall-related injuries and, compared with men, older women are at a higher risk of fall-related fractures (Verma, et al., 2016). Compared with urban elders, rural residents are more prone to unintentional fall injuries, institutionalization, and related mortality (Porell & Carter, 2012). Falls in older adults' daily life have become a major public health concern (Burns, Stevens, & Lee, 2016; Howard et al., 2018).

Alzheimer's Disease and Dementia

One of the common aging stereotypes is that older adults are cognitively impaired, having memory problems, and eventually developing dementia. Yet, a noticeable decline in cognitive capacity may occur to some older adults. The brain loses plasticity with age, making it difficult for older adults to memorize, recall, or learn new skills. Processing slows and it may seem that the person is not understanding, not attending, or confused. These changes are usually not disease processes. Most people remain cognitively intact until death or near death; given time and interest, the older adult engages and understands.

Approximately 10% of people over 65 years develop Alzheimer's disease, a degenerative disease that causes memory loss, forgetfulness, confusion, and behaviors with a potential for harming one's self. Alzheimer's disease involves loss of cognitive ability, decreased motor skills, and reduced functional abilities; it is progressive, irreversible, and incurable. According to the Alzheimer's Association (2019), its prevalence has increased in recent years; it is currently the fifth-leading cause of death among older adults 65+ years and the third-leading cause of death among those 85+ years (Heron, 2019). As population aging expands, the number of older adults likely to be affected by Alzheimer's disease is expected to increase (Alzheimer's Association, 2019).

Older adults in rural areas are at a higher risk of Alzheimer's disease; the death rate due to Alzheimer's disease was 11% higher among nonmetropolitan residents than their metropolitan counterparts (Singh & Siahpush, 2013). Conversely, in some rural areas, the prevalence of Alzheimer's disease and related disorders (ADRD) tended to be lower than for urban residents. A national study of urban and rural older adults using measures of cognition and dementia found that cognitive functioning was lower among the rural participants than for the urban elders (Barth, Nickel, & Kolominsky-Rabas, 2018). Education was a key difference between the two groups. While education among rural elders has been improving, the link between education and cognitive functioning highlights an important area of emphasis for public health messaging regarding the lifelong benefits of education.

The general public is now aware of Alzheimer's disease, although some mythology still surrounds the disease. Both in the disease's folklore, medical practice, and in research, the causal ambiguity of environment vs. heredity is evident (Sharma, Sharma, Fayaz, & Wakode, 2020; Ye, Bai, & Zhang, 2016). Treatment is also a realm of diverging opinions and evidence, likely because different treatments work for some people and not for others. Furthermore, a particular treatment may work for an individual for a period of time but as the disease progresses, the effectiveness may wane, and an alternative must be found. At this time, the direct causes of Alzheimer's disease have not been identified and no medication has been developed that cures it (Ihara & Saito, 2020). However, public health and related disciplines have cultivated public understanding of this devastating disease and the demands it places on the families and caregivers of those living with the disease (Zarit and Eddwards, 2008).

Quality of Life

Quality of life refers to life satisfaction or contentment and has implications for well-being. It is influenced by an array of interacting factors, including demographic and social resources (e.g., age, gender, ethnicity, family size, marital status). Socioeconomic status, health and behavioral status (e.g., chronic illnesses, activities of daily living) are additional factors to be considered in assessing one's quality of life. For example, observing that you are unfairly disadvantaged, economically or socially, can lead to lower life satisfaction. Additionally, sociocognitive status (e.g., memory issues, depression) influence life satisfaction (Tran, et al., 2018). Rural older adults report lower quality of life than their urban counterparts (Peltzer, et al, 2019) [See Michalska-Żylal & Marks-Krzyszkowska, 2018) for an exception in Poland]. Hispanic and African Americans were associated with even poorer quality of life than urban or rural older white adults (Baernholdt, et al., 2012). Thus life satisfaction overarches many aspects of life and varies within and between individuals and communities.

Social Networks/ Relationships: Family and Friends

Social connectedness, also called social engagement, refers to a sense of belongingness within a social milieu. It indicates a social ease within a family and/or community (Buys, et al., 2015).

Through social connectedness, people are involved in planned and unplanned social contact, receiving and giving support and exchanging conversations of significant events. It also involves a sense that support or help, whether emotional or task-related, will be available when needed.

Social well-being is a critical part of overall health for older adults wherever they live. Social functioning of older adults in rural areas tends to be poorer than that of urban older adults (de Koning, Stathi, & Richards, 2017), indicating that rural older adults are at a higher risk of social isolation. These research results must be considered in the context of income levels; social isolation may be a result of poverty which is higher in rural areas and among minority populations.

Contrary to expectations, Henning-Smith, Moscovice, and Kozhimannil (2018) found that older adults in urban areas reported higher levels of loneliness than their rural counterparts. Rather than being more isolated, rural elders were more likely to live nearer relatives and to know more people in their communities; however, differences within the rural elderly were noted.

Specifically, rural black elders were lonelier than their white counterparts. Based on qualitative interviews with minority elderly men living in rural Australia, Rademacher and Feldman (2017) found that retirement contributed to loneliness, particularly when one's work role was the foundation for identity. As more women are engaging in careers as men have in the past, we may see that women also feel lonely when they retire. Alternately, they may have established relationships that foster their well-being through the retirement transition. A limitation of the research on loneliness is that it remains largely cross-sectional. We do not know the extent to which loneliness in late life is a lifelong pattern rather than a condition of old age. Furthermore, Black elders were the only racial/ethnic group included in the investigation by Henning-Smith, et al., (2018). The inclusion of more minority elders as well as gender analysis could test the effects of familism as well as additional racial/ethnic differences in relation to loneliness in late life.

Depression

Finally, public health has an important role to perform in addressing depression. The WHO (2017) reported that 264 million people worldwide suffer from depression. Across the life course, the prevalence of depression is higher for women and girls than it is for men and boys. This worldwide pattern is especially pronounced from 50–75 years of age and then narrows and continues into the 80s (WHO, 2017). Thus, we see that depression can affect people of all ages. Rather than being a function of urban or rural residence, the risk of depression is heightened by poverty, unemployment, illness (mental and physical), and substance abuse. These risk factors may be found in both urban and rural settings and will vary across time, economies, and locations. Furthermore, depression is a risk factor of Alzheimer's disease (Linnemann & Lang, 2020); moreover, depression and Alzheimer's disease can coexist, and informal family caregivers are at high risk of depression. The array of correlates and risk factors related to depression necessitate that the public health professional remain well informed about the community and its culture (Underwood, Jeffery, Muhajarine, & Hackett, 2018).

What Contributes to the Observed Rural/Urban Disparities in Late Life?

Health behaviors, combined with healthcare availability and quality, and geographic characteristics in rural communities, have profound effects on urban vs. rural wellness.

Compared with urban older residents, rural residents are less likely to participate in preventive health services. Moreover, limited transportation, social isolation, lack of quality health care, and financial difficulties all contribute to health disparities (National Healthcare Disparities Report, 2011). Considering these barriers, it is not surprising that rural elders are less likely to have annual checkups (Cohen, Cook, Sando, & Sabik, 2018), more likely to smoke, and tend to overuse drugs and alcohol (Benson, 2019; Kheun & Wierich, 2019; Roberts, et al., 2016).

However, life expectancy must be considered from a life course perspective: infant mortality, maternal death, participation in risky behaviors, and limited access to resources (education, poverty, health care) all contribute to life expectancies and have greater impact on rural people than on those in urban contexts (Crimmens & Zhang, 2019).

Limited Access to Health Care and Services

Greater geographic distances, more traveling costs, and fewer transportation options contribute to urban/rural disparities in accessing the needed healthcare services (CDC, 2019). As rural health care in general, and geriatric health care are less available, rural longevity suffers. The barriers have contributed to the gap in longevity between urban and rural residents and minority elders. Poor African American rural residents now have a life expectancy of 67.7 years, more than 10 years fewer than the national average. In late life, the major causes of death contributing to the urban/rural and racial disparities include heart disease, unintentional injuries, chronic obstructive pulmonary disease (COPD), lung cancer, stroke, suicide, and diabetes (Gopal & Siahpush, 2014). At the time of this writing, COVID-19 is a significant cause of death, particularly among older adults and minorities.

Two important factors undergird disparities in health for older adults: insurance rates and the closure of rural hospitals. Uninsured rates in rural areas are generally higher than in urban areas, particularly for low income elders although Medicaid expansion has eroded the disparity to some degree. For example, the uninsured rate for low-income rural elders declined from 35% to 16% between 2008 and 2016 for those residing in expansion states. For those in nonexpansion states, the decline was noteworthy but dramatically less: 38% to 32%. Comparison with Americans who are less than 65 years old, the rate of uninsured dropped from 18.2% to 10.7% over roughly the same time period (2010–2017). As states decide whether to accept Medicaid expansion, and who will be covered (children, older adults, working age adults), we see a patchwork of insurance coverage that is hard to typify (Hoadley, Alker, & Holmes, 2018).

The rates of uninsured are related to the closure of rural hospitals; the rates of uninsured are higher in rural than urban areas, which may leave the hospital with more unpaid accounts. For clients who are on Medicaid, hospitals must accept the fee established by the state, which tends to be lower than fees for non-Medicaid clients. Thus, rural hospitals operate on smaller margins, in part because their client base includes elderly and low-income persons who are more likely to be uninsured (Ramesh & Gee, 2019). In addition, rural hospitals tend to be smaller, more distal to other hospitals, and to maintain fewer specialties. A rural gynecologist may serve all the local women's reproductive health and deliver four babies per year: this may not be cost-efficient. As a result, a gynecologist may be deemed a business liability, and women will have to travel greater distances to access reproductive health care. The same issues apply to other medical specialties.

Smoking

The use of tobacco products, whether by smoking, chewing, or snuff, is more prevalent in rural areas than in urban areas (Cepeda-Benitoa, et al., 2016). Moreover, rural smokers are less likely to avoid situations of secondhand smoke (Stillman, Tanenbaum, Wewers, Chelluri, & Roberts, 2018). Preventive interventions to curb smoking have found that of men and women, urban and rural, rural women tend to be most resistant to decreasing smoking or quitting entirely (Cepeda-Benitoa, et al., 2016). It is noteworthy that urban/rural disparities by age (especially for older adults) were insignificant; however, race/ethnicity, socioeconomic status (SES), and educational levels were related to differences in smoking.

Substance Abuse

Rural adults use and abuse alcohol, tobacco, marijuana, amphetamines, prescription medications, heroin, and to a lesser degree, cocaine (Lenardson, Race, & Gale, 2009). Of these, alcohol abuse is the most common reason for hospitalization. Rates of substance abuse are higher in the context of less education, low income, unemployment, and social isolation. In rural settings, resources for prevention, treatment, and rehabilitation are sparse. Moreover, privacy issues may inhibit seeking needed treatment. The more rural the area, the more likely that substance abuse will result in death.

Alcohol consumption, fewer years of education, and rural residence are all related to multimorbidities (de Melo, et al., 2019). For many individuals who abuse alcohol as adults and in late life, drinking began when they were young. Lal and Pattanayak (2017) recommend that the treatment of older people who abuse alcohol should be nonconfrontive, tailored to the individual, and age-specific.

Furthermore, alcohol users are more likely to use opioids than nondrinkers. Approximately 1.5 million adults (4.9% of rural adults) misused their prescription pain medication in 2015 (Rural Health Information Hub). Currently, opioid use disorder is a significant and growing problem among older adults. Prescription opioids are intended to ease short-term pain, for example, postsurgery. However, the euphoria that accompanies their use can lead to addiction. Additionally, misinformation, advertising, and overprescribing have led to their overuse and subsequent abuse among young and old, both urban and rural. Initially, opioid use disorder was located largely in urban areas and then spread from cities to rural areas. Presently, rural prescription rates are higher, and treatment options are fewer (Benson, 2019).

The impact of opioid use disorder is impressive. Since 1915, opioid deaths have contributed to a reversal in the trend toward increased life expectancy (Benson, Kuehn, & Weirich, 2019); better management of opioids is expected to be reflected in life expectancy but may be overshadowed by increased obesity, vaping, inactivity, and social inequity. Economic distress is related to increased opioid abuse, and drug use overall (Monnat,

2019). Currently, middle aged adults have the highest overdose rate of all age groups. As they age into late life, will their need for and use of painkillers increase, as suggested by the CDC (2018), or will they taper their usage or even abstain? Will the difference between urban and rural users continue, decrease, or increase across time? Opioid use disorder will continue to challenge users and their healthcare providers in the years ahead. Public health professionals are urged to keep their audiences well informed as new challenges and solutions emerge.

Promoting Aging in Place for Rural Communities

Aging in place is the practice of maintaining residential continuity as one ages. Most older adults, to date, have preferred to live in their current housing even as their abilities to maintain it decline. Worldwide, most older adults prefer to age in place. In the United States, 77% of adults 50+ years wanted to remain in their current communities as they aged. Seventy-six percent hoped to remain in their same home (AARP Report, 2018).

Although it may be more or less costly than moving to a less demanding residence, aging in place can be an antidote to social isolation. Aging in place offers continuity of friend networks and healthcare providers surrounded by neighbors who are more likely to know and check up on each other (Buys, et al., 2015). The older adult stays in a familiar environment structurally as well as socially. Senior centers typically offer an array of opportunities for social connectedness and can be quite effective in helping older adults maintain and develop their sense of belonging.

However, the incentive to move to smaller or more protected housing is typically based on increasing disability and forces a person to face his or her own aging. Many older adults do not want to be viewed as aged and many prefer a multiaged community where they do not experience the still existing stigma surrounding nursing homes and old age (Torres and Cao, 2019). Socially, moving to a different residence or location poses a threat to connectedness in rural areas. Planned communities are also becoming a popular option as middle- to upper-income boomers have been more mobile throughout their lives and demonstrate less attachment to place (Malone-Beach and Langeland, 2011).

Dalmer (2019) argues that the emphasis on individual choice, e.g., aging in place, prioritizes the individual over the collective. Furthermore, it fails to consider the cost (to the individual, the community, and the society) of supporting elderly and possibly frail individuals who choose to age in place. Conversely, White, Evans, Connelly & Caine (1914) argue that the technologies are already available to maintain frail older adults as they age in place. They also highlight the conundrum that those most in need are the least likely to be able to access and afford these technologies.

Rural elders who age in place experience different challenges than urban elders. The rural elders, perhaps widowed, are more likely to reside in a farm home that is more distant from healthcare services, that is larger and perhaps older, and in need of more upkeep than homes in urban settings. Moreover, sources of information may be fewer, particularly in areas of the country that lack broadband access. As they age, they are more likely to rely on informal caregivers, such as family and friends. Indeed, due to the outmigration, informal caregivers tend to be older spouses, family members, or friends. Public transportation may be limited or nonexistent. Recent developments in technology have shed light on how telehealth services can be applied to meet the needs among rural aging communities. In the following sections, we discuss each topic in more detail.

Increased Availability of Health Care and Services

Having a **usual source of health care** is associated with positive health outcomes such as effective preventive care, lower costs, and less use of emergency departments. In evaluating rural health needs, a nationwide study identified access to quality health services as the No.1 priority (Bolin et al., 2015). Considering the shortage of health professionals in rural areas (Council of State Governments, 2011; National Center for Health Statistics, 2012), this assessment appears to accurately depict rural health needs. Other priorities indicated for rural public health included nutrition and weight status, diabetes, mental health and mental disorders, substance abuse, heart disease and stroke, physical activity, and oral health (Bolin et al., 2015).

Recent closures of rural hospitals and the lack of healthcare providers have further exacerbated problems in accessing healthcare services, both preventive and curative, in rural areas (National Center for Health Statistics, 2012). The closure of a rural hospital has immediate and potentially long-term effects on the local economy as well the health and well-being of the community members (Holmes, 2016). Overall, rural residents tend to have less access to health information from a variety of sources, including primary care providers and specialists, and the Internet (Chen et al., 2019). For residents in disadvantaged rural areas, mobile clinics can serve as an alternative to permanent services. In addition, mobile clinics serve those with mobility issues. Tele-dentistry and mobile hearing units, may, to some extent, help provide necessary services.

Support Informal Caregiving for Rural Older Adults

Usually, the first symptom of a dementing illness, particularly Alzheimer's disease, is memory loss. As the disease progresses, family members become suspicious that something is not right. This leads to a consultation with a healthcare provider and potentially years of caregiving for a spouse or parent. Informal family members are estimated to provide 80–90% of long-term care needs. More specifically, over 44 million family members care for their loved ones without remuneration. Their contribution to elder care has an estimated economic value of nearly $500 billion per year (Henning-Smith & Lahr, 2018). Yet, government funding focuses on supporting institutionalized care or home and community-based health services (National Conference of State Legislatures, 2014). On the one hand, because of rapid population aging, higher poverty rates, and health disparities, rural older adults are likely to need more assistance from caregivers. Because access to formal caregiving services is limited and less affordable, their reliance on informal caregivers is becoming greater. Concurrently, fewer caregiver support programs are available in rural areas. The lack of caregiving support threatens the well-being of both the caregiver and elder living with a dementing illness.

Some states and communities have offered day programs to support informal caregivers with respite, intending that this will delay institutionalization or avoid it all together (National Conference of State Legislatures, 2014). In a recent report on rural caregiving challenges and interventions (Henning-Smith & Lahr, 2018), caregiver participants noted limited access to resources (e.g., formal support programs, restricted access to health care, workforce shortage, and less access to home care and respite services. In addition, they are frustrated by long distances to health care and supportive services, lack of public transportation, rural culture, population aging and out-migration, and social isolation. These and other challenges heighten the risk of depression and anxiety for both caregivers and care recipients. At least 43 states have offered cash and/or counseling programs to informal caregivers. For example, rural informal caregivers can be paid for their services jointly by state and federal governments.

Moreover, because 16–20% of American workers serve as family caregivers concurrently (Feinberg & Choula, 2012); they may struggle to maintain a balance between family and work. A subset of caregivers are also supporting children as well as the older generation. Paid workplace leave, affordable health insurance, and/or expanded family leave policies to informal caregivers, may mitigate the strain on caregivers and relieve the care recipient of guilty feelings when receiving support from their working family members (Feinberg & Choula, 2012; Henning-Smith & Lahr, 2018). Additional support is also needed for family caregivers, no longer working and potentially retired, who are themselves quite elderly.

Numerous strategies have been tried in efforts to support family caregivers. Many more ideas have been proposed but not implemented in every state. For example, tax credits are now available to caregivers. For caregivers who can no longer participate in paid work, they might accrue working "credits" in the Social Security program and apply for subsidies for providing care. Many senior centers offer caregiving training, and screening for caregiver depression/isolation/stress. They may also locate resources in the senior center so that access is easier. In addition, senior centers, churches, and women's groups provide caregiver support programs. Alternatively, states may divert more funding to home and community-based services rather than to traditional nursing homes to meet the caregiving needs of current and future rural older adults who prefer aging to relocating to institutions.

Promote Safe and Reliable Transportation in Rural Community

Safe and reliable transportation is critical to a community's livability, including access to food, health care, education, employment, social engagement, and recreational activities (Bayne, Siegfried, Stauffer, & Knudson, 2018). Even more important for rural communities, efficient and affordable transportation is usually coupled with economic growth (Dabson, Johnson, & Fluharty, 2011) and allows people to obtain needed services (Peng & Nelson, 1998).

In terms of transportation mode, rural residents are more likely than urban residents to rely on personal automobiles (cars, trucks, vans, and even golf carts or ATVs) for transportation.

According to the American Public Transportation Association (APTA), although about 20% of the U.S. population lives in rural areas, only 11% of the federal government funding was provided to rural public transportation in 2016. Across the United States, only 60% of rural communities have available public transportation, 28% of which is limited (TRIP, 2019). As a result, it is not surprising that only 0.5% of rural residents use public transportation for work commuting than their urban counterparts (6.3%) (Mattson, 2017). Rural residents tend to drive over the age of 75 years compared with their urban counterparts. However, many rural residents cannot maintain personal vehicles. Those with physical or mobility limitations may not be able to drive themselves, resulting in social isolation and relying on informal caregivers' help. Other transportation options are limited, such as ride-sharing services and commercial taxis, because it is costly to operate in such geographically dispersed rural communities (Smith, 2016). These costs can include longer distances between pick-up locations and longer wait times between passengers, which can increase costs for drivers, which may also be passed down to users.

Limited transportation modes and long distances between places in rural areas may have negative consequences for health. Rural residents are less likely to participate in social services and delay other daily needs such as grocery shopping. They may not be able to receive timely health care, such as miss or delay appointments, medications, or interventions. Moreover, because the primary transportation is personal vehicles, rural older adults are at higher risk of social isolation when they could no longer drive (Baernholdt, et al., 2012). Although medical transport through Medicare is available for rural older adults, nonessential transportation options are still limited (Smith, 2016). A recent study has suggested high cost-benefits in medical services and employment by improving rural and small urban transit (Godavarthy, Mattson, & Ndembe, 2015). To address the rural transportation problems, the U.S. Department of Transportation (2020) distributes 70 million dollars annually to decrease inequities in urban/rural transportation (https://www.transportation .gov/connections/future-rural-mobility) and nongovernment agencies, such as ITNAmerica, have launched volunteer driver programs to assist older adults (https://www.itnamerica.org /#myCarousel).

Apply Technology to Meet the Healthcare and Social Needs

A common stereotype of older adults is that they are computer impaired; they are hesitant to use computers and slow to learn how to use them. A recent meta-analysis auger against the assumption that age and computer use are related. More accurately, older adults are inclined to use a computer when they feel that they will be able to learn how to use it easily and when they see a purpose or benefit from its use. Their learning is enhanced in the context of social support, usually a spouse; education; and frequency of use. They also learn better when the instruction is based on how to perform a task rather than explanations about how the computer works (Hauk, Hüffmeier, & Krumm, 2018). For example, when technology use is a means to stay in contact with one's children and grandchildren, many older adults are eager learners (Hakoyama and

MaloneBeach, 2018. However, the necessary learning can be more challenging in rural areas lacking broadband access (Arcury, Quant, et al., 2017).

The use of patient portals for health care is becoming prevalent; however, its success is related to ethnicity, education, and poverty, all contributing to urban/rural disparities in health care.

Rurality is a factor in portal use: Arcury (2017) found that the use of patient portals is lower when the health care is received from a rural clinic. This can be related to the absence of computers and electronic devices in the homes of low-income elders as well as the lack of broadband access in rural areas. This has the potential to widen the urban/rural gap in **access to services** as broadband investors estimate their costs vis a vis the number of likely users (Kim & Orazem, 2017).

Rural elders leave their homes to engage in social activities more frequently than urban elders whereas urban elders are most likely to host family and friends in their own homes (White, Evans, Connolly, & Cain, 2014). These observations suggest that hand-held portable technologies may be a better fit for rural elders whereas more stationary in-home devices may work well for urban elders. Batsis, et al., (2017) tested the use of the Fitbit Zip device to encourage physical activity in obese older adults who were nonexercisers. Their participants found it difficult to schedule regular exercise time and decreased in exercise self-confidence. The authors suggested that the intervention may have been more successful if the social component of exercise groups was included whether by in-person classes or via the Internet. In-person classes are less likely to be offered in rural areas and Internet support will depend on broadband access.

In addition to the work cited here, numerous studies have examined the effectiveness of innovative technologies to mitigate caregivers' potential for exhaustion and to delay the institutionalization of the care recipient. These efforts are based on the assumption that elders and their families prefer aging in place and strive to help them to do so. Early caregiving research has found that caregiving necessitates some level of hands-on care and nearby support (Silverstein & Litwak, 1993). In many parts of the world, the younger generation is leaving rural areas to find work in urban centers and are, thus, unavailable to provide the physical care that the older generation may need. On the other hand, many labor migrants send money back to their families to sustain them in their absence (Liu, 2014), an activity that is made easy by communication devices. The extent to which formal care systems and technologies can fill the rural care gap remains to be seen.

Overall, older adults' use of communication technologies, particularly strategies for telehealth, are not yet well researched. By default, the COVID-19 pandemic of 2020 stands to provide a plethora of data regarding the effectiveness of telemedicine for both providers and healthcare recipients, including the rural elderly.

Aging Friendly Communities for All Ages: Addressing "Isms" in Late Life

Throughout this chapter and book, we see that marginalization and discrimination harm physical health and cause psychosocial damage. In recent years, the U.S. political and policy climates have been altered by initiatives to decrease discrimination for religious minorities, people of color, older adults, and LGBTQ individuals of all ages (Ard & Makadon, 2016).

Ageism is an "ism" that public policy must confront (Voyles, 2020). Idioms, marketing, film, businesses, and schools all reinforce ageism. Ordinary forgetfulness is referred to as "a senior moment." Greeting cards mock memory loss, incontinence, baldness, wrinkles, and sagging breasts. In film, older men have typically had roles to play but only recently have older women, wrinkles and all, been featured. In business and education, older adults are often considered to be slower and less able to learn despite significant evidence to the contrary. This is especially evident in computer use. Arguably, age is not the determining factor here; interest is likely to play a bigger role.

Ageism assumes that old is bad and the message is ubiquitous. The more this attitude is perpetuated, the more it spreads. Like racism and other "isms," the idea becomes entrenched and resistant to change. Age does not provide immunity: older adults learn that they are inferior and expected to be incompetent regarding specific tasks and activities. As their confidence is eroded, they are less likely to attempt actions that they could learn or are capable of doing. As a result, their competence deteriorates. Ageism has serious negative implications for living a healthy life.

Ageism is just beginning to receive more widespread attention as the last bastion of "ism"s, and in gerontology, attention to LGBTQ persons has been limited: cisgender is assumed (Reczek, 2018). This stands to change. The American Psychological Association (APA) states that there are 35 million older adults in the United States, of whom 2.4 identify as LGBTQ. The APA, like numerous other national organizations (The Gerontological Society of America, American Society on Aging, The National Resource Center n LGBT Aging), are working through publications, interest groups, and formal organizations to decrease disparities in health care between gender identity groups to make aging a positive experience for everyone.

Simultaneously, young people are increasingly vocal about their sexual identities and their intended status as full participants in society. Their voices are calling attention to a previously marginalized segment of the population with the intent to implement more considerate and inclusive public policies. The intersection of ageism and homophobia is just beginning to move from neglect to receive attention.

In bringing elderly LGBTQ persons into the realm of public policy, it will be necessary to examine urban/rural differences. Many of today's older adults who are LGBTQ have lived their entire lives closeted, and with advanced years, find that they are now experiencing age discrimination as well. As LGBTQ persons, their unique health concerns are likely to have been ignored or unnoticed. Their social development may have been altered by limited access to activities and organizations. Their psychological health may have been challenged by exclusion, derogatory language, and blatant discrimination (Reczek, 2018). As such damage accrues across the life course, health and well-being are jeopardized and their unique needs are still unnoticed and are now exacerbated by ageism. Public policy is challenged to educate the public about the damage of living an entire life in secrecy and fear of discovery.

Recommendations and Future Directions

Throughout the literature cited in this chapter, a theme emerged. Overall, the authors consistently emphasized the need for public health policy, program designers, practitioners, and researchers to assume that two cultures, i.e., distinct urban and rural public health disparities, and many co-cultures within each, exist. The cultures are overlapping, yet, each is unique. To be effective, based on the examples of the existing initiatives and programs discussed in the chapter, it is imperative that the voices of the people being served are heard (Bacsu, et al., 2017; McKenzie, 2002: Stoller, et al., 2011; Boggs, et al., 2017).

Conclusion

Ample evidence shows significant health disparities between urban and rural communities in public health and health care; rural elders are lacking in the services needed to ensure the sufficient levels of health care that more urban dwellers have readily available. The disparities are further complicated by race, education, incomes, ethnicities, and by the cultural ethos of local communities. The demographics of rural aging has compelled the needs to support rural elders age in place by improving the availability of rural health care and services, supporting informal caregiving, providing safe and reliable transportation, and adopting technology to meet their healthcare and social needs. We also suggest addressing the pervasive ageism in the society and advocate for an aging-friendly environment for current older adults and future generations. In consideration of the correlates of health and health care, it is unlikely that one shoe will fit all.

Thus, public health professionals will be most effective if they approach rural health care with attention, creativeness, insight, and persistence.

Chapter Summary

Knowledge of normal development in late life is necessary to distinguish it from treatable impairments and/or disease processes. In particular, hearing, vision, and oral health are addressed in this chapter because they are so critical to maintaining one's abilities and autonomy with age. Noteworthy disparities between urban and rural elders were addressed in terms of obesity and physical inactivity, diabetes, and falls. In the realm of quality of life, we focused on mental health, specifically depression, loneliness, and Alzheimer's disease (as the most common form of dementia). Because of the insidious nature of Alzheimer's disease, its prevalence, and resulting dependence on others, informal family and friend caregivers are noted for their contributions and vulnerabilities as the disease takes its toll

on the social setting of those surrounding the person living with Alzheimer's disease. Lifestyle factors also play a complicating role in the health of elderly rural individuals: smoking, alcohol abuse, opioid use disorder, and physical and mental inactivity. All of these factors interact in a rural context of fewer healthcare services, lack of transportation options, absence of local providers, no or intermittent broadband access, and older people's interest in aging in place.

Change is inevitable. At the time of this writing in early 2020, much of the world is sequestered to prevent further spread of COVID-19. Change has been startlingly abrupt, and the vulnerability of the older population has been demonstrated by the death rate among older adults. Moreover, the glaring disparity of income, race, and income has been evidenced by the death rates among marginalized people of all ages. While this pandemic is devastating, it may hold the seeds to ideas for improved public health in rural communities and worldwide.

Case Studies

- Opioid epidemic: A case study in rural Litchfield County, Connecticut https://www.ruralhealthinfo.org/project -examples/1083
- Alzheimer's screening training: A case study in rural Florida https://www.rural healthinfo.org/project-examples/1082
- Depression: A case study with rural older veterans https://www.ruralhealthinfo.org /project-examples/941
- Palliative care: A case study in rural New Hampshire and Vermont https://www .ruralhealthinfo.org/project-examples/956
- Mental health first aid training: https:// www.ruralhealthinfo.org/project -examples/725

Discussion Questions

1. Propose two strategies for assuring that public health messaging successfully reaches rural elders who do not have broadband access.
2. Discuss the pros and cons of aging in place for a) rural elders, b) the families of rural elders, c) rural communities, and d) society.
3. Many people know a number of lifestyle choices that are recommended for health and well-being, yet they choose to be sedentary, overeat, or self-medicate. How can already health-educated older adults in rural areas be motivated to put their information into action?
4. In the wake of rural hospital closings, propose solutions for the delivery of in-person health care, particularly in emergency situations.

References

American Association of Retired Persons (AARP) (n.d.). *Stats and Facts from the 2018 AARP Home and Community Preferences Survey.* http://www.aarp.org/livable-communities/about/info-2018/2018-aarp-home-and-community-preferences-survey.html

Alzheimer's Association (2019). Alzheimer's & Dementia: *The Journal of the Alzheimer's Association November 2019 Journal Digest.* https://www.alz.org/news/2019/alzheimer-s-dementia-the-journal-of-the-alzheim

American Public Transportation Association (APTA) (2017). *2016 Public Transportation Fact Book.* https://www.apta.com/wp-content/uploads/Resources/resources/statistics/Documents/FactBook/2016-APTA-Fact-Book.pdf#page=8

Arcury, T. A., Quandt, S. A., Sandberg, J. C., Miller, Jr., D. P., Latulipe, C., Leng, X., . . . Bertoni, A. G. (2017). Patient portal utilization among ethnically diverse low-income older adults: Observational study. *JMIR Medical Informatics, 5*(4), e47. https://doi.org/10.2196/medinform.8026

Ard, K. L., & Makadon, H. J. (2016). Improving the health care of lesbian, gay, bisexual and transgender (LGBT) people: Understanding and eliminating health disparities. The Fenway Institute: Pennsylvania Department of Health. https://www.lgbthealtheducation.org/publication/improving-the-health-care-of-lesbian-gay-bisexual-and-transgender-lgbt-people-understanding-and-eliminating-health-disparities/

Bae, S., Lee, S., Lee, S., Haradac, K., Makizako, H., Parke, H., & Shimada, H. (2018). Combined effect of self-reported hearing problems and level of social activities on the risk of disability in Japanese older adults: A population-based longitudinal study. *Maturitas, 115,* 51–55. https://doi.org/10.1016/j.maturitas.2018.06.008

Baernholdt, M., Yan, G., Hinton, I, Rose, K., & Mattos, M. (2012). Quality of life in rural and urban adults 65 years and older: Findings from the national health and nutrition examination survey. *The Journal of Rural Health, 28*(4), 339–347. https://doi.org/10.1111/j.1748-0361.2011.00403.x

Bacsu, J., Abonyi, S., Viger, M., Morgan, D., Johnson, S., & Jeffery, B. (2017). Examining rural older adults' perceptions of cognitive health. *Canadian Journal on Aging/La Revue canadienne du vieillissement 36*(3), 318–327. https://doi.org/10.1017/S0714980817000150

Barth, J., Nickel, F., Kolominsky-Rabas, P. L. (2018). Diagnosis of cognitive decline and dementia in rural areas—A scoping review. *International Journal of Geriatric Psychiatry, 33*(3), 459–474. https://doi.org/10.1002/gps.4841

Batsis, J. A., Whiteman, K. L., Lohman, M. C., Scherer, E. A., & Bartels, S. J. (2017). Body mass index and rural status on self-reported health in older adults: 2004-2013 Medicare expenditure panel survey. *Journal of Rural Health, 34*(S1), s56–s64. https://doi.org/10.1111/jrh.12237

Batsis, J. A., Naslund, J. A., Gill, L. E., Masutani, R. K., Agarwal, N., & Bartels, S. J. (2016). Use of a wearable activity device in rural older obese adults: A pilot study. *Gerontology and Geriatric Medicine, 2,* 1–6. https://doi.org/10.1177/2333721416678076

Bayne, A., Siegfried, A., Stauffer, P., & Knudson, A. (2018). *Promising practices for increasing access to transportation in rural communities.* The Walsh Center for Rural Health Analysis. Retrieved from https://www.norc.org/PDFs/Walsh%20Center/Rural%20Evaluation%20Briefs/Rural%20Evaluation%20Brief_April2018.pdf

Biener, A., Cawley, J., & Meyerhoefer, C. (2018). The impact of obesity on medical care costs and labor market outcomes in the US. *Clinical Chemistry, 64*(1), 108–117. https://doi.org/10.1373/clinchem.2017.272450

Benson, W., Kuehn, K., & Weirich, M. (2019). Why are rural older adults turning to opioids? *Generations: Journal of the American Society on Aging, 43*(2), 55–61. https://doi.org/10.2307/26760115

Blustein, J., & Weinstein, B. E. (2016). Opening the market for lower cost hearing aids: Regulatory change can improve the health of older Americans. *American Journal of Public Health, 106*(6), 1032–1035. https://doi.org/10.2105/AJPH.2016.303176

Bolin, J., Bellamy, G., Ferdinand, A. O., Vuong, A. M., Kash, B., Schulze, A., & Helduser, J. W. (2015). Rural healthy people 2020: New decade, same challenges. *The Journal of Rural Health, 31*(3), 326–333. https://doi.org/10.1111/jrh.12116

Boggs, J. M., Portz, J. D., King, D. K., Wright, L. A., Helander, K., Retrum, J. H., & Gozansky, W. S. (2017). Perspectives of LGBTQ older adults on aging in place: A qualitative investigation. *Journal of Homosexuality, 64*(11), 1539–1560. https://doi.org/10.1080/00918369.2016.1247539

Burns, E., & Kakara, R. (2018). Deaths from falls among persons aged ≥65 years—United States, 2007–2016. *MMWR Morbidity and Mortality Weekly Report, 67*(18), 509–514. https://doi.org/10.15585/mmwr.mm6718a1

Buys, L., Burton, L., Cuthill, M., Hogan, A., Wilson, B., & Baker, D. (2015). Establishing and maintaining social connectivity: An understanding of the lived experiences of older adults residing in regional and rural communities. *The Australian Journal of Rural Health, 23*(5), 291–294. https://doi.org/10.1111/ajr.12196

Caldwell J. T., Lee, H., & Cagney, K. A. (2017). The role of primary care for the oral health of rural and urban older adults. *The Journal of Rural Health, 33*(4), 409–418. https://doi.org/10.1111/jrh.12269

Callaghan, T. H., Towne, Jr., S. D., Bolin, J., & Ferdinand, A. O. (2017). *Diabetes Mortality in Rural America: 1999-2015.* Policy Brief. Southwest Rural Health Research Center. https://srhrc.tamhsc.edu/docs/srhrc-pb2-callaghan-diabetes.pdf

Centers for Disease Control and Prevention (CDC). (2018a). CDC: More obesity in U.S. rural counties than in urban counties. US Department of Health and Human Services, Media Statement.

Centers for Disease Control and Protection (CDC). (2018b). *Annual Surveillance Report of Drug-Related risks and Outcomes – United States.* Washington, DC: U.S. Department of Health and Human Services.

Chang, M., Kim, H. J., Mook-Jung, I., & Oh, S. (2019). Hearing loss as a risk factor for cognitive impairment and loss of synapses in the hippocampus. *Behavioral Brain Research, 372,* 112069.

Cepeda-Benito, A., Doogan, N. J., Redner, R., Roberts, M. E., Kurti, A. N., Villanti, A. C., . . . Higgins, S. T., (2018). Trend differences in men and women in rural and urban U. S. settings. *Preventive Medicine, 117,* 69–75.

Cho, S. I., & An, D. H. (2014). Effects of a fall prevention exercise program on muscle strength and balance of the old-old elderly. *Journal of Physical Therapy Science, 26*(11), 1771–1774.

CMS Centers for Medicare and Medicaid Services. (2019). Rural-urban disparities in health care and Medicare. Executive Summary.

Cohen, S. A., Cook, S. K., Sando, T. A., & Sabik, N. J. (2018). What aspects of rural life contribute to rural-urban health disparities in older adults? Evidence from a national survey. *The Journal of Rural Health, 34*(3), 293–303. doi: 10.1111/jrh.12287

Cohen S. A., Greaney, M. L., & Sabik, N. J. (2018). Assessment of dietary patterns, physical activity and obesity from a national survey: Rural-urban health disparities in older adults. *PLoS ONE 13*(12): e0208268. https://doi.org/10.1371/journal.pone.0208268

Crimmins, E. M., & Zhang, Y. S. (2019). Aging populations, mortality, and life expectancy. *Annual Review of Sociology, 45,* 69–89.

Curhan, S. G., Willett, W. C., Grodstein, F., & Curhan, G. C. (2019). Longitudinal study of self-reported hearing loss and subjective cognitive function decline in women. *Alzheimer's & Dementia, 15*(4), 525–533. doi: 10.106/j.jalz.2018.11.004

Dabson, B., Johnson, T. G. & Fluharty, C. W. (2011). *Rethinking federal investments in rural transportation: Rural considerations regarding reauthorization of the Surface Transportation Act.* Rural Policy Research Institute (RUPRI). http://www.rupri.org/Forms/RUPRI_Transportation_April2011.pdf

Dai, W., Gao, J., He, P., Ma, Z., Tian, X., & Zheng, X. (2019). The association between socioeconomic status and visual disability among older adults in China. *International Journal of Ophthalmology, 12*(1), 106–113.

Dalmer, N. K. (2019). A logic of choice: Problematizing the documentary reality of Canadian aging in place policies. *Journal of Aging Studies 48,* 40–49.

Daniel, S. J., & Kumar, S. (2014). Teledentistry: A key component in access to care. *Journal of Evidence Based Dental Practice, 14*(Suppl), 201–208. https://doi.org/10.1016/j.jebdp.2014.02.008

de Groot, R., van den Hurk, K., Schoonmade, L. J., de Kort, W., Brug, J., & Lakerveld, J. (2019). Urban-rural differences in the association between blood lipids and characteristics of the built environment: A systematic review and meta-analysis. *British MJ Global Health, 4*(1). doi:10.1136/bmjgh-2018-001017

De Koning, J., Stathi, A., & Richards, S. (2017). Predictors of loneliness and different types of social isolation of rural-living older adults in the United Kingdom. *Ageing and Society, 37*(10), 2012–2043. doi:http://dx.doi.org.cmich.idm.oclc.org/10.1017/S0144686X16000696

de Melo, L. A., de Castro Braga, L., Leite, F. P. P., Bittar, B. F., de Figueirēdo Oséas, J. M., & de Lima, K. C. (2019). Factors associated with multimorbidity in the elderly: An integrative literature review. *Revista Brasileira de Geriatria E Gerontologia, 22*(1), e180154.

De Trinidad Young, M., León-Pérez, G., Wells, C. R. & Wallace S. (2018). More inclusive states, less poverty among immigrants? An examination of poverty, citizenship stratification, and state immigrant policies. *Population Research Policy Review, 37*, 205–228. https://doi.org/10.1007/s11113-018-9459-3

Dye, B. A., Thornton-Evans, G., Li, X., Iafolla, T. J. (2015). Dental caries and tooth loss in adults in the United States, 2011–2012. NCHS data brief, no 197. Hyattsville, MD: National Center for Health Statistics.

Eke, P. I., Lu, H., Zhang, X., Thornton-Evans, G., Borgnakke, W. S., Holt, J. B., & Croft, J. B. (2019). Geospatial distribution of periodontists and US adults with severe periodontitis. *The Journal of the American Dental Association, 150*(2), 103–110. https://doi.org/10.1016/j.adaj.2018.09.021

Feinberg, L., & Choula, R. (2012). Understanding the Impact of Family Caregiving on Work. Washington, D.C.: AARP Public Policy Institute.

Finney Rutten, L. J., Agunwamba, A. A., Beckjord, E., Hesse, B. W., Moser, R. P., & Arora, N. K. (2015). The relation between having a usual source of care and ratings of care quality: Does patient-centered communication play a role? *Journal of Health Communication, 20*(7), 759–765. https://doi.org/10.1080/10810730.2015.1018592

Ford, A. H., Hankey, G. J., Yeap, B. B., Golledge, J., Flicker, L., & Almeida, O. P. (2018). Hearing loss and the risk of dementia in later life. *Maturitas, 112*, 1–11.

Godavarthy, R. P., Mattson, J., & Ndembe, E. (2015). Cost–benefit analysis of rural and small urban transit in the United States. *Transportation Research Record, 2533*(1), 141–148. https://doi.org/10.3141/2533-16

Singh, G. K., & Siahpush, M. (2016). Inequalities in U.S. life expectancy by area unemployment level: 1990–2010. *Scientifica*. https://doi.org/10.1155/2016/8290435

Hakoyama, M. & MaloneBeach, E. (2018). Grandparental adoption of modern communication technology and its impact on grandparent-grandchild relationships. *Journal of Communication and Media Studies, 3*(4), 21–38. https://doi.org/10.18848/2470-9247/CGP/v03i04/21-38

Hamano, T., Takeda, M., Tominaga, K., Sundquist, K., & Nabika, T. (2017). Is accessibility to dental care facilities in rural areas associated with number of teeth in elderly residents? *International Journal of Environmental Research and Public Health, 14*(3), 327. https://doi.org/10.3390/ijerph14030327

Hauk, N., Hüffmeier, J., & Krumm, S. (2018). Ready to be a silver surfer? A meta-analysis of the relationship between chronological age and technology acceptance. *Computers in Human Behavior, 84*, 304–319.

Henning-Smith, C., & Lahr, M. (2018). *Perspectives on rural caregiving challenges and interventions.* University of Minnesota Rural Health Research Center. http://rhrc.umn.edu/wp-content/files_mf/1535129278UMNpolicybriefcaregivingchallenges.pdf

Henning-Smith, C., Moscovice, I., & Kozhimannil, K. (2019). Differences in social isolation and its relationship to health by rurality. *The Journal of Rural Health, 35*(4), 540–549.

Heron. (2018). Deaths: Leading Causes for 2016. *National Vital Statistics Reports, 67*(6), 1–77.

Hirsch, S. (2019). Rural America by the numbers. *Generations, 43*(2), 9–16. Retrieved from https://www.ingentaconnect.com/contentone/asag/gen/2019/00000043/00000002/art00003

Holmes, M. (2016). How rural communities respond and recover after a hospital closure. *Rural Health Research Gateway.*

Hoadley, J., Alker, J., & Holmes, M. (2018, September 25). Health insurance coverage in small towns and rural America: The role of Medicaid expansion. Center for Children & Families (CCF) of the Georgetown University Health Policy Institute. https://ccf.georgetown.edu/2018/09/25/health-insurance-coverage-in-small-towns-and-rural-america-the-role-of-medicaid-expansion/

Ihara, M., & Saito, S. (2020). Drug repositioning for Alzheimer's disease: Finding hidden clues in old drugs. *Journal of Alzheimer's Disease, 74*(4), 1013–1028. https://doi.org/10.3233/JAD-200049

ITNAmerica (May 1, 2020). https://www.itnamerica.org/#myCarousel

Jeffery, B., Muhajarine, N., & Hackett, P., (2018). Assessing the rural built environment to support older adults' mobility and social interaction. *Innovation in Aging, 2*(S1), 154.

Kim, Y., & Orazem, P. F. (2017). Broadband Internet and new firm location decisions in rural areas. *American Journal of Agricultural Economics, 99*(1), 285–302. https://doi.org/10.1093/ajae/aaw082

Kramarov, E. A. (2019). Dental care among adults aged 65 and over, 2017. *NCHS Data Brief, 337*, 1–8.

Lal, R., & Pattanayak, R. D. (2017). Alcohol use among the elderly: Issues and considerations. *Journal of Geriatric Mental Health, 4*(1), 4–10.

Lee, Y. H., Chen, A. X., Varadaraj, V., Hong, G. H., Chen, Y., Friedman, D. S., . . . Ehrlich, J. R. (2018). Comparison of access to eye care appointments between patients with Medicaid and those with private health care insurance. *JAMA Ophthalmology, 136*(6), 622–629. https://doi.org/10.1001/jamaophthalmol.2018.0813

Lenardson, J., Race, M., & Gale, J. A. (2009). Few and far away: Detoxification services in rural areas. *University of Southern Maine Digital Commons (Research & Policy Brief).*

Lin, F. R., & Ferrucci, L. (2012). Hearing loss and falls among older adults in the United States. *Archives of Internal Medicine, 172*(4), 369–371.

Linnemann, C., & Lang, U. E. (2020). Pathways connecting late-life depression and dementia. *Frontiers in Pharmacology, 11*, 279. https://doi.org/10.3389/fphar.2020.00279

Lui, J. (2014). Aging, migration, and familial support in rural China. *Geoforum, 51*, 305–312.

MacKenzie, P. (2002). Aging people in aging places: Addressing the needs of older adults in rural Saskatchewan. *Rural Social Work, Special Australian/Canadian issue, 6*(3), 74–83. http://dx.doi.org/10.1037/a0016939

MaloneBeach, E. E., & Langeland, K. L. (2011). Boomers' prospective needs for senior centers and related services: A survey of persons 50–59. *Journal of Gerontological Social Work, 54*, 1, 116–123.

Mattson, J. (2017). *Rural Transit Fact Book 2017*. Small Urban and Rural Transit Center. https://www.ugpti.org/surcom/resources/transitfactbook/downloads/2017-rural-transit-fac t-book.pdf

Michalska-Żyła, A., & Marks-Krzyszkowska, M. (2018). Quality of life and quality of living in rural communes in Poland. *European Countryside, 10*(2), 280–299. doi:10.2478/euco-2018-0017

Monnat, S. M. (2019). The contributions of socioeconomic and opioid supply factors to U.S. drug mortality rates: Urban-rural and within-rural differences. *The Journal of Rural Studies, 68*, 319–335.

Morken K., & Warner, W. (2012). Planning for the aging population: Rural responses to the challenge. National Association of Area Agencies on Aging. Centers for Disease Control and Prevention (CDC).

National Council of State Legislatures, 2014. https://www.ncsl.org/blog/2019/09/25/older-adult-falls-a-growing-health-concern.aspx

National Healthcare Disparities Report 2011 AHRQ Publication No. 12-0006 March 2012 https://www.yumpu.com/en/document/view/32078838/national-healthcare-disparities-report-ldi-health-economist

Niigata, K., Fukuma, S., Hiratsuka, Y., Ono, K., Yamada, M., Sekiguchi, M., . . . Fukuhara, S. (2018). Association between vision-specific quality of life and falls in community-dwelling older adults: LOHAS. *PLoS ONE, 4*(13), e0195806.

Owsley, C., & McGwin, G., Jr. (2010). Vision and driving. *Vision Research, 50*(23), 2348–2361.

Painter, J. A., Allison, L., Dhingra, P., Daughtery, J., Cogdill, K., & Trujillo, L. G. (2012). Fear of falling and its relationship with anxiety, depression, and activity engagement among community-dwelling older adults. *The American Journal of Occupational Therapy, 66*, 169–176. http://dx.doi.org/10.5014/ajot.2012.002535

Peltzer, K., Phaswana-Mafuya, N., & Pengpid, S. Rural–urban health disparities among older adults in South Africa. *African Journal of Primary Health Care & Family Medicine, 11*(1), 1–6. a1890. https:// doi.org/10.4102/phcfm. V11i1.1890

Peng, Z. R., & Nelson, A. C. (1998). Rural transit services: A local economic and fiscal impact analysis. *Transportation Research Record, 1623*(1), 57–62. https://doi.org/10.3141/1623-08

Polyakova, M., & Hua, L. M. (2019). Local area variation in morbidity among low-income, older adults in the United States: A cross-sectional study. *Annals of Internal Medicine, 171*(7), 464–473. doi: 10.7326/M18-2800

Prakash, S. J., Bihari, G. S., & Kumar, S. A. (2016). Lifestyle habits and diseases amongst rural geriatrics population. *International Journal of Community Medicine and Public Health, 3*(4), 957–961.

Purtle, J., Nelson, K. L., Yang, Y., Langellier, B., Stankov, I., & Roux, A. V. (2019). Urban–rural differences in older adult depression: A systematic review and meta-analysis of comparative studies. *American Journal of Preventive Medicine, 56*(4), 603–613.

Radermacher, H. & Feldman, S. (2015). Health is their heart, their legs, their back': Understanding ageing well in ethnically diverse older men in rural Australia. *Ageing & Society, 35*, 1011–1031. doi:10.1017/S0144686X14001226

Ramesh, T., & Gee, E. (2019). Rural hospital closures reduce access to emergency care. *Center for American Progress, Washington, DC.*

Reczek, C. (2018). Queering Aging. Policy Brief. The Ohio State University: Aging Studies Institute.

Roberts, M. E., Doogan, N. J., Kurti, A. N., Redner, R., Gaalema, D. E., Stanton, C. A., . . . Higgins, S. T. (2016). Rural tobacco use across the United States: How rural and urban areas differ, broken down by census regions and divisions. *Health & Place, 39*, 153–159.

Rural Health Information Hub. Substance Abuse in Rural Areas Introduction. Retrieved from https://www.ruralhealthinfo.org/topics/substance-abuse

Sharma, P., Sharma, A., Fayaz, F., Wakode, S., Pottoo, F. H. (2020). Biological signatures of Alzheimer's disease. *Current Topics in Medicinal Chemistry, 20*(9), doi: 10.2174/1568026620666200228095553

Silverstein, M. & Litwak, E. (1993). A task-specific typology of intergenerational family structure in later life. *The Gerontologist, 33*(2), 258–264.

Sinclair, A. J., Conroy, S. P., & Bayer, A. J. (2008). Impact of diabetes on physical function in older people. *Diabetes Care, 31*(2), 233–235.

Singh, G. K., & Siahpush, M. Widening rural–urban disparities in all-cause mortality and mortality from major causes of death in the USA, 1969–2009. (2014). *Journal of Urban Health, 91*, 272–292. https://doi.org/10.1007/s11524-013-9847-2

Stillman, F. A., Tanenbaum, E., Wewers, M. E., Chelluri, D., Mumford, E. A., Groesbeck, K. . . . Roberts, M. (2018). Variations in support for secondhand smoke restrictions across diverse rural regions of the United States. *Preventive Medicine, 116*, 157–165.

Smith, A. (2016, May 19). *Shared, collaborative and on demand: The new digital economy*. Pew Research Center. https://www.pewresearch.org/internet/2016/05/19/on-demand-ride-hailing-apps/

Stoller, E., Grzywacz, J. G., Quandt, S. A., Bell, R. A., Chapman, C., Altizer, K. P., & Arcury, T. A. (2011). Calling the doctor: A qualitative study of patient-initiated physician consultation among rural older adults. *Journal of Aging and Health, 23*(5) 782–805. doi:10.1177/0898264310397045

Sinclair, K., Ahmadigheidari, D., Dallmann, D. M., Miller, M., & Melgar-Quiñonez. H. (2019). Rural women: Most likely to experience food insecurity and poor health in low- and middle-income countries. *Global Food Security, 23*, 104–115.

Smith, A. S., & Trevelyan, E. (2019). The older population in rural America: 2012-2016. U. S. Department of Commerce, U. S. Census Bureau.

Strosnider H, Kennedy C, Monti M, & Yip, F. (2017). Rural and urban differences in air quality, 2008–2012, and Community Drinking Water Quality, 2010–2015—United States. *MMWR Surveillance Summaries 66*(13), 1–10. doi:http://dx.doi.org/10.15585/mmwr.ss6613a1external icon

Torres, S., & Cao, X. (2019). Improving care for elders who prefer informal spaces to age-separated institutions and health care settings. *Innovation in Aging, 3*(3), 1–10.

Torres-Gil, J., & Demko, C. (2019). The politics of aging and diversity: Moving toward a majority-minority nation. *Generations, 42*(4), 57-64. Retrieved from https://www.asaging.org/blog/politics-aging-and-diversity-moving-toward-majority-minority-nation

Tran, B. X., Moir, M. P. I., Thai, T. P. T., Nguyen, L. H., Ha, G. H., Nguyen, T. H. T., Truong, N. T., & Larkin, C. A. (2018). Socioeconomic inequities in health-related quality of life among patients with cardiovascular diseases in Vietnam. *BioMed Research International*, Special Issue, 8 pages. https://doi.org/10.1155/2018/2643814

Tremmel, M., Gerdtham, U. G., Nilsson, P., & Saha, S. (2017). Economic burden of obesity: A systematic literature review. *International Journal of Environmental Research and Public Health, 14*(4), 435.

TRIP. (2019, May 22). *Rural connections: Challenges and Opportunities in America's Heartland*. https://tripnet.org/wp-content/uploads/2019/08/Rural_Roads_TRIP_Report_May_2019.pdf #page=6

Underwood, E. A., Davidson, H. P., Azam, A. B., & Tierney, M. C. (2019). Sex differences in depression as a risk factor for Alzheimer's Disease: A systematic review. *Innovation in Aging, 3*(2), 1–7. doi:10.1093/geroni/igz015

U. S. Department of Transportation. The Future of Rural Mobility. https://www.transportation.gov/connections/future-rural-mobility

Timsina, L. R., Willetts, J. L., Brennan, M. J., Marucci-Wellman, H. R., Lombardi, D. A., Courtney T. K., & Verma, S. K. (2016). Circumstances of fall-related injuries by age and gender among community-dwelling adults in the United States. *PLoS One. 11*(3), e0150939. Epub

Voyles, E. C. (2020). Stereotypes: The Incidence and Impacts of Bias. United States: ABC-CLIO, LLC.

White, G., Evans, R., Connelly, K., & Caine, K. (2014). *Designing aging-in-place technologies to reflect the lifestyles and precious artifacts of urban and rural older adults*. Proceedings of the Human Factors and Ergonomics Society, 58th Annual Meeting.

White, G., Evans, R., Connelly, K., & Caine, K. (2014). Designing aging-in-place technologies to reflect the lifestyles and precious artifacts of urban and rural older adults. Proceedings of the Human Factors and Ergonomics Society, 58th Annual Meeting.

WHO (2019, September 19). *Dementia*. https://www.who.int/news-room/fact-sheets/detail/dementia

WHO (2020, January 30). *Depression*. https://www.who.int/news-room/fact-sheets/detail/depression

Ye, Q., Bai, F., & Zhang, Z. (2016). Shared genetic risk factors for late-life depression and Alzheimer's disease. *Journal of Alzheimer's Disease, 52*(1), 1–15.

Yaemsiri, S., Alfier J. M., Moy, E., Rossen, L. M., Bastian, B., Bolin, J., . . . Heron, M. (2019). Healthy People 2020: Rural areas lag in achieving targets for major causes of death. *Health Affairs, 38*(12).

Zarit, S. H., & Edwards, A. B. (2008). Family caregiving: Research and clinical intervention. In R. Woods & L. Clare (Eds.), *Handbook of the clinical psychology of ageing* (p. 255–288). John Wiley & Sons Ltd. https://doi.org/10.1002/9780470773185.ch16

Additional Reading

Boggs, J. M., Portz, J. D., King, D. K., Wright, L. A., Helander, K., Retrum, J. H., & Gozansky, W. S. (2017). Perspectives of LGBTQ older adults on aging in place: A qualitative investigation. *Journal of Homosexuality, 64*(11), 1539–1560. http://dx.doi.org/10.1080/00918369.2016.1247539

Burholt, V., Foscarini-Craggs, P., & Winter, B. (2018). 20 Rural ageing and equality. *Ageing, Diversity and Equality: Social Justice Perspectives*, 311–328.

Caldwell, J. T., Ford, C. L., Wallace, S. P., Wang, M. C., & Takahashi, L. M. (2016). Intersection of living in a rural versus urban area and race/ethnicity in explaining access to health care in the United States. *American Journal of Public Health.* 2016;106(8), 1463–1469. doi:10.2105/AJPH.2016.303212

Chemtob. K., Rocchi, M., Arbour-Nicitopoulos, K., Kairy, D., Fillion, B., & Sweet, S. N. (2019). Using tele-health to enhance motivation, leisure time physical activity, and quality of life in adults with spinal cord injury: A self-determination theory-based pilot randomized control trial. *Psychology of Sport & Exercise, 43,* 243–252.

Cilluffo, A., & Ruiz, N. G. (2019). World's population is projected to nearly stop growing by the end of the century. *Facttank News in the Numbers.* Pew Research Center.

Cohen, A. L. & Bennett, C. R. (2017). Support network connectedness in the lives of community-dwelling rural elders and their families. *Marriage & Family Review 53*(6), 576–588. doi:10.1080/01494929.2016.1247763

DiGilio, D. A., Gatz, M., & Antonucci, T. C. (2017). Addressing issues facing a diverse aging population: Scientific perspectives for practice and policy. *Innovation in Aging, 1*(Suppl 1), 976–977. https://doi.org/10.1093/geroni/igx004.3525

Findlay, A. H., & Nies, M. A. (2017). Understanding social networking use for social connectedness among rural older adults. *Healthy Aging Research, 6*(4), e12.

Galloway, A. P., & Henry, M. (2014). Relationships between social connectedness and spirituality and depression and perceived health status of rural residents. *Online Journal of Rural Nursing and Health Care, 14*(2), 43–79. https://doi.org/10.14574/ojrnhc.v14i2.325

Gaugler, J. E., & Kane, R. L. (2015). *Family caregiving in the new normal* (Vol. 1st). San Diego, CA: Academic Press.

Hamel, L., Wu, B., & Brodie, M. (2017). The health care views and experiences of rural Americans: Findings from the Kaiser Family Foundation/Washington Post survey of Rural America.

Laditka, J. N., Laditka, S. B., Olatosi, B., & Elder, J. T. (2007). The health trade-off of rural residence for impaired older adults: Longer life, more impairment. *The Journal of Rural Health, 23*(2), 124–132.

MacKenzie, P. (2002). Aging people in aging places: Addressing the needs of older adults in rural Saskatchewan. *Rural Social Work, Special Australian/Canadian issue, 6*(3), 74–83.

Skinner, M. W., & Winterton, R. (2018). Interrogating the contested spaces of rural aging: Implications for research, policy, and practice. *The Gerontologist, 58*(1), 15–25. https://doi-org.cmich.idm.oclc.org/10.1093/geront/gnx094

Son, J., Erno, A., Shea, D. G., Femia, E. E., Zarit, S. H., & Parris Stephens, M. A. (2007). The caregiver stress process and health outcomes. *Journal of Aging and Health, 19*(6), 871–887. https://doi.org/10.1177/0898264307308568

Sriram, U., Morgan, E. H., Graham, M. L, Folta, S. C., & Seguin, R. A. (2018). Support and sabotage: A qualitative study of social influences on health behaviors among rural adults. *Journal of Rural Health, 34*(1), 88–97. doi:10.1111/jrh.12232

Whitlatch, C. J., Judge, K., Zarit, S. H., Femia, E. (2006). Dyadic intervention for family caregivers and care receivers in early-stage dementia, *The Gerontologist, 46*(5), 688–694. https://doi.org/10.1093/geront/46.5.688

Williams, S., Bi, P., Newbury, J., Robinson, G., Pisaniello, D., Saniotis, A., & Hansen, A. (2013). Extreme heat and health: Perspectives from health service providers in rural and remote communities in South Australia. *International Journal of Environmental Research and Public Health, 10*(11), 5565–5583.

Wolff, J. L., Mulcahy, J., Huang, J., Roth, D. L., Covinsky, K., & Kasper, J. D. (2018). Family caregivers of older adults, 1999–2015: Trends in characteristics, circumstances, and role-related appraisal. *The Gerontologist, 58*(6), 1021–1032. doi:10.1093/geront/gnx093

CHAPTER 19

Rural Public Health for the LGBTQ Community

Chun-Fang Frank Kuo, PhD, MS
Kathleen Khong Hor Yan, BS

LEARNING OBJECTIVES

At the end of this chapter, readers will be able to:

1. Identify some societal norms and characteristics that contributed to the lived experiences of rural LGBTQ individuals.
2. Compare and contrast the physical and mental health concerns that the rural LGBTQ community faces compared with those living in urban areas.
3. Describe the reasons behind rural LGBTQ individuals' health statuses as well as the key challenges they experience.
4. Distinguish the similarities and differences in experiences that different subgroups and age groups within the LGBTQ community face.
5. Evaluate current efforts and recommendations provided to improve quality of life and reduce discrimination of LGBTQ individuals.

KEY TERMS

Bias among healthcare providers
Disclosure of sexual orientation
Discrimination
Gender identity
Heteronormativity
LGBTQ
Meyer's minority stress model
Prejudice
Stigma

CHAPTER OVERVIEW

The purpose of the chapter is to provide an overview of the current public health issues that are specific to the rural lesbian, gay, bisexual, transgender, and queer (LGBTQ) community. The first section covers physical health concerns, including prevalence of certain physical illnesses and preventative healthcare behaviors. The following section focuses on mental health issues specific to the LGBTQ community, comparing the differences between urban and rural populations. Then the chapter also highlights the challenges the LGBTQ community faces due to the members' geographic locations as well as cultural norms they are expected to adhere to. The next section attempts to address the current challenges by discussing current efforts carried by various organizations within the United States as well as innovative interventions proposed in other countries. Lastly, the chapter ends with a review of current research as well as limitations and implications.

359

Introduction

LGBTQ is an acronym that is commonly used to refer to nonheterosexual or noncisgender individuals and to describe their sexual orientation and **gender identity**. It stands for lesbian, gay, bisexual, transgender, and queer or questioning. Definitions of these terms are presented in **Table 19-1**. Historically, the term "gay" was used, but this was then replaced by LGB, as the original term was not accurately representing the community to which it referred. Over the years, the acronym continued to evolve to be more inclusive and accurately representing the individuals in the community. Other acronyms include LGBT, LGBTI, and LGBTQ2+. Currently, there is not a standardized use of these acronyms. For example, some studies may use the term LGBT, which may or may not represent those who identify as questioning or pansexual, as these new categories may not have been identified when these studies were done. Thus, both LGBT and LGBTQ are used in this chapter to more accurately represent the results reported from various studies, depending on the acronym that was used.

General Statistics

There are no census data on the demographic information of sexual orientation and gender identity in the United States as the U.S. Census Bureau does not include questions to ask about them. Questions regarding sexual orientation and gender identity that were proposed to be in the 2020 U.S. Census were removed. Currently, the only information collected is on same-sex couple households, including information on marital status, age groups, ethnicity, educational and income levels, employment status, home tenure, and presence of children in the household.

Other institutions, however, collected data related to LGBTQ. Gallup, Inc., an American analytics and advisory company, collects data daily and found a steady increase in the number of people identifying as a member of the

Table 19-1 Definitions

Gay	An adjective that is generally used to refer to a person who is physically, romantically and/or emotionally attracted to someone of the same sex or the trait of being a homosexual person. This term is often used with homosexual males.
Lesbian	A female who is physically, romantically and/or emotionally attracted to other females.
Bisexual	A person who is physically, romantically and/or emotionally attracted to both males and females.
Transgender	This is a broad term used for individuals whose gender identity or gender expression does not correspond to their assigned sex at birth. It also includes individuals who do not identify with the male/female binary system and whose gender expression and behavior do not conform to the societal norms.
Queer	An umbrella term used for sexual and gender minorities who do not identify as heterosexual or cisgender.
Questioning	Someone who may be questioning his or her own gender identity or sexual orientation. This person may be uncertain, still exploring, or concerned about using certain labels on themselves.

Note. These individuals often have unique experiences due to their sexual orientation or gender identity, and this is reflected in the following research findings presented in this chapter.

LGBTQ community, starting from 2012 at 3.5%. In 2017, 4.5% of the sample identified as lesbian, gay, bisexual, or transgender, with more females (5.1%) than males (3.9%; Newport, 2018, May 22).

Heteronormative Culture and Stigma

Heteronormativity refers to the belief that heterosexuality is the natural expression of sexuality and normative sexual orientation (Ward & Schneider, 2009). It assumes that sex and gender are natural binaries, where people are categorized as either males or females, with no exceptions. Sex refers to biological differences between males and females, whereas gender refers to the roles males and females are socially expected to have (i.e., gender role) or one's view of himself or herself as a male or female (i.e., gender identity). Heteronormativity describes how society expects, behaves, and normalizes practices based on presumption of heterosexuality and gender roles as the norm of the society. As a result, those of different sexuality or those who adopt gender identity that does not match their sex are seen as unnatural, "deviant" from the norm, or problematic.

Individuals who do not conform to the normative culture, and in this case, the non-heterosexual and noncisgender individuals, are likely stigmatized. **Stigma** is a phenomenon in which a person's attribute, visible or not, is severely discredited by others in the society (Goffman, 1963). When such an attribute is made known in an individual, others are likely to label the difference between themselves and this individual; this person may then be rejected or discriminated against by others as long as he or she is stigmatized. Stigmatization is related to many physical and mental health issues within the LBGTQ community. The following sections cover physical and mental health concerns specific to the rural LGBTQ community.

The Minority Stress Model

Meyer's (2003) minority stress model provides a framework to understand the health risks disparities between LGBTQ and heterosexual individuals. This model posits that the conflicting nature in sexual or gender values between the LGBTQ community and heterosexual individuals creates various stressors in the minority's lives, which accumulates and subsequently leads to long-term health issues in the minority population. This model describes a continuum between two types of stressors, ranging from distal to proximal stressors. Distal stressors represent external and objective circumstances where LGBTQ individuals may experience such **prejudice** and discriminations from society, whereas proximal stressors are more subjective and internalized processes because they depend on the interpretations and meanings formed by the individuals. For example, minorities may hide their sexual orientation due to the fear of **discrimination**. Many past studies often draw upon the minority stress model when describing minority stress and have found this to be especially evident in rural areas (Barefoot, Smalley, & Warren, 2017; Rosenkrantz, Black, Abreu, Aleshire, & Fallin-Bennett, 2017; Swank, Frost, & Frahs, 2012).

According to Meyer's model, being a part of the sexual minority could be a stressor on its own due to associated stigma, and it influences how individuals behave in order to cope with matters associated with the stressor (e.g., sexual status) (Whitehead, Shaver, & Stephenson, 2016). This could be observed in the healthcare setting when a screening process involves disclosure of sexual behavior practices that subsequently leads to the need for sexual orientation disclosure. In order to avoid this process of disclosure, LGBTQ individuals may choose to avoid healthcare screenings or appointments altogether, which may explain the increased health risks compared with heterosexual counterparts (Barefoot, Warren, & Smalley, 2017).

Physical Health

Disclosure of Sexual Orientation to Healthcare Providers

Anticipated stigma, one of the domains of stigma, stands out when understanding health-care behaviors among LGBTQ individuals. Anticipated stigma is reflected when a LGBTQ individual expresses or behaves out of concern for future possible stigma-associated consequences, such as negative reactions or rejections from health caregivers following sexual orientation disclosure (Whitehead, Shaver, & Stephenson, 2016).

This fear of future possible discrimination that then leads to delays in help-seeking behaviors or putting off of healthcare appointments, has been observed among LGBTQ individuals from both rural and nonrural areas (Barefoot, Warren & Smalley, 2017). However, it was found that LGBTQ individuals in rural areas were comparatively less likely to disclose their sexual orientation than their nonrural counterparts. This could be due to the more perceptible heteronormative culture in rural areas, which may have led them to greater anticipation of negative reactions from health caregivers (Barefoot et al., 2017).

Preventative Health Care and Health Screenings

Within the physical healthcare system, health-care providers may enquire about the patients' sexual orientation. This notion potentially places rural LGBTQ individuals at greater discomfort from being "unprepared" to deal with the perceived higher negative risks of disclosure, which may lead to rejection of health care to protect themselves. Consequently, these individuals would then miss opportunities to screen for potential risky health behaviors or symptoms of diseases. In a setting that holds more heteronormative values, rural LGTBQ populations may be more motivated to avoid healthcare screenings than their nonrural counterparts.

Studies have found evidence that suggests that LGBTQ individuals are more likely to opt for tests that do not require the disclosure of their sexual orientation. For instance, within a wide sample of rural LGBT, higher rates of screening uptake were found for tests that did not require patients to disclose their sexual orientations such as for high blood pressure (92% of the sample, N = 1012, took the test) and high cholesterol (92%, N = 207; Whitehead, Shaver, & Stephenson, 2016). Lower uptake rates were found, however, for screenings that potentially require sexual orientation disclosure such as for human papillomavirus (HPV) vaccination (26%, N = 660), human immunodeficiency virus (HIV), (57%, N = 1008) and cervical cancer (69%, N = 357; Whitehead, Shaver, & Stephenson, 2016).

In the lesbian patients recruited by Barefoot, Warren, and Smalley (2017), those aged 40 years and above were significantly less likely than their nonrural counterparts to have received a mammogram in the past 3 years. Low rates of other health screenings such as HIV screening, pap testing, and clinical breast examinations were also reported. Overall, the study demonstrated that rural lesbians are less likely to engage in preventive healthcare behaviors than nonrural counterparts (Barefoot et al., 2017). However, this does not explain the higher number of cervical cancer cases found among both rural-residing women and lesbians, compared with their heterosexual and nonrural counterparts. A patent difference could be that rural areas have less accessibility to these healthcare services and as a result, inhabitants of rural areas delay or miss out on early preventive screening for diseases. Certain screening services may require multiple visits to a clinic, which would require rural inhabitants to travel further into nonrural areas, thus making it less convenient for these individuals to attend appointments (Whitehead, Shaver, & Stephenson, 2016).

Previously, an underlying misconception was that it was often assumed that lesbians had lower chances of contracting the human papillomavirus (HPV; Barefoot et al., 2017), as unprotected sex with multiple male partners has been the promulgated risk factor for HPV. However, this assumption does not take into account past sexual experiences of lesbians with male partners. In a study comparing rural and urban lesbians, Barefoot and colleagues (2017) found that 78.1% of rural lesbians reported at least one sexual experience with a male partner whereas 69.1% of urban lesbians reported such experiences. Moreover, it has been found that HPV infections can be transmitted through sexual experiences between women (Marrazzo & Gorgos, 2012). Despite that, fewer rural lesbians reported having received a recommendation for the HPV vaccination from female healthcare providers compared with their urban counterparts (Barefoot et al., 2017). These combined factors stemming from low understanding of LGBTQ's unique health concerns call for more attention to engage rural LGBTQ populations and their healthcare providers in preventative health care.

Sexually Transmitted Infections

The human immunodeficiency virus (HIV) has been reported to be less prevalent in rural areas (Hubach et al., 2015), where a majority of individuals with an HIV diagnosis lives in urban areas (Centers for Diseases Control and Prevention, 2019). However, rural areas are unique in that HIV-related stigma and discrimination are amplified because of lower levels of awareness and understanding about individuals with HIV. Some individuals in the rural community may be misinformed about how HIV is transmitted or they may assume that all HIV-positive individuals indulge in debauchery acts that are frowned upon. Such an environment provides fewer opportunities to discuss on the taboo topic of HIV, which

maintains or contributes to a greater sense of fear toward HIV-positive individuals. These individuals may then find the need to conceal their HIV-status or avoid situations that require disclosure. Should disclosure be considered, HIV-positive individuals may potentially experience stress from needing to consider if the benefits from disclosure would outweigh potential negative consequences (Hubach, et al., 2015). Thus, the lower prevalence rate of HIV in rural areas could be due to under-reporting.

Generally, disclosure of one's HIV-positive status is important as it allows individuals to receive appropriate help and suggestions on improving lifestyles that may assist in coping with HIV. However, there could also be fear among HIV-positive individuals of unfavorable social consequences that pertain to overall well-being (Hubach et al., 2015). Some frequently reported examples would be sexual segregation, increased likelihood of receiving rejections in relationships, and violation of privacy that could occur when a HIV-status is revealed to a third party without consent. When fulfilled, these risks may be more intensified within rural LGBT communities that are even smaller. LGBT individuals who are HIV-positive risk discrimination not just from the rural community as a whole due to their status and sexual orientation but possibly also from within the LGBT community, resulting in an increased lack of social support. For instance, if HIV-status is disclosed to a sexual partner who does not keep it confidential, the risk of having one's HIV status exposed to one's social connections is relatively high given the small size of LGBT communities in rural areas. In turn, this then limits one's opportunities to form future relationships within a local LGBT community, potentially resulting in social isolation.

On a personal level, LGBT individuals could again be robbed of their choice to disclose, as well as in choosing the timing of disclosure when their HIV-status is exposed through no fault of their own. This could motivate individuals to seek intimacy or to look for opportunities to form relationships outside of their immediate LGBT networks, such as through online platforms (Hubach et al., 2015). A sense of privacy or control could then be regained with regard to HIV-status disclosure especially with a potential partner. Hubach and his colleagues (2015) found that many LGBT individuals do disclose their HIV status and engage in sexual behaviors that are safe for their partners. However, for those who engaged in riskier sexual behaviors, it was not due to a lack in knowledge of HIV transmission or of safe-sex practices. Rather, these individuals could be concerned with pleasing their partners in hopes of developing emotional intimacy and potential romantic relationships.

A study conducted on a sample of African Americans, who identified as gay men and tested HIV-positive, revealed interesting patterns that pointed at higher frequencies of risky sexual behaviors following discriminatory experiences (Jeffries, Marks, Lauby, Murrill, & Millett, 2013). African American gay men who experienced a homophobic incident involving discrimination were significantly more likely to engage in unprotected anal sex with other men. The researchers discussed the possibility of having homophobia experiences interfere with one's ability to cope with HIV-related stigma. This notion is congruent with a qualitative study involving gay participants, who tested HIV-positive, that expatiated on how sex was utilized as a means to suppress feelings of social isolation or loneliness (Hubach et al., 2015). Thus, attention should be given to further understand how social loneliness or isolation could lead to more practices of unsafe sexual behaviors in order to compensate for the lack of social connectedness or intimacy, particularly among LGBTQ individuals in rural areas.

Given the complex nature of stigma surrounding LGBTQ communities in rural areas, there is a need to address HIV-related stigma. Some feasible solutions include, but are not limited to, providing a safe space for LGBTQ individuals who are living with HIV to speak of their experiences to the community. Education programs could be designed and embedded with the intention to normalize discussions on HIV-related issues. By increasing awareness toward HIV risks and fostering understanding toward HIV-related stigma, we could hope to gradually transform the social environments within rural LGBT communities to be more inclusive of LGBT individuals who are HIV-positive (Jeffries et al., 2013). While these suggestions are specific to targeting HIV-related stigma within rural communities, infected LGBT individuals may also possess (initial or added) fear of receiving negative reactions to sexual orientation disclosure from health caregivers. This calls for the need to train health caregivers to be sensitive toward the needs of LGBT patients in addition to being educated on HIV-related stigma.

Mental Health

Comparisons between LGBTQ and non-LGBTQ populations reveal stark mental health disparities in general. Referring once again to the Meyer's (2003) minority stress model, these differences are largely due to exposure to the various distal and proximal stressors that their non-LGBTQ counterparts do not otherwise experience (Swank, Frost & Fahs, 2012). Members of the LGBTQ community are more likely to experience psychological stressors from needing to cope with prejudices or discrimination, as well as suffer from a higher frequency of disconnectedness. Experiences of discrimination coupled with acceptance of LGBT identity more frequently have depressive symptoms (Su et al., 2016). Depending on the support available and specific to the unique needs of LGBTQ individuals, the psychological distress experienced varies, impacting the individual's ability to function and thrive within a hostile environment to different degrees.

Exhibit 19-1 Statistics on LGBTQ Youths

Growing up LGBT in America, an extensive survey completed by over 10,000 LGBT youths in 2012, revealed insightful yet alarming statistics on factors that impact the psychological well-being of LGBT youth (Human Rights Campaign, 2012). Notably, LGBT youth were twice as likely as their non-LGBT counterparts to have encountered hostile experiences of discrimination and prejudice, ranging from verbal harassment to physical assaults. When asked to list their top problems faced in life then, there was a stark difference between issues faced by LGBT youths versus their non-LGBT peers. The most common issue reported by LGBT youths was nonaccepting families (26% of those who responded in the survey), followed by school or bullying problems (21%) and lastly, fear of being out (18%). While the survey did not differentiate results between rural or nonrural areas, at least 60% of the LGBT youths reported their top negative experience to be intolerance in the community due to sexual orientation.

A more recent National Health Survey on LGBTQ Youth Mental Health in 2018 involving 25,896 LGBTQ youths across the United States, a mix of rural and nonrural areas, showed that 71% of LGBTQ youths had experienced feelings of sadness or hopelessness for at least two weeks in the past year. The survey also revealed that similar experiences of discrimination due to sexual orientation or gender identity have been experienced by at least 71% of the LGBTQ youths in the United States (The Trevor Project, 2019). While 80% of these experiences did not involve physical harm, 36% of LGBTQ youths who did experience physical harm also reported to have attempted suicide. An overall 39% of the LGBTQ youths reported to have seriously contemplated suicide while 18% reported that they have attempted suicide; for both these categories, more than half identified themselves as transgender and nonbinary individuals.

Mental Health Disparities in Rural Areas

Hostile experiences could be intensified in the setting of rural areas, with even more discriminative attitudes held against the LGBTQ community. Studies have found rural lesbians and gay men to live with higher levels of overall psychological distress such as stress, anxiety, and depression, compared with their nonrural counterparts (Barefoot et al., 2015; Kauth, Barrera, Denton, & Latini, 2017). Among the transgender individuals, significant differences were also reported across rural and nonrural counterparts; this was particularly evident for rural transgender males who had significantly higher depressive and anxiety symptoms (Horvath et al., 2014). With veterans; however, rural gay, lesbian, and transgender veterans seemed to show significantly higher anxiety symptoms compared with their non-rural counterparts; however, only gay veterans reported higher depressive symptoms comparatively (Kauth et al., 2017). From additional analyses, the researchers also suggested that these greater levels of symptoms exhibited may also be associated to the long distances that some of these rural LGBTQ veterans travel in order to consult their primary care providers.

Connectedness and Loneliness

Given the interconnected nature of networks in rural areas, disclosure of one's own sexual orientation not only raises the concern of being rejected by one's closest social circle but potentially by the community as a whole. This may lead to higher anticipation of risks of disclosure, which may prevent LGBT individuals from engaging in as many meaningful relationships as they would like to (Barefoot, et al., 2015; Swank et al., 2012). In fact, studies found that rural LGBT individuals were more likely to have experienced feelings of isolation and disconnection from communities that accept them than their nonrural counterparts (Swank et al., 2012). Similarly, this was also observed among the LGBT veterans, whereby the rural LGBT veterans reported a lower sense of connectedness to the LGBT community within the rural area (Kauth et al., 2017). Connectedness is important as it may serve as a buffer against the ills of a hostile environment, which may lead to other detrimental psychological effects or to social loneliness.

Closely related to connectedness is the degree to which LGBTQ individuals form positive LGBT identities as well as "outness." Outness refers to how open these individuals are about their sexual orientation. Positive identification with the LGBTQ community enables individuals to feel that they belong or are connected to a group of social support, which may reduce the risk of social isolation resulting in loneliness. Outness requires the **disclosure of sexual orientation** that may expose LGBTQ individuals to more events of discrimination, as highlighted in the literature (Kauth et al., 2017). However, it may also come with opportunities to form meaningful relationships outside of the LGBTQ community, thus increasing the individual's limited social network.

The risk of social loneliness paired with a need to cope with a hostile environment due to discrimination may cause too much psychological strain on LGBTQ individuals who may also be dealing with internalized stigma associated to sexual orientation or gender identity. This, in turn, may also lead to mental disorders such as anxiety, depression, and substance abuse, which are associated with suicide behaviors.

Suicide Behaviors Among Rural LGBTQ

Are all LGBTQ individuals with mental disorders bound to engage in suicide behaviors? Studies reveal that factors of suicide risk are not as clear cut as they are perceived to be although mental disorders have been found

to be significantly associated with greater risks for suicide behaviors (Irwin, Coleman, Fisher, & Marasco, 2014). Even in the absence of mental disorders, the risk for suicide behaviors was still significantly higher among LGBTQ individuals than those who are non-LGBTQ. However, this is not to say that suicide behaviors are tied to the identity of LGBTQ.

The terms associated with suicide behaviors comprise suicide attempt, suicidal ideation (serious consideration of committing suicide), and completed suicides (Irwin et al., 2014). Other newer classifications of suicidal behavior include interrupted and aborted suicide. Gender differences reveal that rural females are more likely to possess suicidal thoughts and attempts, whereas rural males are more likely to complete suicide attempts.

As depicted in aforementioned paragraphs, most national surveys conducted in the United States have focused on suicide risk among the LGBTQ youth. However, studies have shown that suicidal thoughts are not age-dependent although age has been posited as a risk factor to suicide behaviors. Older ages have been found to be significantly related to increased suicidal thoughts with many rural LGBT adults in Nebraska who reported to have considered suicide in the past (Irwin et al., 2014). When asked to list the ages at which these rural LGBT adults seriously considered suicide, some reported the ages of 16, 30s, and the 60s. Going back in time, most of these LGBT adults would have encountered negative experiences while growing up as the environment then may have considered sexual diversities apart from the heterosexual norm to be an illness. This goes on to reiterate that experiences of discrimination could lead to increased suicide ideation among rural LGBTQ individuals. Individuals who identified themselves as transgender were also more likely to report having experienced suicide ideation, especially when stressors unique to LGBTQ identity such as outness and perceived discrimination were considered (Irwin et al., 2014; Su et al., 2016).

Substance Use

The avoidance of healthcare appointments also reduces the chances of detecting risky behaviors such as substance use. In 2014, surveys reported prevalent substance use among rural LGBTQ individuals although there were no differences found compared with their nonrural counterparts (Horvath et al., 2014). Transgender individuals in rural areas were more likely to consume higher amounts of marijuana but engage in lesser binge drinking activities relative to those in nonrural areas (Horvath et al., 2014). A more recent study revealed that homosexual males in rural areas were more likely to engage in more tobacco use than their nonrural counterparts (Kauth et al., 2017; Whitehead et al., 2016).

Discrimination

Meyer's minority stress model depicts that LGBT individuals often experience distress due to distal stressors such as stigma, enacted discrimination, and disconnectedness from the LGBT community (Meyer, 2003; Su et al., 2016). Other studies posit that heterosexism and homophobia are the two most common forms of discrimination in the United States (Rosenkrantz et al., 2017). Some discovered that discrimination that the LGBT community experiences are physical or sexual assaults, workplace discrimination (e.g., not allowed promotion, lower pay, and others), verbal harassment, as well as hostile attitudes from both family members and strangers (Rosenkrantz et al., 2017; Swank, Frost & Fahs, 2012; Szymanski & Henrichs-Beck, 2014). Following the minority stress model, these distal stressors could transition into proximal stressors when LGBT individuals begin to anticipate these hostile incidences, and in some instances, internalize negative attitudes. Both external events and internalized heterosexism have been found to predict psychological distress in LGBT individuals (Szymanski & Henrichs-Beck, 2014).

Age is a notable factor following that older LGBT individuals would have more lifetime experiences of discrimination across years compared with younger counterparts who may experience more recent discrimination (Irwin et al., 2014; Swank, Frost & Fahs, 2012). Lifetime discrimination could be accumulated, especially during the years when homophobia and heterosexism were more evident, which may explain the comparative difference for older LGBT adults (Irwin et al., 2014; Swank et al., 2012). The surveys, albeit less representative of rural areas, also showed that LGBT individuals who reported a household income below $25,000 have higher odds of attempting suicide and reported more depressive symptoms (Irwin et al., 2014; Su et al., 2016). The authors postulated that the suicide attempts could be due to gender-based discrimination. An older study posited the notion that poorer LGBT individuals may have lesser access to resources that could help avoid instances of discrimination (Swank, Frost & Fahs, 2012). In contrast, LBG individuals who have a higher income reported greater connections to the LGB community, which could serve as a protection against discrimination (Swank et al., 2012). This is possible as these individuals also reported fewer experiences of long-term discrimination.

Swank, Frost, and Fahs (2012) also found that those in the southern United States reported higher levels of recent and lifetime enacted discrimination along with a lesser connection to the LGBTQ community than those in other parts of the United States. Lower levels of connectedness to the LGB community were also frequently reported among rural inhabitants compared with their nonrural counterparts. Gender differences were also found in that gay and bisexual men experienced more discrimination compared with lesbian and bisexual women (Swank et al., 2012).

Sociology studies on the differences in traditional values and openness to diversity, across geographical locations, suggest that individuals living in rural areas may be less

---

Exhibit 19-2 The Case of Rich

At the time of the study, Rich was an 80-year-old gay man who had resided in rural communities in a Midwestern state for his entire life (Rowan, Giunta, Grudowski, & Anderson, 2013). The researchers found Rich to be a unique case. His experience as a gay man in rural environments is antithetical to the hostility that is commonly purported in literature. Physically, Rich's lifestyle is healthy and active as he exercises daily even after having undergone a pacemaker surgery. As for his social relationships, Rich is described as a social butterfly with large and diverse social networks. Once a week, he meets with a group of friends consisting of both gay and straight individuals. When asked about his closest friends, Rich shares about a heterosexual couple he contacts not just for casual interactions alone but for when he needs assistance as well. Rich also frequently relates to his late partner for 37 years with whom he shared a respectful relationship despite their individual differences in matters like clothing choices. Having adapted to living alone, Rich appears to have moved past his grief and continues to live his life that he considers to be free of discrimination or isolation. While literature typically reflects young gay individuals encountering discrimination or rejection from families, Rich described his relationships growing up to be positive as well. He also remarked that his parents may have never openly acknowledged that he was a gay although he was certain that everybody knew. At this, the researchers noted that it could be a conditional acceptance by Rich's parents depending on Rich's discretion in managing disclosure of his sexual orientation. Rich's discretion was also observed in the way he referred to his two gay friends who lived together as, "two guys" who lived together. It would seem that this discretion not only directly applied to managing his own disclosure, but it pervaded his language as well. This may explain why Rich never described having encountered discrimination but instead only spoke of largely positive social experiences. Upon entering adulthood, he expressed having met more gay and lesbian friends through his antique business. This provided him with both enjoyment and a sense of social support that must have bolstered his resilience and added to the sense of life satisfaction.

Note. Rich is the selected pseudonym by the participant who was interviewed for this study.

---

accepting or adaptable to diversity in sexual orientation (Swank, Frost & Fahs, 2012). This could be due to the economic distribution that is less diverse in rural areas, with lower percentages of individuals with liberal values, thus rendering individuals who live or grew up in rural areas more likely to perceive diversity as a potential form of threat. Other possible reasons such as strongholds in orthodox fundamentals may consist of religious beliefs that homosexuality would induce heavenly wrath as it is believed to be an act of sin. These purported understandings on the prevalence of discriminating attitudes in rural areas are often used to explain any mental health disparities observed. While there are studies that indicate that environments in rural areas may be more hostile, there is little actual support for

this, leading to the notion that only a few rural areas may hold especially hostile attitudes and that it is not so common.

Another study reported significant differences in heterosexism and bipositivity attitudes among rural, suburban, and urban areas (Casazza, Ludwig, & Cohn, 2015). They had found that most rural inhabitants believed heterosexuality is "the right way" compared with homosexuality (heterosexism) and scored the lowest on having positive attitudes toward bisexuality (bipositivity). Additional insights are drawn when merely comparing the scores reported from rural inhabitants alone to that of the actual range of scales. The rural individuals still scored relatively low on the scale rating for heterosexism and relatively high on the bipositivity scale. This provides an interesting notion in that while rural inhabitants may have more discriminative attitudes compared with nonrural counterparts, they may still lean toward being accepting of diversity in sexual orientation. Another possibility is that perhaps only some or a few rural inhabitants are actually averse and hostile toward the LGBT community.

Other antithetical findings reveal no significant difference in negative attitudes or experiences of discrimination among LGBT individuals when rurality of a location was considered (Anderson et al., 2015; Wienke & Hill, 2013). Swank, Frost, and Fahs (2012) also discovered that LGB individuals from rural and small-town areas did not differ in their experiences of recent discrimination. This is possible as there could be improvements in mindsets toward accepting LGB individuals with higher exposure to social issues within rural communities in the past decade. However, methodological technicalities such as types of samples or discrimination reported could also be potential factors of the distinctive outcomes. In particular, most studies seem to have sampled from LGBT communities where individuals are connected to one another through their shared identity. This could lend support against external discriminative events and individuals are likely to be more accepting of their LGBT identities, serving as a protective buffer against psychological distress (Kauth et al., 2017; Su et al., 2016).

Barriers to Health Care for Rural LGBTQ Populations

The previous sections have explored individual-level barriers to health care for rural LGBTQ individuals pertaining to issues surrounding disclosure of sexual orientation stemming from the need to be wary of potential hostile reactions. Given the inconsistent findings in confirming the purported hostile environments across different rural areas,

other barriers to health care on the systemic level are important to discuss.

Geographical Barriers and Healthcare Expertise

Rural areas provide unique geographic barriers as healthcare services and expertise are generally more accessible in nonrural areas with denser populations. This, in turn, creates an additional challenge requiring rural inhabitants to travel long hours to nonrural areas for treatment. Taxing arrangements that require long, draining hours of transportation coupled with potentially poorer transportation infrastructures may elicit more harm in the long term, especially for chronically ill individuals. Indeed, longer travel hours has been associated with higher depression and anxiety levels as well (Kauth et al., 2017).

Rural and small-town LGBT individuals reported making long trips to consult with their primary care providers (Kauth et al., 2017). This suggests that there is a lack of healthcare services for rural LGBT individuals, especially compared with nonrural counterparts. Some specialized healthcare services such as health care for HIV and HIV-risk reduction services, are less available in rural areas (Horvath et al., 2014). These services are comparatively more available in populated, nonrural areas and it has been suggested that these services be made available to rural areas through online platforms or mobile applications.

Unique Experiences Among Lesbians

Studies were done to compare lesbians in rural and nonrural areas, where similarities and differences were found in their experiences with the healthcare system. A similar number of rural and nonrural lesbians reported having a woman healthcare provider (WHCP) whom they primarily go to for both physical and mental health services (Barefoot, Warren & Smalley, 2017). This study reported no differences between rural ($N = 278$) and nonrural ($N = 617$) lesbians in having experienced a WHCP: ask for their sexual orientation (Rural = 61.2%, Non-rural = 55%), provide safe-sex education appropriate to their orientation (Rural = 21.4%, Non-rural = 25.4%), initiate HIV screening (Rural = 15.7%, Non-rural = 19.5%), and seem knowledgeable about lesbian health concerns (Rural = 56.5%, Non-rural = 54.6%). However, they discovered a difference in recommendation of HPV vaccination; with rural lesbians significantly less likely to have received a recommendation compared with nonrural lesbians. In this case, lesbians in rural areas are at a higher risk of getting HPV and begs the question if healthcare providers are fulllty equipped to serve the lesbian population in both rural and nonrural settings.

Bias Among Healthcare Providers

Studies have found that rural members of the LGBTQ community have frequently encountered discrimination from healthcare providers (e.g., Austin, 2013; Barefoot, et al., 2015). Their experiences include negative reactions such as being questioned about their personal relationships, being made fun of due to their sexual orientation or gender identity, and being turned away from receiving services due to their statuses. As a result, these individuals were more likely to avoid seeking physical or mental health care due to fear of rejection and unfair treatment. In addition, rural lesbians were more likely to have negative attitudes toward sexual orientation disclosure to their WHCP than urban lesbians (Barefoot, Smalley, & Warren, 2017). Findings such as these are not uncommon, considering that there were also qualitative interviews with healthcare providers who reported access to care being denied to LGBT patients and of LGBT patients being discouraged from discussing their sexuality or gender (Rosenkrantz et al., 2017). Such

bias against the LGBT community is shown at both individual and institutional levels.

One might ponder if the heightened vigilance among rural LGBTQ attitudes toward health caregivers stemmed from a general sense of anticipated stigma or from recurring negative healthcare experiences. This is important to consider as LGBTQ members from rural areas may choose to terminate treatment and display avoidance due to anticipated fears and mistreatment. Overall, while a common need for general training in LGBTQ-specific health concerns could be observed across both rural and nonrural areas, there seem to be a lack of LGBT-friendly healthcare providers and LGBT-supportive policies in rural areas (Rosenkrantz et al., 2017). This is an evident notion as some rural LGBTQ individuals may opt to travel further into urban areas having perhaps obtained a recommendation of a LGBTQ supportive health caregiver, through a LGBTQ network.

The importance of creating a safe space for clients to speak their troubles is common knowledge among healthcare providers. Self-reflective exercises are involved whereby practitioners are responsible in observing and noting their attitudes, beliefs, and potential biases. Some of these biases could be micro-aggression tendencies (i.e., intentional or unintentional hostile communication toward marginalized groups) or even projected heterosexist assumptions. Encounters tinted with implicit micro-aggression would prove to be uncomfortable for LGBTQ individuals who may then be less motivated to seek help again. In an already (perceived or actual) hostile environment, services or attitudes that are LGBTQ-supportive may in turn be less visible. As most research reveals that a majority of rural LGBTQ individuals fall within the lower ranges of income and education level, complexity of health processes could be a barrier as well (Hughto, Reisner, & Pachankis, 2015). In these instances, rural LGBTQ individuals may be further discouraged from seeking to understand or comply, thus rendering these services inaccessible.

Financial Constraints and Insurance Coverage

Closely tied to care accessibility are distribution of income levels. Similar to the patterns of lower income levels distributed in rural areas, surveys demonstrate a similar pattern across LGBTQ individuals who, compared with their non-LGBTQ counterparts, tend to have a lower income (Barefoot, et al., 2015; Rosenkrantz et al., 2017). These findings could partly be explained by economic discrimination faced at work, whereby LGBTQ individuals are less likely to be employed or are often not granted a pay raise. With a lower income, LGBTQ individuals are less able to afford to pay for healthcare services and other important privileges such as insurance. Indeed, lesbians reported being unable to afford healthcare costs to be one of the main reasons they do not seek care (Barefoot, et al., 2015; Ward, Dahlhamer, Galinsky, & Joestl, 2014).

As for being able to afford insurance, there are mixed findings in the coverage differences across rural and nonrural areas. A review reported significant differences found with fewer rural LGBT community members having insurance coverage than individuals in nonrural areas (Rosenkrantz et al., 2017), whereas one study reported a roughly equal amount of rural and nonrural lesbians with insurance coverage (Barefoot, et al., 2015). Across rural and nonrural areas, more bisexuals are likely to be insured compared with their lesbian, gay, queer, or questioning counterparts (Macapagal, Bhatia, & Greene, 2016).

More recent studies seem to suggest that transgender individuals face more challenges in accessing proper health care that is insured than other LGBT members (Hughto, Reisner, & Pachankis, 2015; Macapagal, Bhatia, & Greene, 2016; Ranji, Beamesderfer, Kates, & Salganicoff, 2014). Transgender-specific care

such as hormone therapy and sex change surgeries are not insured as they are labeled cosmetics. A qualitative study had participants relating to their knowledge or having known other transgender women who engage in sex work in order to be able to afford these services (Romanelli & Hudson, 2017). Some others seek cheaper alternatives that are available on the black market and these often involve unsafe procedures with negative physiological side effects (Hughto, Reisner, & Pachankis, 2015). They share similar experiences of not receiving support from insurance companies. Furthermore, another complication arises when it comes to accurate or consistent reflection of the insured's gender identity in insurance documents. Only a small percentage of transgender people has been found to update their identity documents, which suggests that this could be a potential barrier to affording future healthcare services when needed.

While some barriers are similarly shared between rural and nonrural LGBTQ individuals, a discrepancy exists in insurance coverage and actual resources available for rural communities. Quality and type of insurance coverage may differ as the providers that are actually available in rural areas may not be included in the panel networks offered by the insurance company (Barefoot, et al., 2015). Rural LGBTQ individuals are also more likely to possess public insurance such as Medicare, Medicaid, or other types of insurance that may not necessarily be accepted by the limited providers available in rural areas. When confined by financial insecurities, rural LGBTQ individuals may then delay or neglect seeking healthcare services (Ward et al., 2014). This contributes to the health disparities mentioned in previous sections. As such, support is vital for policy efforts such as The Patient Protection and Affordable Care Act (ACA) to improve access to health insurance and coverage for rural LGBTQ individuals (Barefoot, et al., 2015). Acts such as the ACA ensures that healthcare parties are prohibited from refusing LGBTQ individuals care based on their gender identity or sexual orientation. For low-income transgender individuals, this act also provides the support for these individuals to undergo gender affirmation therapy with Medicaid (Hughto, Reisner, & Pachankis, 2015).

Recommendations and Efforts

Training for Healthcare Professionals

Misconceptions and lack of knowledge about LGBTQ among healthcare providers could potentially explain, in part, the reported inadequate and improper care for the rural LGBTQ community (Romanelli & Hudson, 2017; Rosenkrantz et al., 2017; Su et al., 2016). The purported hostile environment in rural areas also warrants reviewing the health problem corollary of social issues surrounding homophobia or heterosexism (Romanelli & Hudson, 2017).

A common recommendation is to integrate LGBTQ-specific healthcare knowledge into medical curricula. This integration should extend beyond mandating attendance for short lectures or workshops that review common health problems for LGBTQ individuals. Rather, trainers should be trained to recognize culturally appropriate terminology and guided in practicing interview questions that facilitate disclosure of sexual orientation.

Another systemic approach would be to include LGBTQ cultural competency training as a mandatory training program requirement to gain a state license for healthcare providers. All these could help create a nonheterocentric and LGBTQ-friendly space. This allows LGBTQ individuals to feel more comfortable approaching providers for healthcare services as well as reducing fear of rejection surrounding sexual orientation disclosure (Barefoot, Smalley & Warren, 2017; Rosenkrantz et al., 2017).

LGBTQ-Appropriate Services

In addition to appropriate training, healthcare providers should also be made aware of the need to increase visibility of LGBTQ-friendly services available in rural areas (Romanelli, & Hudson, 2017). With rural lesbians especially, where screening rates and HPV vaccination uptake rates are reported to be lower (Barefoot, Smalley & Warren, 2017), delivery of gynecologic and behavioral health care that are LGBTQ-friendly should be made available. Small environmental changes that showcase availability of services catered to LGBTQ populations would help indicate that the healthcare provider is LGBTQ-supportive. This could be implemented by placing office signs, posting in web pages, advertising, and including LGBTQ-associated professional experiences in profiles of providers.

Other suggestions from the growing body of literature include conducting online training modules, live webinars, and cyber-based supervision for rural healthcare providers. However important, interventions pertaining to provider contact with LGBTQ rural patients may only be effective on the individual level and after actual contact is initiated. This calls for intentional involvement of community-level efforts such as working closely with support groups for rural LGBTQ individuals. Knowledge of LGBTQ-friendly services can then be dispersed to many individuals at once in rural areas.

Support Groups

Support groups also serve as a space whereby rural LGBTQ individuals could easily access information pertaining to physical and mental healthcare services that are LGBTQ-friendly. It may also help if services to facilitate or navigate through the complex healthcare processes are offered. This helps to make it less daunting for rural LGBTQ individuals to access these services as the complicated processes involved in accessing healthcare services often deter individuals from seeking help in the first place.

Involvement in support groups has also been shown to create a collective sense of identity, which may lead to an accumulation of self-esteem among LGBTQ individuals (Hughto, Reisner, & Pachankis, 2015; Woodford et al., 2018). These groups act as support for LGBTQ individuals in coping with internal struggles such as loneliness, self-acceptance, or rejection from family members. Opportunities such as preparing individuals or family members with coping skills to deal with external systems (e.g., discrimination and violence) could also be provided (Hughto et al., 2015).

Over the years, there seems to be an increase in support groups for LGBTQ youth but with little appearance of groups catered toward older LGBTQ adults (Irwin et al., 2014). An example would be the Trevor Project that focuses on preventive measures for suicide ideation among LGBTQ youth. Such an effort is important to provide a safe space for LGBTQ individuals to connect with others in their community. However, there are little available that caters to the older LGBTQ individuals who are twice as likely to possess suicidal thoughts in a lifetime. Thus, there is also a need to increase the support available for older LGBTQ adults, especially within their community.

Community Efforts

Our review of the detrimental effects corollary of hostile environments shows a need for interventions that cultivate attitudes of openness and acceptance of LGBTQ diversity in rural areas. For instance, community outreach programs could be implemented to promote understanding and acceptance of sexual and gender diversity in rural communities (Barefoot, et al., 2015). Discussions should be held on the disparities in mental health among rural LGBTQ individuals and how hate crimes or discrimination have contributed to this.

Allport's (1954) contact hypothesis posits that appropriate interactions between different groups of individuals who are in conflict could reduce prejudice held between these groups. Studies based on contact hypothesis have reported changes in attitudes toward LGBTQ populations to be more positive following actual contact with an individual of opposing attitudes (Galarza et al., 2017; Woodford et al., 2018). A mixed method study collected quantitative and qualitative responses from a sample of rural students from helping professions after they had attended a presentation focused on older LGBTQ populations (Galarza et al., 2017). The students reported greater awareness of issues pertaining to LGBTQ populations that they were unaware of previously and expressed considerations of practicing culturally appropriate language afterward. As such, awareness-based efforts could tailor outreach programs in similar ways by creating opportunities for rural communities to experience positive encounters or collaborations with LGBTQ-supportive counterparts or LGBTQ individuals themselves.

Changes in Legislations

Throughout the literature, there are high levels of discrimination consistently reported across LGBTQ populations and some specifically in rural areas (Rosenkrantz et al., 2017). Awareness targeted at changing community attitudes could also be strengthened with improved hate crime legislations (Su et al., 2016). This could be used to identify sources of discrimination and act as a form of protection for rural LGBTQ individuals from violence or rejection.

Changes in existing policies toward becoming more LGBTQ-inclusive have been found to promote a safer environment, especially within educational institutions (Woodford et al., 2018). Institutions that included sexual and gender orientation in their antidiscrimination policies were found to have lower incidences of victimization, micro-aggressions, and perceived stress (Woodford et al., 2018). The indirect protection received from heterosexism under these inclusive policies has been discussed to contribute to lower levels of psychological distress and greater identity acceptance among LGBTQ students. Researchers also discussed how implementing inclusive policies may have possibly encouraged a greater number of initiatives or forming of student organizations that are LGBTQ-supportive. This posits that interventions targeted at a policy-level provide opportunities for systemic changes that, in turn, impact initiatives on the individual level.

With insurance and healthcare acts such as the ACA, there is a constant need to review how inclusive these policies are (Romanelli & Hudson, 2017). Anti-discriminatory policies should include explicit protection against discrimination based on sexual and gender orientation. Transgender individuals may face a unique challenge in that they could inevitably be more reliant on health services in undergoing gender-affirming procedures (Hughto, Reisner, & Pachankis, 2015). An increase in coverage or policy protection may also increase awareness among healthcare providers of this need. This may spur an increase in relevant training on gender-affirming processes as well as other LGBTQ-specific needs among healthcare providers. If implemented specifically within rural areas, this could also compensate for the lack of healthcare providers who are competent in LGBTQ-specific needs. As such, it is important to support funding or initiatives that are inclusive of sexual and gender orientation needs.

Initiatives in Foreign Countries

Over the years, the United Kingdom government has made significant progress in their effort to protect the rights of and to promote equality for the LGBTQ community. A national LGBT survey was launched in 2017 by the United Kingdom's Government Equalities Office (2018) to gather data on this population. This is important as there is a lack of representative data that could be used to fuel initiatives that address the specific needs of the LGBTQ population. A total of 108,100 responses were analyzed (Government Equalities Office, 2018). These individuals who identified as LGBT provided basic demographic information such as sexual orientation, gender identity, age, education, income level, and relationship status. Furthermore, they were also asked specific questions in several areas of their life, including life satisfaction, openness about their sexual orientation or gender identity, different experiences in education, experiences in the workplace, physical and mental health concerns, and experiences with LGBT-related services. Some qualitative information was also collected. Such governmental effort is commendable and encouraged as it provides valuable information that helps to better guide future research and interventions for this population.

In addition to surveys, some countries such as France have launched an action plan that combats discrimination against LGBTQ individuals. According to ILGA-Europe (2017), this action plan was proposed following the Orlando attacks in the United States in 2016. The French government has allocated an annual budget of €1.5 million for the implementation of this action plan and to support LGBT organizations. There is a wide range of strategies proposed within this action plan, and it is composed of activities such as having physical and mental health campaigns, streamlining protocols in case of discrimination, providing education and training to prevent discrimination, increasing LGBT-friendly services, and training the media in handling LGBT issues. Among these broad areas, there were also plans to raise awareness on LGBT issues in rural areas.

At the state level, Victoria State Government in Australia has established Safe Schools to create a safe space in a school environment for students who identify as LGBTQ members (Victoria State Government, 2018). This program focuses on providing a safe environment that is supportive, inclusive, and free of discrimination. The Department of Education and Training directly manages and delivers this program, mainly for educators and school communities. Support could be delivered in the form of training and development programs for school staffs, reviewing of school policies, and forming students' associations within the school system (Victoria State Government, 2018).

These initiatives are formed based on research findings that point to a need to address inequalities and discriminatory practices that LGBTQ individuals face. Addressing this need is imperative as it contributes to a systemic change that eventually transforms the society into one that is more inclusive and tolerant of diversity.

Research Needs

There are increasingly more studies that specifically focus on LGBTQ individuals compared with decades ago when the status of LGBTQ community was mostly neglected or dismissed. Studies reviewed in this chapter investigated various physical and mental health concerns, as well as barriers faced by LGBTQ individuals. Some focused on comparing rural and nonrural communities, whereas others focused on subgroups within the LGBTQ community, highlighting unique challenges and needs of specific subgroups of the community.

As more research is done, it has become clear that there is a lack of standardization in the way that these studies were conducted. For example, although some studies attempted to study LGBTQ as a whole, the distribution of the samples recruited are often skewed in that the majority of the participants could be gays and lesbians, with little to no representation of the transgender population. This is not uncommon as it is likely more difficult to recruit transgender individuals than gays or lesbians. However, this makes it difficult to generalize the findings of the studies as the results are likely more reflective of the majority of the sample instead of the minority

within the LGBTQ community itself. Despite that, some studies may have neglected this point and generalized results to the community as a whole. Thus it is difficult to compare studies that are said to focus on LGBTQ individuals when some subgroups are not at all or less represented. For such studies, it would be helpful for researchers to make clear to what extent the results of their study could be generalized. Future research could also be more careful with the conclusions made based on their results after taking into account the generalizability of their sample.

In addition, there is also a lack of studies done on the rural LGBTQ community as many of the studies either did not specify if their sample is composed of both urban or rural samples or if they mostly focused on urban samples. Needless to say, as the challenges and needs of rural and urban LGBTQ individuals are different, the results of many studies cannot be applied to the rural community. As a result, some members of the rural LGBTQ community may end up feeling neglected, misrepresented, or unsupported. As such, more studies could be done with the rural community for a more accurate representation of this community.

Conclusion

There are similarities and differences in terms of physical and mental health behaviors and patterns between LGBTQ and non-LGBTQ individuals. Many such differences appear to be contributed by societal norms and beliefs that emphasize heteronormativity, sometimes at the expense of the rights of sexual and gender minorities in the society. As a result, LGBTQ individuals may be stigmatized and discriminated against, which leads to poorer mental health; the impact on their physical health becomes apparent when these individuals avoid seeking out a healthcare provider for fear of being ridiculed or worse, rejected. Cases like this may be more prevalent in rural areas with more prominent heteronormative culture than urban areas.

Furthermore, the geographic distribution of rural LGBTQ communities also sometimes put them at a disadvantage where a lack of access to appropriate services and insurance network coverage create additional obstacles for them in seeking health care. With a lower income, they are also sometimes unable to afford to pay for medical or mental health treatment. As such, policy efforts for public insurance such as Medicaid or Medicare become vital to improve access to health insurance and coverage for rural LGBTQ individuals.

Conversations among professionals and advocacy work have helped to raise awareness among the public of the disparities in physical and mental health observed between rural and non-rural LGBTQ communities. To further this effort in improving healthcare services for rural LGBTQ individuals, all members of the society could come together to contribute whether it is in the form of training young healthcare professionals, providing LGBTQ-friendly services, being a part of the community outreach programs, or advocating for their rights through changes in the legislations.

Chapter Summary

LGBTQ stands for lesbian, gay, bisexual, transgender, and queer or questioning. Very few statistics are known about this population in the United States as there ares no census data on the demographic information of sexual orientation and gender identity. Surveys from private institutions showed that there is a steady increase in the number of people who have identified as LGBTQ over the years, with 4.5% of the population in 2017 identified as a LGBTQ member.

The society mainly holds the idea that heterosexuality is natural and is considered a normal sexual orientation, and those who do not conform to that standard in such heteronormative cultures are seen as unnatural and problematic. As a result, LGBTQ individuals are likely to be stigmatized and discriminated against. According to the Meyer's (2003) minority stress model, the conflicting nature in sexual or gender values between the LGBTQ and heterosexual individuals creates various stressors in the minority's lives. When accumulated, these stressors lead to long-term health issues in the minority population and affect future preventative healthcare behaviors.

Rural LGBTQ individuals were found to be more motivated to avoid healthcare screenings than urban LGBTQ individuals, which puts them at a higher risk of not detecting the presence of certain infections and diseases. A reason that is often attributed to this is the fear that they may need to disclose their sexual orientation to healthcare providers, where they may be discriminated against, especially when rural areas tend to have a more heteronormative culture than urban areas. Stigma and misinformation about certain illnesses in rural areas also make it more difficult for the LGBTQ community to access appropriate services when needed.

In general, studies have found that rural LGBTQ individuals have higher levels of overall psychological distress such as stress, anxiety, depression, and suicidality than their nonrural counterparts. This pattern is consistently seen among different groups of individuals—e.g., youth, men, women, and veterans, among others. Some individuals gain support from others and are able to feel connected, whereas others experience loneliness when they are not able to form meaningful relationships. Discrimination is one of the central themes in various LGBTQ studies, and although some found that it is more prevalent in rural areas, others found that there is no difference in experiences of discriminations between rural and urban LGBTQ communities.

Various barriers contributed to rural LGBTQ's physical and mental health statuses, and these include the lack of access to healthcare services due to geographic barriers, **bias among healthcare providers** that discouraged rural LGBTQ individuals to seek help, as well as financial constraints and the lack of insurance coverage in rural communities. Based on the barriers identified, some recommendations were offered. Specific LGBTQ-oriented training could be provided to reduce bias and discrimination among healthcare providers as well as bridge their knowledge on common health problems for LGBTQ individuals. The increase in LGBTQ-appropriate services, support groups, and community outreach efforts as well as changes in legislations are also important to improve the physical and mental health of LGBTQ individuals.

Finally, future research with the LGBTQ community could focus on specific populations such as rural LGBTQ individuals, bisexuals, or transgenders, where research is more scarce to effectively identify the similarities and differences among different subgroups within the LGBTQ community.

Discussion Questions
Self-Test Questions

1. What is heteronormativity?
2. Describe two types of stressors identified in Meyer's (2003) minority stress model.
3. Identify the physical health concerns experienced by the rural LGBTQ community.
4. What are some of the main mental health disparities between rural and nonrural LGBTQ individuals that are covered in this chapter?
5. What are the unique challenges that rural LGBTQ individuals face compared with their nonrural counterparts?
6. Explain why LGBTQ individuals may experience more discrimination in rural areas than in a city.
7. How can Meyer's minority stress model explain why there are often health disparities between heterosexual and homosexual individuals?
8. How can one reduce prejudice against LGBTQ members among healthcare providers?
9. Describe the recommendations and current efforts that are in place to improve the health of rural LGBTQ community.

Group Discussions

1. If you are a legislator, what are the pros and cons that you will have to consider when it comes to improving the physical and mental health of LGBTQ individuals in rural areas through public policies?
2. Imagine that you are in a committee overseeing grants for LGBTQ research; what do you think is lacking in current LGBTQ research and what kind of research will most likely earn a grant from your committee?
3. As healthcare providers may have biases against and negative attitudes toward LGBTQ individuals, what are some strategies that could help promote acceptance or awareness among healthcare providers? Discuss.

Student activities and worksheets are available inside the Navigate eBook, included with the printed text. Simply redeem the access code found at the front of the book at www.jblearning.com.

References

Allport, G. W. (1954). *The nature of prejudice.* Cambridge, MA: Perseus Books.

Anderson, R. K., Kindle, P. A., Dwyer, A., Nowak, J. A., Callaghan, T. A., & Arkfeld, R. (2015). Rural perspectives on same-sex marriage. *Journal of Gay & Lesbian Social Services, 27*(2), 201–215. doi:10.1080/10538720.2015.1022274

Austin, E. L. (2013). Sexual orientation disclosure to health care providers among urban and nonurban southern lesbians. *Women & Health, 53*(1), 41–55. doi: 10.1080/03630242.2012.743497

Barefoot, K. N., Smalley, K. B., & Warren, J. C. (2015). Psychological distress and perceived barriers to care for rural lesbians. *Journal of Gay & Lesbian Mental Health, 19*(4), 347–369. doi:10.1080/19359705.2015.1041629

Barefoot, K. N., Smalley, K. B., & Warren, J. C. (2017). A quantitative comparison of the health-care disclosure experiences of rural and nonrural lesbians. *Stigma and Health, 2*(3), 195. doi:10.1037/sah0000052

Barefoot, K. N., Warren, J. C., & Smalley, K. B. (2017). Women's health care: The experiences and behaviors of rural and urban lesbians in the USA. *Rural & Remote Health, 17.* Retrieved from https://pdfs.semanticscholar.org/58a5/44482e4ebf5576149711e0e2be48186a4661.pdf

Casazza, S. P., Ludwig, E., & Cohn, T. J. (2015). Heterosexual attitudes and behavioral intentions toward bisexual individuals: Does geographic area make a difference? *Journal of Bisexuality, 15*(4), 532–553. doi:10.1080/15299716.2015.1093994

Centers for Diseases Control and Prevention. (2019). *HIV in the United States by region.* Retrieved from https://www.cdc.gov/hiv/statistics/

Dentato, M. P. (2012). The minority stress perspective. *Psychology & AIDS Exchange, 37,* 12–15. American Psychological Association. Washington, D.C. (Spring Issue).

Galarza, J., Bourassa, D., Shupp, M., & Lane, C. (2017). Serving our (in)visible elders: The impact of a LGBTQ+ aging presentation on a rural college campus. *Journal of Gay & Lesbian Social Services, 29*(1), 25–40. doi:10.1080/10538720.2016.1261748

Goffman, E. *Stigma: Notes on the Management of Spoiled Identity.* Englewood Cliffs, NJ: Prentice-Hall; 1963.

Government Equalities Office. (2018). *National LGBT Survey* (Reference: GEO – RR001). Retrieved from https://www.gov.uk/government/consultations/national-lgbt-survey

Haas, A. P., Eliason, M., Mays, V. M., Mathy, R. M., Cochran, S. D., D'Augelli, A. R., . . . Russell, S. T. (2010). Suicide and suicide risk in lesbian, gay, bisexual, and transgender populations: Review and recommendations. *Journal of Homosexuality, 58*(1), 10–51. doi:10.1080/00918369.2011.534038

Horvath, K. J., Iantaffi, A., Swinburne-Romine, R., & Bockting, W. (2014). A comparison of mental health, substance use, and sexual risk behaviors between rural and non-rural transgender persons. *Journal of Homosexuality, 61*(8), 1117–1130. doi: 10.1080/00918369.2014.872502

Hubach, R. D., Dodge, B., Schick, V., Ramos, W. D., Herbenick, D., Li, M. J., . . . Reece, M. (2015). Experiences of HIV positive gay, bisexual and other men who have sex with men residing in relatively rural areas. *Culture, Health & Sexuality, 17*(7), 795–809. doi:10.1080/13691058.2014.994231

Hughto, J. M., Reisner, S. L., & Pachankis, J. E. (2015). Transgender stigma and health: A critical review of stigma determinants, mechanisms, and interventions. *Social Science & Medicine, 147,* 222–231. https://doi.org/10.1016/j.socscimed.2015.11.010

Human Rights Campaign. (2012). *Growing up LGBT in America.* Retrieved from https://assets2.hrc.org/files/assets/resources/Growing-Up-LGBT-in-America_Report.pdf?_ga=2.101024705.1960619500.1563097801-1373569779.1563097801

ILGA-Europe. (2017). *French government launches action plan to fight hate against LGBT people.* Retrieved from https://www.ilga-europe.org/

Irwin, J. A., Coleman, J. D., Fisher, C. M., & Marasco, V. M. (2014). Correlates of suicide ideation among LGBT Nebraskans. *Journal of Homosexuality, 61*(8), 1172–1191. doi:10.1080/00918369.2014.872521

Jeffries, W. L., Marks, G., Lauby, J., Murrill, C. S., & Millett, G. A. (2013). Homophobia is associated with sexual behavior that increases risk of acquiring and transmitting HIV infection among black men who have sex with men. *AIDS and Behavior, 17*(4), 1442–1453. doi:10.1007/s10461-012-0189-y

Kauth, M. R., Barrera, T. L., Denton, F. N., & Latini, D. M. (2017). Health differences among lesbian, gay, and transgender veterans by rural/small town and suburban/urban setting. *LGBT Health, 4*(3), 194–201. doi:10.1089/lgbt.2016.0213

Macapagal, K., Bhatia, R., & Greene, G. J. (2016). Differences in healthcare access, use, and experiences within a community sample of racially diverse lesbian, gay, bisexual, transgender, and questioning emerging adults. *LGBT Health, 3*(6), 434–442. doi:10/1089/lgbt.2015.0124

Marrazzo, J. M., & Gorgos, L. M. (2012). Emerging sexual health issues among women who have sex with women. *Current Infectious Disease Reports, 14*(2), 204–211. doi:10.1007/s11908-012-0244-x

Meyer, I. H. (2003). Prejudice, social stress, and mental health in lesbian, gay, and bisexual populations: Conceptual issues and research evidence. *Psychological Bulletin, 129*(5), 674–697. doi:10.1037/0033-2909.129.5.674

Newport, F. (2018, May 22). In U.S., estimate of LGBT population rises to 4.5%. *Gallup.* Retrieved from https://news.gallup.com/poll/234863/estimate-lgbt-population-rises.aspx

Ranji, U., Beamesderfer, A., Kates, J., & Salganicoff, A. (2014). Health and access to care and coverage for lesbian, gay, bisexual, and transgender individuals in the U.S.

Romanelli, M., & Hudson, K. D. (2017). Individual and systemic barriers to health care: Perspectives of lesbian, gay, bisexual, and transgender adults. *American Journal of Orthopsychiatry, 87*(6), 714–728. https://doi.org/10.1037/ort0000306

Rosenkrantz, D. E., Black, W. W., Abreu, R. L., Aleshire, M. E., & Fallin-Bennett, K. (2017). Health and health care of rural sexual and gender minorities: A systematic review. *Stigma and Health, 2*(3), 229–243. doi:10.1037/sah0000055

Rowan, N. L., Giunta, N., Grudowski, E. S., & Anderson, K. A. (2013). Aging well and gay in rural America: A case study. *Journal of Gerontological Social Work, 56*(3), 185–200. doi:10.1080/01634372.2012.754813

Su, D., Irwin, J. A., Fisher, C., Ramos, A., Kelley, M., Mendoza, D. A. R., & Coleman, J. D. (2016). Mental health disparities within the LGBT population:

A comparison between transgender and nontransgender individuals. *Transgender Health, 1*(1), 12–20. doi:10.1089/trgh.2015.0001

Swank, E., Frost, D., & Fahs, B. (2012). Rural location and exposure to minority stress among sexual minorities in the United States. *Psychology & Sexuality, 3*(3), 226–243. doi:10.1080/19419899.2012.700026

Szymanski, D. M., & Henrichs-Beck, C. (2014). Exploring sexual minority women's experiences of external and internalized heterosexism and sexism and their links to coping and distress. *Sex Roles, 70*(1–2), 28–42. https://doi.org/10.1007/s11199-013-0329-5

The Trevor Project. (2019). *National survey on LGBTQ mental health.* Retrieved from https://www.thetrevorproject.org/survey-2019/?section=Conversion-Therapy-Change-Attempts

Victoria State Government. (2018). *Safe schools.* Retrieved from https://www.education.vic.gov.au/

Ward, J., & Schneider, B. (2009). The reaches of heteronormativity: An introduction. *Gender & Society, 23*(4), 433–439. doi:10.1177/0891243209340903

Whitehead, J., Shaver, J., & Stephenson, R. (2016). Outness, stigma, and primary health care utilization among rural LGBT populations. *PloS one, 11*(1), e0146139. doi:10.1371/journal.pone.0146139

Wienke, C., & Hill, G. J. (2013). The relationship between multiple roles and well-being among gay, lesbian, and heterosexual adults. *Journal of GLBT Family Studies, 9*(4), 305–329. https://doi.org/10.1080/1550428X.2013.799417

Additional Reading

- Institute of Medicine (U.S.). (2011). *The health of lesbian, gay, bisexual, and transgender people: Building a foundation for better understanding.* Washington, D.C.: The National Academic Press.

- Smalley, K. B., Warren, J. C., & Barefoot, K. N. (Eds.). (2018). *LGBT Health: Meeting the needs of gender and sexual minorities.* New York, NY: Springer Publishing Company, LLC.

PART 5

Advancing Rural Health: Assessment, Planning, and Interventions

CHAPTER 20

Community Needs and Asset Assessment

Mary L. Kushion, MSA

LEARNING OBJECTIVES

At the end of this chapter, readers will be able to:

1. Define community scope and describe the attributes and assets of a rural community.
2. Articulate how to identify and engage stakeholders.
3. Identify at least three methods to collect both qualitative and quantitative data necessary to assess community needs.
4. Describe the skills and strategies necessary to lead a community dialog on building a healthy community.

KEY TERMS

Alignment
Assessment
Asset mapping
Assets
Collaboration
Community
Healthy community
Public Health 3.0
Qualitative
Quantitative
Stakeholder

CHAPTER OVERVIEW

This chapter will discuss the **community** needs and asset assessment process. It will provide the reader with the methods and skills necessary to engage the community and stakeholders. It will also inform the reader of data resources for both **qualitative** and **quantitative** data collection. It will provide real-world examples from rural public health agencies on lessons learned during the **assessment** process and provide health professional expert advice.

Introduction to Community Health Needs and Assets Assessment

The Patient Protection and Affordable Care Act of 2010 (ACA) includes a mandate for nonprofit hospitals throughout the United States to conduct community health needs assessments every three years starting in 2012. Furthermore, the ACA requires the hospitals to work in **collaboration** with public health

383

entities (The Patient and Affordable Care Act 2010).

The national Public Health Accreditation Board (PHAB), requires that any local, state, Tribal, or territorial health department that desires to become accredited must either lead, or actively participate in a community health needs assessment process every three years (PHAB 2019).

The community health needs assessment requirement for both healthcare systems and governmental public health agencies seeking national accreditation has resulted in collaborative efforts to complete the work that the nation had not experienced previous to the mandates. At the local level, governmental health department officials were aware of their hospital administration counterparts, but it was the exception, rather than the rule to have both entities engaged in an assessment and health improvement planning process together. Stoto wrote, "The similar requirements from PHAB and the IRS provide an opportunity to catalyze stronger collaboration and better shared measurement systems among hospitals and health departments" (Stoto, 2015).

Historically, governmental public health agencies did not have the resources to engage in assessment activities and as such, were not motivated to pursue them due to lack of a funding mechanism. However, when the ACA mandated that hospitals conduct community health needs assessment and demonstrate participation by governmental public health on their IRS reporting forms, suddenly, public health was invited to the table.

Similarly, local health departments who were eager to pursue PHAB accreditation took the lead in their jurisdictions and leveraged the resources available from healthcare systems and other community partners to conduct the assessment process. Health departments have access to data that the hospitals may not and, in many communities, are the lead agencies to address both communicable and chronic diseases.

In 2016, Dr. Karen DeSalvo, while serving as the Acting Assistant Secretary for Health at the U.S. Department of Health and Human Services, authored a white paper titled "Public Health 3.0, A Call to Action to Create a 21st Century Public Health Infrastructure." A white paper is a report, traditionally written by a government agency to inform readers outside of the organization of an issue and potential solutions. The illustration provided from another of Dr. DeSalvo's publications titled, **Figure 20-1** provides a clear illustration of "The Evolution of Public Health Practices" since its beginnings in the late 1800s. It had been a number of years since the role of governmental public health had been reviewed and updated to reflect the current and necessary roles for public health related to the engagement of multiple community sectors through collective impact with the goal of improving the social determinants of health that include, but are not limited to, employment; education; equity and access to care; and safe, affordable housing.

The DeSalvo white paper has five key themes for PH 3.0:

1. Strong leadership and workforce
2. Strategic partnerships
3. Flexible and sustainable funding
4. Timely and locally relevant data, metrics, and analytics
5. Foundational infrastructure

DeSalvo articulates in her paper that public health needs to be the chief health strategist (CHS) in its community. Interpretations of this statement vary. Some view the CHS as the local public health leader while others contend it is the entity as a whole that serves the role. According to DeSalvo, "public health departments should engage with community stakeholders from both the public and private sectors—to form vibrant, structured, cross-sector partnerships designed to develop and guide **Public Health 3.0**-style initiatives and to foster shared funding, services, governance, and collective action (U.S. Department of Health and Human Services, n.d.)."

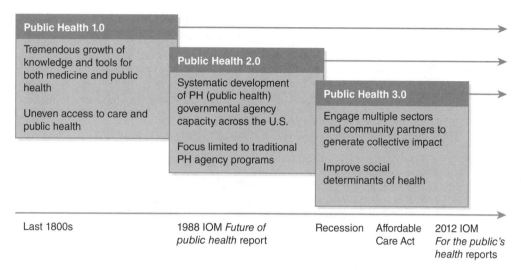

Figure 20-1 Evolution of Public Health Practices.

Data from DeSalvo et al. (2016). Public Health 3.0: Time for an Upgrade. AJPH.

Regardless of how one interprets the concept of chief health strategist, the skills and abilities required to carry out the function remain the same:

- Ability to engage the community, leverage assets, and foster collaboration
- Ability to interpret and present data
- Ability to develop, implement, and monitor policies, plans, and processes

These skills and abilities are necessary to conduct a community needs and **asset mapping** assessment.

Understanding and Describing the Rural Community

Dictionary.Com defines "Community" as "a social group of any size whose members reside in a specific locality, share government, and often have a common cultural and historical heritage" (Dictionary.com, 2019) and while that is true, the definition alone does not describe a community, but it does start to develop the parameters to understand it.

Prior to starting a community health assessment and asset mapping process, a core group needs to be convened by the CHS. The assembled core team will begin the work of defining and describing the community to be assessed. Is it a city? A county? Multiple counties? What are the geographic boundaries of the assessment area? In rural areas, data may not be as readily available due to the size of the population compared with its urban counterparts. Therefore, it is important when defining the community to be able to have access to the data that is available, which may be at best at the county level and at least on a regional or statewide level.

Once the "community" to be assessed has been determined, the core team will begin the assessment process by gathering demographic data. The Community Commons website (CommunityCommons.org) is a helpful source to collect both demographic and health details on a community. If the community has been defined as one or more counties, the County Health Rankings (CHR) website is also useful (CountyHealthRankingsandRoadmaps.org). The assessment process needs to include the demographics of the population within the community. These include but are not limited to population size (age group, gender, race) and socioeconomic factors that include income levels (mean, median), transportation availability, educational attainment, home ownership, and employment status. Both of these websites provide general information related to population size, economy, education, and housing, among others.

The core team will also need to gather locally available information on their community such as governmental structure and representation as well as cultural norms, beliefs, disparities, and values to be able to accurately describe the community.

One tool for community teams to use are windshield or walking surveys. As the name implies, this type of assessment takes place either in a moving car or by walking around the community. The Community Tool Box developed by the University of Kansas cites the following benefits:

- Windshield or walking surveys give an objective view of the community.
- They can be adapted to community-based participatory action research, inviting community participation.
- They may allow you to see assets that community members take for granted or don't see.
- They can be the easiest and quickest way to get an overview of the entire community.
- They allow clear comparisons among different neighborhoods in a city, villages in a rural area, etc.
- They can be very useful in understanding specific aspects of a community.
- They give you a "feel" for the community. (ctb.ku.edu)

Conducting one of these two surveys (or both, if possible), allows the core team and coalition members to take a really close look at the conditions within their community. It is also important to conduct the assessments at critical times. For example, to determine if the community has safe walking and bicycling routes to schools, the survey should be conducted during the times when students are walking to and from school rather than in the middle of the day. This will determine if streetlights are working at those times, if crossing guards are necessary, the amount of traffic, and perhaps if dogs are out in the neighborhood yards and need to be restrained.

Identifying Stakeholders

The Core Team will be responsible for identifying and bringing additional stakeholders and community representatives to the assessment table. One method of identifying potential members is to conduct a **stakeholder** analysis to determine who needs to be invited and included in the assessment process. The County Health Rankings and Roadmap Action Cycle illustrated in **Figure 20-2** provides examples of the various sectors that could and should be brought into the assessment process. The sectors identified on the graphic should not be considered an exhaustive list and it will vary based on the individual community. What is important to consider when developing the stakeholder list is to include community members who are in the center of the CHR model but can be overlooked or underrepresented. Community members are often the people who can tell stakeholders the "why" or the root cause of the data results.

MindTools Ltd developed a Power/Interest Grid to identify stakeholders by level of interest and level of power and is illustrated in **Figure 20-3**. During the stakeholder analysis process, coalitions need to identify the individuals and organizations who have:

- Both a high level of interest and power in the community
- A high level of interest but do not have a high level of power
- Both a low level of interest and power in the community

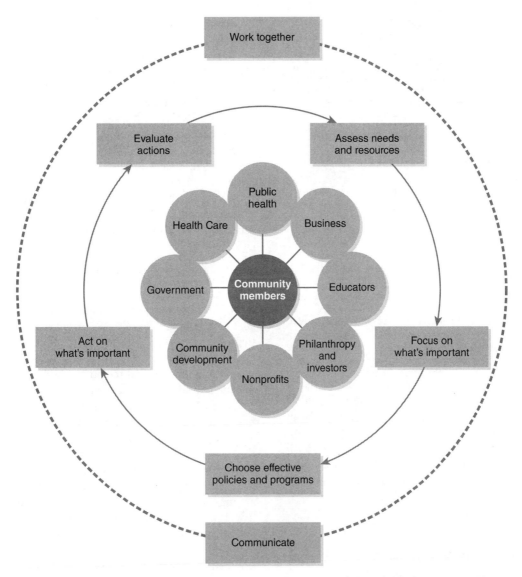

Figure 20-2 County Health Rankings and Roadmap.

Robert Wood Johnson Foundation.

- A high level of power but do not have a high level of interest

Potential Assessment Team members will fall into one of the four quadrants. It is imperative to have, either by design or default, representation in each quadrant and all four of the quadrants should have a mix of community members, partners, and opponents identified to be able to acknowledge and identify how to engage and inform each group. Conducting a stakeholder analysis early in the process allows the team to create the strategies needed to garner support both from those who are supportive of the work but also from those in the community who may be negatively impacted. Knowing the interests, concerns, and resources that each stakeholder brings to the table, or refuses to

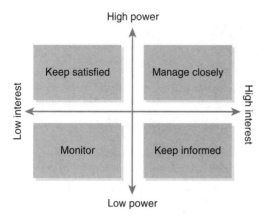

Figure 20-3 Power/Interest Grid for Stakeholder Prioritization.

Mind Tools Ltd. Adapted from Mendelow, A. L. (1981). 'Environmental Scanning - The Impact of the Stakeholder Concept,' ICIS 1981 Proceedings, 20.

bring to the table, will be key in the development and implementation phases of health improvement efforts.

The Center for Creative Leadership, in cooperation with the County Health Rankings and Roadmaps program at the University of Wisconsin's Population Health Institute, also provides a template and guidance for stakeholder mapping and analysis. A link is provided here: https://www .countyhealthrankings.org/sites/default/files /media/document/resources/Stakeholder %20Mapping.pdf

Stakeholder Engagement and Monitoring

Bringing stakeholders to the table to work collaboratively to improve the health within the community is relatively easy; keeping them there is more complex. It is important to establish and gain a consensus at the initial meetings on the charge, scope, responsibilities, and time frame that will apply to the work. Stakeholders want to know what will be involved in the health improvement process and exactly what is expected of them.

Stakeholder engagement and sustaining membership can be accomplished by having a common goal and purpose that aligns with the work that the members do outside of the coalition as well as with their values. Having a call to action where everyone at the table is engaged and plays an active role in resolving the problem creates a sense of ownership in achieving the goal. Periodically asking the members questions like, "How does the work we are doing in this group relate to other aspects of your world?" and "Where and how can the work we are doing be shared outside of these meetings?" will prompt and remind the members that they often wear a variety of hats and the information and actions taken to improve health in the community can and should be brought to all civic organizations, houses of worship, little leagues, and other points of contact.

Setting the tone and providing a welcoming and safe space is critical when establishing a new coalition. It is recommended but not mandatory to develop with the team members a set of ground rules or code of conduct for the members. Again, this will ensure that the members know what is expected of them and helps avert any negative behaviors or conflicts among members before they occur. Although it will seem simplistic, it is important to start and end the meetings on time, have consistent meeting dates and locations and provide an orientation session to new members as they are added to the group. Ending each meeting on a positive note by asking "What did we create today?" allows the members to reflect and share what was accomplished. Periodically, survey the members to make sure they are satisfied with the content and direction of the meetings and make changes based on their input.

Stakeholder engagement is often enhanced and sustained when members are recognized for their actions and contributions. Sending thank you letters to the members—and one to their boss to thank them for the commitment of time and talents is usually appreciated. Ask the members to participate in photo opportunities and use their quotes in press releases and publications. Everyone likes to see their name in print so share their success stories in presentations and on traditional and social media.

While it is preferable to have all of the members stay on the coalition for an extended period, there will be times when a member will need or choose to leave. It is a fact that life gets in the way and people may change jobs, move out of the area, or perhaps the priorities of the coalition do not align with their personal or professional identity. When this occurs, recognize, and appreciate the member's efforts and thank him or her for his or her time. Offer to maintain communication and perhaps, in certain cases, the person will be able to stay engaged through an email membership option or as a subject matter expert, as appropriate.

> "Be inclusive rather than exclusive. Set expectations up front. The stakeholders and partners will then be making decisions and giving input rather than spinning wheels because nothing has been done between meetings."
> Carol Moehrle, District Director, Idaho North Central District

Asset Mapping

Once the stakeholders have been identified and oriented, the team can start to focus on the available community **assets** to address the health issues that will be identified during the assessment process. This is called **Asset Mapping**. Community assets come in many forms and include:

- Human resources—staffing, coalition members, community champions, and data collectors
- Financial resources—designated funding, grants, donations, and contributions

- Physical resources—meeting location, bike paths, community gardens
- Existing programs and interventions—services provided by healthcare, public health, mental health, and other community sectors
- Policymaker resources—local, state, and national policymakers or their aids who can advocate for and implement health policies

(Healthycommunities.org)

The CHS will need to work with the team to seek out these community resources. Most people and organizations want to help but may not know what is needed so they are just waiting to be asked specific requests for support. Not everyone is able to provide financial support, but perhaps they have talents in grant writing or graphic design that are useful. Others may have conference room space and are willing to host the team meetings or open spaces for physical activities or community gardens. Still others may indeed have the ability to provide start-up funds to launch the initiative or have the ability to enact a policy. It is imperative to assess and assemble the time, talents, and treasures within the community that comprise its assets as these will be the resources needed to address the health issues identified. Local public health officer Marcus Cheatham recommends,

> "Look for the right people. You want people who understand the connections between public health and other parts of the community and who are excited to collaborate with each other."

Having the right people at the table who are enthusiastic and excited will launch and sustain the process further and faster. It has been said to not let a lack of time or money be the excuse to NOT do something and this also applies to the assessment process. If you have the right people at the table, they will find the time and the money.

Quantitative Data Collection

Quantitative data are data that can be counted or measured. The collection efforts of local data in rural areas, while challenging, has become better in recent years due to the annual County Health Rankings provided by the University of Wisconsin's Population Health Institute. The County Health Rankings provide county-specific quantitative health data for nearly every county, in every state in the nation. Assessment teams are also able to collect and analyze primary (data the team collects) and secondary data (collected by others) from local and state sources. These include, but are not limited to:

- Hospital discharge data
- State health agency data (immunization rates, communicable and chronic disease rates, behavioral risk factor surveillance surveys)
- School data (free and reduced lunches, high school graduation rates)
- 2-1-1 data on types of assistance requested

At the outset, assessment teams need to determine what data they want and need to collect, the data sources to be used, who will collect the data, and how often the data will be reviewed and updated. It is also important to have a starting and ending date for data collection.

Figure 20-4 illustrates how, once your criteria for data collection has been

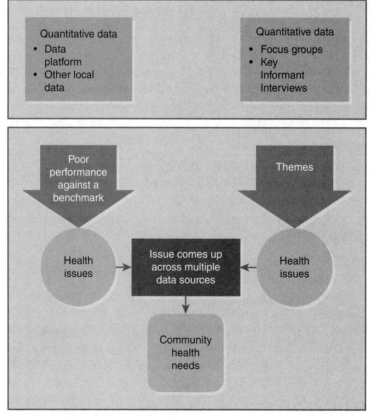

Figure 20-4 Process for Identifying Needs.

determined, data is analyzed to identify health issues and health needs.

As data become timelier and readily available through the Internet and in increasing abundance, it is important for the team to decide which types of data they want to collect, both quantitative and qualitative data, and the sources that will be used to assure the data are credible and relevant. State health departments are a good source for health-related data, but communities may also want to seek out data from federal sources such as the Centers for Disease Control and Prevention and the Health Resources and Services Administration.

The data collection process can be completed by a subset of the team or the team may wish to utilize graduate students, independent contractors, or a specific organization. The primary data collectors will need to assure that the data obtained are from reputable sources and the most current available as well as to cite the sources for future reference and updating as necessary.

Kaiser Permanente's Community Health Needs Assessment Toolkit, developed for its healthcare system identified seven questions when determining the strength of a data source:

1. Is the sample size large enough?
2. Does it represent the broader population?
3. How recent are the data?
4. How granular are the data?
5. Do the data allow you to examine health needs by subgroups?
6. Are the data complete enough to allow an examination of all health needs?
7. Are the data sources reliable?

(Kaiser Permanente 2015)

Qualitative Data Collection

Quantitative health data at a local level is often difficult to find due to the small sample sizes associated with rural areas. However, that only provides a part of the assessment. Qualitative

data, which are data that are observed and recorded, must also be collected through key informant interviews, surveys, and focus groups or listening sessions to determine the root causes for the quantitative data results. The observations from the windshield or walking surveys mentioned previously are an example of qualitative data collection at the local level.

UCLA's Center for Health Policy Research defined Key Informant interviews as "qualitative in-depth interviews with people who know what is going on in the community. The purpose of key informant interviews is to collect information from a wide range of people— including community leaders, professionals, or residents—who have firsthand knowledge about the community. These community experts, with their particular knowledge and understanding, can provide insight on the nature of problems and give recommendations for solutions." (UCLA, nd.) Key Informant interviews can be either in person or over the phone, but typically, are one-on-one conversations with the community expert. Questions should be prepared in advance, but one of the benefits of the interview is the ability to ask follow-up questions or additional questions depending on where the conversation leads. In rural communities, key informants may wear many hats and fill multiple roles. For example, a local school superintendent may also be a youth soccer coach or a member of the rotary club. Interviewers should be aware and prepared to discuss all aspects of the Key Informant's community contributions rather than solely focusing on their paid profession.

Conducting electronic and paper surveys with open-ended questions is another way to collect qualitative data. Surveys are often used to solicit a large amount of qualitative data in a short time. They are typically anonymous and the process allows for the participants to be candid and open about the health issues and concerns in their community. They can be used to generate ideas and solutions to resolve health issues within the community such as obesity, teen pregnancy, or any other health issue that was identified in the quantitative data. Surveys can also bring out community perceptions regarding the culture of the community with regard to safety, discrimination, and the physical and natural environment that may not be evident from the quantitative data.

Community assessment teams should also conduct focus groups during the data collection process. In her article, "Involving the Communities in Community Assessment," Dr. Mary Jo Clark stated, "A focus group is a group of people who have personal experience of a topic of interest and who meet to discuss their perceptions and perspectives on that topic (Urden, 2003; Webb, 2002). Put more simply, it is, "a group of people focused on a particular discussion topic" (Jayanthi & Nelson, 2002; p. 2; emphasis added). Focus groups differ from individual interviews as a method of data collection in that they capitalize on the interaction between and among participants to stimulate and refine thoughts and perspectives (Owen, 2001). Perspectives may be formulated or changed in response to those of other participants (Webb, 2002), and the nature of the interaction between participants is itself considered data (Owen, 2001)" (Clark et al., 2003).

Focus groups and community listening sessions are excellent data collection tools to be able to speak to and to hear directly from persons impacted by a health condition. For example, when conducting an assessment on the prevalence of opioids in a community, the team may want to conduct focus groups with both healthcare providers and those who are in treatment facilities.

Conducting Public Focus Groups and Listening Sessions

The successful collection of qualitative data relies on the skills and abilities of the facilitator or interviewer and the composition of the questions. The atmosphere, setting, and attitude of the convener will either make or break the public forum. It is crucial for the participants to believe they are in a trusted and safe space to share their opinion. They will also want to feel as though their contributions are valued and important.

The team will want to utilize a neutral, credible convener who can provide an overview of the process, present the quantitative data if available, and engage the participants in discussion by asking open-ended questions such as "What do you believe are the biggest health issues in our community?" and "What do you believe should be done to address these health issues?" It is not the convener's role to provide input or responses during the session but rather to seek information and ask follow-up questions as appropriate. The convener may also have to engage in conflict management if differing opinions are expressed during the discussions that become heated or argumentative among the participants. Knowing how to diffuse the situation and continue the conversation is a key skill for the forum's facilitator.

The Association for Community Health Improvement created a Community Health Assessment Toolkit for the CHA process. The toolkit contains guiding principles to consider when seeking community input and some include:

- Involve community members in the survey development to ensure the questions are culturally appropriate. Do not use healthcare jargon.
- Assure the questions accurately and directly address what is being measured.
- Train individuals who are conducting interviews and focus groups to be consistent and neutral.
- Make the location easily accessible for community members.

(Association for Community Health Improvement)

If possible, a second neutral person should attend the session to serve as a scribe to capture the information shared and record the session to assure all comments are captured.

This person will also not contribute to the discussion but rather serve in a supportive role to the facilitator. He or she may also serve as a timekeeper to keep the session on track.

Leading a Community Dialogue on Building a Healthy Community

Once the quantitative and qualitative data have been collected and assembled in the proposed community health needs assessment document, the materials need to be widely disseminated for public consumption and comment. After a reasonable review period, the CHS will need to bring together stakeholders, partners, and interested members of the community to discuss and decide on the priority areas to be addressed in the community, the strategies that will be employed, and both the assets available and the barriers that will need to be overcome to improve the health status of the community.

The role of the CHS is to outline the findings from the data, present a proposed list of health issues to be addressed, and provide potential evidence-based strategies to resolve them. However, the CHS should be open and receptive to innovative, community-driven interventions too. For example, if the community members believe the best way to improve physical activity is to paint the sidewalks purple, the team should seriously consider the assets and resources within the community to acquire purple paint. Every evidence-based program started out as an innovative idea. Former Polk County, Wisconsin, Health Department Director Gretchen Sampson reflected on their assessment and said,

> "having a successful CHA process pays dividends in terms of public awareness about the health of the community and is a good springboard for others to want to get involved in the community health improvement plan."

It may be necessary to host more than one community dialog session at various times of the day or evening to be able to include representation from different population groups and organizations. In her article in the Stanford Social Innovation Review article, Barnes wrote "One of the biggest mistakes that social change leaders make is failing to differentiate between mobilizing and organizing. Mobilizing is about recruiting people to support a vision, cause or program. In this model, leaders or an organization is the subject that makes decisions, and community members are passive object of those decisions. Organizing, of the other hand, is about cultivating leaders, identifying their interests, and enabling them to lead change. Here, community members are the subject of the work: They collaborate on making decision. At its best community engagement involved working with a variety of leaders – those at the grass tops and those at the grass roots – to ensure that an effort has the support necessary for long-term success." (Barnes and Schmitz, 2016). She continued by stating "It's important, in other words, to view community members as producers of outcomes, not just as recipients of outcomes. Professional leaders must recognize and respect the assets that community members can bring to an initiative" (Barnes, 2016).

> "Your community is hungry for leadership and direction. By undertaking a community health ASSESSMENT, you provide an opportunity for the organizations in your community to establish that direction. Use the process to bring forward their best ideas and seek ways together to put them into practice"
> Marcus Cheatham, Health Officer, Mid-Michigan District health department

Prioritizing Health Issues

After receiving community input as to what they believe the health issues are and adding them to the list of issues identified during the data collection process, the coalition team will need to determine the best method to prioritize all health issues identified during the assessment process. A structured and democratic process should be employed to prioritize the issues and determine which ones will be addressed in the community health improvement plan. It does not matter which method is selected. Coalitions should opt for the one that makes the most sense to the members, making sure it is documented in the final report.

The first step in the prioritization process is to determine the set of criteria to be used in the prioritization process. The criteria should have the consensus of the coalition members and developing criteria will avoid subjectivity among the members. One example of prioritization criteria developed by the American Heart Association includes:

- Magnitude of the problem
- Severity of the problem
- Need among vulnerable populations
- Community's capacity and willingness to act on the issue
- Ability to have a measurable impact on the issue

- Availability of community resources
- Existing interventions focused on the issue
- Whether the issue is a root cause of other problems
- Trending health concerns in the community
- Importance of each problem to community members

(American Hospital Association)

It is a good practice for the coalition members to review the identified assets and interventions before commencing the prioritization process. Prioritization methods range from being relatively simple to complex. The National Association of City and County Health Officials (NACCHO) developed "First Things First: Prioritizing Health Problems" to provide health departments with a guide on the decision-making process of which method to use. **Table 20-1** provides a brief description of NACCHO's prioritization techniques.

After all of the health issues or problems have been prioritized and the final set for interventions has been decided, it will be necessary to indicate and justify why some of

Table 20-1 National Association of City and County Health Officials (NACCHO) Prioritization Techniques

NACCHO Prioritization Techniques	
Multi-Voting Technique	Good technique to use when many issues have been identified and the list needs to be narrowed down.
Strategy Grids	Utilizes only two select, broad criteria to categorize and prioritize through use of a four-quadrant grid.
Nominal Group Technique	The Nominal Group Technique (NGT) priorities are developed as a result of brainstorming, list generation, and anonymous ranking. Many groups also use the multi-voting technique in combination with the NGT to reduce the list generated and in lieu of the anonymous ranking.
Hanlon Method	A complex method developed by JJ Hanlon. It provides a rating method of the health problems based on defined criteria and feasibility factors.
Prioritization Matrix	A complex method that utilizes weighted criteria and ratings by the team to determine priority scores of health needs.

Data from National Association of County and City Health Officials. (n.d.) *First things first: Prioritizing Health Problems.*

the health issues will not be addressed in the improvement planning process.

Collaboration Through Direction, Alignment, and Commitment

To enhance the success of building a **healthy community**, all persons and all sectors will need to know the direction of the process. They need to be informed and take ownership in the areas in which they can see **alignment** with their personal, family, and organizational goals and values. The alignment will create commitment, collaboration, and dedication to achieving a healthy community as illustrated in **Figure 20-5**.

More information on the various community health needs assessment models is available in Chapter 23.

Conclusion

Public health departments will need to take the lead in the community health needs assessment and recognize that it must be done with the participation and support of the community it serves. They need to be able to define the community and identify its assets and challenges. To accomplish this, they need to be able to identify, engage, support, and develop relationships with stakeholders, those who possess the power to make change as well as those who possess enthusiasm and commitment to improve the health status within their community.

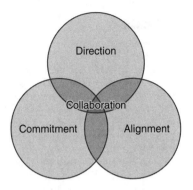

Figure 20-5 Direction, Alignment, Commitment, Collaboration.

Modified from the Center for Creative Leadership, "Direction + Alignment + Commitment (DAC) = Leadership", retrieved from https://www.ccl.org/articles/leading-effectively-articles/make-leadership-happen-2/

Given the limited resources available, it is crucial to make data-driven decisions prior to embarking on new interventions or policies. Data collection and analysis are the primary and key elements of the assessment process. These include both quantitative and qualitative collection efforts.

The importance of sharing the results of the assessment process and gathering feedback from those who are impacted and those who can have an impact cannot be overlooked. The CHS will need the interpersonal skills, communication skills, and listening skills to be able to articulate the findings and garner feedback. The CHS needs to be seen as a credible and trusted source of information within the community as well as a motivating force to move the assessment findings into improvement action plans for building a healthy community.

Discussion Questions

1. Which of the various skills do you believe is the most important for a CHS to possess when engaging in the assessment process and why?
2. Discuss specific communication methods for keeping each of the four groups or quadrants of stakeholders informed.
3. What are three ways or sources of both quantitative and qualitative data?
4. What are possible solutions or alternatives when the public health leader does not possess the necessary skills and abilities of a CHS? Who else can fill this role in the community?

References

American Hospital Association, Association for Community Health Improvement *"Community health assessment toolkit"* https://www.healthycommunities.org/resources/community-health-assessment-toolkit

Barnes, M and Schmitz. 2016. *Community engagement matters (now more than ever)* Stanford Social Innovation Review.

Clark, M. J., Cary, S., Diemert, M. S., Ceballos, R., Sifuentes, M., Atteberry, F. V., & Trieu, S. (2003). Involving communities in community assessment. *Public Health Nursing, 20*(6), 456–463.

Community Tool Box https://ctb.ku.edu/en/table-of-contents/assessment/assessing-community-needs-and-resources/windshield-walking-surveys/powerpoint

Dictionary.com. Accessed July 2019.

Jayanthi, M., & Nelson, J. S. (2002). *Savvy decision making: An administrator's guide to using focus groups in schools.* Thousand Oaks, CA: Corwin Press.

Kaiser Permanente 2015. *Community health needs assessment toolkit Part II: Completing the CHNA report.* MindTools.com.

National Association of County and City Health Officials. (n.d.) *First things first: Prioritizing Health Problems.*

Owen, S. (2001). The practical methodology and ethical dilemmas of conducting focus groups with vulnerable clients. *Journal of Advanced Nursing, 36*(5), 652–658.

Public Health Accreditation Board 2019. http://phaboard.org

Stoto, M. A., and Smith, C. Ryan 2015. *Community health needs assessments – Aligning the interests of public health and the health care delivery system to improve population health.* Discussion Paper, Institute of Medicine, Washington, DC. https://nam.edu/perspectives-2015-community-health-needs-assessments-aligning-the-interests-of-public-health-and-the-health-care-delivery-system-to-improve-population-health/

The Patient and Affordable Care Act: Pub Law 111–148, Section 9007, 2010.

Urden, L. D. (2003). Don't forget to ask: Using focus groups to assess outcomes. *Outcomes Management, 7*(1), 1–3.

U.S. Department of Health and Human Services. ND. *Public health 3.0 A call to action to create a 21st century public health infrastructure.*

Webb, B. (2002). Using focus groups as a research method: A personal experience. *Journal of Nursing Management, 10*(1), 27–35.

Additional Reading

- Assessing and Addressing Community Health Needs https://www.chausa.org/docs/default-source/community-benefit/2015-cbassesmentguide.pdf?sfvrsn=2
- Asset-Based Community Development Institute https://resources.depaul.edu/abcd-institute/Pages/default.aspx
- Centers for Disease Control and Prevention. (2018). Health impact in 5 years (HI-5) Retrieved from https://www.cdc.gov/policy/hst/hi5
- Collective Impact Forum – Community Engagement Toolkit Version 2.2, March 2017.
- Kaiser Permanente. (n.d.). Community Commons—Community Health Needs Assessment Toolkit http://assessment.communitycommons.org/CHNA
- Centers for Disease Control and Prevention. (2015). Community Health Navigator. Retrieved from http://www.cdc.gov/chinav/
- County Health Rankings & Roadmaps. (n.d.). What works for health. Retrieved from www.countyhealthrankings.org/roadmaps/what-works-for-health

CHAPTER 21

Program Planning Models and Theories

Osayande Agbonlahor, MD, MPH
Governor Ameh, BDS
Joseph N. Inungu, MD, DrPH, MPH

LEARNING OBJECTIVES

At the end of this chapter, readers will be able to:

1. Appreciate the need for health theories in the design of health programs and interventions in rural health.
2. Understand the health theories described and the associated constructs.
3. Appreciate the similarities and differences in the constructs of various theories described.
4. Identify instances where application of individual or collective theories are desirable.
5. Recognize the limitations of the theories described.

KEY TERMS

Diffusion of Innovation Theory, Precede-
    Proceed, MAPP
Health Belief Model (HBM)
MAP-IT
Model
Precede-Proceed, Mobilizing for Action
    through Planning and Partnerships
    (MAPP)
Theory
Transtheoretical Model

CHAPTER OVERVIEW

At the inception of any rural health community intervention, public health practitioners principally ask themselves two key questions that guide in framing the scope of the problem and increasing the effectiveness of program design, implementation, and evaluation. The questions that are generally asked include:

- What model can a given community use to improve the health of a rural community?
- Which theories and models have other successful, culturally sensitive interventions used for similar community and rural environments?

The answers to this pattern of questions drive rural health intervention design and implementation. Models and theories are used in program planning to identify, understand, and explain health behavior, provide a framework for program planners in selecting constructs, and guide the development and implementation of interventions. Theories provide a framework for generating testable hypotheses and integrating empirical evidence and, over time, a road map for the design and implementation of intervention strategies (Rothman, 2009), while models are a mixture of ideas or concepts taken from any number of theories and used together (Hayden, 2009).

A planning **model** is different from a **theory**. A theory is a set of testable propositions that help us to explain and predict phenomena, such as health behaviors. Planning models are not composed of a set of testable propositions, they serve as a blueprint for building and improving intervention programs. Planning models are much broader than theories, and they, in fact, are inclusive of theories. Theories are used in attempts to change the phenomena that they help us to understand, as it is widely believed that theory-based interventions are more successful than those that are not based on theory (Crosby & Noar, 2011).

In identifying a model or theory to guide rural health intervention, program planners must take into consideration the multifarious range of factors that can influence an individual's or community's desire and/or ability for positive behavioral change. Factors such as the community being served, specific public health issue being addressed, sociocultural and economic context must be considered, as different theories or models are best suited for different situations, individuals, and communities.

No one model or theory is perfect or dominates research and practice; each individual or community requires effective interventions tailored specifically to their needs. In addressing rural community needs, interventions use the framework of existing models and theories to design and implement culturally sensitive programs resulting in positive community behavior.

This chapter discusses six selected existing models and theories that are needed to guide the design of rural health interventions. These include: **Diffusion of Innovation Theory, Precede-Proceed, MAPP, Health Belief Model**, Transtheoretical Model, and MAP-IT.

Need for Rural Tailored Health Programs

Across the spheres of rurality, a wide range of factors will determine the design and implementation of public health programs. The rural urban dichotomy is not just reflected in the way of living, pattern of settlement, or infrastructural deficit; it is evident across a list of social inequalities and health disparities. To assume, therefore, that similar health promotion models and theories will fit both settings, may result in shortened expectations or desired intentions.

Rural populations are not only culturally heterogeneous and diverse but they also occupy large geographic expanses in the United States and reflect varying demographics (Douthit, Kiv, Dwolatzky & Biswas, 2015). Mitigating factors faced by healthcare providers and patients are likewise different from urban areas. Economic factors, low literacy levels, cultural and social delineations, neglect by legislators and the sheer isolation from living in remote rural areas all conspire to impede rural Americans in their quest for better living (NRHA, 2020). Because of these challenges, rural health promotion programs must be tailored to the needs of individual communities, using evidence-based health promotion models and theories.

However, many theories and models with underlying constructs, which are generally suited for urban populations with individual autonomy and purpose, have limited applications in the rural populations with smaller, more traditional communities. (Elder et al., 2001). Additionally, certain constructs of theories require remarkable attention to detail in the execution and measurement of impact. Rural communities with a large unlettered population, and limited measurement tools may fall short in perfect delivery of the intended health promotion programs. Therefore, health planners must examine the peculiarities of individual communities and health needs before deploying evidence-based theory informed interventions.

Models or theories discussed in this chapter have been shown to provide a successful framework for designing culturally sensitive rural health programs in the United States.

Diffusion of Innovation Theory

Diffusion of Innovation (DOI) Theory is a research theory that describes how a novel, innovative idea, product, or positive health behavior (Innovation) spreads through a community or social structure (Diffusion). The theory, developed by E. M. Rogers in 1962, is one of the oldest social science theories and has its origin in communication and social marketing. However, the framework has recently been popularly adopted in public health and medical care in achieving effective disease prevention. **Diffusion of Innovation theory** has been applied in different fields to understand how people translate new ideas, such as new treatment skills, disease knowledge or educational strategies, into real-world applications (Shin-Yu Lien & Jiang, 2016). It has also been applied to improve effective outcomes by disseminating intervention strategies and encouraging the application of high-technology media and mass media with rapid transmission characteristics to meet the demand of health needs, such as diabetes care and other chronic diseases in rural communities and globally (Shin-Yu Lien & Jiang, 2016) (De Civita & Dasgupta, 2007).

DOI identifies several factors that influence how quickly an idea or behavior is adopted. There are four elements of diffusion that influence the adoption of a new idea, and they include: (1) characteristics of the innovation, (2) communication channels, (3) time, and (4) social system. Adoption of a new idea means that an individual or community does something differently from what they had done previously (i.e., purchase or use a new product, and/or perform a new behavior). This theory highlights the uncertainties associated with new behaviors and helps public health program implementers consider ways to resolve these uncertainties.

In simple terms, the diffusion of innovation refers to the process that occurs as people adopt a new idea, product, practice, philosophy, and so on. Adoption of a new idea, product, or positive health behavior is a process rather than a simultaneous action, with some individuals and communities more disposed to new ideas. Rogers mapped out this process, stressing that in most cases, an initial few are open to the new idea and adopt its use. As these early innovators "spread the word," more and more people become open to it, which leads to development of a critical mass. Over time, the innovative idea or product becomes diffused among the population until a saturation point is achieved. Rogers (Kaminski, 2011) distinguished five categories of adopters of an innovation: innovators, early adopters, early majority, late majority, and laggards. **Figure 21-1** shows the adopter categories. They are:

1. **Innovators:** These are the pioneers, risk takers, the first to be interested in testing

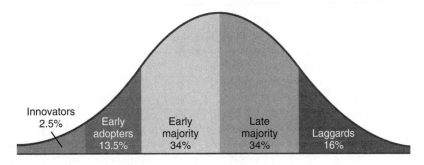

Figure 21-1 The Diffusion of Innovations (DOI) Theory.

Shin-Yu Lien, A., & Jiang, Y.-D. (2017). Integration of diffusion of innovation theory into diabetes care. *Journal of Diabetes Investigation, 8*(3), 259–260.

and developing new ideas. The individuals with the most courage to adopt innovation. Marginal or zero intervention or promotional efforts are required to convince them of the need for positive change. They make up 2.5% of the social system.

2. **Early Adopters:** These are stakeholders and opinion leaders. They seek information and advice from pioneers. They are aware of the need to change and are receptive to adopting new ideas. Strategies to appeal to this population include the provision of how-to manuals and information sheets on implementation. They make up 13.5% of the social system.

3. **Early Majority:** These people are rarely leaders, more risk-averse, but they have a higher interest in and adopt new ideas before the average person. They observe close associates, successful experiences, and typically need to see evidence that the innovation works before they are willing to adopt it. Strategies to appeal to this population include evidence of successful interventions, data-driven messages showing the effectiveness of the innovation. They make up 34% of the social system.

4. **Late Majority:** These people are more conservative, skeptical of change, and cautious. They tend to only adopt an innovation after it has been safely tried by the majority, and in most cases, are still reluctant regardless. Strategies to appeal to this population include information on how many other people have tried the innovation and have adopted it successfully. They make up 34% of the social system.

5. **Laggards:** These people are very conservative or vulnerable groups with limited information and unstable incomes. They are very skeptical of new ideas and change and are the hardest group to bring on board. Strategies to appeal to this population include fear-based appeals and pressure from other adopter groups. They make up 16% of the social system.

The five main factors influencing the adoption of an innovation (i.e., new health product or positive health behavior) shown in **Table 21-1** include:

1. Relative Advantage: Refers to how much better, time-saving, and cost-effective an innovation is compared with the traditional ideas or product it replaces.

2. Compatibility: Refers to the consistency of the innovation with the needs, values, and experiences of the target population.

Table 21-1 Factors Influencing Innovation Adoption

Relative Advantage	Compatibility	Complexity	Trialability	Observability
How much better?	Does it work for me?	Is it simple to understand?	Can I test it out?	How visible is it?
A novel product or idea that saves time and cost is of the most appeal to adopters	Word of mouth, radio discussions increase familiarity and appeal of new product	Mass media and social advertising increases understanding of innovation	Testing a product or watching someone on tv or the Internet go through the experience and can influence use	Seeing in person or hearing someone on tv or social media speak positively about a product and can positively influence use

3. Complexity: Refers to the simplicity or difficulty of understanding and using the innovation.
4. Trialability: Refers to the degree to which the innovation can be experimented on or tested before adoption.
5. Observability: Refers to the degree of visibility and prominence of innovations producing tangible results.

Characteristics of Innovation

It is important to emphasize the importance of community leaders (opinion leaders) as channels of communication in rural communities in the United States. As trusted members of the community, they can increase the diffusion of an innovation or prevent it. As such, it is critical for program planners to share information about new ideas, educate them about the innovation, and ensure their support is gained before attempting to apply the framework of the diffusion of innovation theory to promote positive behavioral change. Mass media, specifically radio and tv, are important channels of communication in rural communities. Also, understanding the rural environment in which the intervention is planned and its constituents are important, as connecting the laggards/skeptics to the early adopters and/or innovators is crucial to the success of the program and promoting diffusion.

The diffusion of innovation theory has been used successfully in reducing the incidence of chronic diseases in communities in the United States and globally (Owen, Glanz, Sallis, & Kelder, 2006) (Shin-Yu Lien & Jiang, 2016). As such, it is suitable as an intervention framework depending on the target community and time required, for future program implementers and public health practitioners to adopt in promoting positive healthy behavioral change in rural communities in the United States. The most successful adoption of the public health programs will result from understanding the target population and the factors influencing their rate of adoption, and successfully incorporating the community leaders in diffusion strategies.

Limitations of Diffusion of Innovation Theory

1. It does not encourage a participatory approach to adoption of a public health program.
2. It is more suitable for interventions involving adoption of behaviors rather than cessation or decreasing negative behavior.
3. It does not take into consideration an individual's resources or social system.
4. Sustained change depends on how fast the new behavior can be obtained or observed, with individuals more likely to relapse if tangible outcome or benefit from the new behavior is not seen.
5. The theory did not originate from public health and was not developed explicitly to adopt new behavior or health innovations.

PRECEDE-PROCEED Model

The PRECEDE-PROCEED model is a comprehensive evaluation framework for assessing health needs for designing and implementing public health promotion or disease prevention programs. The PRECEDE-PROCEED Model focuses on the community as the nucleus for health promotion. In this framework, health behavior is believed to be influenced by both individual and environmental factors. When determining the utility of the PRECEDE-PROCEED model as an intervention framework for health promotion or disease prevention programs, it is important to consider the target population, needs of the population, and the resources available to support successful implementation. In the case of rural communities in the United States, this model can be very useful, as it emphasizes community mobilization and engagement, which is critical in having long-lasting, positive behavioral and health outcome in rural areas, as citizens feel an affinity and community toward their local area.

PRECEDE-PROCEED are both acronyms with PRECEDE standing for Predisposing, Reinforcing, and Enabling Constructs in Educational/Environmental Diagnosis and Evaluation. PROCEED stands for Policy, Regulatory, and Organizational Constructs in Educational and Environmental Development. The model literally breaks down the process of planning and implementing an intervention, with "PRECEDE" representing the process that leads up to an intervention, and "PROCEED" describes how to initiate and evaluate the intervention.

The PRECEDE-PROCEED model has eight phases (4 each) shown below in Figure 21-2 that assess community factors, identify desired outcomes, and program implementation. The phases include: PRECEDE

- **Social Assessment.** This phase involves identifying the needs, and social problems of a given population that affect quality of life and identify the desired results. Community organization and mobilization are the goals for this phase, and this is achieved by developing a planning community and conducting focus groups, surveys, interviews, and community forums to gain a good understanding of the target population, their strengths and weaknesses, resources and attitudes toward change.

- **Epidemiological, Behavioral, and Environmental Assessment.** This phase involves identifying the behavioral, genetic,

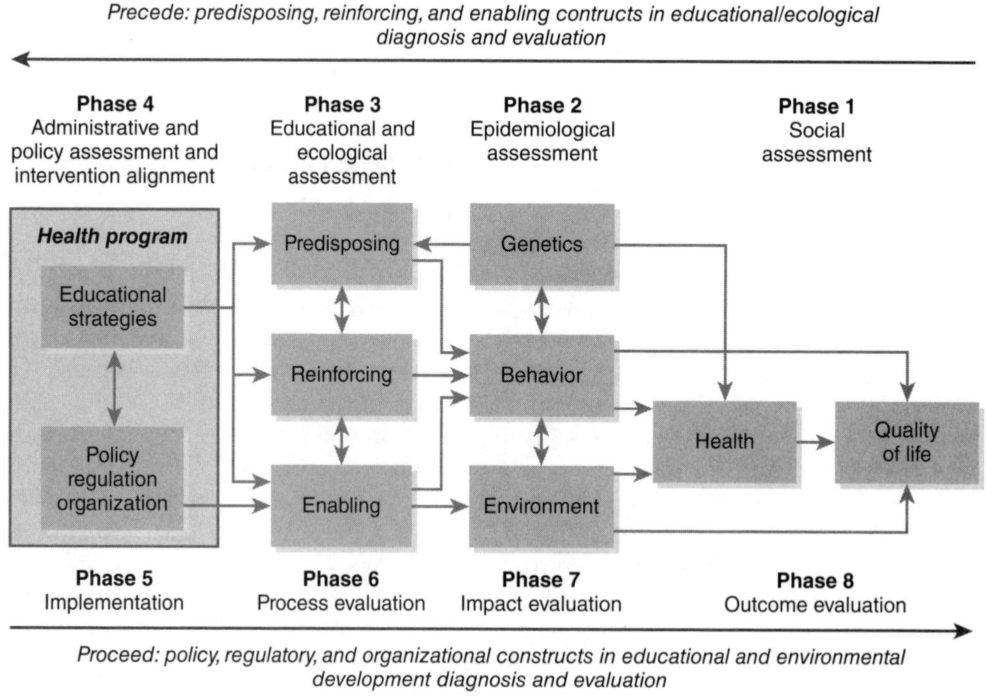

Precede: predisposing, reinforcing, and enabling contructs in educational/ecological diagnosis and evaluation

Figure 21-2 The PRECEDE-PROCEED Model.

Reproduced from Porter, C. M. (2016). Revisiting Precede-Proceed: A leading model for ecological and ethical health promotion. *Health Education Journal, 75*(6), 753–764.

and environmental determinants most likely to influence the identified priority health problems. It may include collecting original data or secondary data through medical and administrative records, state, and national health surveys. It is important in this phase to assess how the behavior of an individual can directly affect the health of another individual (e.g., second-hand smoking or parents of teens who keep alcohol accessible at home), and it is also important to understand how the actions of community leaders affect the environment of the individuals at risk (e.g., policies that restrict access to e-cigarettes for teens).

- **Educational and Ecological Assessment.** After identifying the behavioral and environmental determinants that influence health outcomes in the community, program planners can select and analyze factors that predispose, reinforce, and enable the behaviors and lifestyle. If modified, these factors can result in sustainable positive behavioral change.

Predisposing factors refers to the characteristics of an individual such as beliefs, values, and attitudes that influence behavior. Enabling factors refers to the characteristics of the environment such as availability and access to resources and services that influence specific behavioral and skills attainment, and, reinforcing factors refers to the rewards or punishments such as peer and social support, which strengthen or weaken motivation for a behavior.

- **Administrative and Policy Assessment and Intervention Alignment.** This phase involves assessing the compatibility of program goals and objectives with community goals, resources available, budget development and allocation, policies that could facilitate or hinder program development, and implementation. Program planners must identify the policies

that influence implementation and match appropriate interventions that result in sustained change. They must focus on the macro (organizational and environmental systems) and micro levels (individual, peer, and family) of alignment between the assessment and selection of determinants (Green & Kreuter, 2005).

PROCEED

- *Implementation of the Program.* This phase may involve designing the intervention, assessing availability, and like the name implies, implementing program interventions. In this phase, program planners must ensure that data collection plans are in place for evaluating the program

- *Process Evaluation.* This phase involves determining the extent to which the program reaches the target community and achieves desired goals and objectives, modifications needed to improve the program, and the extent to which protocol was implemented accordingly.

- *Impact Evaluation.* This phase is used to assess any change in behavior due to successful implementation of program intervention. Program effectiveness is assessed with regard to changes in predisposing, reinforcing, and enabling factors, as well as in behavioral and environmental factors.

- *Outcome Evaluation.* This phase involves measuring the effectiveness of the program in increasing positive behavior or decreasing negative behavior resulting in a significant positive effect on the health and quality of life of the community.

The PRECEDE-PROCEED model has been shown to be successful in communities in the United States and globally (Binkley & Johnson, 2013) (Li, et al., 2009), and consequently, can be a good model framework to use for program planners when designing culturally sensitive interventions in rural and urban communities.

How Do You Use PRECEDE-PROCEED? An example of Addressing Childhood Obesity

This nine-step model puzzles people when they first look at the model. The arrows point from left to right, yet the steps are numbered from right to left. This is actually a key point of the planning model. This layout necessitates that you plan "backward"—working from the end goal to produce objectives and sub-objectives that, if met, will culminate in the realization of that goal (Crosby & Noah, 2011).

Phase 1

Defining the Outcome. Program planners focus on community needs and discovering the most important and/or urgent health issue as determined by the community. This could range from lack of access to health care, homelessness, obesity, poverty, poor water, and air quality, and so on. Program planners can do this by conducting one of the following: community surveys, phone interviews, face-to-face interviews, questionnaires, and focus groups. Community member involvement (which includes decision making and providing significant input) in all phases of the PRECEDE-PROCEED model is crucial for the successful use of this model in public health intervention programs.

Phase 2

Identifying the Issue. It is important for program planners to pinpoint issues and factors with the greatest influence on the outcome identified in Phase 1. For example, if, after conducting a community survey and a face-to-face interview, addressing obesity in children is identified as the most urgent health issue in a rural community, program planners in this phase will then choose to: (1) Focus on issues directly related to the outcome they are seeking e.g., building food banks and food pantries to prevent obesity and address food insecurity. (2) Focus on the issues indirectly related to the outcome, e.g., implementing mandated nutrition standards for children's school meals, vending machines in schools, and physical education requirements to control for obesity in children in the community. (3) Identify the behavioral, lifestyle, and/or environmental factors that influence the issue or outcome.

Using the example of the outcome of addressing obesity in children in a rural community, it is important for program planners to identify which behaviors, lifestyles, or environmental factors to focus on in addressing obesity, and this is where critical thinking and analysis comes in. Questions such as "What are children in the community eating?", "What are the factors in the environment that lead to, maintain, or prevent addressing childhood obesity in the community?", and "Why?" These questions help the program planner to narrow down the factors that influence childhood obesity, and this stage is crucial as the majority of public health intervention is designed to change behavior, lifestyle, and environmental determinants of health. Changes in these factors and issues identified in Phase 2 result in the attainment of the outcome identified in Phase 1.

It is known that behavioral factors (poor diet, physical inactivity, lack of self-control of satiety) and environmental factors (family, neighborhood, school, politics, and economy) working in combination, increase the risks of childhood obesity in a rural community. A realistic assessment is made by program planners in this stage to measure the extent of change in caloric imbalance, lifestyle patterns, and self-control/self-efficacy required to address childhood obesity in the community.

To limit the chances in this phase of selecting ineffective behaviors to change the intervention, the possible behavioral influences on childhood obesity are identified by program planners, and one or more selected for change that are most strongly related to obesity; while paying close attention to possible compensatory efforts, with some evidence that a) the behaviors are amendable to change; b) there are mediating variables for why people show these behaviors; c) changes in the behavior can be measured to evaluate the outcome (Baranowski, Cerin, & Baranowski, 2009). Program planners then address how the intervention channels (e.g., the elementary school) influences the behavior (e.g., foods ordered in school, vending machines), the environment of the channels (e.g., proximity of the schools to fast food stores, lack of sidewalks or safe bike trials to walk or bike to the store), and especially the common behaviors exhibited in this environment (Baranowski, Cerin, & Baranowski, 2009).

Phase 3

Examining Predisposing, Enabling, and Reinforcing Factors that Influence Behavior and Responses to the Environment. In this phase, program planners begin by examining the influence of predisposing factors such as knowledge, attitudes, beliefs, and values. For instance, parents who know that obesity increases the risks of type 2 diabetes, asthma, bone fractures, and low quality of life in children are more likely to avoid giving them sugar-sweetened beverages and high-calorie dense meals and are more likely to encourage physical activity in their kids. Also, children who have an affinity for sports and athletics are more likely to adopt regular exercise as an integral part of life and so on. These factors can be influenced by implementing educational intervention strategies to increase knowledge and positive attitudes, and as such, program planners may use that in the model after acquiring the knowledge, beliefs, and values of the target community. Enabling factors such as the availability of resources, accessibility of services, government laws, and policies are next examined by program planners.

For example, obese children in schools in near proximity to healthy food stores, are more likely to start eating healthier foods as those are readily available and, more importantly, accessible. Also, implementation of state mandated policies such as the Texas Senate Bill 19 to increase physical activity in elementary schools have been useful in addressing childhood obesity in the state (Kelder, et al., 2009). Taking this into consideration, the program planner devise strategies incorporated into the model that creates environments suitable for physical activity engagement and healthy eating for children in the community. Finally, in this phase, reinforcing factors, such as peer and family support, influence of teachers, pediatricians, and social media are examined by program planners to determine which groups or communication channels are the best to aim intervention toward, so as to effectively reach and sustain healthy-lifestyle behavior change in children in the community.

Phase 4

Examining Administrative and Policy Issues that Can Influence Intervention Outcome. This phase is important as an analysis done by program planners enables them to select, map, and match organizations to the best proposed intervention, and alert an organization to an internal or external policy that needs to be changed for an intervention to proceed effectively. For example, elementary school organizational structures may be hierarchical, democratic, or collaborative. Depending on the rigidity of the structure, the obesity prevention intervention proposed may be easy or difficult to implement; however, such adjustments will need to be made. One of the unique advantages of using a PRECEDE-PROCEED model as an intervention framework is that it allows for adjustments in intervention as a response to community needs and changes in the situation. Organizational procedures, cultures, internal policies (how are employees in the community treated, professional ethics, and so on), and external policies (state laws, community policies, and so on) are examined in this phase to ensure successful implementation of the program. The four phases discussed are part of PRECEED.

Phase 5

Implementation. The majority of the intervention is designed in Stages 3 and 4, based on the findings of analysis. This stage is about setting up and implementing the intervention designed.

Phase 6

Process Evaluation. The first phase of evaluation is performed as intervention is going on. Process evaluation requires answering the question, "Is my program offering the services, my proposed intervention suggested." Using the example of childhood obesity prevention intervention, if the intervention proposed provides food banks three days a week for kids in the rural community, are those services being offered?

Phase 7

Impact Evaluation. This next phase involves program planners answering the question, "How successful are my intervention efforts?" Is the intervention having the desired effect on behavioral patterns, self-efficacy, social and political environment, and increasing healthier lifestyles? The answers to these questions help program planners to evaluate how effective the intervention has been and if it requires any adjustments and modifications.

Phase 8

Outcome Evaluation. This final phase involves program planners answering the question; "Did my intervention result in the outcome identified by the community in phase 1." As an example, intervention programs aimed at addressing childhood obesity may take some time to show long-term health benefits; in this

case, it will be important for program planners to continue to monitor the process and impact evaluations, as these are good predictors for the eventual outcome realization.

Advantages of Using PRECEDE-PROCEED Model

1. Allows the intervention to be monitored and adjusted to respond to community needs and situations
2. Structured as a participatory model and encourages community engagement, incorporating the ideas of the community, and help in decision making
3. Provides a framework for designing, implementing, and evaluating community interventions
4. Incorporates ecological, ethical, administrative, and policy guidelines in its design by examining how they can hinder or shape an intervention

MAPP Model

Mobilization for Action through Planning and Partnerships (MAPP) is a community-driven strategic planning process for improving the health of the community. The MAPP process was developed as a joint project of the National Association of County and City Health Officials (NACCHO) and the Centers for Disease Control and Prevention (CDC). The concept of health that MAPP embraces is that health is not just an absence of disease or medical treatment but must be viewed from a community perspective. MAPP is not an agency-focused assessment process but rather an interactive process that can enhance the performance, efficiency, and effectiveness of local public health systems. MAPP has seven underlying principles that are important to the successful implementation of the model in the community. These principles include:

- *Systems Thinking*. This involves investigating community health issues and systems to create long-term positive change on a community level.
- *Strategic Thinking*. Proactive approach to systems, issues, and decision making.
- *Dialogue*. This encourages all voices of stakeholders to be heard in the MAPP process and the integration of diverse perspective and ideas.
- *Shared Vision*. Having a vision shared by everyone concerned in the MAPP process ensures full approval and ownership, increasing the likelihood of success.
- *Data*. Using evidence-based data rather than beliefs, intuitions, or preconceptions, provides a firm basis for planning and successful implementation.
- *Partnership*. Collaboration is key as it increases the likelihood of success, shared responsibility, and fairness.
- *Celebration of Successes*. This is important as it highlights individual and community achievements, as well as keep everyone motivated.

The MAPP process ensures community participation and as a result, the following individuals and institutions, at a minimum, must be involved in the process and in decision making to assure complete community participation in the process: 1) local and state public health agencies, e.g., health departments, safety inspectors, health boards, human service agencies, and so on, 2) health practitioners, 3) first responders, e.g., EMTs, paramedics, firefighters, and so on, 4) educational institutions, 5) human service organizations, 6) local and state elected or appointed officials, 7) faith-based institutions, 8) community organizations e.g., athletic clubs, youth organizations, rotary services clubs, and so on, 9) local/individual businesses, and 10) community members. The MAPP process is driven by all of their contributions and not solely by public health agencies.

Advantages of Using MAPP Model

1. MAPP model is based on collaboration and partnership among all relevant public health bodies and between the community and public health system, resulting in shared goals and responsibilities.
2. MAPP focuses on strengthening the local public health system.
3. MAPP uses strategic planning, which is important in achieving desired results.
4. MAPP process was developed using information obtained from previous planning efforts.
5. MAPP is a participatory process, which ensures stakeholder involvement in assessment, planning, and implementation.
6. MAPP (using the forces of change assessment) helps the community to anticipate and manage change.
7. MAPP takes a community perspective by the creation of a healthy community as the main goal.

The MAPP model has six phases as shown in **Figure 21-3**, which provide a framework for intervention. These include:

Phase 1

Organize for Success and Partnership Development. The first phase of the MAPP process involves recruiting a core support team (to recruit participants), steering committee (broadly representative of the community and local public health system to guide and oversee the process), and community involvement.

Phase 2

Visioning. The second phase of MAPP involves a collaborative, creative process in which members of the community and the steering committee recruited in Phase 1 work together to develop a shared community vision, with the overarching goal of a healthy

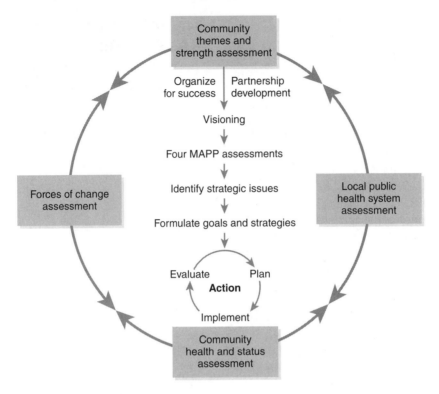

Figure 21-3 The MAPP Model.

Reproduced from NACCHO & CDC. (2000). *A strategic approach to community health improvement: MAPP.*

community. This phase also helps to bringing the community together and build enthusiasm for the intervention process.

Phase 3

The Four Assessments. This phase involves employing four community assessments that yield important information for improving the health of the community. However, these assessments are connected, with the value of its whole four times greater than each individual assessment. As such, conducting all four assessments are important to prevent an incomplete understanding of the factors that affect the local public health system and the community.

- **Community Themes and Strength Assessment.** Aims to fully understand the

health issues that community members feel are most important. Questions such as: "What is important to your community?," "What resources already exist in the community that can be used to improve community health?," and "How do you feel about the community and its health?," are discussed and answered to provide a deep understanding of the issue.

- **Local Public Health System Assessment (LPHSA).** Examines all the elements of the public health system, organizations, and entities that contribute to public health. LPHSA aims to answer the questions: "What are the components, activities, competencies, and capacities of the local public health system?" and "How are essential services being provided to the community." The LPHSA used in the MAPP model was developed by the National Public Health Performance Standards (NPHPS).

- **Community Health Status Assessment.** Examines the health of the community members, community, and quality of life by identifying community health issues of most priority. This assessment aims to answer the questions: "How healthy are the community members?", "What does the health of the community look like?", and "How does the health of the community affect employment, housing, environment, and so on?"

- **Forces of Change Assessment.** This aims to identify novel forces such as technological and legislative changes and their effects on the relationship between the community and its public health system. The assessment aims to answer the questions: "What is happening or might happen in the future that will have an impact on community health?" and "What specific opportunities or threats will result from these situations?" This is crucial as it helps the community to anticipate and manage change adequately.

Phase 4

Identifying and Prioritizing Strategic Issues. This phase involves employing a participatory approach where participants are asked to develop a list in order of the most important issues facing the community. The community and committee can collaboratively examine data obtained from the results of the four assessments in Phase 3 and determine the priority issues that must be addressed to achieve the community-shared vision.

Phase 5

Formulate Goals and Strategies. In this phase, members of the community involved in the MAPP process set goals for each strategic

issue identified in Phase 4. Then broad strategies are formulated to reach these set goals related to the community vision. This will result in a mapped route in the form of strategy statements.

Phase 6

Action Cycle. The action cycle involves planning, implementation, and evaluation of the actions of the community in achieving its set goals, with each of these activities building upon the other. It is seen as a cycle despite this being the final phase of the model; it is not the end of the process, as action is continually evaluated and modified to achieve greater effectiveness.

Implementing the MAPP model can be useful at any time for a community; however, there are circumstances that occur that are uniquely suited to employing the MAPP model instead of other model or theories: this includes:

1. When there has been an issue or crisis previously mishandled. For example, the start of the COVID-19 pandemic tested local and global public health systems and found them wanting in some states and countries, despite the best efforts of those involved. When situations like this occur, they can lead to an increase in community engagement toward a healthier community, calls for restructuring of the public health systems, and for more government funding to be focused on the public health sector as a proactive approach.

2. When there is no money available for public health systems.

3. When health issues surfaces, either in the media or among health practitioners.

4. When there is a government push to reevaluate public health system.

5. It is useful in a rapidly growing community.

6. When there is money available for public health improvement.

How to Conduct a MAPP Model Intervention

Phase 1

Organize for Success and Partnership Development. This phase involves organizing the planning process and developing the planning partnerships. It is the phase in which the MAPP committee (which should be representative of diverse community members and sectors of the community), core support team (convening local or state public health agency responsible for recruiting participants and designing the planning process), and community members. For this phase to be successful the following steps must be taken by program planners:

1. **Determine the necessity of undertaking the MAPP process by answering the questions:** "Does the community really need the intervention?", "What are the benefits of the MAPP process to the community?", and "What are the potential barriers to the set goals?"
2. **Identify and organize participants.** This step involves consulting with community members about who key participants are, the individuals and groups that should be included in the MAPP committee, and the organizations whose support is critical to the success of the intervention. By offering strong support early on, certain key individuals and/or organizations give the intervention legitimacy in the eyes of the community. Participants involved in the process must be representative of all members of the community, and they are organized in a manner highlighting their roles and responsibility.
3. **Design the planning process.** The MAPP committee that is chosen will then establish the ground rules for the process and design the process through which the planning for action will occur. This process aims to answer the questions: "What will the planning process entail?", "How

long will it take?", "How long do you have?", "Who is responsible for each task?", "What results are we expecting?" and "How would we know when we are done?"

4. **Make an assessment of resources needed such as money (for travel costs, printing, supplies, consultant fees, and so on), meeting space, transportation, reliable volunteers, and so on, for the planning process.** In some communities, all resources required for the intervention are readily available and in some communities they are not. Therefore, it is important to know what the community has and where you will get what you need before beginning. Approaching private and public funders for the intervention may be a solution, among others.
5. **Conduct a readiness assessment to ensure community readiness for successful implementation of the intervention.** This stage helps determine if all of the elements needed for successful intervention are in place by examining how much members of the community know and care about the issue at hand, how much they know about the benefits of the intervention proposed, and how well organizations and individuals effectively collaborate with another.
6. **Develop a work plan** and guiding assumptions that will help you determine how well the process will be managed by laying out what has to be done in a specific timeline to complete the planning process.

Phase 2

Visioning. Vision and value statements are important as they provide purpose and guidance for participants in the MAPP model to collectively achieve a shared community vision. This process can result in community unity toward striving for MAPP intervention success. For this phase to be successful, the following steps must be taken by program planners:

1. Identify other visioning efforts by looking at what has been done in previous community initiatives and connecting them. If other visionary efforts focused on a community approach like you plan to do, you then make the connections and link both efforts. If it relates to only a separate area, you can consider incorporating their efforts and vice versa.

2. Design the visioning process and select an expert facilitator who is perceived in the community as neutral and fair. It is the job of the facilitator to help the visioning group identify shared values and goals that should be included in the final statement. The facilitator is key in the visioning process as the help with conflict resolution among participants.

3. Conduct the visioning process. This stage involves identifying a vision that can be universally agreed upon by all participants; the group also agrees on the shared values that guide vision. Some ways to achieve this involve brainstorming and asking questions such as: "Looking 5-10 years in the future, what would you like to see?" and "What does a healthy community mean to you?"

4. Formulate the vision and values statement based on the results of the other stages.

Phase 3

The Four Assessments. One uniqueness of the MAPP process is its detailed assessment phase focused on collecting and analyzing data for improving community health. For this phase to be successful the following steps must be taken by program planners:

1. **Assessment of community themes and strengths.** Using data collection techniques such as surveys, community forums, focus groups, face-to-face interviews and so on, the MAPP committee are able to determine from the community members what issues they care about, their perception of the community environment, and the resources available.

2. **Assessment of the local public health system.** This is done using the National Public Health Performance Standards Program (NPHPSP) local instrument and examines the state of the local public health system. This assessment aims to answer the question: "Are the Ten Essential Public Health Services being provided by the public health system in the community?"

3. **Assessment of community health status.** The next stage involves again using data collection techniques such as surveys, face-to-face interviews and so on, depending on the target community to assess quality of life and community health. It aims to answer questions such as: "What is the general health status of the community?" and "How does the quality of life affect the health of individuals in the community?"

4. **Assessment of forces of change.** This assessment involves measuring and anticipating the effects economic fluctuations, technology, and population shifts may have on the health of the community. Although they may be some overlap, not all four assessments have to take place at the same time, as such it is important to be orderly, and conduct them in an arrangement that increases the chances of one assessment informing the other, thereby saving time and effort.

Phase 4

Identifying and Prioritizing Strategic Issues. The MAPP process to this point has developed a shared community vision and collected data (through the four assessments). This phase involves analyzing and integrating the results of the four assessments. Systems thinking is employed in this stage to identify the strategic issues that will help the community realize its shared vision. For this phase to be successful, the following steps must be taken by program planners:

1. Identify potential strategic issues by reviewing the results of the four MAPP assessments and information obtained during the visioning process.
2. Develop an understanding of why certain issues are strategic by asking questions such as: "Can something be done about the issue in a cost-effective and reasonable way?" and "Is the issue important in multiple ways?" An understanding can also be gained by considering the findings of the assessments altogether.
3. Determine the consequences of not addressing certain issues by considering the urgency or priority of the issue.
4. Consolidate overlapping or similar issues in an organized manner that can be managed. The final list should include no more than 12 issues. MAPP suggests choosing three to five strategic issues to address.
5. Arrange issues in an orderly list based on priority and/or the most likely to help you achieve your vision. This list becomes the beginning of your action plan as it guides you on what you need done and when.

Phase 5

Formulate Goals and Strategies. The next stage involves deciding what the goals of the intervention are and what you plan to do to achieve them. This stage aims to answer questions such as: "What can I do that will enable me to achieve my goal?" and "What reasonably set goals can I achieve in this issue?" The answers to these questions give you a better understanding of why those issues were chosen initially and what the best strategy is to use. For this phase to be successful, the following steps must be taken by program planners:

1. Create goals related to the identified strategic issues and shared community vision.

2. Generate novel and innovative alternative strategies to help achieve community vision and meet set goals, taking into consideration current strategies in place.
3. Identify and consider potential factors that will hinder implementation, such as technological difficulties, lack of community support, legal or policy guidelines, and insufficient resources. Knowledge of these barriers should not result in elimination of strategy, but this step is done to determine your ability to do what is necessary to overcome such barriers.
4. Explore implementation details by considering actions that need to be taken, key organizations and individuals whose involvement are necessary, resources required, and implementation time.
5. Select and adopt strategies (through formal or informal processes) that are feasible, effective, and a good fit. Questions such as: "Do the strategies work together effectively to achieve a community-shared vision?" and "Will the overall strategy result in long-term positive change?"
6. Draft and adopt the planning report. An individual or small group is tasked with the responsibility of putting together a written documentation communicating the vision, goals, and strategies of the MAPP process to stakeholders, as well as informing the community about the process. This provides a source of reference for future work, and once the MAPP committee has reviewed and modified, if necessary, can be formally adopted as the action plan and can then be implemented.

Phase 6

Action Cycle. The final phase of the MAPP model involves planning, taking, and sustaining action. For this phase to be successful, the following nine steps (divided into three stages) must be taken by program planners:

A. *Planning for Action.* This stage involves the following three steps:

1. **Organization for action by assembling the key participants.** A subcomittee is created to oversee implementation activities, ensure smooth coordination of the process, and prepare the implementation.
2. Develop specific, measurable, relevant, and achievable objectives, as well as establishing accountability by allocating responsibility to an individual or group to achieve a specific objective as it relates to each strategic goal.
3. Generate action plans geared toward achieving outcome objectives and addressing the selected strategies.

B. *Implementation.* This stage involves the following two steps:
   1. Action plans are reviewed for opportunities to coordinate and combine resources, operations, address more than one objective, avoid duplication of services/efforts, and maximize efficiency and effectiveness
   2. Implement and monitor action plan progress. This involves putting action plans in practice in the real world and keeping a thorough and careful documentation of the process, steps, and what is being done.

C. *Evaluation.* This stage involves the following three steps:
   1. Prepare for evaluation through stakeholder engagement. Also take stock and review all community member responses collected during the process, notes of the meetings, names of stakeholders, MAPP committee members and participants as this provide raw material for evaluation, and help in describing the activities to be evaluated.
   2. Design for the evaluations of each strategy/action plan are developed, with evaluation design focus involving methodology, evaluation questions, evaluation action plan, and strategy for reporting results.

3. Assemble and analyze credible evidence-based data to answer the evaluation questions, and after, justify conclusions.
4. Ensure the usage and distribution of evaluation results, and celebrate the successes of the MAPP process.

Health Belief Model

The Health Belief theory, depicted in **Figure 21-4**, is derived from numerous psychological and behavioral theories in an attempt to understand possible reasons for widespread failure of people to accept disease preventive or screening tests for early detection of asymptomatic disease (Rosenstock, 1974). The model posits that health behavior of an individual is premised on (A) the desire to avoid illness or if ill, to get well and (B) the belief that a specific health action will prevent or ameliorate the illness or the belief that a course of action is available to them that would be beneficial in reducing either their susceptibility to or severity of the condition (Janz & Becker, 1984). The constructs of the theory include:

- Perceived Susceptibility: This construct describes the individual's belief about the likelihood of getting a disease or condition. For instance, a woman is likely going to go for a mammogram if she believes that there is a possibility of getting breast cancer.
- Perceived Severity: Feelings about the seriousness of contracting an illness or leaving an already contracted illness untreated varies from person to person. This includes evaluations in both medical and clinical consequences such as death, disability, injuries, and pain. The social consequences that precipitate such feelings are effects on conditions of work, family life, and social relations. The combined concepts of susceptibility and severity make up the construct of the "perceived threat."

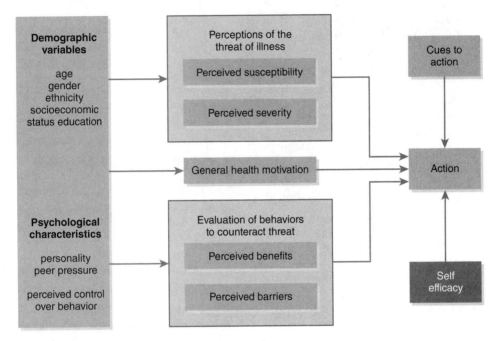

Figure 21-4 Health Belief Model.

Data from Rosenstock, I. M. (1974). Historical origins of the health belief model. *Health Education Monographs, 2*(4), 328–335.

- Perceived Benefits: While the perception of threat is likely to establish a force that may lead to behavior change, a sufficiently threatened individual would not be expected to accept the recommended health action unless it was perceived as feasible and efficacious (Champion & Skinner, 2008). For example, an individual may come to terms with the consequences of having sexually transmitted diseases (STDs) from unprotected sex; his determination to use a condom will likely be influenced by the protection that the condom provides against STDs.

- Perceived Barriers: This construct highlights the belief about the tangible and psychological costs of the recommended action. The potential negative aspects such as cost, potential side effects, inconvenience, and time-consumption may act as impediments to undertaking recommended behaviors. For example, one common cost that may be perceived by

many people is the mistaken belief that being vaccinated for HPV will lead to death or serious illness. Thus, "combined levels of susceptibility and severity provide the energy or force to act and the perception of benefits (less barriers) provide a preferred path of action" (Rosenstock, 1974).

- Cues to Action: This construct is regarded as the required stimulus needed to potentiate the decision to accept a recommended health action. Cues to action may be internal; symptoms such as chest pain, sneezing, or wheezing; or external such as posters, hospital reminders, or watching a celebrity's throat cancer broadcast and how it stemmed from HPV infection. (Salazar, Crosby, Noar, Walker & Diclemente, 2013).

- Self-efficacy: Self-efficacy has been described as the conviction that one can successfully execute the behavior required to produce outcomes (Bandura, 1997). It is the confidence in one's ability to take action or change health-related behavior. People will not try a new behavior unless they are confident that they can perform the behavior.

Numerous Health Belief Model (HBM) studies have been conducted. Janz and Becker (1984) reviewed 18 prospective studies. Analysis of results showed that of the four constructs reviewed (perceived severity, perceived susceptibility, benefits, and barriers), perceived severity was the least consistent predictor and barriers the most consistent. Similarly, Kamran et al., (2015) explored the determinants of patients' adherence to hypertension medication using the health belief model among rural Ardabil, Iran, residents.

Transtheoretical Model of Change

The **transtheoretical model** was developed from comparative review and analysis of psychotherapy and behavioral change theories. The conceptual framework for this model was developed from careful observations of how people quit smoking on their own compared with smokers in professional treatments. The common denominator was that individuals move through a series of stages of change in their efforts to quit (Prochaska & Diclemente, 1983). Identification of the stages allows "stage-matched" interventions to be developed and provides practitioners the reasons for targeting their interventions on those most likely to change. From its earliest application to the smoking cessation program, the model has since evolved to include investigations and applications for a broad range of health and mental health issues, including addictions to alcohol and substance abuse, anxiety and panic disorders, depression, eating disorders and obesity, HIV/AIDS prevention and condom use, mammography, and other cancer screenings (Prochaska, Redding & Evers, 2015).

Core Constructs

The transtheoretical model has stages of change, process of change, decisional balance, and self-efficacy at the heart of its framework.

- *Stages of Change.* The stage construct is important because it is a temporal dimension that represents when specific changes occur (Prochaska et al., 2015). This model proposes that five distinct stages in behavior change exist (**Figure 21-5**). These are: Precontemplation: characterized by unwillingness to make behavior changes anytime soon. Contemplation: intending to change within 6 months. Preparation: Actively planning to change within the next 30 days. Action: making changes. Maintenance: taking steps to sustain changes made and resist temptation of relapse (Prochaska, Redding, Harlow, Rossi & Velicer, 1994). It is instructive to note that the Stages of change are a dynamic process that is often described as a cycle in lieu of linearity. Thus, individuals can relapse or enter the cycle at any given stage before successfully reaching maintenance (Prochaska & Diclemente, 1998).

- *Processes of Change.* The processes of change are covert and overt activities people use to progress through stages. They are stage-matched interventions designed to facilitate progression through various stages. To ensure successful progression through the stages of change, a person's stage of change must first be identified, and then appropriate processes of change should be tailored and applied. For example, consciousness raising has been seen as important for moving an individual from the precontemplation to contemplation stage. The 10 processes of change (as shown in **Table 21-2**) are consciousness raising, dramatic relief, self-reevaluation, environmental reevaluation, self-liberation, social liberation, counterconditioning, stimulus control, reinforcement management, and helping relationships.

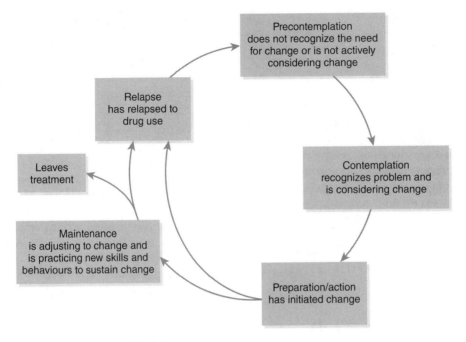

Figure 21-5 Transtheoretical Model.

Data from Prochaska, J. O., & Velicer, W. F. (1997). The transtheoretical model of health behavior change. *American Journal of Health Promotion, 12*(1), 38–48.

Description of the Processes of Change

Cognitive processes such as consciousness raising, dramatic relief, environmental reevaluation, and self-evaluation tend to be used in the early stages (Prochaska et al., 2008). The later stages of preparation to maintenance, self-liberation, counter conditioning, helping relationships, reinforcement management, and stimulus control are commonly applied. Social liberation has not been associated with a specific stage movement. (Prochaska et al., 2008).

- *Decisional Balance.* Adapted from the work Janis and Mann (1977), decisional balance refers to the relative weight given to the pros and cons of changing behavior. Several studies have allied decision balance construct with the stage of change. Increasing the pros and decreasing the cons of making behavior change underscores the progression from precontemplation to contemplation stage

and shifts the decision balance in favor of behavior change (Prochaska & Velicer, 1997; Prochaska et al., 1994).

- *Self-efficacy.* This construct consists of two components: confidence and temptation (Diclemente, Crosby & Salazar, 2013). Confidence describes an individual's perceived ability to cope with a high-risk situation without relapsing to unhealthy behaviors. It is the principal construct in self-efficacy. The amount of confidence that influences an individual to change behavior is directly correlated with stage. Temptation, the other construct upon which self-efficacy stands describes the intensity of urge to engage in a specific behavior when confronted with challenging situations. The interaction of these two constructs determines the eventual behavior adoption or change. High confidence and low temptation interact to enhance the individual's self-efficacy to a

Table 21-2 Transtheoretical Model Process of Change

Processes of Change	Definition	Examples
Consciousness	Increasing awareness and information about health behavior adherence	Education Brochures, Online Materials, Behavior
Dramatic Relief	Experiencing strong negative emotions that come along with not practicing healthy behaviors	Allowing time to talk about recent life changes, Personal testimonials
Environmental Reevaluation	Realizing the impact that one's healthy behaviors has on other people	Asking others about their feelings about a person's behavior
Self-Reevaluation	Emotional and cognitive reappraisal of values and self-image related to healthy behaviors	Value Clarification, personal narratives
Reinforcement Management	Increasing intrinsic and extrinsic rewards for adopting healthy behaviors	Self-rewards, Overt and covert reinforcement
Counterconditioning	Relaxation or desensitization exercises, or replacement of unhealthy behaviors with healthy substitutes.	Positive statements, Nicotine replacement therapy for cigarette smokers
Stimulus Control	Adding cues or reminders to adhere to the health behavior adoption	Avoiding high-risk cues, posting notes, Planning ahead

Adapted from Prochaska, J. M., Prochaska, J. O., & Johnson, S. S. (2006). Assessing readiness for adherence to treatment. In W. T. O'Donohue & E. R. Levensky (Eds.), *Promoting adherence: A practical handbook for healthcare providers* (pp. 35–46). Thousand Oaks, CA: Sage.

lasting behavior change. Conversely, the reduced confidence and high temptation may influence the individual, negatively resulting in relapse.

Pullen & Walker (2002) applied the theory in examining adherence to U.S. dietary guidelines among older rural American women. Similarly, Hawkins et al., (2001) surveyed overweight and obese African American women to determine whether the transtheoretical stages of the change model was generalizable to weight loss intention among. Schorling (1995) analyzed the smoking behavior of rural African American smokers and concluded that 51% of respondents were in precontemplation stage, 28% in contemplation stage, 17% in the preparation stage, and 4% in the action stage.

MAP-IT Model

The process of creating a healthy community is a collective responsibility, which often requires time, effort, and dedication. The **MAP-IT** tool provides a guide to health professionals and community stakeholders. Adapted from the United States Department of Health and Human Services, this tool is intended to help communities plan and evaluate public health interventions that aim to address Healthy People 2020 objectives. It leverages existing structures and evokes generalized community participation in addressing the health issues of the community. The guide recommends that you MAP-IT (Mobilize, Assess, Plan Implement and Track). This step-by-step approach (**Table 21-3**) will help individuals

Table 21-3 MAP-IT Model

M	Mobilize key individuals and organizations who care about the health of the community into a coalition.
A	Assess community needs, strengths, and resources to address the targeted issue.
P	Plan your approach and create an action plan with concrete steps to achieve the vision of the coalition.
I	Implement your plan using concrete action steps that can be monitored and will make a difference.
T	Track your progress over time.

Department of Health and Human Services. (2001, February). *Healthy people in healthy communities*. Washington, DC: U.S. Government Printing Office.

and communities appreciate and remember the specific steps to be taken and in what order. However, there is no "singular" path in following the recommended approach as the needs of communities are diverse and some of these steps may need to be taken multiple times. (Guidry, Vischi, Han & Passons, 2001)

How to Use the MAP-IT Approach

1. *Mobilize*

Begin by mobilizing key individuals and organizations into forming a coalition. In most communities, there are healthcare centers and government agencies that routinely provide health services. Coalitions also exist to address concerns of the communities such as security and community development. These groups typically have members with diverse interests and resources that can be pulled to address health concerns of the community. It is generally easier to engage potential coalition members around issues that are of special concern to the community. HIV/AIDS, substance abuse, maternal and child health, teenage pregnancy, and domestic violence are common rallying points for community coalitions. (Guidry, 2001). In order to build an effective and thriving coalition, it is often advisable to work with specific individuals and organizations over a period of time to promote their interests and ensure commitment to work with you and others in the coalition.

Individuals: As with many organizations in the health sector, effective coalitions are built around the core of certain individuals with demonstrable commitment. Members of a coalition are more eager to work when they are in sectors that directly affect their lives. When a coalition has its members with similar passion, zest, energy, and willingness to collaborate with each other, success is almost certain.

Organizations: Many community organizations such as hospitals, clinics, religious institutions, schools, businesses, community unions, and groups command substantial respect and provide valuable resources to the community. Similarly, several individuals in effective coalitions are members of these organizations within the community. Therefore, it is important to liaise with them to mobilize resources in furthering the action plan.

It is important to note that sustaining the commitment of individuals and groups in any coalition is vital in achieving the set goals. A recommended way is to create and share a vision that originates from the community's most important needs, values, and goals (USHDDS, n.d.).

The vision should be descriptive of the coalition's ideals of how the community should be and must equally represent the goals and values of the members of the coalition.

2. *Assess Community Needs and Resources*

To ensure that the priorities of a community are met, it is always best to first determine the health issues of greatest importance to the communities and the resources available to help address these health issues.

Assessment not only helps to uncover the needs and resources of the program but will also help you understand how to utilize resources that are already available to your program. (Buns, Pettitt & Blanton, 2017). The second step of MAP-IT aims to determine the real needs of the community as opposed to what people assume them to be and provides a sense of what is realistically attainable given the strengths and resources that can be mobilized. The coalition members can then set priorities by identifying what community members and key stakeholders see as the most important issues. As coalition members work together to set priorities and allocate resources, their interest grows and they are far more likely to continue to participate in the process and to achieve measurable results.

Data gathering and evaluation: Data gathering is a crucial process in the design of health programs. Whenever possible, gather and evaluate available information about the predominant health issues in a community. Data can be collected from the state, county, or city. In some instances, these data may not be readily available. When this is the case, it will be incumbent upon you to gather these data yourselves. The information collected during the assessment stage, before initiating a program will serve as baseline data. By comparing these data with those collected after the program had started, you can determine the progress made and measure the success recorded.

Make a list of resources: Following a comprehensive assessment, coalition members can develop a list of resources. This list may include available infrastructure (housing, hospitals, roads, supermarkets, bus lines, and office space) technology, communication, funding, professional expertise, and data. (Guidry et al., 2001). We must look beyond money as our only resource. Every community has a rich reserve of nonmonetary resources that can only be discovered when

an assessment is done. These resources will be invaluable in designing programs.

3. *Plan*

Plan to achieve the vision and goals of the program in line with the views of the members of the coalition. A good plan includes clear objectives with steps and timelines to achieve them. Objectives should be specific and tailored to reflect the issues of the community, address goals of the program, resources to achieve set goals, and a yardstick for measuring progress. Typically, a plan of action will include:

Action Steps: Specific efforts that are made to reach desired goals set by the coalition. They must be detailed and should explain the program, to what extent these actions will occur, who will carry out specific duties, when they should be done, and designated timeframes.

Assignment of Responsibilities: Assigning specific individuals of the coalition to well-defined and agreed upon roles. This will encourage active participation from members as they will begin to see themselves as part of the project with duties and responsibilities to fulfill for the overall interest of the community.

Information Collection: Information collected either prior to the commencement or during the program will be important in measuring progress.

Feasible Timeline: Timelines must be realistic. Consider how much time will be necessary to complete each part of the plan, as well as the schedules of the members of the coalition.

4. *Implement*

Following the establishment of the action plan, coalition members who have duties assigned to them can begin the implementation of the strategies described in the action plan within the stipulated timeframe. To ensure compliance, regular monitoring is advocated. Monitoring will also ensure that specific duties are carried out in line with the goals and objectives of the action plan. It is important to point out that monitoring is most effective if it is planned before the commencement of the program. (Guidry et al., 2020). Similarly, monitoring gives for feedbacks and cross information from existing partners. Appropriate indicators—measurable landmarks—will be useful guides in monitoring the progress of the program.

Ensure that responsibilities and duties are shared across coalition members. The addition of new coalition members brings in energy, additional resources, and fresh ideas. (U.S. Department of Health and Human Services, 2020). It is also vital to communicate progress to the community. Get the word out by developing a communication plan, and relay kick-off events, activities, and community meetings to showcase your progress and accomplishments. (UDHHS, 2020)

5. *Track*

Evaluation and tracking are crucial to the long-term success of the coalition's efforts. Tracking entails two steps, which are data analysis and progress report. Data analysis ensures a comprehensive account of the program implementation. Efficient and accurate data collection also allows for transparent monitoring of the performance indicators.

Communities can leverage the presence of local universities and statistical centers and partner with them for development of tools to track data. Take note of the following when evaluating data over time.

- Quality of Data: standardization of data collection, analysis, and structure of questions.
- Data Validity and Reliability: Revisions in data collection tools may affect the validity of responses over time. A statistician will help with the validity and reliability testing.
- Limitations of Self-Reported Data: A potential issue with relying on self-reported

data such as income or dietary consumption is reporting bias.
- Data availability: Data collection efforts are not always performed on a regular basis.

A progress report guarantees effective communication with the other team members on the progress made in the program. This can be achieved by scheduling periodic meetings to brief members' details of the extent of the program implementation, changes made, challenges encountered, and what percentage of goals was achieved. Positive trends in data, reflective of success in the program must be announced with emphasis. This promotes enthusiasm among members and will keep them involved.

Conclusion

Program planning models and theories are important in guiding and implementing public health interventions in rural communities in the United States and globally. They provide a framework for program planners to plan their program, and organize thinking and actions so that health interventions are well thought-out, coherent, and effective processes. Each model and/or theory discussed in this chapter has its uniqueness, advantages, limitations, and in most cases, shared similarities with other another model or theory.

Community participation, stakeholder engagement, data collection, and analysis are the most common themes found in the models or theories that are discussed in this chapter. Therefore, before beginning a public health model-designed intervention in rural communities, program planners must take this into consideration. No one model or theory is perfect or dominates research and practice; each individual or rural community requires effective evidence-based, data driven interventions tailored specifically to their needs.

Discussion Questions

1. Why are theories and models important in health promotion?
2. Discuss the difference between planning models and theories.
3. Critically evaluate the strengths and weaknesses of the Diffusion of Innovation Theory.
4. Describe the phases of the PRECEDE-PROCEED Model.
5. How could PRECEDE-PROCEED be used to address the problem?
6. If one were assessing the acceptability of a HIV counseling and testing center, what would one need to know before implementing the service? Use an HBM framework to develop your answer.
7. List and describe the different stages of the transtheoretical model.
8. Discuss the four assessments conducted in MAPP.
9. What does MAP-IT stand for in health education?

References

Baranowski, T., Cerin, E., & Baranowski, J. (2009). Steps in the design, development and formative evaluation of obesity prevention-related behavior change trials. *International Journal of Behavioral Nutrition and Physical Activity*, 6.

Binkley, C. J., & Johnson, K. W. (2013). Application of the PRECEDE-PROCEED planning model in designing and oral health strategy. *Journal of Theory and Practice of Dental Public Health*.

Buns, M. T., Pettitt, C., & Blanton, J. (2017). Using the MAP-IT framework for implementing a home-school physical education program at a university campus. *International Journal of Physicl Education, Sports and Health, 4*(3), 84–88.

Champion, V. L., & Skinner, C. S. (2008). The health belief model. Health behavior and health education: *Theory, Research, and Practice, 4*, 45–65.

Crosby, Richard ; Noar, Seth M. (2011). What is a planning model? An introduction to PRECEDE-PROCEED. *Journal of Public Health Dentistry, 71*, S7–S15.

De Civita, M., & Dasgupta, K. (2007). Using diffusions of Innovations theory to guide diabetes management program development: An illustrative example. *Journal of Public Health, 29*(3), 263–268.

DiClemente, C. C., & Prochaska, J. O. (1998). Toward a comprehensive, transtheoretical model of change: Stages of change and addictive behaviors. In Miller W. R., & Heather, N. (Eds.), *Applied Clinical Psychology. Treating Addictive Behaviors* (p. 3–24). Plenum Press. https://doi.org/10.1007/978-1-4899-1934-2_1

DiClemente, R. J., Salazar, L. F., & Crosby, R. A. (2013). Health behavior theory for public health: Principles, foundations, and applications. Jones & Bartlett Publishers.

Douthit, N., Kiv, S., Dwolatzky, T., & Biswas, S. (2015). Exposing some important barriers to health care access in the rural USA. *Public health, 129*(6), 611–620.

Green, L. W., & Kreuter, M. W. (2005). Health Program Planning: An Educational and Ecological Approach. 4th Edition. New York: McGraw Hill.

Guidry, M. (2001). Healthy people in healthy communities: A community planning guide using healthy people 2010. Office of Disease Prevention and Health Promotion, Office of Public Health and Science, Department of Health and Human Services.

Guidry, M., Vischi, T., Han, R., & Passons, O. (2001) Healthy people in healthy communities: A community planning guide using healthy people 2010 Retrieved from http://www.healthypeople.gov/Publications .HealthyCommunities2001/default.htm

Hartley, D. (2004). Rural health disparities, population health, and rural culture. *American Journal of Public Health, 94*(10), 1675–1678.

Hawkins, D. S., Hornsby, P. P., & Schorling, J. B. (2001). Stages of change and weight loss among rural African American women. *Obesity Research, 9*(1), 59–67.

Hayden, J. (2009). Health belief model. Introduction to health behavior theory. Surdbury, MA: Jones and Bartlett.

Janz, N. K., & Becker, M. H. (1984). The health belief model: A decade later. *Health Education & Behavior, 11*(1), 1–47.

Kaminski, J. (2011). Diffusion of Innovation Theory. *Canadian Journal of Nursing Informatics, 6*(2).

Kamran, A., Ahari, S. S., Biria, M., Malpour, A., & Heydari, H. (2014). Determinants of patient's adherence to hypertension medications: Application of health belief model among rural patients. *Annals of Medical and Health Sciences Research, 4*(6), 922–927.

Kelder, S. H., Springer, A. S., Barroso, C. S., Smith, C. L., Sanchez, E., Ranjit, N., & Hoelscher, D. M. (2009). Implementation of Texas Senate Bill 19 to increase physical activity in elementary schools. *Journal of Public Health Policy, 30*, S221–S247.

Li, Y., Cao, J., Lin, H., Li, D., Wang, Y., & He, J. (2009). Community health needs assessment with precede-proceed model: A mixed methods study. *BMC Health Services Research, 9*, 181.

NRHA. (n.d.). Retrieved July 06, 2020, from https://www.ruralhealthweb.org/about-nrha/about-rural-health-care

Owen, N., Glanz, K., Sallis, J. F., & Kelder, S. H. (2006). Evidence-based approaches to dissemination and diffusion of physical activity interventions. *American Journal of Preventive Medicine, 31*(4), 35–44.

Porter, C. M. (2016). Revisiting Precede-Proceed: A leading model for ecological and ethical health promotion. *Health Education Journal, 75*(6), 753–764.

Prochaska, J. O., Redding, C. A., & Evers, K. E. (2015). The transtheoretical model and stages of change. In Glantz Rimer, B. K., & Viswanath, K. *Health behavior: Theory, research, and practice*, 125–148. John Wiley & Sons.

Prochaska, J. O., & Velicer, W. F. (1997). The transtheoretical model of health behavior change. *American Journal of Health Promotion, 12*(1), 38–48.

Prochaska, J. O., Velicer, W. F., Rossi, J. S., Goldstein, M. G., Marcus, B. H., Rakowski, W., . . . Rossi, S. R. (1994). Stages of change and decisional balance for 12 problem behaviors. *Health Psychology, 13*(1), 39–46.

Pullen, C., & Noble Walker, S. (2002). Midlife and older rural women's adherence to U.S. dietary guidelines across stages of change in healthy eating. *Public Health Nursing, 19*(3), 170–178.

Rosenstock, I. M. (1974). Historical origins of the health belief model. *Health Education & Behavior, 2*(4), 328–335.

Rothman, A. J. (2009). Capitalizing on opportunities to refine health behavior theories. *Health Education & Behavior, 36*(S5), 150S–155S.

Salazar, L. F., Crosby, R. A., Noar, S. M., Walker, J. H., & DiClemente, R. (2013). Models based on perceived threat and fear appeals. Health behavior theory for public health principles, foundations, and applications. America: Jones & Bartlett Learning, 83–104.

Schorling, J. B. (1995). The stages of change of rural African-American smokers. *American Journal of Preventive Medicine, 11*(3), 170–177.

Shin-Yu Lien, A., & Jiang, Y.-D. (2017). Integration of diffusion of innovation theory into diabetes care. *Journal of Diabetes Investigation, 8*(3), 259–260.

(U.S), I. o. M. (2002). The Future of the Public's Health in the 21st Century. Washington: National Academic Press.

CHAPTER 22

Rural Public Health Policy

Richard G. Greenhill, DHA, PMP, FACHE
James A. Johnson, PhD, MPA, MSc

LEARNING OBJECTIVES

At the end of this chapter, readers will be able to:

1. Explain the implications of federal, state, and local health policy on rural health.
2. Explain the organization of the healthcare system related to access to care and social determinants of health.
3. Identify the impact of health reform on rural public health policy.
4. Discuss opioids and their emergence as a public health concern.
5. Describe and discuss migrant workers and rural health.
6. Identify relevant state public health agencies and programs.
7. Describe emerging challenges.

KEY TERMS

Accountable care organizations
Affordable Care Act (ACA)
Assessment
Assurance
Federalism
Health data
Hospital closures
Opioid
Patient Protection and Affordable Care Act (PPACA)
Policy development
Public health
Public health policy
Social Security Act (SSA)

Introduction

As stated by **public health policy** scholar James Johnson, "Public health by its very definition and practice is shaped by public policy (Johnson, 2013)." Furthermore, **public health** agencies and their funding are established by federal and state policy in the form of legislation. Additionally, public health agencies are central to the regulatory functions of the government. This is especially evident at the federal level with the Department of Health and Human Services (HHS), the U.S. Food and Drug Administration (FDA), and the Centers for Disease Control and Prevention (CDC) and in the states with health agencies, bureaus, and commissions. As delineated by the American Public Health Association (APHA) and others, one of the core functions of public health is policy development, which is often done through the provision of **health data** and population-based information policymakers. Furthermore, Johnson asserts that public health education increasingly requires students to study health policy in order to see the big picture and to understand the constraints and enhancements placed on public health agencies by legislative entities (Johnson, 2013).

Public Health Policy Overview

As further elaborated by Johnson, public health policy is an attempt by the government at all levels to address a public health issue, problem, or concern (Johnson, 2013). The government, whether it is city, county, state, or federal, develops public policy that is manifested in laws, regulations, codes, and actions. The three fundamental parts to public policymaking include: 1) problems, 2) stakeholders, and 3) the policy itself. What is referred to as the *problem* is the issue that needs to be addressed, such as access to health care in rural communities. The *stakeholders* are the affected individuals or communities along with those who are influential in forming a plan to address the problem in question, such as a town or county. *Policy* is the finalized course of action decided upon by the government, perhaps in the form of opening a rural health clinic or enlisting mobile health units to come to the area. In most cases, policies are widely open to interpretation by nongovernmental actors, including those in the private sector. This often leads to the infusion of *politics* before the policy is formulated and after it is implemented. As such, most public policies have a life cycle and are subject to modification as events and opinions change (Rural Health Programs, 2019).

As mentioned earlier in this book, the three core functions of public health are:

1) **assessment**—the delineation of health problems, their nature, and the means of dealing with them; 2) **policy development**—the formulation and advocacy of what should be done about health problems; and 3) **assurance**—the implementation of policy, either by activities of others or by direct public health activities. Each of these functions is designed to address the needs of communities, families, individuals, and the society.

Schulz and Johnson described that the primary objective of a public health service is to improve the health of the population for which it is responsible, such as a state or local community (Johnson, 2013). A second objective is to protect public interests, such as occupational safety, sanitation, safe food, clean water, and air. A third objective of public health services is to implement expectations and policies of elected officials. Furthermore, public policy is central to the accomplishment of societal and community goals; this is especially true when the goal pertains to the public's health. Policy is the mechanism whereby resources are allocated or distributed, regulations are refined and enforced, and organizational missions are deployed. In fact, one of the core functions of public health is policy formulation.

Furthermore, the Constitution established two levels of government, the federal and the state. This is often called **federalism** and represents a system of government where two or more levels (i.e., national, state, and local) have certain powers and authority. For example, the United States Constitution ensured that there would be shared power between the federal government and the state and local governments. In general, a federal system allows powers that concern the whole nation to be granted to the federal government whereas state power is more focused on issues that directly affect its residents only; Michigan, for example, cannot dictate what laws Indiana or Illinois enacts. Sometimes, the state-level governments have to work through problems together. For example, Georgia, Alabama, and

Florida have had to work out a water-sharing agreement and West Virginia and Kentucky have worked together on **opioid** abuse.

In public health policy, there are many examples of intergovernmental programs where all levels of the system—federal, state, and local—are involved, such as the control of air pollution, opioids, or vaccination programs.

As described by the Association of State and Territorial Health Officers (ASTHO), rural America is as diverse as its people, reflecting the unique geography, culture, and history of each location. Well over 40 million people live in rural areas of the United States, accounting for nearly 15% of the population. People in rural areas have fewer resources and opportunities available to them in their communities, so local health departments are an important resource, serving as the frontline providers in many rural regions.

Rural Health Policy Challenges

This section of the chapter focuses on three very challenging issues and how they are being addressed. Included are 1) access to care; 2) opioid epidemic; and 3) farm-worker health.

Hospital Access and Reform

The fractured healthcare system in the United States continues to struggle to provide timely access to patients across the nation. The most recent attempt to rectify this was the passage of the **Patient Protection and Affordable Care Act (PPACA)** of 2010, commonly known as the **Affordable Care Act (ACA)**. Rural areas in the United States are strained for resources more often than most urban centers. Issues with access are best highlighted by the steady and increasing rate of rural **hospital closures** over the past decade. Between January of 2010 and January 2019, there were 95 rural hospital closures across the United States, of which 32 were Critical Access Hospitals (Rural Report, 2019). **Figure 22-1** illustrates a 13-year trend of closures that was steady through 2009 but rapidly accelerated after 2010. These closures are linked to financial pressures as well as pressures from other factors linked to staffing and resources.

Public health and access to care are inextricably linked. When individuals do not have access to preventive care, they will experience declines in health that further erode their circumstances. While it is

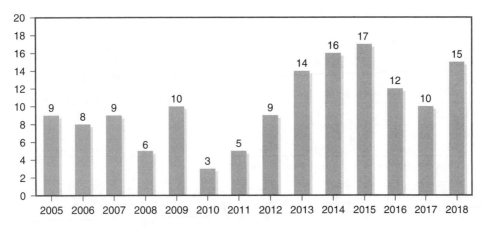

Figure 22-1 Rural Hospital Closures in the United States.

Data from NC Rural Health Research Program. (2018). 95 Rural Hospital Closures: January 2010 – Present. The Cecil G. Sheps Center for Health Services Research, University of North Carolina; www.shepscenter.unc .edu/programs-projects/rural-health/rural-hospital-closures/ (Note: In cases where closures occurred in Medicaid expansion states prior to their expansion, those closures are considered "non-expansion.")

acknowledged that the attributes that contribute to health exist outside of the acute care setting, access to these services is important for maintaining health.

The Federal government has offered a host of programs and initiatives to support rural hospitals and rural health research and policy programs. Under Section 1102(b) of the **Social Security Act (SSA)**, the foundations were laid for regulatory impact analyses from rules passed down related to rural health (Rural Hospital Programs, 2019). These rules were an acknowledgement of the sensitivity of rural health to broader policy decisions on health. Section 1102(b) gave rise to the Federal Office of Rural Health Policy (FORHP). The FORHP extends technical assistance and support for rural health hospitals through a host of programs. **Table 22-1** gives a glimpse into the key programs and their purposes.

Table 22-1 Federal Office of Rural Health Policy (FORHP) Programs

Program	Key Purpose
State Offices of Rural Health Program	A focal point for state issues linking communities with state, federal, and nonprofit resources to discover long-term solutions.
Medicare Rural Hospital Flexibility Program Evaluation	Mechanism to monitor and evaluate the program in support of quality, financial, and operational improvement.
Medicare Rural Hospital Flexibility Grant	Supports Critical Access Hospitals promoting quality and performance improvement. Other areas include: financial stabilization, emergency medical services integration, population health integration, and fostering an environment for innovative care models.
Small Rural Hospital Improvement Program	Provides funding for state governments in support of rural hospitals with 49 beds or fewer. Helps them: join or become **accountable care organizations**; participate in shared savings programs; purchase health information technology (both soft and hardware).
Rural Quality Improvement Technical Assistance Cooperative	Assists Critical Access Hospitals through funding for quality initiatives through supporting data driven improvement (tracking, analysis, & benchmarking).
Small Rural Hospital Transitions Project	Helps small rural hospitals bridge the gaps between the current healthcare system and emerging systems of delivery and payment. Provides technical assistance that includes: financial assessment, aligning organizational quality; & service alignment to community need.
Rural Veterans Health Access Program	Funds states in partnerships with providers and other entities to improve access to mental health and coordination of care for veterans in rural areas.
Vulnerable Rural Hospitals Assistance Program	Gives assistance to rural hospitals struggling to maintain and provide essential healthcare services.
Delta Region Community Health Systems Development	Enhances healthcare delivery targeting the Mississippi Delta region through multiyear onsite technical assistance.

Data from Rural Hospital Programs. Health Resources & Services Administration (HRSA). https://www.hrsa.gov/rural-health/rural-hospitals/index.html. Published September 5, 2019. Accessed November 3, 2019.

On the reform side, FORHP funds a host of rural health research and policy programs that helps to carry out its roles of advisory and compliance (Rural Hospital Programs, 2019). The Rural Health Research Center (RHRC) Program is the only federal program whose research is solely dedicated to the production of policy-relevant research in rural areas on healthcare and population health. Projects for this program are determined yearly by FORHP leaders and RHRC directors (Rural Health Research and Policy Programs, 2019). Like the programs under FORHP, the RHRC contains a plethora of programs that integrate various aspects of research together to discover challenges and come up with solutions. Each of the RHRC programs work in together to inform FORHP programs, and vice versa. This permits a system of learning, collaboration, and improvement. **Table 22-2** outlines the various programs and their contribution to RHRC programs.

Table 22-2 Rural Health Research and Policy Programs, Initiatives, and Projects

Program	Background
Frontier Community Health Integration Project	A demonstration project to test and develop new models for the delivery of healthcare services in frontier areas. Foci were to: explore means to increase access and improve adequacy of payment; evaluate regulatory challenges facing frontier providers and their communities served. https://www.ruralhealthinfo.org/new-approaches/frontier-community-health-integration-program
Rapid Response to Requests for Data Analysis	Initiative supports rapid data analysis on specific issues to inform national, state, and local policymakers.
Rural Health Clinic Policy and Clinical Assessment	Provides support for identification and analysis of key issues facing rural health clinics.
Rural Health Research Dissemination Cooperative Agreement	Aids stakeholders, rural policy and decision makers through the dissemination of policy-oriented information.
Rural Health Research Grant Program	Provides grants to research centers that work in consultation with FORHP to conduct policy-focused research on rural health services.
Rural Health Innovation and Transformation Technical Assistance Program	Supports the analysis of changes to Federal policy related to healthcare delivery, finance, and organization in rural health areas. This also assists rural health providers in navigating requirements of health system reform.
Rural Policy Analysis Cooperative Agreement	Supports identification of trends and challenges through research and analysis of key healthcare issues in rural areas.
Telehealth Focused Rural Health Research Center Cooperative Agreement	Goals to improve and increase the amount of policy-oriented research linked to telehealth.
National Rural Health Information Clearinghouse Program	Serves as a national clearinghouse for information on rural health in support of access to health care and improvement of population health in rural areas.

(continues)

Table 22-2 **Rural Health Research and Policy Programs, Initiatives, and Projects** *(Continued)*

Program	Background
National Rural Health Policy, Community, and Collaboration Program	Program that encourages policy and practice collaboration with rural health stakeholders through identification, education, and engagement.
Rural Health and Economic Development Analysis Program	Program that works to quantify the impact of rural health care on the economies (national, state, and local) and to improve awareness of such impact. Also analyzes the link between local rural economies and the health outcomes of their residents.
Rural Health Residency Planning and Development Program	Expands the physician workforce in rural areas through the development of new residency programs in family medicine, internal medicine, and psychiatry.
Rural Residency Planning and Development Technical Assistance Program	Provides technical assistance to grantees in the Rural Residency Planning and Development Program.

Data from Rural Health Research and Policy Programs. Health Resources & Services Administration. https://www.hrsa.gov/rural-health/research/index.html. Published September 4, 2019. Accessed November 3, 2019.

There is a fine line between rural public health and general rural healthcare delivery. These two areas overlap in ways that are either positively or negatively synergistic for these affected populations. This means that unresolved public health issues can quickly become issues needing to be addressed by the healthcare delivery system and vice versa. Additionally, a lack of access to services on the healthcare delivery side can contribute to poor public health. The American Hospital Association issued a report in 2019 detailing the plethora of issues facing rural health communities (Overview of the Rural Health Research Gateway, 2019). The issues facing rural health communities on the healthcare delivery side include: low patient volume, challenging payer mix, challenging patient mic, geographic isolation, workforce shortages, limited access to essential services, aging infrastructure, and access to capital.

Passage of the ACA was poised to mitigate some of these issues, particularly through Medicaid expansion; however, this was a choice at the state level. While Medicaid expansion might have been the right choice, for many, it was not politically expedient. Many of the states that chose not to expand Medicaid coverage under the law had higher numbers of uninsured citizens (Rural Report, 2019). Uninsured individuals may delay or not receive preventive care, which means that once problems arise, they will usually be more advanced; and therefore, more costly. The expenses from the uninsured are passed on to the public as well as being absorbed by hospitals. Interestingly, researchers found positive associations between Medicaid expansion and hospital financial performance in the rural setting (Garfield et al., 2018). Thus, the states that did not expand Medicaid for their uninsured population experienced 80% of the rural hospital closures that occurred since 2014 (Lindrooth et al., 2018). The impact of hospital closures on the rural communities further complicates a delicate situation for access to care for essential services. This compounds cost pressures to operations and, when combined with the aforementioned list, contribute to rural hospital closures as seen in Figure 22-1. Another phenomenon

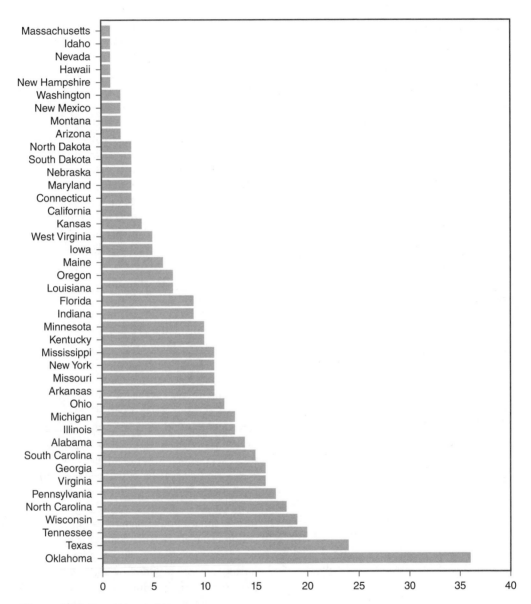

Figure 22-2 Rural Hospital Mergers.

Data from Rural Health Research Gateway Study. https://www.ruralhealthresearch.org/alerts/249

that emerged in the rural setting was mergers of rural hospitals. **Figure 22-2** illustrates rural hospital mergers by state in the United States over an 11-year period. Some of these were likely due to attempts to reduce operational costs and remain viable in a cost-prohibitive environment. Interestingly, states that had more mergers tended to be those that may have rejected Medicaid expansion.

While there are a host of interlinked public health issues in rural communities as discussed throughout this book, in addition to hospital access, this chapter also highlights the scope of two very concerning emergent rural health challenges.

Opioid Epidemic

Over the past few years, an epidemic of great magnitude hit the United States in terms of opioid use. Opioids are chemicals that may be natural or synthetic, which were created to interact with opioid receptors in the body and brain to reduce pain (NC Rural Health Research Program, 2018). The American Medical Association (AMA) estimated that 3–19% of individuals who take prescription pain medicines such as opioids had the potential to develop an addiction to them (NC Rural Health Research Program, 2018). Recent statistics noted that upwards of 115 deaths occur daily linked to opioid overdoses (Opioid Use Disorder, 2018).

The use of opioids in the United States spiked due to an increase in prescribing patterns and sales (Centers for Disease Control and Prevention, 2016). Opioid use disorder has been described in the literature as opioid use that is associated with a host of physical, social, mental, and legal issues; often leading to clinically significant distress or impairment (Kolodny et al., 2015; World Health Organization, 2018; American Psychiatric Association, 2013; Charlson et al., 2016). Data from 2017 illustrated that more than 11 million people used prescription opioids for other than medical purposes (Olfson et al., 2018). The trend with usage outside of the medical milieu is a cause for concern, as these drugs are particularly known to be habit-forming. Thus, the use of prescription opioids is likely a significant factor in the overall epidemic due to the potential for dependence.

Rural data suggested that opioid use disorder is more prevalent in rural settings (SAMHSA, 2017). National challenges with opioid use are compounded in the rural setting to a greater degree due to the limitations mentioned earlier in the chapter (e.g., access to care, etc.). In rural areas, the opioid epidemic is manifested via a host of disorders: perinatal opioid use disorder (Sun, et al., 2016) and opioid use disorder (Higgins, et al., 2019). Opioid use disorder may mimic other substance disorders, but its characteristics make it unique in some regards. Opioids have been known to lead to physical dependence within as little as four to eight weeks (NC Rural Health Research Program, 2018). This and a host of other attributes makes these particular drugs dangerous. Opioid use disorder is a chronic, lifelong endeavor that may result in negative consequences from disability up to death (NC Rural Health Research Program, 2018).

In rural health communities, the ramifications of opioid use are magnified exponentially. Rural populations are noted to be more vulnerable to health-related disparities and disease burden as seen in social epidemiology (Diagnostic and Statistical Manual of Mental Disorders DSM-5, 2013). Thus, disease burden risk is greater in rural areas due to the other social constraints of this community. While some of the health disparities in the rural community are linked to demographic composition (e.g., poverty and age), there are consistent findings that the context of rural areas is also an independent risk factor (Diagnostic and Statistical Manual of Mental Disorders DSM-5, 2013). Therefore, opioid misuse is a major public health concern for rural areas, more so than many metropolitan populations in the United States (Lutfiyya et al., 2012). Other studies illustrate findings that rural communities were more engaged in opioid misuse than urban or metropolitan populations in the United States (Palombi et al., 2018). Thus, the prevailing notion is that the crises associated with opioid misuse are compounded by additional factors that impact rural communities and even the very fact of being rural.

Migrant Farm Workers

American farmers and the corresponding workforce demographic (immigrants and migrants) are at the center of the discussion on rural public health. Historically, farming is known to be a hazardous line of work with frequent dangerous potential hazards (e.g., tools, machinery, and livestock) (Keyes et al., 2014).

Many farms in the United States are run by large-scale farmers who draw from a cheap labor pool, primarily immigrant labor. Thus the agriculture industry in the United States is mostly dependent on seasonal and migrant farmworkers, who are both documented and undocumented (Graber et al., 2001). These groups emerge as one of the most disadvantaged groups in the United States: legally, socially, and economically (Ramos et al., 2017). The risk to these workers is immense, in particular due to their legal status. Many of these workers originate from Mexico or Central American countries (Arcury et al., 2009; National Agricultural Workers survey, 2017) and reside below the federal poverty levels (Arcury et al., 2009; Robinson et al., 2011) in part due to their pay and lack of legal documented status (Arcury et al., 2009; Ingram et al., 2014). The health challenges for migrant workers in the United States are numerous. These workers live in the shadows of typical American life and work under conditions that are less than optimal or safe as depicted in **Exhibit 22-1**. This compounded by the already noted dangers of the farm industry complicate the health and wellness of this population. Some reports estimate injury rates for this population of workers to be as high as 12.5 per 100 individuals (Reid et al., 2016), with underreporting likely. Underreporting may be linked to fears of deportation, job loss, inability to provide for loved-ones, and cultural norms related to being hard working (Thierry & Snipes, 2015; Lopez-Cevallos, et al., 2014; McCullagh et al., 2015). Thus the actual impact on the migrant farm worker group may go vastly underestimated. Additionally, personal protective equipment (PPE) may be inaccessible (Reid et al., 2016), as well as safety and health information that is translated properly (Shannon et al., 2015). The lack of these resources adds greater risk of exposure to other factors. Without PPE, farmworkers may be exposed to harsh chemicals or pesticides that further add to poor health outcomes. Thus, the conditions to which migrant farmworker populations are subjected perpetuate an ongoing public health disaster for rural communities.

The social determinants of health are related to long-term viability of individuals and their communities. These factors or determinants directly impact populations in terms of how a population thrives and are based on many attributes, including social policies and access to care (Graber et al., 2001). Migrant workers in the U.S. agricultural industry often suffer with the greatest health issues (Ramos et al., 2016). The transient nature of these workers in order to maintain earning potential often contributes to a lack of access to timely needed care (Thierry & Snipes, 2015; Holmes, 2013; Thompson et al., 2015). From a policy standpoint, the federal government recognized the needs of this population and other indigent groups through the establishment of primary care centers. Federally qualified health centers (FQHC's) were established to serve the indigent and migrant workers, however, many may not be able to physically access them (Holmes, 2013). Thus these workers may go without a regular source of care. This initiates a cycle, since when illness occurs from exposure, the outcomes are worse and costlier. This adds financial and resource pressure to the rural healthcare delivery system, which, in turn, may contribute to closures, etc.

Policies create or influence the systems that determine the extent of individual's livelihood. With health insurance tied to employment, one's legal immigration status determines their access to health insurance (Ingram et al., 2014), thereby directly linking legal to health status. Therefore, immigration policy determines the social determinant of immigration legal status (Padilla et al., 2014), being that migrant workers may be documented or undocumented. Agricultural exceptionalism adds to the negative influence of policies on farmworkers and the lack of protections afforded to other work groups (e.g., workers' compensation, minimum wage, and unemployment insurance) (Thompson et al., 2015; Castañeda et al., 2015). Suffice it to say, migrant farmworkers continue to be a vulnerable population. Their status and location (primarily rural) adds to the complexity to properly assess and provide needed preventive as well as acute health services.

Exhibit 22-1 Perspectives from the Field

Contributed by Carrie Shaver, University of Indiana

The Hoosier state is popularly imagined as flat and homogenous, populated by more corn and soybean fields than folks, yet the rolling fields, sharp hills, and valleys of southern Indiana were once more densely wooded than any other area east of the Rocky Mountains. Yes, there are corn and soybeans, but the region is also home to leading advanced manufacturing and logistics companies, the flagship campus of the Indiana University system and regional campuses, and one of the world's best cities for modern architecture.

In order to improve health equity within this mixed rural region, significant health disparities necessitate a robust public health response, including commitment to a separate field of practice, study of, and investment in its communities. The confluence of geographic, demographic, cultural, and economic factors greatly influence wellness and life expectancy. While there is substantial variation among counties, rural residents of southern Indiana are more likely than their urban peers to live in poverty, lack a higher educational, practice self-destructive health behaviors, have poor healthcare access, and experience adverse health outcomes. Given the evidence of disparities, it is clear that a social justice agenda must include rural southern Indiana.

Dispersed, Dwindling, Aging, and Diversifying Population

Geographic challenges of the region include poor access to transportation and high-speed Internet. There are many miles between home, the grocery store, school, town governmental offices, primary and acute care centers, nonprofit social support agencies, and work. The rural setting can and often does restrict economic and social opportunities. For elderly and poor rural Hoosiers, the challenges posed by distance may not be surmountable without significant public support.

Following the Baby Boom generation, comparatively low birth rates and rising life expectancy have created a dwindling and aging population. In Indiana's rural counties, accelerating outmigration of the working-age population for education and employment opportunities in Indianapolis has generated a labor supply shortage. For example, an internationally renowned mountain biking destination with flowing trails, hilly and densely wooded scenic vistas, and challenging terrain, Brown County, has a replacement rate percentage of 58% and a median age of 46.7 years (Waldorf & McKendree, 2013).

Since 2000, the population's insufficient replacement rates and net domestic migration losses have been offset by positive net international migration (Waldorf & Ayres, 2013). In Johnson County, 60 Central and South American countries are represented by newcomers. A significant demographic shift is happening and the existing white, non-Hispanic residents are largely unaccustomed to immigration and unprepared for their arrival.

Rural Skepticism of Higher Education

Secondary students in southern Indiana's rural communities graduate from high schools at rates comparable to the state and the nation; however, higher educational attainment rates are remarkably low. While 38% of Indiana residents have earned associate degrees, in Switzerland and Crawford counties, only 17% of adults have. Nearly 60% of Orange County's workforce is in low-skilled occupations without formal training (Indiana Business Research Center, 2011).

At the beginning of my career in higher education, I served as a liaison for Indiana University, a state-wide tuition scholarship program, and southcentral Indiana's low-to-moderate income middle school students and families. Tuition-free, post-secondary education was often not significant enough to overcome additional financial barriers, including institutional fees (parking, technology, printing, and textbooks), transportation, food, and housing. In addition, limited local employment prospects lower the perceived value of postsecondary credentialing, especially when federal students loans are needed to supplement scholarships. Young adults who receive bachelor's degrees often do not return to their home communities, further exacerbating community skepticism of the value of higher education.

Limited Economic Prospects

Increasing levels of poverty in southern Indiana are detrimental to the overall wellness and viability of rural life in the region. Rural and rural mixed counties have higher levels of unemployment than urban counties. County to county, there are striking inequalities. For instance, on the southeastern Ohio boarder, Switzerland County has a 22.2% poverty rate while their neighbor to the north, Ohio County, has an 8.3% rate. Children account for one-third of the poor in rural southern Indiana and concentrated areas of poverty, like those in Switzerland County, have the potential to influence the educational outcomes for all children (Waldorf & Carriere, 2013). Being poor and rural has outsized consequences as access to social services designed to assist is restricted by the very nature of rural living.

Self-Destructive Health Behaviors

Researchers of premature death in rural America have begun calling mortality due to self-destructive health behaviors "despair deaths," positing the likelihood of their occurrence due to underlying social and economic factors (Stein, Gennuso, Ugboaja, & Remington, 2017). Rural southern Indiana mirrors the national trends among middle-aged, white, non-Hispanic Americans with shorter lifespans than their parents and grandparents. In Bartholomew County, the prevalence of mortality due to cancer, diabetes, heart disease and stroke, kidney disease, respiratory disease, and substance abuse disorder account for the bulk of age-adjusted death rates. In Jefferson County, the suicide rate grew from 11.2 per 100,000 in 2013 to 41.8 in 2016, more than 3.2 times higher than the national rate (Kings' Daughters' Health, 2018).

Substance Abuse

While alcohol and tobacco continue to be the most widely used substances, Hoosiers are more likely to die from an overdose than a car accident (Indiana University School of Medicine, 2019). In the community health needs assessment of Bartholomew County, substance abuse was the most cited, by 83.2% of respondents, as a major health issue. Of those informants, heroin or other opioids were identified as the most problematic substance abused in the community, followed by methamphetamine/other amphetamines, alcohol, and prescription medications. In addition, respondents who rated substance abuse as a major problem most identified substance abuse treatment, behavioral health care, and primary care as the most difficult to access in the community (Professional Research Consultants, 2018).

While 79 of the 92 counties in Indiana have a county-wide response to the opioid epidemic, none provide comprehensive prevention, treatment, and recovery support services. Of southern Indiana counties, five have overdose response projects, four have nonsyringe harm reduction programs, and three have syringe exchange programs (Indiana State Department of Health, 2019).

In 2015, Scott County received national attention when a public health emergency was declared due to an HIV epidemic. From November 18, 2014, to November 1, 2015, 181 residents were diagnosed with HIV and 92.3% were coinfected with the hepatitis C virus (Peters, Pontones, Hoover, Patel, Galang, Shields, . . . Conrad, 2016). Young adults who were dependent on prescription opiates had switched to injectable opioids or heroin, sharing syringes with one another. Recent computer simulation research found that earlier action in 2010 would have limited the number of infections

(continues)

Exhibit 22-1 **Perspectives from the Field** (*Continued*)

to 10 of the 215 actual (Gonsalves & Crawford, 2018). While a syringe exchange program was finally established, state law is still conflicted. Exchanges reduce needle sharing and HIV incidence and yet needle possession remains illegal in Indiana.

Farm Family Domestic Violence

The remoteness of the home and lack of community resources for survivors of domestic violence in southern Indiana compound the effects of intimate partner violence. Although prevalence rates are roughly the same in rural, mixed, and urban counties, there are distinct barriers. Isolation in rural communities is literal. Neighbors and others who in other settings would be able to identify and report signs of abuse are not physically proximate. Survivors may not have access to a phone or Internet connection, a sole vehicle may be accessed only by the abuser, and work outside of the home may be prohibited.

Even when domestic abuse is recognized and reported, other community members, including law enforcement, may not acknowledge the violence as serious or criminal. Cultural norms of the community may conceptualize the abuse as a private family matter, allowing abusers to continue their behavior and marginalizing the survivors' experience. Economic and familial concerns may also prevent survivors from prioritizing their own health concerns.

There are only 29 domestic violence shelters in Indiana, of which six are located in rural southern counties. Community challenges for rural residents (housing, employment opportunities, education, health care) are especially difficult for this vulnerable population. Healthcare providers, police, educators, and social service professionals must work together to create and sustain appropriate prevention and treatment programs for rural domestic violence survivors.

Health Professions Shortage

The aging population of southern Indiana is creating a rising demand for elder goods and services, including health care. The outmigration of working-age adults not only impacts local employers trying to fill open positions but its rural residents also face healthcare access problems because communities do not have a sufficient number of healthcare professionals. In addition to registered nurse, primary care provider, and specialist shortages, there is limited access to mental health professionals. Critical and hard-to-fill positions also include certification-only employees such as certified medical assistants (CMA), medical lab technicians, certified nursing assistants (CNA), and licensed practical nurses (LPN).

State-wide healthcare workforce development initiatives seek to provide rural residents with education through the community college and employers for stackable credentials leading to higher educational attainment (for instance, CNA to LPN to ASN). In addition, the Indiana Health Care Professional Recruitment and Retention Fund Program (IHCPRRF) provides healthcare professionals a loan repayment to incentivize psychiatric and mental health counselor practice in a specific, federally designated Indiana region experiencing high numbers of opioid deaths.

References

Gonsalves, G., & Crawford, F. W. (2018). Dynamics of the HIV outbreak and response in Scott County, IN, USA, 2011–15: A modelling study. *The Lancet, 5*(10), e569–e577. doi: 10.1016/S2352-3018(18)30176-0

Indiana Business Research Center at the Kelley School of Business, Indiana University & Strategic Development Group, Inc. (2011). *Orange County benchmarking and target industry analysis: Spotlight on a changing region*. Retrieved from https://www.ibrc.indiana.edu/studies/OrangeCountyBenchmarkStudy2011.pdf

Indiana State Department of Health. (2020). *Indiana drug overdose dashboard: County response*. Retrieved from https://www.in.gov/isdh/27393.htm

Indiana University School of Medicine. (2019). *Opioids abuse crisis*. Retrieved from https://medicine.iu.edu/expertise/indiana-health/opioid-crisis/

King's Daughters' Health. (2018). *Healthy communities of Jefferson County*. Retrieved from https://www.kdhmadison.org/media/1916/community-meeting-april-2018.pdf

Peters, P. J., Pontones, P., Hoover, K. W., Patel, M. R., Galang, R. R., Shields, J., . . . Gentry, J. (2016). HIV infection linked to injection use of oxymorphone in Indiana, 2014–2015. *New England Journal of Medicine, 375*(3), 229–239.

Professional Research Consultants, Inc. (2018). *2018 Community Health Needs Assessment Report: Columbus Regional Health Service Area*. Retrieved from https://www.crh.org/docs/default-source/pdf/2018-prc-chna-report-crh-service-area.pdf

Waldorf, B., Ayres, J., & McKendree, M. (2013). Population trends in rural Indiana. *Purdue Extension Center for Rural Development*. Retrieved from https://www.extension.purdue.edu/extmedia/EC/EC-767-W.pdf

Waldorf, B. & Carriere, D. (2013). Poverty in rural Indiana. *Purdue Extension Center for Rural Development*. Retrieved from https://www.extension.purdue.edu/extmedia/EC/EC-771-W.pdf

Waldorf, B., & McKendree, M. (2013). The aging of rural Indiana's population. *Purdue Extension Center for Rural Development*. Retrieved from https://www.extension.purdue.edu/extmedia/EC/EC-769-W.pdf

Courtesy of Carrie Shaver.

State Public Health Agencies

There are numerous state-level agencies involved in public health and policy. To provide some examples, we have developed **Table 22-3**. These agencies are specifically in states with large rural populations and as such have a major role in rural health.

Public Health Official Interview

To provide students and other readers of this book with some visibility into the mindset and work of a senior public health official, James Johnson conducted an interview that focuses on several of the challenges addressed in this chapter (**Exhibit 22-2**).

Table 22-3 Sample of State Organizations that Support Rural Health

State	Agency/Organization	Website
Michigan	Michigan Center for Rural Health	https://www.mcrh.msu.edu/index.html
	Michigan Rural Council	http://cedamichigan.org/rpm/
	USDA Rural Development Michigan State Office	https://www.rd.usda.gov/mi
Alabama	Alabama Office of Primary Care and Rural Health	http://www.alabamapublichealth.gov/ruralhealth/
	Alabama Rural Coalition for the Homeless	https://www.archconnection.org/
	Alabama Rural Health Association	https://arhaonline.org/
	Institute for Rural Health Research at the University of Alabama	https://cchs.ua.edu/research/#irhr
	USDA Rural Development Alabama State Office	https://www.rd.usda.gov/al
Indiana	Indiana Office of Community and Rural Affairs	https://www.in.gov/ocra/

(continues)

Table 22-3 Sample of State Organizations that Support Rural Health　　　　*(Continued)*

State	Agency/Organization	Website
	Indiana Rural Health Association	https://www.indianaruralhealth.org/
	Indiana State Office of Rural Health	https://www.in.gov/isdh/24432.htm
	Richard G. Lugar Center for Rural Health	https://www.lugarcenter.org/
	Rural Health Innovation Collaborative	https://therhic.org/rhic
	USDA Rural Development Indiana State Office	https://www.rd.usda.gov/in
Tennessee	Rural Health Association of Tennessee	http://www.rhat.org/
	Tennessee Office of Rural Health	https://www.tn.gov/health/health-program-areas/rural-health.html
	USA Rural Development Tennessee State Office	https://www.rd.usda.gov/tn
Texas	A&M Rural and Community Health Institute	https://architexas.org/
	Texas Association of Rural Health Clinics	http://www.tarhc.org/
	Texas Organization of Rural & Community Hospitals	https://www.torchnet.org/
	Texas Rural Health Association	http://trha.org/
	Texas State Office of Rural Health	https://www.texasagriculture.gov/GrantsServices/RuralEconomicDevelopment/StateOfficeofRuralHealth.aspx
	USDA Rural Development Texas State Office	https://www.rd.usda.gov/tx
Montana	Montana Office of Rural Health	http://healthinfo.montana.edu/morh/index.html
	Montana Rural Health Association	http://healthinfo.montana.edu/morh/mrha/
	Montana Rural Health Initiative	http://montanaruralhealthinitiative.info/
	USDA Rural Development Montana State Office	https://www.rd.usda.gov/mt
West Virginia	Robert C. Byrd Center for Rural Health	http://crh.marshall.edu/

	West Virginia Center for Rural Health Development	http://wvruralhealth.org/
	West Virginia Rural Health Association	https://wvrha.org/
	USDA Rural Development West Virginia State Office	https://www.rd.usda.gov/wv
Mississippi	Mississippi Office of Rural Health	https://msdh.ms.gov/msdhsite/_static/44,0,111.html
	Mississippi Rural Health Association	https://msrha.org/
	USDA Rural Development Mississippi State Office	https://www.rd.usda.gov/ms
Arkansas	Arkansas Division of Rural Services	https://www.arkansasedc.com/Rural-Services
	Arkansas Office of Rural Health & Primary Care	https://www.healthy.arkansas.gov/programs-services/topics/rural-health-and-primary-care
	USDA Rural Development Arkansas State Office	https://www.rd.usda.gov/ar

Exhibit 22-2 Public Health Interview

Scott Harris, MD, MPH, FACP, FIDSA
State Health Officer, Alabama Department of Public Health
Interview conducted by Dr. James A. Johnson
November 5, 2019

NOTE: This interview was conducted prior to the COVID-19 epidemic

Dr. Johnson: What are the leading public health challenges in rural communities in Alabama?

Dr. Harris: Rural areas in Alabama face many public health challenges. As younger people leave rural areas for urban ones, the residents of rural areas become relatively older on average and bear disproportionate burdens of chronic diseases and diseases of aging. Since employment opportunities may be lacking in many rural communities, there are often lower numbers of residents with employer-sponsored health insurance, and it is not surprising that rural residents are less likely overall to have private health insurance than urban residents. This combination of increased disease burden and lower insurance coverage means that local hospitals and providers often provide care that is uncompensated, which in turn can lead to economic stresses on local hospitals and providers (and, not least, the patients themselves!). Those providers who remain in rural communities are also more likely to be older and in later stages of their careers, and many rural communities find themselves dreading the inevitable retirements of older providers, since it is increasingly more difficult for small rural areas to recruit replacements. Younger providers, who are just completing their training and entering the workforce, are increasingly attracted to urban areas with better educational opportunities and more amenities. This is particularly true for medical specialists, who require larger population bases in order to see sufficient numbers of patients. Healthcare

(continues)

Exhibit 22-2 Public Health Interview   *(Continued)*

---

challenges are not the only ones faced by rural communities, of course; it has become difficult for rural communities to recruit potentially high-earning professionals of any kind: attorneys, engineers, high technology workers, and others are simply not interested in relocating to rural areas.

Besides the problems of increased disease burden and lack of providers, the residents of rural areas have additional challenges. They are more likely than urban residents to have lower levels of educational attainment, contributing to lower health literacy. Many may lack reliable transportation, making it difficult to travel to relatively distant providers and healthcare facilities. And all of these issues are compounded by a lack of health insurance!

Dr. Johnson: Does this differ from what is happening in other states? If so, please provide a few examples.

Dr. Harris: The demographic shifts that are occurring now in Alabama are similar to those in other states, as young people leave rural communities for opportunities of education and employment. However, Alabama has some special challenges that are not found everywhere. For example, the passage of the Hill-Burton Act in 1946 made federal dollars available to states for the construction of hospitals. Over the next several years, Alabama took advantage of this program to build dozens of new hospitals in rural parts of the state. Since these facilities, which were state of the art at the time of construction, are now several decades old, attempts at renovation may face prohibitive costs, making it difficult for these "Hill-Burton hospitals" to modernize their facilities or add updated technology.

Alabama's Black Belt is a region of about a dozen counties across the midsection of the state that is so named for its black fertile soil that attracted many farmers and planters in our state's early years. The subsequent enslavement of African Americans in Alabama and throughout the Old South has created a legacy of poverty in these rural Black Belt counties, which even today remain impoverished and geographically isolated. The nonmedical determinants of health in these low-income, African American communities are associated with significant health disparities and poor health outcomes. Alabama's history of enslavement still occupies a significant place in today's public health landscape.

Dr. Johnson: In your role as State Health Officer, how do you interface with policymakers to address these challenges? Please provide some examples.

Dr. Harris: Our department has worked diligently to develop personal relationships with members of the Governor's staff, key legislators, and colleagues who serve in other state agencies. For example, one physical aspect of Alabama's Black Belt is the relative impermeability of its soil to water, which creates difficulty in trying to manage residential wastewater. While rural residents in many places use a conventional septic tank to handle sewage and wastewater, these inexpensive systems do not function well in Black Belt soil, which necessitates much more expensive engineered solutions. Sadly, these are often not feasible to many impoverished residents of the Black Belt. The Alabama Department of Public Health (ADPH) has worked closely with state and local officials from these areas to find federal grants to enable the construction of wastewater systems that can be accessed by residents, and to develop and implement legislation that creates a legal framework for this initiative.

Also, ADPH enlists state legislators to assist us with local issues, whenever possible. For example, our county health departments are primarily funded through the clinical revenue that they earn themselves by the provision of clinical services, but because of the amount of uncompensated care they provide, local health departments also rely on local financial support from city and county governments. ADPH works with state legislators in their districts to help approach local officials with requests for resources. This helps us to build relationships with legislators while improving our credibility with local officials. As the saying goes, all politics is local.

Dr. Johnson: What are some of the obstacles or barriers you face in this regard?

Dr. Harris: Because ADPH is a regulatory agency, we sometimes find ourselves in conflict with those we regulate. If a facility receives a poor inspection score, many restaurants, nursing homes, hospitals, tattoo facilities, or other businesses are quick to reach out to local government or state legislators to register their displeasure with ADPH. Legislators generally understand the dilemma we face in our mission to protect the health of the public, but they ultimately answer to the wishes of their constituents, which may create uncomfortable situations on occasion.

Similarly, as the state agency charged with the inspection and regulation of abortion clinics, there is almost no action we can perform that avoids antagonizing at least some of those who are engaged with this polarizing issue. But sometimes, the opposite may be true: public health may be interested in a particular health concern that is of little or no interest to policymakers. A good example is in the area of sexually transmitted infections. While ADPH works hard to explain the public health impact of our state's increasing STI rates, and frequently seeks resources to assist our mission of reducing them, lawmakers are unlikely to hear from constituents who support this, and subsequently, we have a difficult time convincing legislators to provide additional support.

A number of issues would seem to be very straightforward from a scientific standpoint, like restrictions on the sale of tobacco or the benefits of syringe service programs in reducing transmission of hepatitis C virus and HIV. However, science does not always triumph, and political calculations are often the deciding factor. This can certainly create frustrating interactions when public health goals conflict with political decisions.

Dr. Johnson: Please provide a short description of three health improvement or prevention initiatives your Department is currently leading.

Dr. Harris: ADPH is working through our Governor's Children's Cabinet (comprised of other health service agencies and state legislators) to implement a pilot project in three central Alabama counties that have rates of infant mortality above the state average. Our state government partners include the Department of Human Resources, the Department of Mental Health, Medicaid, the Department of Early Childhood Education, and the Governor's Office of Minority Affairs. The pilot is focused on home visitation programs, safe sleep initiatives, utilization of the SBIRT (screening, brief intervention, and referral to treatment) screening tool to identify substance use, depression and domestic violence, breastfeeding, preconception and interconception health care for women who may potentially have high-risk pregnancies, and the use of 17-alpha-hydroxyprogesterone (17P) in women with previous preterm births. Additional ideas include working with insurance payers to make long-acting reversible contraceptives (LARC) available immediately after delivery, and further strengthening of Alabama's perinatal regionalization guidelines.

The Children's Health Insurance Program (CHIP) in Alabama is administered through ADPH and the Centers for Medicare & Medicaid Services (CMS) offers the opportunity to states to draw down federal administrative funds, within the federal administrative cap for states, to be used for demonstration projects that improve the health care of children. ADPH has designed a program to use CHIP coverage that is provided to an "unborn child," effectively providing services to an expecting mother who is determined to be at high-risk for a poor fetal outcome. The project will provide a variety of evidence-based case management/ wraparound support services that may include care by nurses, social workers, community health workers or others.

Preventing new cases of HIV infection in our state is a major priority. Given that effective antiretroviral treatment of persons who are living with HIV eliminates the possibility of transmission of the disease to others, the concept of treatment of prevention has added an additional sense of urgency to our goal of ensuring that all infected persons receive appropriate medical therapy. ADPH is currently developing a program to identify persons living with HIV who are not receiving medical care and attempting to re-engage them with the medical community

(continues)

Exhibit 22-2 Public Health Interview   *(Continued)*

---

by connecting them to providers. Using laboratory data that identifies HIV-positive persons who do not have evidence of additional follow-up lab studies (e.g. HIV viral loads or T-cell profiles), public health social workers will attempt to contact these persons who are not in care and identify any barriers that may be preventing them from access to providers.

Dr. Johnson: Please provide any websites developed by your Department that may be helpful to the reader in their understanding of your rural public health efforts.

Dr. Harris: The Office of Primary Care and Rural Health at the ADPH maintains a list of important rural health resources and programs, which may be found at our website: http://alabamapublichealth.gov/ruralhealth/index.html

Dr. Johnson: How has the postgraduate medical training you received in public health, specifically the MPH, been helpful to you in your current leadership role?

Dr. Harris: My professional background and training are in the realm of clinical medicine, and I began to pursue a Master's in Public Health degree only after changing my career to begin working in public health. I originally saw the degree as the standard credential that I thought I ought to obtain, in order to be on par with my new colleagues. However, my studies in my MPH graduate program opened my eyes to the wider world of public health and has informed everything that I currently do in my role as State Health Officer. Public health is a vast discipline that contains many diverse technical subject matters, from disease control to maternal child health to environmental regulation. My exposure to these areas was tremendously helpful to me as I began to work with public health experts across many different professional fields. My MPH program also introduced me to the theoretical underpinnings of public health, with instruction in areas like public health law, medical economics, and medical ethics. I literally developed a new vocabulary, which was necessary for me to understand and communicate in my new profession. Finally, my graduate program helped me to develop many administrative skills that I had never formally studied in my previous career, such as management and finance.

Courtesy of Scott Harris, MD, MPH, FACP, FIDSA.

Chapter Summary

This chapter provides an overview of key policy processes and actions that seek to address public health challenges in rural America.

Specifically, rural providers and practitioners are discussed as are overarching topics of Medicaid, access, regulation, and social determinants. Furthermore, the opioid epidemic and farm family health are discussed.

Discussion Questions

1. What are the benefits and challenges in mobilizing the human resources in rural America to improve access to health care?

2. How does rural geography influence opioid abuse? Is it a good idea to avoid prescription opioids on a regular basis

   for the prevention of abuse and decrease its contribution to the overall epidemic?

3. As a public health practitioner, which of the challenges mentioned in the chapter should be addressed for the improvement in health care in rural America?

4. By providing better access to health care, do you think the population in rural America would take advantage of the opportunity? How many of you know that most of the rural Americans take pride in self-care and not visiting a primary care physician for their health concerns?

5. Did you ever live in a rural community? Did you experience any major challenges in health care? Do you think innovation is easier in rural America?

6. Where do patients without insurance get opioid abuse services?

7. Enumerate the various barriers to care in rural America? What are the healthcare services that are most difficult to access in rural America?

Student activities and worksheets are available for use inside the Navigate eBook, included with the printed text. Simply redeem the access code found at the front of the book at www.jblearning.com.

References

American Psychiatric Association. Diagnostic and Statistical Manual of Mental Disorders, 5th edition. Washington, DC: American Psychiatric Association, 2013.

Arcury TA, Quandt SA, eds. Latino Farmworkers in the Eastern United States. New York: Springer; 2009.

Castañeda H., Holmes, S. M., Madrigal, D. S., DeTrinidad Young, M. E., Beyeler, N., Quesada, J. (2015). Immigration as a social determinant of health. *Annual Reviews of Public Health, 36,* 375–392.

Centers for Disease Control and Prevention (CDC). Wide-ranging online data for epidemiological research (WONDER). Atlanta, GA: CDC, National Center for Health Statistics; 2016. Available at: http://wonder.cdc.gov

Charlson, F. J., Baxter, A. J., Dua, T., Degenhardt, L., Whiteford, H. A., & Vos, T. (2015). Excess mortality from mental, neurological, and substance use disorders in the Global Burden of Disease Study 2010. In Patel, V., Chisholm, D., Dua, T., Laxminarayan, R., Medina-Mora ME, (Eds.) Mental, neurological, and substance use disorders: disease control priorities, 3rd Ed. (Volume 4). Washington, DC: The International Bank for Reconstruction and Development/The World Bank, 41–66.

Garfield R, Damico A, & Orgera, K. (2018 June). The Coverage Gap: Uninsured Poor Adults in States that Do Not Expand Medicaid. Kaiser Family Foundation. Retrieved from https://www.kff.org/report-section /the-coverage-gap-uninsured-poor-adults-in-states -that-do-not-expand-medicaid-issue-brief/view /print/

Graber, D. R., Jones, W. J. (2001). Health care for family farmers and Women Involved in Farm Economics (WIFE). *Journal of Agromedicine, 7*(4), 29–38. doi:10.1300/j096v07n04_03

Han, B., Compton, W. M., Blanco, C., Crane, E., Lee, J. L., & Jones, C. M. (2018). Prescription opioid use, misuse, and use disorders in U.S. adults: 2015 National survey on drug use and health. *Annals of Internal Medicine, 168,* 383–384.

Health Resources & Services Administration (HRSA). Rural Health Research and Policy Programs. https:// www.hrsa.gov/rural-health/research/index.html. Published September 4, 2019.

Health Resources & Services Administration (HRSA). Rural Hospital Programs. https://www.hrsa.gov /rural-health/rural-hospitals/index.html. Published September 5, 2019.

Higgins, T. M., Goodman, D. J., & Meyer, M. C. (2019). Treating perinatal opioid use disorder in rural settings: Challenges and opportunities. *Preventive Medicine, 128,* 105786. doi:10.1016/j .ypmed.2019.105786

Holmes, S. M. (2013). Fresh fruit, broken bodies: Migrant farmworkers in the United States. Berkeley, CA: University of California Press, Ltd.

Ingram, M., Schachter, K. A., Guernsey de Zapien, J., Herman, P. M., & Carvajal, S. C. (2015). Using participatory methods to enhance patient-centered mental health care in a federally qualified community health center serving a Mexican American farmworker community. *Health Expectations, 18*(6), 3007–3018.

Johnson, J. A. (2013) Introduction to public health management, organizations, and policy, Clifton Park, NY: Delmar Cengage.

Jones, C. M. (2017). The paradox of decreasing nonmedical opioid analgesic use and increasing abuse or dependence—an assessment of demographic and substance use trends, United States, 2003–2014. *Addictive Behaviors, 65,* 229–235.

Keyes, K. M., Cerdá, M., Brady, J. E., Havens, J. R., & Galea, S. (2014). Understanding the rural-urban differences in nonmedical prescription opioid use and abuse in the United States. *American Journal of Public Health, 104*(2), e52–e9.

Kolodny, A., Courtwright, D. T., Hwang, C. S., Kreiner, P., Eadie, J. L., Clark, T. W., & Alexander, G. C. (2015). The prescription opioid and heroin crisis: A public health approach to an epidemic of addiction. *Annual Review of Public Health, 36*(1), 559–574. doi:10.1146 /annurev-publhealth-031914-122957

Liebman, A. K., & Augustave, W. (2010). Agricultural health and safety: Incorporating the worker perspective. *Journal of Agromedicine, 15*(3), 192–199.

Lindrooth, R. C., Perraillon, M. C., Hardy R. Y., & Tung G. J. (2018). Understanding the relationship between Medicaid expansions and hospital closures. *Health Affairs, 37*(1). Retrieved from https://www .healthaffairs.org/doi/abs/10.1377/hlthaff.2017.0976

Lopez-Cevallos, D. F., Lee, J., & Donlan, W. (2014). Fear of deportation is *not* associated with medical or dental care use among Mexican-origin farmworkers served by a federally-qualified health center—faith-based partnership: An exploratory study. *Journal of Immigrant Minority Health, 16,* 706–711.

Lutfiyya, M. N., McCullough, J. E., Haller, I. V., Waring, S. C., Bianco, J. A., & Lipsky, M. S. (2012). Rurality as a root or fundamental social determinant of health. *Disease-a-Month, 58*(11), 620–628.

McCullagh, M. C., Sanon, M. A., & Foley, J. G. (2015). Cultural health practices of migrant seasonal farmworkers. *Journal of Cultural Diversity, 22*(2), 64–67.

National agricultural workers survey. U.S. Department of Labor Web site. https://www.dol.gov/agencies/eta /national-agricultural-workers-survey/data. Published January 13, 2017.

NC Rural Health Research Program. (2018). 95 Rural Hospital Closures: January 2010 — Present. The Cecil G. Sheps Center for Health Services Research, University of North Carolina; www.shepscenter.unc.edu /programs-projects/rural-health/rural-hospital -closures/

Olfson, M., Crystal, S., Wall, M., Wang, S., Liu, S. M., & Blanco, C. (2018). Causes of death after nonfatal opioid overdose. *JAMA Psychiatry 75*(8), 820–827.

Oquendo, M. A., & Volkow, N. D. (2018). Suicide: A silent contributor to opioid-overdose deaths. *New England Journal of Medicine, 378,* 1567–1569.

Padilla, Y. C., Scott, J. L., & Lopez, O. (2014). Economic insecurity and access to the social safety net among Latino farmworker families. *Social Work, 59*(2), 157–165.

Palombi, L. C., St. Hill, C. A., Lipsky, M. S., Swanoski, M. T., & Lutfiyya, M. N. (2018). A scoping review of opioid misuse in the rural United States. *Annals of Epidemiology, 28*(9), 641–652. doi:10.1016/j .annepidem.2018.05.008

Patel, K., Watanabe-Galloway, S., Rautiainen, R., Haynatzki, G., & Gofin, R. (2016). Surveillance of non-fatal agricultural injuries among farm operations in the Central States region [dissertation]. Omaha: University of Nebraska Medical Center.

Ramos, A. K. (2018). A human rights-based approach to farmworker health: An overarching framework to address the social determinants of health. *Journal of Agromedicine, 23*(1), 25–31. doi:10.1080/1059924x .2017.1384419

Ramos, A. K., Fuentes, A., & Trinidad, N. (2016). Perception of job-related risk, training, and use of personal protective equipment (PPE) among Latino immigrant hog CAFO workers in Missouri: A pilot study. *Safety, 2*(4), 1–10. doi:10.3390/safety2040025

Reid, A., & Schenker, M. B. (2016). Hired farmworkers in the US: Demographics, work organisation, and services. *American Journal of Industrial Medicine, 59*(8), 644–655.

Robinson, E., Nguyen, H. T., Isom, S., Quandt, S. A., Grzywacz, J. G., Chen, H., & Arcury, T. A. (2011). Wages, wage violations, and pesticide safety experienced by migrant farmworkers in North Carolina. *New Solutions, 21*(2), 251–268.

Rural Health Research Gateway. Overview of the Rural Health Research Gateway. https://www.rural healthresearch.org/about. Published 2019.

Rural Report: Challenges Facing Rural Communities and the Roadmap to Ensure Local Access to High-quality, Affordable Care. American Hospital Association. https://www.aha.org/system/files/2019-02 /rural-report-2019.pdf. Published February 2019.

SAMHSA 2017: Substance Abuse and Mental Health Services Administration. Key Substance Use and Mental Health Indicators in the United States: Results from the 2017 National Survey on Drug Use and Health (HHS Publication No. SMA 18-5068, NSDUH SeriesH-53) (2018). Rockville, MD: Center for Behavioral Health Statistics and Quality, Substance Abuse and Mental Health Services Administration.

Shannon, K. L., Kim, B. F., McKenzie, S. E., & Lawrence, R. S. (2015). Food system policy, public health, and human rights in the United States. *Annual Review of Public Health, 36,* 151–173.

Sigmon, S. C. (2019). Innovations in efforts to expand treatment for opioid use disorder. *Preventive Medicine, 128,* 105818. doi:10.1016/j.ypmed.2019.105818

Sun, E. C., Darnall, B. D., Baker, L C., & Mackey, S. (2016). Incidence of and risk factors for chronic opioid use among opioid-naive patients in the postoperative period. *JAMA, 176*(9), 1286–1293.

Thierry, A. D., & Snipes, S. A. (2015). Why do farmworkers delay treatment after debilitating injuries?

Thematic analysis explains if, when, and why farmworkers were treated for injuries. *American Journal of Industrial Medicine, 58*(2), 178–192.

Thompson, R. H., Snyder, A. E., Burt, D. R., Greiner, D. S., & Luna, M. A. (2015). Risk screening for cardiovascular disease and diabetes in Latino migrant farmworkers: A role for the community health worker. *Journal of Community Health, 40,* 131–137.

World Health Organization (WHO). International Classification of Diseases 11th revision. Disorders due to substance use. December, 2018. https://icd.who.int /browse11/l-m/en#/http%3a%2f%2fid.who.int%2ficd %2fentity%2f499894965

CHAPTER 23

Leadership

Donald J. Breckon, PhD, MPH

LEARNING OBJECTIVES

At the end of this chapter, readers will be able to:

1. Define leadership and coleadership and discuss the similarities and differences.
2. Discuss leadership and management, to include how they overlap and how they differ.
3. Articulate three commonly accepted elements of leadership.
4. Identify two or three leadership styles and describe situations in which various leadership styles are most appropriate.
5. Describe their preferred leadership style and describe how that is affected by their personality and experiences, as well as elements that might need to be adapted to meet specific group needs.
6. Describe strategies for mobilization of various target groups in rural health settings.
7. Discuss methods for identifying existing coalitions or partnerships as well as forming new ones.
8. Describe strategies that work effectively with various subcultures in rural health settings.

KEY TERMS

Coalition
Coleadership
Community
Leadership
Leadership styles
Partnership
Power structure
Readiness to change
Resistance to change
Target group

CHAPTER OVERVIEW

This chapter will discuss the concept of leadership and its components and discuss their application to rural health settings. It will encourage self-analysis and identification of personal traits and skills that might need more or less emphasis to best lead in a variety of rural health settings.

The Nature of Leadership

There are many definitions of *leadership* in the literature, with much overlap but also with different emphases. That is true in part because the concept of **leadership** has changed over time but also because that which is required of leaders will depend on the setting or group that a leader is in.

This chapter will focus on leadership in a **community** setting, not organizational leadership. Again, there will often be overlap, because an organizational leader may well see community leadership as an important part of job responsibilities. To illustrate, one might hold the title of director or administrator or chief executive officer and have a job description that includes management and/or leadership responsibilities for that agency or organization. The individual or board that the administrator reports to may see leadership within the community as a key component of job responsibilities. Of course, the director may see leadership within the community as essential to advancing the interests of the employer.

There is also overlap and differences between the concepts of *management* and leadership. Most definitions of management cite the elements of supervising, directing, controlling, and manipulation of what exists, and imply the person in that position has the inherent authority and power to make things happen by staffing or budgeting changes, changing job descriptions, etc. However, managers usually also have the responsibility to achieve organizational goals through planning, organizing, deploying staff, and budget, etc. Setting and achieving goals is also a part of leadership, and organizational goals may involve the role of community leader. Although there is overlap and subtle differences, some with the title of manager will also be leaders, but certainly this will not always be the case. Managers sometime think of themselves as focusing mostly on status quo, trying to do the best possible job running their organization, rather than producing community change.

Worth noting, one does not necessarily need a title to be a leader. While leadership can come from an employee with leadership responsibilities, it can also come from a community activist, a citizen with a passion. Parents who have lost a child due to gun violence are one such example of people who informally get other concerned citizens involved with pressuring more formal leaders to work for change.

Leadership within a community emphasizes working with other community leaders, guiding, coordinating, inspiring, and motivating them to set and achieve common goals. As one meets with known community leaders, a simple yet effective step is to ask who else has or should have programming in the area of interest, as well as if there are any groups of agencies already working on the problem. Asking six to a dozen community leaders these two questions will usually produce a fairly reliable assessment of who should be involved. Of course, doing an Internet search of agencies interested in the problem within a specific geographical boundary can yield useful information.

Leadership within a community is more democratic than autocratic and implies participative consensus building in setting goals and deciding on strategies to achieve those goals.

Visioning what will be is a key task of leaders. Visioning involves thinking of an ideal scenario, an understanding of how several sectors of the community can contribute toward a more effective future, one that will be ideally more efficient and more cost-effective as well. Visioning will not usually be done alone, although an individual's vision of what can be is often a precursor to formation of a **coalition** or **partnership**.

After the *partnership or coalition* is formed, however, members must either buy into the vision or be involved in modifying it. A very simple element of leadership is that to be a leader, one must have followers, and others are not likely to follow someone else's vision unless they thoroughly understand it and agree that it is worth pursuing.

Once community leaders agree to goals, they each can work toward change within their organization or sphere of influence that contributes to the accomplishment of the larger goal. This can be thought of as **coleadership**, which can involve shared expertise and resources that their organization can provide.

While *coleadership* has similarities to delegation, coleadership is more likely to be spontaneous and voluntary, rather than executing an assigned task, which is implied in delegation. Both concepts imply coordination to varying degrees.

Leadership within a community obviously has a much broader focus than leadership of an organization and involves coordination and even compromise between other community leaders and organizations. Leadership within a community health setting always involves participative and creative visioning of what might be better for the community. It involves team-building and teamwork, focused on achieving a common goal.

Leadership in community settings involves meetings, (some but not all of the time via technology), and a great deal of listening and empathy. It involves effective group leadership skills to ensure that all points of view are understood. It may well involve being open-minded, and may require compromise, but always involves consensus building.

Leadership in a community involves sensing *readiness* of the community and how willing its organizations are to change. Readiness can be determined by thinking about how concerned the community is about the issue, and if there are feasible, cost-effective solutions available. It might also be due in part to media support. How aware segments of the community are of the issue and the passion of those advocating change is another indicator of readiness to pursue change.

The readiness of a community to change also involves an assessment of how much *resistance to change* there is and the status of those resisting change. If resistance is widespread and among the **power structure** of the community and no obvious ways to overcome it come to mind, producing change may be exceedingly difficult. One needs to think about whether resistance is resistance coming from religious groups, political groups, or elsewhere? Is resistance coming from mainline groups or fringe groups? One need only think of opposition to vaccinations to know that resistance can be very intense. Whatever the proposed program, assessing the level of readiness and **resistance to change** is critical to success.

There are numerous *leadership styles*, and each has a use, but in mobilizing rural community health groups, the more democratic and participatory the style, the more commitment is likely. It may be necessary to use a more autocratic style at times to keep the process moving, by suggesting goals for the next meeting, making assignments, etc. The best leadership style is the one that gets results and will definitely vary from situation to situation. Readers will likely encounter situations where varying **leadership styles** are needed.

Chapter 20 in this book focuses on Community Need's and Assets Assessment and understanding the concepts are an essential part of the leadership process.

Community Mobilization

For purposes of this discussion, the term *community* will be used to describe a group of people in rural settings with common interests. *Mobilization* is widely used in the military and has the inherent assumption of organizing troops prior to action. *Community mobilization*, therefore, involves preparing for purpose-driven community action.

An initial thought on the nature of community might start with citizens in a rural unit of government, and geopolitical boundaries may be a defining characteristic. A county health department, for example, would logically focus on rural problems affecting families within that political jurisdiction. Yet, some stakeholders might be in nonprofit agencies that serve several counties, or at the state or national level. Moreover, the common interests may not be that wide, as for example, it might be young mothers in one area of the county as part of an immunization campaign, isolated seniors who lack access to medical care, or those interested in reducing teenage suicide rates.

If a community is going to be mobilized to improve some aspect of rural health, a considerable amount of time needs to be invested in defining the stakeholders. In earlier years, the term *target group* was used to help define the community of interest. For many reasons, knowing whose programs are being specifically designed will facilitate planning and delivery. It is, therefore, a good place to start, by defining the community and the various subgroups that will need to be mobilized. In short, who will be the beneficiaries of any new programming?

Another early step in this process is to identify all of the groups who have some level of programming in place that serves the **target group**, as they will also have to be mobilized. Appraisal of existing services and unmet needs is part of the need's assessment process and is critical to establishing new goals and objectives. Of course, getting to know peers in relevant agencies is essential as is discussing existing programming and coordination efforts. Sharing the vision and the need for additional coordination will usually lead to at least an informal assessment of their interest in being part of an envisioned group. Part of the message should be that more coordination may well result in more efficiency and will likely free up resources within member groups

to meet unmet needs. In short, all groups who may be the providers of needed services will need to be identified and mobilized for action. Asking about existing programming and coordinating efforts of several peers will usually identify potential members of any coordination group that is envisioned.

Analysis of the *power structure* within the target group, within the provider groups, and extraneous to both groups is also important. Identifying who has influence, prestige, budget, and other resources will become increasingly important as the process develops. Staff in senior citizen programs, transportation agencies, tribal councils, health department personnel, rural hospital administrators, radio or television talk show hosts, and newspaper editors. Nonprofit community health groups such as those focused on substance abuse or other specific health problems may well be part of the community mobilization process.

Communication among the relevant communities is vital, although how that will occur will likely vary from group to group. Using existing *preferred channels of communication,* such as joining groups and attending meetings and hearings, is a basic part of most public health strategies. Exchanging emails, texts, and other forms of electronic communication may all be used appropriately with a variety of groups.

To mobilize a community requires an understanding of an unmet need, especially if it is reaching the crisis stage, and if obvious programming steps can affect an improvement. Collecting statistics from local, state, and national organizations, as well as case studies of programming efforts that are actually in place elsewhere should occur, as well as any relevant situations that have made the media. To mobilize a community, other community leaders must be aware that a need exists and that something can be done about it. Of course, if one's peers are already motivated to effect lasting change, an advantage of coordinating groups in some form is that studying needs and potential programs can be a shared task.

A generation or two ago, the term *community organization* was used for what is now called *community mobilization*. While there are subtle differences, the processes have much in common.

Coalition and Partnership

Significant progress toward achieving rural community health goals usually requires a cooperative approach that includes providers and opinion leaders. That usually starts informally but often progresses toward a more formal organization, especially if external funding is anticipated. A *coalition* is the more informal, loosely knit group of organizations with a common interest, while a *partnership* is more formal and usually includes negotiated roles and responsibilities. It often involves a signed Memorandum of Understanding, which is similar to a contract.

One place to start is identifying and understanding existing interested organizations, both formal and informal, and especially with relevant programming. Whether the initiator of this proposed partnership is new or established within a community, discussions focused on who should be involved in this problem-oriented community action is critical; as many stakeholders as possible will be involved.

Creating enhanced awareness and interest in the problem and potential solutions is also important prior to discussing the need for a coalition or partnership. Often, it is feasible to establish a coordinating mechanism under the umbrella of an existing agency such as the local health department, council on aging, etc. The coalition or partnership can be formal or informal and can evolve over time. There simply needs to be a format for numerous focused discussions to occur. Keeping the structure as simple as possible by working as part of an existing organization is usually a productive strategy.

Of course, a community-based group can have ties to state and federal organizations, but they would not usually be part of the coalition of partnership. In fact, a search for relevant state and federal agencies is an important early stage because of the many resources they can provide. Such agencies may have consultative services, printed and electronic resources, and perhaps even grant money that can be accessed. Both tax-based and voluntary health agencies should be explored.

The specifics of how to mobilize and/or organize a group will vary from location to location, problem to problem, and individual to individual. Regardless, people cannot avoid the use of social media and still be as successful as they might be without it. It is simply too pervasive in today's society, as much of our discourse and engagement takes place over electronic media.

Communication strategies within public health have always emphasized using channels of communications preferred by the target groups, to include traditional media such as radio, television and newspapers, emails, texting, etc. In an extreme example, think of media usage by teens, young professionals, and senior citizens, and how they get information. The essential step to communicate effectively is to use channels that the target group already uses, regardless of if it is one-on-one, a small group, or a very large group.

Social media can be used to create awareness and interest, announce decisions or events, encourage involvement and consensus building, and raise money. It can be used to connect, educate, seek expertise, or recruit volunteers. In addition to carefully selecting which media are appropriate, carefully crafting the message is essential to success. Obviously, messages to raise money or recruit volunteers would vary significantly from messages designed to create awareness or motivate action.

While it won't eliminate face-to-face meetings or telephones, social media can surely reduce them and facilitate decision making in a timely fashion. Email and texting are basic, and links to websites such as YouTube, Facebook, Instagram, Twitter, and Snapchat are useful tools. Other forms of emerging social media are likely to be valuable resources in most rural community health settings.

It will usually be appropriate in the early stages of an organization to discuss preferred communication channels within the group and between the group and the community at large. It may be appropriate to appoint a social media manager and perhaps even explore use of social media management software. A leader does not have to be a hands-on social media manager but needs to be sure it is used effectively and appropriately.

Building consensus on goals and strategies is important because it facilitates coleadership. At its basic, coleadership involves committee chairs and delegation of task to individuals or committees. However, in community-wide coalitions or partnerships, it must be shared, with member groups thoroughly understanding the goals and the role their agency can play.

In review, communities and the component subgroups will need to be identified. Data will need to be gathered. Individuals and organizations who will become part of the solution need to be identified, educated, and motivated. Needs will need to be established and prioritized, in part by impact and in part as to feasibility. Of course, it will be necessary to create awareness and interest, as well as build consensus on which needs to address and what specific goals to tackle first. Communication strategies will have to be addressed. Budget needs and potential funding sources are essential. It will also be essential to motivate action, how to measure progress, and how to move the community forward.

Forms and Styles of Leadership

There are a variety of forms and styles of leadership in the literature. People tend to focus on one style of leadership (**Exhibit 23-1** Styles of Leadership) and may change their beliefs through the years from their personal

---

Exhibit 23-1 Styles of Leadership

Transformational Leadership: Motivates others to reach their potential, be creative, and foster team spirit.

　　Transactional Leadership: Uses exchanges in the way of promotions, promises, titles, etc., to encourage employees.

　　Authentic Leadership: Seems to develop from an intrapersonal perspective. The life experiences of the leader assist in creating the leadership style often based on strong ethical standards.

　　Servant Leadership: Wants to serve and assist others to reach their full potential. They try to eliminate barriers for others in their daily work.

　　Adaptive Leadership: Helps others to develop skills to adapt to changes within an ever-changing environment. They may set a vision to guide people through the change process.

Greenleaf, R. K. (1970). The servant as leader. Westfield, In: Greenleaf Center for Servant Leadership; Hale, J. R., & Fields, D. L. (2007). Exploring servant leadership across cultures: A study of followers in Ghana and the USA. *Leadership, 3*(4), 397–417; Northouse, P. (2019). *Leadership: Theory and practice.* (8th ed.). Los Angeles: Sage; Notgrass, D. (2014). The relationship between followers' perceived quality of relationship and preferred leadership style. *Leadership & Organizational Development Journal, 35*(7), 605–621; Shamir, B., & Eilam, G. (2005). "What's your story?" A life-stories approach to authentic leadership development. *The Leadership Quarterly, 16*(3), 395–417; Walumbwa, F. O., Avolio, B. J., Gardner, W. L., Wernshing, T. S., & Peterson, S. J. (2008). Authentic leadership: Development and validation of a theory-based measure. *Journal of Management, 34*(1), 89–126.

experiences and development. As discussed, there are many styles of leadership administrators can select from. Working in a rural public health setting has its own unique challenges in serving its constituents. It should be noted that people observe the behaviors of their leaders to draw conclusions of their effective or ineffective leadership. Leaders should never stop learning and growing in how they can best serve the people they are guiding.

Cultural Competence

The term *culture* in this chapter refers to traditions, beliefs, values, attitudes, and behaviors shared by a specific group of people. It may be based on ethnicity, religion, gender, age, and a whole host of other factors. It is more than merely being aware of the various cultures or even making diversity a part of the group's membership, although both are important. It involves understanding the elements of various cultures, being open-minded, accepting, respectful, and empathetic.

 Cultural competence usually takes time but starts with spending time with members of that culture, observing, asking questions, and listening with both ears and heart. Gaining such understanding prevents unintentional offenses and even resistance and is essential to gaining support.

 Developing cross-cultural skills and using them effectively may well be the difference between success and failure, and that is increasingly more so as community diversity is increasing at the local, state, national, and global levels. It involves being sensitive, making eye contact, respecting customs and preferences, and building trusting, comfortable relationships. It means being comfortable in that setting and making all cultures present feel comfortable. Building comfortable, trusting relationships greatly increases the probability of creating buy-in for the project. In fact, developing cultural competence and cross-cultural skills is often a key to career advancement and a valued part of one's resume.

Review

In review, to effectively address a rural health issue, directly affected communities and component subgroups will need to be identified. Data will need to be gathered. Individuals and organizations who will become part of the solution need to be identified, educated, and motivated. Needs must be established and prioritized, in part by impact and in part as to feasibility. Of course, it will be necessary to create awareness and interest, as well as build consensus on which needs to address and what specific goals to tackle first. Communication strategies will have to be addressed. Budget needs and potential funding sources are essential. It will also be essential to motivate action and learn how to measure progress while moving the community forward.

 A familiar quote by Margaret Meade, the world-famous sociologist, seems a fitting way to conclude this chapter. She said, "Never doubt that a small group of thoughtful, committed citizens can change the world; indeed, it's the only thing that ever has."

Discussion Questions

1. Identify two or more effective leaders you know. Think about what elements of leadership they seem to possess. Think about how much of these characteristics are personality based, and how many of them are learned behaviors. Identify leadership traits that would have enhanced their effectiveness. Discuss how these behaviors may be learned. Analyze your own leadership skill strengths and

weaknesses and think about how they can be improved. Discuss in large or small groups or online groups.

2. Think of a specific rural community near where you live or have lived. What ethnic groups live there? Is the community high or low income? Would you consider the rural community you chose highly educated? Which religions play a prominent role? Would you guess the community is elderly or predominantly young families? Is the community predominantly Republican or Democrat or Liberal or Conservative? What are the major media sources used by them to obtain information? Where might you go to obtain data on these matters? What do you need to learn to work more effectively with these subgroups? Identify how these and other factors can affect readiness or resistance to change.

3. Identify a group advocating change in a community with which you are familiar, for example, Black Lives Matter. Think about how it was affected by leadership. Think about **readiness to change** as well as where resistance was coming from, what motivations were present, and how it was overcome. What might be done to assist groups that have not fared so well to improve their situations? Discuss in either large, small, or online groups.

4. Google or otherwise search for community health groups, organizations, coalitions, or partnerships that serve that community. Which of these do you think are most influential and why? Is credibility built up over time, is it budget factors, is it membership, or other factors?

5. What do you think the top three to five health problems are in this community? What sources might you contact to obtain data to substantiate or invalidate your opinion?

6. Pick one of these health problems in that community and investigate if any agencies or group of agencies are already addressing that issue. Do you see ways that working together might help create solutions to this problem rather than working alone?

7. What people (or positions if you do not know names) would logically be involved if a coalition or partnership would emerge? Do any of these already engage in interorganizational planning?

8. What state and federal agencies could bring resources to assist in the mobilization? Visit their websites.

9. Do some online research about the *ice bucket challenge*, *crowd sourcing*, and *GoFundMe*. Also investigate rules and traditions associated with them. Discuss whether these might apply to the rural health community and to the problem identified above.

10. Think of specific examples where other forms of social media have been used. What has worked well?

11. Do an online search of leadership styles and make a list. Think about what styles fit your personality.

Student activities and worksheets are available for use inside the Navigate eBook, included with the printed text. Simply redeem the access code found at the front of the book at www.jblearning.com.

References

Greenleaf, R. K. (1970). The servant as leader. Westfield, In: Greenleaf Center for Servant Leadership.

Hale, J. R., & Fields, D. L. (2007). Exploring servant leadership across cultures: A study of followers in Ghana and the USA. *Leadership, 3*(4), 397–417.

Northouse, P. (2019). *Leadership: Theory and practice.* (8th ed.). Los Angeles, Sage.

Notgrass, D. (2014). The relationship between followers' perceived quality of relationship and preferred leadership style. *Leadership & Organizational Development Journal, 35*(7), 605–621.

Shamir, B., & Eilam, G. (2005). "What's your story?" A life-stories approach to authentic leadership development. *The Leadership Quarterly, 16*(3), 395–417.

Walumbwa, F. O., Avolio, B. J., Gardner, W. L., Wernshing, T. S., & Peterson, S. J. (2008). Authentic leadership: Development and validation of a theory-based measure. *Journal of Management, 34*(1), 89–126.

Additional Reading

Readers will likely benefit from an online review of:

- The literature on organizational change theory as there is much overlap.
- The literature on community organization.
- The literature on organizational change theory as there is much overlap.
- The Flint, Michigan, Lead Contamination of Drinking Water, to ascertain how the various concepts in this chapter were used or not used.

CHAPTER 24

Services to Support Rural Health

Heather Craig Alonge, PhD, MPH, CHES

LEARNING OBJECTIVES

At the end of this chapter, readers will be able to:

1. Describe how availability of transportation impacts access to care in rural areas.
2. Explain the challenges around rural emergency preparedness and response.
3. Identify modalities of health communication and how they contribute to the emergence of new models of rural health care.
4. Describe the capacity of telehealth to improve access to care and support the rural workforce and community.

KEY TERMS

Emergency preparedness
Emergency response
Health communication
Telehealth
Transportation

CHAPTER OVERVIEW

As healthcare delivery and services to support rural health care continue to evolve and change, there has been a broader focus on those services that extend beyond the traditional scope of clinical practice. There has been a concerted effort to build out the public health infrastructure that supports rural health. While resources and services are a concern for many communities in America, these concerns are pronounced in rural areas where local health departments and medical centers are operating on limited budgets, limited staff, and in isolation. This infrastructure includes services that aim to address barriers to access to care and important health education to include **transportation**, **health communication**, and new technologies such as **telehealth**. Additionally, rural communities and their leaders need to be prepared to respond to a disaster, whether it be natural or man-made, or other emergencies in a manner that protects the health and safety of the community while operating on limited resources and in isolation.

Transportation

Rural public transportation systems vary in type, access, management, and need. In rural communities, the types of transportation can include: demand–response public transportation; fixed bus routes; and vanpools and shuttles operated through nonprofits, municipalities, or reimbursement programs. Access to transportation in rural communities is essential in order to link citizens to essential employment, shopping, and health care, particularly those persons with disabilities, low income, and older adults. The American Public Transpiration Association (APTA) reported that from 2000 to 2005, close to 9% of public transportation trips for those areas with a population less than 200,000 were for medical purposes. Healthcare providers, health educators, local government officials, and rural communities themselves understand the necessity of transportation to access health care.

Barriers to transportation in rural communities can result in delays in seeking medical care, missed appointments, and lack of medication compliance because of not being able to access facilities. These barriers lead to both negative health consequences and influence how those who live in rural communities make decisions regarding their medical care (Syed, Gerber, & Sharp, 2013). Even if public transportation or other transportation services are available, the schedules do not always meet the need of the resident. For example, fixed-route bus services in rural communities do not run early or late routes. If residents need to make an early appointment or the appointment goes over the expected time, they may be without transportation to and from the medical office. Additionally, residents may also have challenges, such as physical limitations or safety concerns, which prevent them from utilizing the public transportation services.

Tips from the Field: Health Professional Expert Advice

What happens when the nearest doctor who takes your insurance is an hour away? Or when you don't have regular access to a car or bus? It is frustrating and can be hazardous to your health when the right care is out there, but you can't get to it. Patients often experience this scenario, which is why patients frequently do not keep appointments or delay receiving care.

In some situations, patients who live in rural communities without transportation access may wait for a medical emergency just to be able to access care by ambulance. Even with public transportation, some patients may find it difficult to utilize, so they have been waiting until they are short of breath, passing out, or in a very frail condition and then calling an ambulance because there are simply no other options.

For healthcare providers, missed appointments mean that we can't address our patients' questions and concerns, or update any changes to the patient's health history or life circumstances, a situation that can be particularly worrisome for patients with diabetes, cancer, and other chronic diseases that require ongoing active care.

Some providers, clinics, and hospitals in both rural and urban areas are using community health workers (CHWs), people who help patients navigate the healthcare system to assist in coordinating transportation for at-risk patients. CHWs, who generally are not licensed healthcare professionals, will coordinate transportation for patients to and from appointments, motivate them to take their medications, and help them implement positive lifestyle habits. Some hospitals and physicians also use care coordinators: people who, unlike CHWs, are trained in a health-related field, most often social workers or nurses. These coordinators support groups of low-income or chronically ill patients, helping them to understand their care plans and schedule primary-care visits instead of making trips to the Emergency Room.

Although a significant number of patients, especially those with few resources, struggle to find consistent and reliable transportation, there are some options for those in certain areas. Each state has a benefit for people with Medicaid for non–emergency-related visits, covering a certain number of rides per month, and some Medicare Advantage plans also cover a limited number of trips each year. Some states contract with local companies and transportation network companies to provide rides; others enlist volunteers or hire taxis. Some private insurers take similar steps to make transportation more accessible for their clients, although this may involve copays or preapprovals to prove their need for the benefit. In many cases, nonemergency rides must also be requested several days in advance.

For healthcare providers, access to care is a major concern when it comes to delivering timely and needed care to patients living in rural communities. This access to care determines health outcomes for patients and quality of care. **Figure 24-1** shows the flow model for the relationship between transportation and health outcomes for Americans living in rural communities.

Recent events, including Hurricane Katrina, California wildfires, and the September 11, 2001, attacks have proven that disasters can occur anywhere at any time. Disaster managers face different challenges and opportunities when handling **emergency preparedness**

in rural regions versus urban and suburban regions.

Various research has been conducted showing the susceptibility of urban communities but far less data exist on how rural populations respond to disasters and emergencies (Brennan & Flint, 2007). In general, rural communities have a smaller pool of financial resources to support disaster response and clean-up/rebuilding efforts. Besides having limited fiscal resources and manpower, rural communities also face scarce communication systems, which pose challenges when disseminating important messages regarding evacuation and execution of plans (Janssen, 2007).

The four phases of a disaster are: prevention or mitigation, preparedness, response, and recovery (Federal Emergency Management Agency, 2019). A prevention or mitigation plan decreases the severity of the disaster, whether natural or manmade. By focusing on preparedness efforts, communities and responders can build capacity and identify resources to be utilized during a response. Preparedness plans should include actions that will protect citizens, responders, and facilities during the event and recovery. A prepared community routinely exercises, debriefs, and alters the plan according to changing needs. Routine and direct communication is important when responding to the disaster and during the recovery phase. Communication should include multiple modalities, the ability to reach the appropriate government officials, responders and providers and the scope to

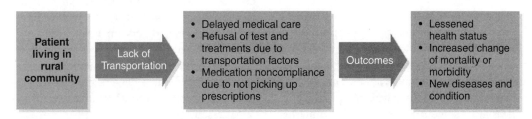

Figure 24-1 Emergency Preparedness.

communicate the important information to the public to ensure that they are prepared, know what to expect, and know how to act, especially at-risk populations such as the elderly and disabled (Savoia, Lin, & Viswanath, 2013).

Almost always, rural communities are geographically distant from major urban areas and resources. Geographic challenges for rural areas may include broad deserts, mountain ranges, rivers, and marshy areas, which make travel and communication difficult (Brennan & Flint, 2007). Rural communities often find it difficult to attract qualified personnel and as a result, shortages in healthcare personnel and responders create challenges. Subsequently, professional and volunteer staff in rural communities may also have limited experience with major disasters, emergency preparedness, surveillance, or outbreak monitoring. Time and distance also impact the ability of urban professionals and responders to get to the rural communities in the time of emergency and disaster.

Public health and healthcare infrastructure also present limitations to rural communities. In rural communities, emergency first responders are often volunteer-based; therefore, they have less training on emergency preparedness equipment and protocols such as the ability to decontaminate, isolate, and quarantine in the time of a disaster. Decontamination abilities are severely inadequate in rural hospitals and clinics and there is virtually no local experience with decontaminating procedures, except for rural communities located near nuclear plants.

Communications also present a special challenge to rural communities given the lack of reliable communication systems. While many rural communities were among the first to use telecommunications technologies in health care and communication, some forms of communication are not available or simply do not work. Some rural areas still lack Internet capacity, which could support notification in the event of a health alert or bioterrorism emergency. Other rural areas find that telephone connectivity is interrupted (Savoia et al., 2013).

In general, fiscal resources for rural hospitals and health departments are far more limited than those in major urban areas. Despite the numerous federal and state-level emergency preparedness compliance standards, rural communities have fewer financial monies. The lack of money makes it difficult for rural communities to comply. Rural communities have smaller public health departments and law enforcement agencies, which also present limited resources. There are likely to be fewer healthcare providers overall and, specifically, few specialists who are most needed, like trauma care, infectious disease specialists, and mental health experts. Rural hospitals are less likely to have both the space and equipment to handle the shear demands of the community. In these situations, the rural hospital emergency departments often must stabilize and transfer the most critical patients to larger facilities. The challenges faced by rural communities can impact their ability to both prepare and react to emergencies and disasters. In summary, rural communities face significant challenges.

Tips from the Field: Health Professional Expert Advice

Both operational size and geographic location determine when and how well a medical center can respond to disasters. Rural medical centers, often smaller in size, tend to have fewer resources and personnel compared with centers located in urban populations. Due to these constrictions, rural medical centers should activate the emergency preparedness plans earlier than those communities with larger resources.

In times of disaster and emergency, health professionals should modify preparedness plans to fit scope, resources, and surroundings. Rural health professionals should take regular inventory of supplies and the skill sets of their staff to determine what they are lacking and how they would access these resources in the event of an emergency or disaster. Telehealth capabilities are one available resource that is highly valuable in assisting rural communities in tapping into resources and staff during times of need and crisis. Additionally, health professionals working in rural medical centers should maintain their ability to function as ancillaries as they do during normal times of operation.

In addition to identifying resources, it is essential that health professionals also need to be able to identify a strong incident command system. A good incident command system includes strategies for patient evacuations; where to relocate patients; and what equipment, care, and medications need to go with the patient or to be received by the patient at the new center where they are relocated.

An essential part of disaster preparedness is conducting routine drills in preparation for big disasters. The Joint Commission currently necessitates accredited hospitals to conduct several disasters drills annually. Accredited hospitals are then assessed by how well they performed at the drill and where areas of opportunity exist. By conducting routine drills, the health center, health professionals, and community members are prepared for a variety of disasters and emergencies, and all involved parties are actively and successfully communicating and working together (Federal Emergency Management Agency, 2019). Due to our role as health professionals in emergency preparedness, it is important to pursue disaster training through Federal Emergency Management Agency (FEMA). It is imperative that rural health professionals understand the role they play in emergency preparedness within their communities (See **Figure 24-2**).

New Technologies: Health Communication and Telehealth-Case Study

Telehealth is defined as the use of electronic-based telecommunication technologies, including computer systems and smartphone applications, to support and promote long-distance clinical health care, related to patients and health professionals. Technologies include video conferencing, the Internet, store-and-forward imaging, streaming media, and terrestrial and wireless communication (Raths, 2018).

Telehealth services are especially critical in rural areas that lack sufficient healthcare services, including specialty care. The range and use of telehealth services have expanded over the past decades, along with the role of technology in improving and coordinating care. Traditional models of telehealth involve care delivered to a patient at an originating (or spoken) site from a specialist working at a distant (or hub) site. A telehealth network consists of a series of originating sites receiving services from a collaborating distant site, (Marcin, Shaikh, & Steinhorn, 2016). With increased smartphone and tablet uses, application services also expand telehealth services (List, Saxon, Devon, & Toole, 2018).

Telehealth-Case Study

With over 17 years of experience with utilizing telehealth services for in-home patient care, MaineHealth Care at Home (MHCAH) was one of the earliest adopters of the telehealth in the United States. For MHCAH, the

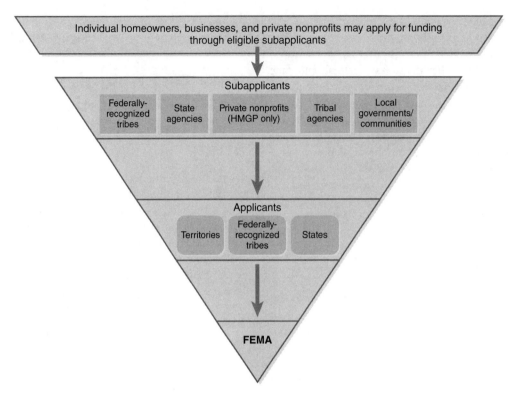

Figure 24-2 Flow Chart for Emergency Preparedness.
https://www.fema.gov/sites/default/files/images/pdm_application_flow_chart.jpg

discovery that the state's demographic could benefit from telehealth due to a large and predominantly elderly population living in a rural service region served as the justification for telehealth delivery.

According to the U.S. Census, Maine has the oldest population in the country, with a median age of 43 years compared with 37 years for the United States (United States Census Bureau, 2018). Maine faces challenges with increased trends in chronic disease, a predominantly rural population, and significant levels of poverty. America's Health Rankings' 2017 annual report found that cardiovascular deaths in Maine increased from 215.4/100,000 to 227.4/100,000 over three years, from 2014 to 2017. Maine is also among the poorest states in the country. Maine seniors, ages 85 year and older, have poverty rates 50% higher than

younger Maine seniors (United States Census Bureau, 2018).

In 2001, MHCAH launched southern Maine's first telehealth demonstration project with grant support from Rural Utilities Services-USDA. This pilot introduced interactive video monitoring units, coupled with traditional home health services, to patients diagnosed with advanced congestive heart failure in rural areas of Maine. Baseline data showed reductions in hospital readmissions for those patients with congestive heart failure. Despite the success of improved patient outcomes, it was determined that acceptance and use of the technology from providers presented obstacles. To improve telehealth utilization among providers, the MHCAH implemented an outreach campaign to the medical community and employed a new platform that was more intuitive to use for both patient and provider (MaineHealth Care at Home, 2019).

MHCAH continued to sustain its telehealth utilization and expansion with grants from federal and local foundations from 2007–2011. During this timeframe, those patients who received routine telehealth care experienced significantly lower rates of hospitalization and emergency care, and improved capability to manage their chronic conditions compared with home health patients who did not utilize telehealth (MaineHealth Care at Home, 2019). MHCAH also collaborated in a pilot project with MaineHealth, a not-for-profit health system in Maine, on a Home Diuretic Protocol for Heart Failure. The findings from this pilot indicated lower hospital readmission rates from 20.5% to 10% (MaineHealth Care at Home, 2019). Telehealth delivery was an essential element to the success of this program as it provided caregivers with the ability to assess patients early, often, and eliminated distance barriers between facility and patient. This project also marked a milestone for solidifying a telehealth partnership between the agency and affiliated healthcare providers that mandated the provision of telehealth in its protocol.

In 2015, MHCAH transitioned to Health Recovery Solutions (HRS), a platform designed for an Internet-enabled tablet, wireless monitoring devices, self-assessment features, medication compliance modules, disease-specific educational video clips, and the ability for patients to quickly connect via voice or video to monitoring nurses. Additionally, MHCAH combined electronic medical records (EMR) capabilities with their telehealth delivery model to share with MaineHealth data. In its first year of utilizing EMR and HRS, MHCAH saw a 75% reduction in 30-day hospital readmission rates. Due to the success in reduced hospital readmissions, MHCAH expanded its telehealth efforts, enrolled 725 patients, and cited 30-day hospital admissions in the range of .07%–5% per quarter compared with nontelehealth patients with 17% readmission rates. The average daily adherence for patients taking part in this cohort was 85%. Patient satisfaction scores were in ranges of 3.35–4.0 (four highest) for responses related to ease of use, willingness to recommend, and how telehealth is helping manage disease (MaineHealth Care at Home, 2019).

Tips from the Field: Health Professional Expert Advice

When patients living in rural communities are diagnosed with illnesses and medical conditions that require care from specialists, they are faced with the reality that they must spend additional time and resources on traveling to healthcare systems that have the needed resources and staff. This could include treatment, tests, consultations, and routine medical appointments. Rural hospitals now have quite a number of options when it comes to providing telemedicine to their patients and all are helpful in allowing patients to receive the care they need without being displaced from their communities and expending mass amounts of time traveling to access that care.

With telehealth, more can be done than just monitoring conditions and health status. Telehealth is an excellent option to educate and engage with patients. Checking in and educating patients at home on a daily basis, in bite size pieces, is transformative. Telehealth providers have the means to intervene immediately when patients have a serious or potentially serious concern, such as a routine blood pressure check.

Providers can expect to see a rise in the number of rural patients receiving treatment right from the comfort of their home or being a part of a medical home, which houses many patients with similar symptoms and diseases for better treatment as a result of telehealth technologies. Additionally, patients can start to use telehealth apps that can be customized to their individual case but also offer the flexibility to specify what sort of information should be displayed.

Telehealth serves as means to connect rural patients to needed care without travel and costs. Telehealth also serves to connect rural providers to urban and metropolitan providers in order to ensure better education, consultations, and community of care.

- Access to specialists without need for travel
- Reduced costs in travel fees and medical care
- Early detection of diseases and conditions
- Reduction of morbidity and mortality

Conclusion

The obstacles that healthcare providers and patients face in rural areas are vastly different from those in urban areas. Economic factors, cultural and social differences, educational barriers, and the isolation of living in remote areas all combine to generate healthcare disparities and hinder rural communities in their ability to lead normal, healthy lives.

Chapter Summary

Rural residents face many barriers to accessing appropriate medical care, including lower income, lower rates of private health insurance coverage, and a lower supply of primary and specialty medical care providers. They must often try to coordinate care across long distances with few supportive resources. Taken in combination with rural residence, certain characteristics such as poverty and racial or ethnic minority status may place a rural person at particularly heightened risk of not receiving adequate preventive screenings or treatment for acute or chronic conditions. Because of these barriers, the health and well-being of rural populations may be compromised. In recognition of the challenges that rural areas face in terms of medical care access, multiple federal agencies have targeted rural residents as a "priority" population and programs such as critical access hospitals, rural health clinics, and community health centers/FQHCs exist to augment the medical care infrastructure of rural communities. Other strategies aimed at using mobile vans and technology to reduce the geographic distance between rural areas and better-resourced urban and suburban areas show some promise and should be investigated further.

Discussion Questions

1. How does telehealth improve healthcare access in rural communities, and what types of services have proven to be effective?
2. What are the challenges related to telehealth services in rural communities?
3. How does the use of telehealth impact rural healthcare providers?
4. What are some of the challenges in emergency management in rural communities?
5. What is the difference between emergency preparedness and **emergency response**?

6. What are some ways that rural communities can utilize resources for communication planning during times of emergency response?
7. How can local legislators work with stakeholders and partners to improve access to transportation for rural communities?

Link for questions 1-3: https://www .ruralhealthinfo.org/topics/tele health#improve-access

Student activities and worksheets are available for use inside the Navigate eBook, included with the printed text. Simply redeem the access code found at the front of the book at www.jblearning.com.

References

America's Health Rankings (2017). Annual Report. Retrieved from https://www.americashealthrankings .org/learn/reports/2017-annual-report

American Public Transportation Association. (2019). *Public transportation fact book*. Retrieved from https://www.apta.com/research-technical-resources /transit-statistics/public-transportation-fact-book/

Brennan, M. A., & Flint, C.G. (2007). Uncovering the hidden dimensions of rural disaster mitigation: Capacity building through community emergency response teams. *Journal of Rural Social Sciences, 22*(2), 111–126.

Federal Emergency Management Agency. (2019). Retrieved from www.fema.org

Janssen, D. (2006). Disaster planning in rural America. *Public Manager, 35*(3), 40–43. Retrieved from https:// search.proquest.com/docview/236296849?pq -origsite=gscholar

List, B. A., Saxon, R., Lehman, D., Frank, C., & Toole, K. P. (2019). Improving telehealth knowledge in nurse practitioner training for rural and underserved populations. *Journal of Nursing Education, 58*(1), 57–60. http://dx.doi.org.library.capella.edu/10 .3928/01484834-20190103-10

Marcin J. P., Shaikh U., & Steinhorn R. H. (2016). Addressing health disparities in rural communities using telehealth. *Pediatric Research, 79*, 169–176. http://dx.doi.org/10.1038/pr.2015.192

MaineHealth Care at Home. (2019). *Annual Report*. Retrieved from https://mainehealth.org/about/annual -report

Raths, D. (2018). Telehealth put to use in rural America: Convenient connections can help reduce relapse rates. *Behavioral Healthcare Executive, 38*(1), 32–35.

Savoia, E., Lin, L., & Viswanath, K. (2013). Communications in public health emergency preparedness: A systematic review of the literature. *Biosecurity and Bioterrorism: Biodefense Strategy, Practice, and Science, 11*(3), 170–184. http://dx.doi.org/10.1089 /bsp.2013.0038

Syed, S. T., Gerber, B. S., & Sharp, L. K. (2013). Traveling towards disease: Transportation barriers to health care access. *Journal of Community Health, 38*, 976–993. http://dx.doi.org/10.1007/s10900-013-9681-1

Additional Reading

American Red Cross: http://www.redcross.org.

Centers for Disease Control and Prevention. (2016). Gateway to Health Communication. Retrieved from http:// www.cdc.gov/healthcommunication/Campaigns /index.html

CERT programs by state: https://community.fema.gov /PreparednessCommunity/s/cert-find-a-program

The Commonwealth Fund: https://scorecard.common wealthfund.org/

FEMA: http://training.fema.gov

Federal Office on Rural Health Policy: https://www.hrsa .gov/rural-health/index.html

Kaiser Family Foundation. The Affordable Care Act and Insurance Coverage in Rural Areas. https://www.kff .org/uninsured/issue-brief/the-affordable-care-act -and-insurance-coverage-in-rural-areas/

Rural Health Information Hub: https://www.ruralhealth info.org/

United States Census Bureau (2018). Quick Facts Maine. Retrieved from: https://www.census.gov/quickfacts /fact/table/ME/PST045218

Glossary

A

Access to care The timely use of personal health services to achieve the best health outcomes.

Access to services A service that provides access to a network.

Accountable care organizations A healthcare organization that connects provider reimbursements to quality metrics and cost-of-care reductions.

Acute Very serious or dangerous; requiring serious attention or action.

Adiposity Containing fat.

Adolescents A transitional stage of physical and psychological development that generally occurs from puberty to legal adulthood.

Affordable Care Act (ACA) Formally known as the Patient Protection and Affordable Care Act, and commonly known as Obamacare, ACA is a United States federal statute enacted by the 111th United States Congress and signed into law by President Barack Obama on March 23, 2010. Together with the Health Care and Education Reconciliation Act of 2010 amendment, it represents the U.S. healthcare system's most significant regulatory overhaul and expansion of coverage since the passage of Medicare and Medicaid in 1965.

Ageism Stereotyping and/or discrimination against individuals or groups on the basis of their age.

Aging in place The ability to live in one's own home and community safely, independently, and comfortably, regardless of age, income, or ability level.

Agribusiness The business of agricultural production that involves the production, protection, sales, and marketing of the product to satisfy the customer's need.

Air Pollution The presence of substances in the atmosphere that are harmful to the health of humans and other living beings or cause damage to the climate or to materials.

Alignment A position of agreement or alliance.

Allied Health Decrease in cost and improvement in quality of patient care.

Anthropometry Measurements of the body, such as height, weight, head circumference, fat mass, etc.

Aquifer An underground layer of water-bearing permeable rock, rock fractures, or unconsolidated materials (gravel, sand, or silt).

Artificial Intelligence (AI) Intelligence demonstrated by machines, unlike the natural intelligence displayed by humans and animals.

Assessment The evaluation or estimation of the nature, quality, or ability of someone or something.

Asset A useful or valuable thing, person, or quality.

Asset mapping A tool that relies on a core belief of asset-based community development; namely, that good things exist in communities and that those things can be highlighted and encouraged—these are assets suited to advancing those communities.

Assurance A statement, affirmation, etc., intended to inspire confidence or give encouragement.

Atherosclerosis The process of plaque or fatty streaks building up in blood vessels, decreasing the diameter and obstructing blood flow. Atherosclerotic plaque can also break off, forming a clot, which can lodge in vessels, causing heart attack (heart), stroke (brain), peripheral vascular disease (legs), and/or pulmonary embolism (lungs), depending on where it blocks blood flow.

B

Barriers to access health services Factors that prevent an individual from gaining access to health, social care, and early years' services.

Behaviors The actions or reactions of a person or animal in response to external or internal stimuli.

Bias among healthcare providers Associations or attitudes that subconsciously change one's perceptions and, therefore, often go unrecognized by the individual, whereas conscious bias is an definitive form of bias that is based on one's discriminatory beliefs and values and can be targeted in nature.

Body composition Different body compartments have a variety of substrates. The human body is between 60 and 70% water. The rest is fat and protein, carbohydrates, and dissolved micronutrients.

Body Mass Index BMI is the ratio of weight to height in kg/meters^2. Specific cutoffs exist for the diagnosis of underweight (<18), normal (18–25), overweight (25–30), obese (30–40), and morbid obesity (>40).

Built environment The spaces in which people live, work, and play.

C

Cancer A disease caused when cells divide uncontrollably and spread into surrounding tissues.

Cancer cluster A geographic area with a statistically higher-than-average occurrence of cancer among its residents.

Cardiovascular disease Disease affecting the heart or blood vessels. Cardiovascular diseases include arteriosclerosis, coronary artery disease, heart-valve disease, arrhythmia, heart failure, hypertension, orthostatic hypotension, shock, endocarditis, diseases of the aorta and its branches, disorders of the peripheral vascular system, and congenital heart disease.

Chronic Continuing or occurring over and over for a long time.

Coalition A bringing together into a whole.

Coleadership A model of operating a business where there are two people who are in charge instead of just one.

Collaboration The process of two or more people or organizations working together to complete a task or achieve a goal.

Community A unified body of individuals such as the people with common interests living in a particular area or the area itself.

Community Outpatient Hospital (COH) A provider type that was proposed in legislation in the Save Rural Hospitals Act in the 114th Congress (2015–2016) and again in the 115th Congress (2017–2018). The Rural Emergency Acute Care Hospital Act (REACH) was considered by the 115th Congress (2017-2018).

Confidentiality The ethical principle or legal right that a physician or other health professional will hold secret all information relating to a patient, unless the patient gives consent permitting disclosure.

Contraception Prevents pregnancy by interfering with the normal process of ovulation, fertilization, and implantation.

Contributing factors Something that helps cause a result.

Coronary Heart Disease (CHD) A condition and especially one caused by atherosclerosis that reduces blood flow through the coronary arteries to the heart and typically results in chest pain or heart damage.

Critical Access Hospital A designation given to eligible rural hospitals by the Centers for Medicare & Medicaid Services (CMS).

D

Delta-9-tetrahydrocannabinol (THC) Primary psychoactive component of marijuana.

Dental therapists A licensed oral care professional who works in conjunction with a dental care team, providing clinical and therapeutic care. These oral care professionals typically work with uninsured, low-income, and underserved populations to help them get necessary dental care.

Developmental changes Improves on previously established processes and procedures and does not necessarily have to be of a large scale. While not necessarily being an extensive change, they are the most frequent type of organizational change.

Diaphragm A body partition of muscle and connective tissue specifically; the partition separating the chest and abdominal cavities in mammals.

Diffusion of Innovation Theory A hypothesis outlining how new technological and other advancements spread throughout societies and cultures, from introduction to wider adoption.

Disclosure of sexual orientation Revealing a person's emotional, romantic, and/or sexual attraction to persons of the opposite, same, both, or neither sex. "Heterosexuality" is a sexual attraction to persons of the opposite sex. "Homosexuality" is a sexual attraction to persons of the same sex. "Bisexuality" is a sexual attraction to both sexes.

Discrimination The unjust or prejudicial treatment of different categories of people or things, especially on the grounds of race, age, or sex.

Disparities The condition or fact of being unequal, as in age, rank, or degree.

Disproportionate Share Hospital A significantly disproportionate number of low-income patients who receive payments from the Centers for Medicaid & Medicare Services to cover the costs of providing care to uninsured patients.

DRI-Daily Recommended Intakes The nutrient recommendations of the U.S. Department of Agriculture that covers the needs of 95% of the healthy population.

Dysbiosis The presence of pathogenic or detrimental microorganism strains in the gastrointestinal tract. These strains displace the good bacteria and cause multiple processes in the human body to become abnormal, thus resulting in disease over time.

E

Emergency preparedness Emergency planning is the intended response to an unexpected, serious, and dangerous occurrence. Emergency planning may involve preparation and planning for a natural or manmade disaster, accidents, breach of security, terrorism, medical emergencies, food, or other essential service chain breakdowns and other disruptive catastrophes.

Emergency response The phase of the disaster-management cycle that often attracts the most attention and resources.

Endemic Diseases that are generally found in a particular area; malaria, for example, is said to be endemic to tropical and subtropical regions.

Energetics Energy is the capacity to do work. Food can be metabolized for energy using Adenosine triphosphate, the body's cellular currency. The measure of energy is the kilocalorie, which is often just called a "calorie." The macronutrients have calories.

Energy Density Measure of energy contained in a specific amount of food, e.g., kilocalories/gram.

Environment The surroundings or conditions in which a person, animal, or plant lives or operates.

Environmental context A type of context that is composed of the aspects directly related to the infrastructure, physical properties, and restrictions regarding the environment.

Ethics The discipline dealing with what is good and bad and with moral duty and obligation.

Exercise The act of bringing into play or realizing in action.

F

Farm hazards Every farm is different, but hazards common to most farms include: injuries inflicted by animals including bites, kicks, crushing, ramming, trampling, and transmission of certain infectious diseases such as giardia, salmonella, ringworm, and leptospirosis.

Federal government agencies Special government organizations set up for a specific purpose such as the management of resources, financial oversight of industries, or national security issues.

Federal health policy The decisions, plans, and actions that are undertaken to achieve specific healthcare goals within a society.

Federalism A mixed or compound mode of government that combines a general government with regional governments in a single political system.

Fluoridation The addition of fluorides to the public water supply to reduce the incidence of tooth decay.

Food desert Geographic locale characterized by limited access to affordable and nutritious foods.

Food insecurity The state of being without reliable access to a sufficient quantity of affordable, nutritious food.

Frontier Community Health Integration Project A project that develops and tests new models of integrated, coordinated health care in the most sparsely populated rural counties with the goal of improving health outcomes and reducing Medicare expenditures.

G

Gender identity A person's internal sense of being male, female, some combination of male and female, or neither male nor female.

H

Hazardous waste A waste that is capable of causing harm to humans and organisms when mismanaged or released into the environment.

Health The condition of the body or mind and the degree to which it is free from illness, or the state of being well.

Health Belief Model (HBM) A tool that scientists use to try and predict health behaviors.

Health care The maintenance and improvement of physical and mental health, especially through the provision of medical services.

Health communication The study and practice of communicating promotional health information, such as in public health campaigns, health education, and between doctor and patient.

Health data Epidemiology information related to health conditions, reproductive outcomes, causes of death, and quality of life.

Health disparities Preventable differences in the burden of disease, injury, violence, or opportunities to achieve optimal health that are experienced by socially disadvantaged populations.

Health Information Technology Information technology applied to health and health care. It supports health information management across computerized systems and the secure exchange of health information between consumers, providers, payers, and quality monitors.

Healthy community Information technology applied to health and health care. It supports health information management across computerized systems and the secure exchange of health information between consumers, providers, payers, and quality monitors.

Heart failure A chronic, progressive condition in which the heart muscle is unable to pump enough blood to meet the body's needs for blood and oxygen.

Heat stress Occurs when the body cannot get rid of excess heat. When this happens, the body's core temperature rises and the heart rate increases. As the body continues to store heat, the person begins to lose concentration and has difficulty focusing on a task, may become irritable or sick, and often loses the desire to drink.

Heroin Illegal and highly addictive drug composed of morphine.

Heteronormativity Of, relating to, or based on the attitude that heterosexuality is the only normal and natural expression of sexuality.

High Density Lipoprotein (HDL) Referred to as "Good Cholesterol," the HDL cholesterol particle picks up excess fats and cholesterol, making high levels an indicator of decreased risk for cardiometabolic disease.

Hill-Burton Act A U.S. federal law passed in 1946, during the 79th United States Congress. It was sponsored by Senator Harold Burton of Ohio and Senator Lister Hill of Alabama. In November 1945, President Harry S. Truman delivered a special message to Congress in which he outlined a five-part program for improving the health and health care of Americans.

Hormonal contraception Birth control methods that act on the endocrine system.

Hospital closures The closing of any health facility.

I

Infant mortality The death of children under the age of one year.

Insulin resistance The diminished ability of cells to respond to the action of insulin in transporting glucose (sugar) from the bloodstream into muscle and other tissues.

Interventions The act or fact or a means of interfering with the outcome or course especially of a condition or process (as to prevent harm or improve functioning).

L

Leadership The action of leading a group of people or an organization.

Leadership styles A leader's method of providing direction, implementing plans, and motivating people.

LGBTQ Lesbian, gay, bisexual, transgendered, and queer (or questioning).

Low birth weight A birth weight of an infant of 2,499 grams or less, regardless of gestational age.

Low Density Lipoprotein (LDL) Referred to as "Bad Cholesterol," the LDL cholesterol particle traffics cholesterol and is implicated in cholesterol buildup and narrowing of the arteries.

M

Macronutrients Nutrients needed in large quantities (grams) comprising carbohydrates, proteins, fats, and water. Each of these categories can be further subdivided into categories, e.g., monounsaturated fats, polyunsaturated fats, saturated fats, and trans fats.

Malnutrition Any condition caused by over- or undernutrition, imbalance of nutrients, or excess or deficiency of calories.

MAP-IT MAP-IT (Mobilize, Assess, Plan, Implement, Track) is a framework that can be used to plan and evaluate public health interventions in a community.

Maternal morbidity Any short- or long-term health problems that result from being pregnant and giving birth.

Maternal mortality The death of a woman while pregnant or within 42 days of termination of pregnancy, irrespective of the duration and the site of the pregnancy, from any cause related to or aggravated by the pregnancy or its management, but not from accidental or incidental causes. The death of a woman from complications of pregnancy or childbirth that occur during the pregnancy or within six weeks after the pregnancy ends.

Medicaid A public health insurance program in the United States that provides healthcare coverage to low-income families or individuals.

Medicare A U.S. federal government program that subsidizes healthcare services for individuals over age 65, as well as younger people who meet specific eligibility criteria.

Medicare-Dependent Hospital A Medicare-dependent hospital is a hospital that has at least 60% of its inpatient days or discharges attributable to Medicare beneficiaries.

Medication-Assisted Treatment (MAT) Comprises behavioral therapy and medications to treat substance use disorders, including opioid, alcohol, and tobacco abuse.

Meikirch model A new concept of health that puts the whole human being into the center. Its components and the functional relationships include society and natural environment. This allows viewing all aspects of health in a new light and leading to interesting new concepts. The consequences: more health at lower costs.

Mental health A person's condition with regard to their psychological and emotional well-being.

Metropolitan area A region consisting of a densely populated urban core and its less-populated surrounding territories under the same administrative division, sharing industry, infrastructure, and housing.

Metropolitan counties There are six metropolitan counties, which each cover large urban areas, with populations between 1 and 3 million. They were created in 1974 and are each divided into several metropolitan districts or boroughs.

Meyer's minority stress model Minority stress processes in lesbian, gay, and bisexual populations—is based on factors associated with various stressors and coping mechanisms and their positive or negative impact on mental health outcomes.

Microbiome The collection of different strains of bacteria that reside in the human gastrointestinal tract. These microbes digest constituents that are nondigestible by humans and their metabolites regulate many processes in the human body.

Micronutrients Nutrients needed in small quantities, often in milligrams, or micrograms. This category can be further subdivided into water-soluble vitamins, fat-soluble vitamins, trace minerals, and electrolytes.

Migrant worker A person who either migrates within their home country or outside of it to pursue work.

Model A three-dimensional representation of a person or thing or of a proposed structure, typically on a smaller scale than the original.

Morbidity The presence of and/or occurrence of disease in an individual or in a population.

N

Naloxone A medication, which can be injected into the muscle, vein, or under the skin or via a nasal spray. Naloxone can safely reverse the potentially fatal effects of an opioid overdose.

National Institute for Occupational Safety and Health (NIOSH) A U.S. federal agency responsible for conducting research and making recommendations for the prevention of work-related disease and injury.

Nonhormonal contraceptives A birth-control option for individuals who do not tolerate or who wish to avoid the use of hormones. These methods include behavioral methods, barrier methods, spermicides, and surgical sterilization.

Nutrient density Measure of the amount of micronutrients present in a specific amount of food, e.g., milligrams/gram.

Occupational Safety and Health Act (OSHACT) A U.S. law that enforces workplace standards to ensure that employees are protected from hazards that compromise their safety and health. The act established the Occupational Safety and Health Administration (OSHA) and the National Institute for Occupational Safety and Health (NOSH).

Occupational Safety and Health Administration (OSHA) The Occupational Safety and Health Administration, more commonly known by its acronym OSHA, is responsible for protecting worker health and safety in the United States.

Opioids Classification of drugs comprising prescription pain medications (e.g., oxycodone, hydrocodone, codeine, morphine, etc.) and illegal drugs such as heroin and synthetically created fentanyl.

Opioid Use Disorder (OUD) Problematic pattern of *opioid use* leading to clinically significant impairment or distress.

Oral health A key indicator of overall health, well-being, and quality of life. It encompasses a range of diseases and conditions that include dental caries, periodontal disease, tooth loss,

oral cancer, oral manifestations of HIV infection, orodental trauma, noma, and birth defects such as cleft lip and palate.

Partnership An association of two or more people as partners.

Patient Protection and Affordable Care Act (PPACA) PPACA, also called Affordable Care Act (ACA) or Obamacare, in the United States, healthcare reform legislation signed into law by U.S. Pres. Barack Obama in March 2010, which included provisions that required most individuals to secure health insurance or pay fines, made coverage easier and less costly to obtain, cracked down on abusive insurance practices, and attempted to rein in the rising costs of health care.

Pesticide exposure When chemicals intended to control a pest affect nontarget organisms such as humans, wildlife, or bees.

Physical health Health can be defined as physical, mental, and social well-being, and as a resource for living a full life. It not only refers to the absence of disease but also to the ability to recover and bounce back from illness and other problems. Factors for good health include genetics, the environment, relationships, and education.

Policy development Policy development includes the advancement and implementation of public health law, regulations, or voluntary practices that influence systems development, organizational change, and individual behavior to promote improvements in health.

Policymaking High-level development of policy, especially official government policy. Of, relating to, or involving the making of high-level policy: policymaking committees; policymaking decisions.

Population health The health outcomes of a group of individuals, including the distribution of such outcomes within the group.

Population health centers An interdisciplinary, customizable approach that allows health departments to connect practice to policy for change to happen locally.

Poverty The state of one who lacks a usual or socially acceptable amount of money or material possessions.

Power structure The hierarchy that encompasses the most powerful people in an organization.

Precede-Proceed, Mobilizing for Action through Planning and Partnerships (MAPP) A community-wide strategic planning process developed by NACCHO and CDC.

Prejudice Preconceived opinion that is not based on reason or actual experience.

Prenatal care Health care that a pregnant woman receives from an obstetrician or a midwife. Services needed include dietary and lifestyle advice, weighing to ensure proper weight gain, and examination for problems of pregnancy such as edema and preeclampsia.

Preterm birth The presence of uterine contractions of sufficient frequency and intensity to affect progressive effacement and dilation of the cervix prior to term gestation (between 20 and 37 weeks).

Prevention The act or practice of stopping something bad from happening.

Primary prevention Primary prevention aims to prevent disease or injury before it ever occurs. This is done by preventing exposures to hazards that cause disease or injury, altering unhealthy or unsafe behaviors that can lead to disease or injury, and increasing resistance to disease or injury if exposure occurs.

Privacy The state or condition of being free from being observed or disturbed by other people.

Public health The science of protecting the safety and improving the health of communities through education, policymaking, and research for disease and injury prevention.

Public Health 3.0 A new era of enhanced and broadened public health practice that goes beyond traditional public department functions and programs.

Public health policy The science and art of preventing disease, prolonging life, and promoting human health through organized efforts and informed choices of society, organizations, public and private communities, and individuals.

Q

Qualitative of, relating to, or involving quality or kind

Quality of life The general well-being of individuals and societies, outlining negative and positive features of life.

Quality-adjusted life year A generic measure of disease burden, including both the quality and the quantity of life lived. It is used in economic evaluation to assess the value of medical interventions. One QALY equates to one year in perfect health.

Quantitative of, relating to, or expressible in terms of quantity.

R

Readiness for change Change readiness means that all of the obstacles that prevent people from changing have been removed, so the only thing left for them to do is change.

Resistance to change The unwillingness to adapt to altered circumstances. It can be covert or overt, organized, or individual. Employees may realize they don't like or want a change and resist publicly, and that can be very disruptive.

Rural Of, pertaining to, or characteristic of the country, country life, or country people; rustic:rural tranquility.

Rural America A deceptively simple term for a remarkably diverse collection of places.

It includes nearly 72% of the land area of the United States and 46 million people. Farms, ranches, grain elevators, and ethanol plants reflect the enduring importance of agriculture.

Rural area A geographic area that is located outside of towns and cities.

Rural Freestanding Emergency Departments (RFEDs) An existing model that has been used in some communities to maintain emergency services. These facilities offer outpatient and emergency services and do not offer inpatient beds or surgical services.

Rural health care In medicine, rural health or rural medicine is the interdisciplinary study of health and healthcare delivery in rural environments.

Rural Health Clinic A clinic located in a rural, medically underserved area in the United States that has a separate reimbursement structure from the standard medical office under the Medicare and Medicaid programs.

Rural older adults Important service recipients because of their economic and social needs. However, studies indicate that rural older adults received certain services, such as home-delivered meals, less frequently than urban older adults.

Rural Referral Center High-volume, acute-care rural hospitals that treat a large number of complicated cases.

S

Screening The evaluation or investigation of something as part of a methodical survey, to assess suitability for a particular role or purpose.

Sealants Material used for sealing something so as to make it airtight or watertight.

Secondary prevention The effort aimed at reducing or halting the progression of the disabling condition after the initial injury has occurred.

Sewer system A facility consisting of a system of sewers for carrying off liquid and solid sewage.

Sexually transmitted infection Infections that can be transferred from one person to another through any type of sexual contact.

Social Determinants The social factors and physical conditions of the environment in which people are born, live, learn, play, work, and age.

Social determinants of health The conditions in which people are born, grow, live, work, and age.

Social Security Act (SSA) A law enacted in 1935 to create a system of transfer payments in which younger working people support older retired people.

Sole Community Hospital A hospital that is located more than 35 miles from other hospitals or is located in a rural area.

Stakeholder A person with an interest or concern in something, especially a business.

Stigma A mark of shame or discredit.

Stroke The sudden death of brain cells in a localized area due to inadequate blood flow.

Structural racism The silent opportunity killer. It is the blind interaction between institutions, policies, and practices that inevitably perpetuates barriers to opportunities and racial disparities.

Surveillance According to the World Health Organization, the continuous, systematic collection, analysis, and interpretation of nutrition and health-related data needed for the planning, implementation, and evaluation of public health nutrition practice.

T

Target group The primary group of people that something, usually an advertising campaign, is aimed at appealing to.

Telehealth The distribution of health-related services and information via electronic information and telecommunication technologies.

Telehealth Services Provides healthcare education, entertainment, and communication systems for the healthcare industry in the United States.

Tertiary prevention A reduction in morbidity, complications, or mortality related to an acute or chronic disease that has recently been diagnosed and partially or entirely treated.

Theory A supposition or a system of ideas intended to explain something, especially one based on general principles independent of the thing to be explained.

The Rural-Urban Continuum Codes, (RUCC) A classification scheme that distinguishes metropolitan counties by the population size of their metro area and nonmetropolitan counties by degree of urbanization and adjacency to a metro area.

Tobacco Products comprising cigarettes, cigars, dissolvables, nicotine gels, hookah tobacco, pipe tobacco, roll-your-own tobacco, smoke tobacco (including dip, snuff, snus, and chewing tobacco), vapes, e-cigarettes, hookah pens, and other Electronic Nicotine Delivery Systems (ENDS).

Transition A movement, development, or evolution from one form, stage, or style to another.

Transportation The movement of humans, animals, and goods from one location to another.

Transtheoretical model An integrative theory of therapy that assesses an individual's readiness to act on a new healthier behavior and provides strategies or processes of change to guide the individual.

U

Unintended pregnancy A pregnancy that is mistimed, unplanned, or unwanted at the time of conception.

Urban cluster (UC) A Census-designated urban area with at least 2,500 residents and no more than 49,999 residents.

Urbanized area (UA) A continuously built-up area with a population of 50,000 or more. It comprises one or more places—central place(s)—and the adjacent densely settled surrounding area—urban fringe—consisting of other places and nonplace territory.

Usual source of health care A place where one usually goes when one is sick such as a physician's office or health center but not an emergency department.

V

Value-based programs Programs that reward healthcare providers with incentive payments for the quality of care they give to people with Medicare.

W

Water contaminants Hazardous materials of any kind that are polluting a source of water.

Well Water Underground water that is held in the soil and in pervious rocks.

Z

Zoonotic diseases A disease that can be transmitted from animals to people or, more specifically, a disease that normally exists in animals but that can infect humans.

Index

Page numbers followed by *e*, *f*, or *t* indicate material in exhibits, figures, or tables, respectively.

O

R

Q

S